Parsons and Wiene

before

CRITICAL CARE

CRITICAL CARE

SECRETS

Fourth Edition

Polly E. Parsons, MD
Professor, Department of Medicine
University of Vermont College of Medicine
Director, Pulmonary and Critical Care Medicine
Chief of Critical Care Services
Fletcher Allen Health Care
Burlington, Vermont

Jeanine P. Wiener-Kronish, MD
Professor of Anesthesia and Medicine
Vice-Chairman, Department of Anesthesia and Perioperative Care
Investigator, Cardiovascular Research Institute
University of California at San Francisco
San Francisco, California

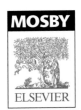

MOSBY

ELSEVIER

MOSBY
ELSEVIER

1600 John F. Kennedy Boulevard, Suite 1800
Philadelphia, PA 19103-2899

Critical Care Secrets
Fourth Edition

ISBN-13: 978-1-4160-3206-9
ISBN-10: 1-4160-3206-1

NOTICE

Knowledge and best practice in this field are constantly changing. As new research and experience broaden our knowledge, changes in practice, treatment and drug therapy may become necessary or appropriate. Readers are advised to check the most current information provided (i) on procedures featured or (ii) by the manufacturer of each product to be administered, to verify the recommended dose or formula, the method and duration of administration, and contraindications. It is the responsibility of the practitioner, relying on his or her own experience and knowledge of the patient, to make diagnoses, to determine dosages and the best treatment for each individual patient, and to take all appropriate safety precautions. To the fullest extent of the law, neither the Publisher nor the Editor assumes any liability for any injury and/or damage to persons or property arising out or related to any use of the material contained in this book.

Library of Congress Cataloging-in-Publication Data

Critical care secrets / [edited by] Polly E. Parsons, Jeanine P. Wiener-Kronish. – 4th ed.
     p. ; cm. – (Secrets series)
  Includes bibliographical references and index.
  ISBN-13: 978–1–4160–3206–9   ISBN-10: 1–4160–3206–1
  1. Critical care medicine–Examinations, questions, etc. I. Parsons, Polly E., 1954 -
II. Wiener-Kronish, Jeanine P., 1951 - III. Series.
  [DNLM: 1. Critical Care–Examination Questions. WX 18.2 C93432007]
  RC86.9.P3752007
  616.02´8076–dc22

                                                                          2006046876

Senior Acquisitions Editor: James Merritt
Developmental Editor: Stan Ward
Project Manager: Mary Stermel
Marketing Manager: Alyson Sherby

Working together to grow
libraries in developing countries

www.elsevier.com | www.bookaid.org | www.sabre.org

ELSEVIER   BOOK AID International   Sabre Foundation

Printed in China.

Last digit is the print number: 9   8   7   6   5   4   3

DEDICATION

To our husbands, Jim and Daniel, and our children, Alec, Chandler, Jessica, and Samuel, for their patience and support and for allowing us to take the time to complete this edition.

CONTENTS

III. PULMONARY MEDICINE

IV. CARDIOLOGY

V. INFECTIOUS DISEASE

VI. RENAL DISEASE

XI. NEUROLOGY

XII. SURGERY AND TRAUMA

XIII. PERIOPERATIVE CARE

XIV. SEDATION AND PAIN MANAGEMENT

XIX. ETHICS

XX. ADMINISTRATION

CONTRIBUTORS

Hasan B. Alam, MD, FACS
Director of Research and Program Director for Surgical Critical Care Fellowship, Division of Trauma, Emergency Surgery and Surgical Critical Care, Massachusetts General Hospital; Associate Professor of Surgery, Harvard Medical School, Boston, Massachusetts

Gil Allen, MD
Assistant Professor, Department of Medicine, University of Vermont College of Medicine, Burlington, Vermont

Carolyn E. Bekes, MD, MHA, FCCM
Senior Vice President of Academic and Medical Affairs, Cooper University Hospital; Professor of Medicine, Robert Wood Johnson Medical School, Camden, New Jersey

Jonathan Berry, MD
Chief Resident, Department of Psychiatry, University of Colorado, Denver; Colorado Department of Psychiatry, Denver, Colorado

Philip E. Bickler, MD, PhD
Professor, Department of Anesthesia, University of California at San Francisco, San Francisco, California

Joshua Blum, MD
Assistant Professor of Medicine, University of Colorado Health Sciences Center, Denver, Colorado

James P. Bonar, MD
Chief, Clinical Investigations Branch, United States School of Aerospace Medicine, Brooks City-Base, San Antonio, Texas

David C. Bonovich, MD
Associate Professor of Neurology, Fellowship Program Director, Neurovascular and Neurocritical Care Service, University of California at San Francisco; Associate Director, Neurocritical Care and Stroke Service, San Francisco General Hospital, San Francisco, California

Mark W. Bowyer, MD, FACS, DMCC, COL, USAF, MC
Chief, Division of Combat and Trauma Surgery, Norman M. Rich Department of Surgery, Uniformed Services University, Bethesda, Maryland; Attending Trauma Surgeon, Washington Hospital Center, Washington, DC

Dan Burkhardt, MD
Department of Anesthesia and Perioperative Care, University of California at San Francisco, San Francisco, California

David G. Burris, MD, FACS, DMCC, COL, USA, MC
Professor and Chairman, Norman M. Rich Department of Surgery, Uniformed Services University, Bethesda, Maryland; Attending Surgeon, Walter Reed Army Medical Center, Washington, DC

Lundy J. Campbell, MD
Department of Anesthesia, University of California at San Francisco, San Francisco, California

E. Michael Canham, MD
Associate Professor of Medicine, National Jewish Medical and Research Center, University of Colorado Health Sciences Center, Denver, Colorado

Stephen V. Cantrill, MD
Associate Director, Department of Emergency Medicine, Denver Health Medical Center; Associate Professor, Division of Emergency Medicine, University of Colorado Health Sciences Center, Denver, Colorado

Lee-lynn Chen, MD
Clinical Fellow in Critical Care Medicine, Department of Anesthesia and Perioperative Care, University of California at San Francisco Medical Center, San Francisco, California

Glenn M. Chertow, MD, MPH
Professor, Division of Nephrology, Department of Medicine and Department of Epidemiology and Biostatistics, University of California at San Francisco, San Francisco, California

Deborah R. Cook, MD
Geriatric Oncology Fellow, University of Colorado Health Sciences Center, Denver, Colorado

John W. Crommett, MD
Assistant Professor, Department of Neurosurgery/Critical Care, University of Texas at Houston Health Science Center, Houston, Texas

Bruce Crookes, MD
Director of Trauma, Fletcher Allen Health Care; Assistant Professor of Surgery, University of Vermont College of Medicine, Burlington, Vermont

Pajman A. Danai, MD
Fellow, Division of Pulmonary, Allergy, and Critical Care, Department of Medicine, Emory University School of Medicine, Atlanta, Georgia

Clifford S. Deutschman, MS, MD, FCCM
Professor, Departments of Anesthesiology and Critical Care and Surgery, University of Pennsylvania School of Medicine, Philadelphia, Pennsylvania

Anne Dixon, MD
Assistant Professor, Department of Pulmonary and Critical Care, Fletcher Allen Health Care, Colchester, Vermont

Thomas J. Donnelly, MD
Assistant Clinical Professor, Department of Internal Medicine, Wright State University; Pulmonary and Critical Care Consultants, Inc., Dayton, Ohio

Rachel H. Dotson, MD
Fellow, Pulmonary and Critical Care Medicine, University of California at San Francisco, San Francisco, California

Enrique Fernandez, MD
Professor of Medicine, University of Colorado Health Sciences Center; National Jewish Center; Denver Health Hospital, Denver, Colorado

Patrick F. Fogarty, MD
Assistant Professor of Medicine, Division of Hematology/Oncology, University of California at San Francisco, San Francisco, California

Michael T. Ganter, MD
Assistant Clinical Professor, Department of Anesthesia, University of California at San Francisco; San Francisco General Hospital, San Francisco, California

Joel A. Garcia, MD
Division of Cardiology, University of Colorado Health Sciences Center, Denver, Colorado

Carlos E. Girod, MD
Associate Professor, Division of Pulmonary and Critical Care Medicine, University of Texas Southwestern Medical Center, Dallas, Texas

Noah E. Gordon, MD
Resident, Department of Anesthesia and Perioperative Care, University of California at San Francisco, San Francisco, California

Michael A. Gropper, MD, PhD
Professor and Director, Critical Care Medicine, Department of Anesthesia and Perioperative Care, University of California at San Francisco, San Francisco, California

Jacob T. Gutsche, MD
Fellow in Critical Care and Cardiac Anesthesiology, Department of Anesthesiology and Critical Care, Hospital of the University of Pennsylvania, Philadelphia, Pennsylvania

Katherine Habeeb, MD, FCCP
Clinical Assistant Professor of Medicine, University of Vermont College of Medicine, Burlington, Vermont

James Haenel, RRT
Department of Surgery, Denver Health Medical Center, Denver, Colorado

Derek Haerle, MD
Critical Care Fellow, Department of Anesthesia and Perioperative Care, University of California at San Francisco, San Francisco, California

Matthew J. Haight, DO
Critical Care Medicine Fellow, Department of Anesthesia and Perioperative Care, University of California at San Francisco, San Francisco, California

Michael E. Hanley, MD
Professor of Medicine, University of Colorado Health Sciences Center; Staff Physician, Pulmonary and Critical Care Medicine, Denver Health Medical Center, Denver, Colorado

C. William Hanson, III, MD
Professor of Anesthesia, Surgery, and Internal Medicine, Chief, Critical Care Medicine, University of Pennsylvania School of Medicine, Philadelphia, Pennsylvania

Andrea Harzstark, MD
Fellow in Hematology/Oncology, University of California at San Francisco, San Francisco, California

Kathryn L. Hassell, MD
Associate Professor of Medicine, University of Colorado Health Sciences Center, Denver, Colorado

John E. Heffner, MD, FACP, FCCP
Professor of Medicine and Executive Medical Director, Medical University of South Carolina, Charleston, South Carolina

Richard Jacobs, MD, PhD
Acting Division Co-Chief, Division of Infectious Disease, Clinical Professor of Medicine and Clinical Pharmacy, University of California at San Francisco, San Francisco, California

James L. Jacobson, MD
Associate Professor, Department of Psychiatry, University of Vermont College of Medicine, Burlington, Vermont

James C. Jeng, MD
Associate Director of Burn Center, Washington Hospital Center; Clinical Associate Professor of Surgery, Georgetown University, Washington, DC

David A. Kaminsky, MD
Associate Professor of Medicine, Department of Pulmonary Disease and Critical Care Medicine, University of Vermont College of Medicine, Burlington, Vermont

Shannon Kasperbauer, MD
Division of Infectious Diseases, University of Colorado Health Sciences Center, Denver, Colorado

Dinkar Kaw, MD
Assistant Professor, Department of Medicine, Medical University of Ohio at Toledo, Toledo, Ohio

Benjamin A. Kohl, MD
Assistant Professor, Department of Anesthesiology and Critical Care, Section of Cardiothoracic Anesthesia and Critical Care, University of Pennsylvania School of Medicine, Philadelphia, Pennsylvania

Rosemary A. Kozar, MD, PhD
Associate Professor of Surgery, University of Texas at Houston, Houston, Texas

Ken Kulig, MD
Associate Clinical Professor, Division of Emergency Medicine and Trauma, Department of Surgery, University of Colorado Health Sciences Center; Toxicology Associates, Prof. LLC, Denver, Colorado

Rondall Lane, MD
Department of Anesthesia, University of California at San Francisco, San Francisco, California

Stephen E. Lapinsky, MB, BCh, MSc, FRCP(C)
Site Director, Mount Sinai Hospital; Associate Professor of Medicine, University of Toronto, Toronto, Ontario, Canada

William Eng Lee, MD
Northern Hematology-Oncology, Thornton, Colorado

Stuart L. Linas, MD
Professor of Medicine, Division of Renal Diseases and Hypertension, Department of Medicine, University of Colorado Health Sciences Center, Denver, Colorado

Kathleen D. Liu, MD, PhD
Fellow, Division of Nephrology, Department of Medicine, University of California at San Francisco, San Francisco, California

Linda L. Liu, MD
Associate Professor, Department of Anesthesia and Perioperative Care, University of California at San Francisco, San Francisco, California

Theodore W. Marcy, MD, MPH
Professor of Medicine, University of Vermont College of Medicine, Burlington, Vermont

Brian T. Marden, PharmD
Critical Care Pharmacy Clinician, Fletcher Allen Health Care; Clinical Assistant Professor of Medicine, University of Vermont College of Medicine, Burlington, Vermont

Vincent J. Markovchick, MD, FAEEM, FACEP
Director, Emergency Medical Services, Denver Health Medical Center; Professor of Surgery, Division of Emergency Medicine, Department of Surgery, University of Colorado Health Sciences Center, Denver, Colorado

John A. Marx, MD
Department of Emergency Medicine, Carolinas Medical Center, Charlotte, North Carolina

Michael T. McDermott, MD
Director, Endocrinology Practice, University of Colorado Hospital, Aurora, Colorado

Philip S. Mehler, MD
Professor of Medicine, University of Colorado Health Sciences Center, Denver, Colorado

John Messenger, MD
Director of Cardiovascular Intervention, Department of Cardiology, University of Colorado Hospital and Health Sciences Center, Denver, Colorado

Stanley L. Minken, MD, FACS, DMCC
Charles A. Rob Professor of Surgery, Norman M. Rich Department of Surgery, Uniformed Services University, Bethesda, Maryland

Benoit Misset, MD
Medical Surgical Intensive Care Unit, Hôpital Saint-Joseph, Paris, France

Frederick A. Moore, MD
Professor of Surgery, University of Texas at Houston, Houston, Texas

Amy E. Morris, MD
Senior Fellow, Division of Pulmonary and Critical Care Medicine, University of Washington, Seattle, Washington

Marc Moss, MD
Professor of Medicine, Division of Pulmonary Sciences/Critical Care Medicine, University of Colorado Health Sciences Center, Denver, Colorado

Victor Ng, MD
Division of Anesthesia, Department of Medicine, University of California at San Francisco, San Francisco, California

Claus U. Niemann, MD
Division of Anesthesia, Department of Medicine, University of California at San Francisco, San Francisco, California

Alan C. Pao, MD
Clinical Fellow, Division of Nephrology, Department of Medicine, University of California at San Francisco, San Francisco, California

Manuel Pardo, Jr., MD
Sol Shnider Endowed Chair for Anesthesia Education, Department of Anesthesia and Perioperative Care, University of California at San Francisco, San Francisco, California

Polly E. Parsons, MD
Professor, Department of Medicine, University of Vermont College of Medicine; Director, Pulmonary and Critical Care Medicine; Chief, Critical Care Services, Fletcher Allen Health Care, Burlington, Vermont

Kapilkumar Patel, MD
Department of Pulmonary and Critical Care Medicine, Fletcher Allen Health Care, Burlington, Vermont

Jon Perlstein, MD
Assistant Professor of Surgery, Uniformed Services Health Sciences University; Program Director, General Surgery Residency; Director, Trauma and Critical Care, David Grant Medical Center, Travis Air Force Base, California

Kullada O. Pichakron, MD
Assistant Program Director, General Surgery Residency, David Grant Medical Center, Travis Air Force Base, Fairfield, California

Ryan P. Peirson, MD
Clinical Instructor, Department of Psychiatry, University of Vermont College of Medicine, Burlington, Vermont

Jean-François Pittet, MD
Professor in Residence, Departments of Anesthesia and Surgery, University of California at San Francisco; San Francisco General Hospital, San Francisco, California

Louis B. Polish, MD
Associate Professor of Medicine, Division of Infectious Diseases, University of Vermont College of Medicine, Burlington, Vermont

Peter T. Pons, MD
Professor, Division of Emergency Medicine, Department of Surgery, University of Colorado Health Sciences Center, Denver, Colorado

Jill A. Rebuck, PharmD, BCPS
Surgical Critical Care Clinician, Fletcher Allen Health Care; Assistant Professor of Surgery, University of Vermont College of Medicine, Burlington, Vermont

Randall Reves, MD
Denver Public Health Department, Denver, Colorado

E. Matt Ritter, MD, MAJ, USAF, MC
Assistant Professor, Norman M. Rich Department of Surgery, Uniformed Services University; Chief, Laparoscopic Surgery, National Naval Medical Center, Bethesda, Maryland

Jeanne M. Rozwadowski, MD
Assistant Professor of Medicine, University of Colorado Health Sciences Center, Denver, Colorado

Jack Sava, MD
Assistant Professor of Surgery, Georgetown University; Attending Surgeon, Washington Hospital Center, Trauma/Critical Care Section, Washington, DC

Richard H. Savel, MD
Associate Director, Surgical Intensive Care Unit, Maimonides Medical Center; Assistant Professor of Medicine, Mt. Sinai School of Medicine, New York, New York

Lynn M. Schnapp, MD
Associate Professor, Division of Pulmonary and Critical Care Medicine, Harborview Medical Center, Seattle, Washington

Peter M. Schulman, MD
Assistant Clinical Professor, Department of Anesthesia and Perioperative Care, University of California at San Francisco, San Francisco, California

Joseph I. Shapiro, MD
Department of Medicine, Medical College of Ohio at Toledo, Toledo, Ohio

David Shimabukuro, MDCM
Assistant Professor, Department of Anesthesia and Perioperative Care, University of California at San Francisco, San Francisco, California

Stuart F. Sidlow, MD
Department of Anesthesiology and Critical Care, University of Pennsylvania School of Medicine, Philadelphia, Pennsylvania

Antoinette Spevetz, MD, FCCM, FACP
Co-Director for ICU Operations, Director of Intermediate Intensive Care Unit, Cooper University Hospital, Camden, New Jersey

Annette Stralovich-Romani, RD, CNSD
Adult Critical Care Nutritionist, Department of Nutrition and Dietetics, University of California at San Francisco Medical Center, San Francisco, California

John M. Taylor, MD
Assistant Clinical Professor, Department of Anesthesia and Perioperative Care, University of California at San Francisco, San Francisco, California

Marshall Thomas, MD
Vice Chair and Medical Director, Department of Psychiatry, University of Colorado, Denver, Colorado

Madhulika G. Varma, MD
Assistant Professor of Surgery, Section of Colon and Rectal Surgery; Director, UCSF Center for Pelvic Physiology, University of California at San Francisco, San Francisco, California

Fernando Velayos, MD, MPH
Department of Medicine, University of California at San Francisco, San Francisco, California

Jennifer Y. Wang, MD
Surgery Resident, University of California at San Francisco, San Francisco, California

Carolyn H. Welsh, MD
Professor of Medicine, Division of Pulmonary Sciences and Critical Care Medicine, University of Colorado Health Sciences Center and Denver Veterans Affairs Medical Center, Denver, Colorado

James E. Wiedeman, MD
Department of Surgery, Sacramento Veterans Affairs Medical Center, Mather, California

Jeanine P. Wiener-Kronish, MD
Professor of Anesthesia and Medicine, Vice-Chairman, Department of Anesthesia and Perioperative Care, University of California at San Francisco; Investigator, Cardiovascular Research Institute, San Francisco, California

Danny C. Williams, MD, FRCPC, FACP, FACR
Division of Rheumatology, University of Colorado Health Sciences Center, Denver, Colorado

Jon Yang, MD
Department of Medicine, University of San Francisco at California, San Francisco, California

Michael Young, MD
Associate Professor of Medicine, Division of Pulmonary and Critical Care, University of Vermont College of Medicine, Burlington, Vermont

Martin R. Zamora, MD
Division of Pulmonary Sciences and Critical Care Medicine, University of Colorado Health Sciences Center, Denver, Colorado

PREFACE

Over the course of now four editions of *Critical Care Secrets,* critical care medicine has become increasingly complex. The fundamentals and clinical skills required to care for critically ill patients continues to transcend subspecialties, so in this edition we have again included chapters from a wide range of specialists, including pulmonologists, surgeons, anesthesiologists, psychiatrists, pharmacists, and infectious disease experts. We have asked these experts to pose the key questions in critical care and formulate the answers so practitioners can identify effective solutions to their patients' medical and ethical problems.

A broad understanding of anatomy, physiology, immunology, and inflammation is fundamentally important to being able to effectively care for critically ill patients. For example, it is hard to imagine understanding the principles of mechanical ventilation without being aware of the principles of gas and fluid flow, pulmonary mechanics, and electronic circuitry. Accordingly, the authors have incorporated these key elements into this edition as well. Finally, critical care medicine requires knowledge of protocols and guidelines that are continuously evolving and that increasingly dictate best practices.

In this fourth edition of *Critical Care Secrets,* we have again been fortunate in having many of the leaders in critical care contribute chapters in their areas of expertise. These experts have expanded the *Secrets*® format to include Top Secrets and Key Points, which readers can use to identify those concepts that experienced clinicians consider to be the most important.

We would like to sincerely thank all of the authors who contributed their time and expertise to this endeavor. We believe they have captured the essence of critical care medicine and presented it in a format that will be useful to everyone from students to experienced clinicians.

Polly E. Parsons, MD
Jeanine P. Wiener-Kronish, MD

TOP 100 SECRETS

These secrets are 100 of the top board alerts. They summarize the concepts, principles, and most salient details of critical care medicine.

1. Except in cardiac arrest, IV epinephrine should be administered carefully via IV drip infusion to minimize the risk of a severe sympathomimetic response.

2. Treat ventricular fibrillation (VF) with early defibrillation: 360 joules with a monophasic defibrillator, 200 joules with a biphasic defibrillator, or at the level the manufacturer recommends. You should know which kind of defibrillator you have. If the initial countershock is not successful in a patient with VF, administer vasopressin or epinephrine with 2 minutes or five cycles of cardiopulmonary resuscitation, and then give another countershock.

3. The absorption pattern of methemoglobin is interpreted by the pulse oximeter as 85% saturation; thus, progressively higher levels of methemoglobin cause the SpO_2 value to converge on 85% regardless of the actual SaO_2.

4. Mixed venous oxygen saturation gives you an idea of adequacy of the perfusion of the whole body. When the mixed venous saturation is <60%, perfusion is inadequate, probably due to congestive heart failure.

5. There is little evidence to support the use of sophisticated monitoring tools such as the pulmonary artery catheter. These devices may be useless or even harmful when used without proper expertise and judgment.

6. Pulse oximetry is good for monitoring, but arterial blood gas (ABG) analyses are best for diagnosis and acute management. If oximetry does not fit the clinical picture, obtain an ABG with co-oximetry. Use the alveolar gas equation to help understand mechanisms of hypoxemia—it's worth the effort!

7. Maintenance IV fluid therapy replaces sensible and insensible losses and amounts to 30–35 mL/kg in an adult patient. Crystalloid remains the fluid of choice for acute volume resuscitation.

8. The respiratory quotient (RQ) is the ratio of the patient's carbon dioxide production to oxygen consumption. The RQ is helpful in guiding the planning of nutritional therapy.

9. For patients with acute exacerbations of chronic obstructive pulmonary disease (COPD), noninvasive ventilation is associated with decreased need for tracheal intubation and improved survival rates. Do not use noninvasive ventilation for a patient with an urgent need for tracheal intubation.

10. When setting up a mechanical ventilator, minimize tidal volumes and airway pressures, even tolerating respiratory acidosis to do so.

11. Daily sedation and analgesia should be minimized or interrupted so patients will be awake, breathing, and protecting their airways and so they can be weaned from mechanical ventilation.

12. In most patients, it is possible to maintain a patent airway without tracheal intubation. The five main indications for tracheal intubation are upper airway obstruction, inadequate oxygenation, inadequate ventilation, elevated work of breathing, and airway protection.

13. The presence of gastric distention, frequent belching, or recurrent aspiration in a ventilated patient with a tracheotomy suggests the possibility of a tracheoesophageal fistula.

14. Chest tube alone is the sole therapy needed for up to 85% of all cases of penetrating chest trauma. Blood drained from a chest tube can be autotransfused without further processing.

15. Flexible bronchoscopy is most commonly used in the intensive care unit (ICU) to diagnose and guide antibiotic choices for ventilator-associated pneumonia. Chest physiotherapy appears to be as effective as bronchoscopy in treating atelectasis, although bronchoscopy has a role in retained, inspissated secretions or foreign bodies.

16. The most common cause of temporary transvenous pacemaker failure is loss of contact between electrical wires and the heart; to restore pacing, advance the electrode until it again contacts the myocardium so as to "capture" or pace the heart.

17. Circulatory assist devices are indicated as a bridging therapy only. They are used for bridge to recovery, bridge to revascularization, and bridge to transplant.

18. Severe community-acquired pneumonia can be recognized by abnormalities described by the acronym *CURB:* confusion, urea, respiratory rate, blood pressure.

19. A normal PCO_2 in acute asthma is a warning sign of impending respiratory failure.

20. Minimizing minute ventilation, even to the point of allowing the development of hypercapnia, is the best strategy to reduce dynamic hyperinflation and the subsequent risk of hemodynamic compromise and barotrauma in mechanically ventilated patients with acute, severe asthma.

21. Noninvasive mechanical ventilation reduces the need for intubation in patients with a COPD exacerbation and impending respiratory failure. In patients mechanically ventilated for a COPD exacerbation, antibiotics decrease morbidity and mortality.

22. Cor pulmonale is right ventricular hypertrophy due to diseases of lung vasculature or parenchyma. Long-term oxygen therapy is the mainstay of treatment.

23. Treatment of hypoxic respiratory therapy should aim to achieve a PaO_2 of about 50 mmHg. Daily weaning should be attempted as soon as the patient is stable physiologically and can maintain adequate oxygenation and carbon dioxide with supplemental oxygen. Weaning from mechanical ventilation is optimally achieved using a protocol.

24. Acute respiratory distress syndrome (ARDS) cannot be prevented. The only therapy that has decreased mortality in ARDS is low-tidal-volume ventilation.

25. Critically ill patients in the ICU are at risk for more frequent aspiration and grave consequences after aspiration. The consequences of aspiration depend on both the volume and nature of aspirated material, as well as the host response to the insult.

26. Death in massive hemoptysis more commonly results from asphyxiation and acute respiratory failure than exsanguination. The immediate management of massive hemoptysis is to protect the healthy lung by placing the patient in a position with the bleeding lung dependent if bleeding is focal or in the Trendelenburg position if it is occurring diffusely.

27. Because there are no specific clinical, radiographic, or laboratory findings for pulmonary embolism, it should be considered in any critically ill patient with deterioration of cardiopulmonary status.

28. Anginal equivalents are atypical symptoms that still represent myocardial ischemia; they include nausea, dizziness, and dyspnea and are brought on and alleviated by the same activities as angina.

29. The immediate goal during acute myocardial infarction is to reestablish blood flow. This can be done by percutaneous coronary intervention or by pharmacologic thrombolysis.

30. With acute-onset tachycardia, begin by measuring blood pressure, either with invasive or noninvasive instruments, to verify that the patient has adequate systemic perfusion. If the patient's blood pressure is inadequate, perform a synchronized cardioversion maneuver.

31. When managing acute aortic dissection, adequate beta blockade must be established *before* the initiation of nitroprusside to prevent propagation of the dissection from a reflex increase in cardiac output.

32. Surgery should be considered before or at the time when pulmonary hypertension occurs in patients with mitral stenosis because mortality increases significantly in patients with established pulmonary hypertension.

33. Critically ill patients with severe aortic stenosis and severe left ventricular dysfunction can benefit from careful administration of nitroprusside.

34. The electrocardiographic (ECG) change most often observed with acute pericarditis is upsloping ST elevation in all leads except aVR and V1 (termed *electrical alternans*).

35. *Severe sepsis syndrome* (SSS) is defined as sepsis plus acute sepsis-induced organ dysfunction. Early diagnosis and therapeutic interventions in patients with SSS are associated with better outcomes.

36. Between 60% and 80% of cases of endocarditis are due to streptococcal infection. *Staphylococcus aureus* tends to be the most common etiologic agent of infective endocarditis in IV drug users.

37. Adjunctive dexamethasone given before or simultaneously with antibiotic therapy reduces mortality in adults with bacterial meningitis from 15% to 7%. The clear benefit is in patients with pneumococcal meningitis, but one cannot delay steroid initiation pending a confirmed etiologic diagnosis.

38. If you suspect disseminated fungal infection, do not wait for culture results to treat. Fungal infections must be considered early in all critically ill patients because failure to treat will result in high mortality rates.

39. Approximately 1% of the population is colonized with methicillin-resistant *S. aureus* (MRSA). Percentages are higher in crowded living conditions with poor hygiene, making community-acquired MRSA infections fairly commonplace.

40. When selecting a central vein for catheterization, consider the subclavian vein because it has a lower risk of catheter-related infection and bacteremia. Peripheral-inserted central venous catheters are as likely to develop catheter-associated infections as standard subclavian or internal jugular central lines.

41. Smallpox lesions involve the palms and soles, whereas chickenpox does not. Smallpox is painful; chickenpox is pruritic.

42. The finding of paresis and paralysis in an afebrile patient without sensory changes is diagnostic of botulism.

43. Only 15% of wound infections have systemic fever and rigors. Blood cultures are not useful in cellulitis.

44. Necrotizing fasciitis can appear as slowly spreading cellulitis, with woody induration. Treatment is rapid surgical débridement.

45. Hypertensive crisis (or hypertensive emergency) is the turning point in the course of hypertension when immediate management of elevated blood pressure plays a decisive role in limiting or preventing damage to the four main target organ systems: eye, brain, heart, and kidneys.

46. The serum creatinine may not change much during acute renal failure in patients with decreased muscle mass. Urinalysis, a simple and easy test, often provides the specific diagnosis.

47. In patients with rhabdomyolysis, the life-threatening complications to watch for are hyperkalemia and hypocalcemia.

48. Hypokalemia can be caused by low potassium (K) intake, intracellular K redistribution, gastrointestinal K loss (diarrhea), and renal K loss. Hyperkalemia can be caused by high K intake, extracellular K redistribution, and low renal K excretion.

49. Overly rapid correction of hyponatremia or hypernatremia can result in devastating long-term neurologic sequelae.

50. Bleeding or rebleeding during hospitalization is associated with high mortality rates. Critically ill patients are at risk for gastrointestinal bleeding from stress-induced ulcers and hypotension-induced ischemia of the colon.

51. Tests of serum amylase and lipase levels are helpful only in making the diagnosis of acute pancreatitis. The degree of elevation has no correlation with disease severity.

52. Variceal bleeding is due to portal hypertension. After resuscitation, move quickly to decrease portal venous pressure with somatostatin. If pharmacology fails, move to portosystemic shunt (transjugular intrahepatic portosystemic shunt versus operative).

53. In patients in whom a history and physical may not be reliable (e.g., patients with head injury or paraplegia, elderly persons, or patients taking steroids), diagnostic peritoneal lavage may be a useful method of determining the presence of peritonitis that requires surgery.

54. Successful treatment of diabetic ketoacidosis (DKA) is defined by normalization of the anion gap. IV insulin given at 0.1 units/kg/h, fluids, and potassium supplementation are the cornerstones of therapy for DKA.

55. In patients with hyperglycemic hyperosmolar syndrome, insulin should not be given until after adequate volume resuscitation.

56. Stress-dose steroids should be given to most patients with severe sepsis/septic shock and relative adrenal insufficiency. Critically ill patients in the ICU who recently received a prednisone equivalent of ≥ 5 mg/day for ≥ 7 days should receive stress-dose steroid coverage.

57. Thyroid storm is treated with antithyroid drugs, cold iodine, beta blockers, stress glucocorticoid doses, and management of any precipitating factors. Myxedema coma is treated with rapid repletion of the thyroid hormone deficit, stress glucocorticoid doses, and treatment of any precipitating causes.

58. In a bleeding patient, stop the hemorrhage! This is more important that replacing the losses. Replace blood carefully.

59. All patients (with or without thrombosis) with heparin-induced thrombocytopenia (type II) must be anticoagulated because the risk of thrombosis is >50% without anticoagulation. Prophylactic platelet transfusion should be avoided in patients with heparin-induced thrombocytopenia because it may worsen thrombotic complications.

60. Use of blood products in the treatment of disseminated intravascular coagulation should be reserved for patients with active bleeding, those requiring invasive procedures, or those otherwise at high risk for bleeding. Heparin, via its ability to reduce thrombin generation, may be useful in some patients with disseminated intravascular coagulation and bleeding that has not responded to the administration of blood products.

61. Pulse oximetry may be inaccurate in patients with sickle cell disease, so undertaking an arterial blood gas measurement and direct measurement of PO_2 is the best way to assess hypoxia. The absence of tachycardia may be a clue that the actual PO_2 and adequacy of oxygenation is better than expected based on pulse oximetry.

62. Maintaining adequate hydration of hypercalcemic patients is critical.

63. A "red hot" joint indicates septic arthritis until proven otherwise, especially in immunocompromised patients with established arthritis.

64. The first step in the clinical assessment of a patient in coma is to determine whether it is a result of bihemispheric dysfunction or brain stem dysfunction. Rapid assessment combining history and physical examination findings with neuroimaging is important in determining the cause and possible treatment options.

65. Demonstration of the loss of all brain stem reflexes including respiration on two examinations separated by 24 hours, after all toxic and metabolic causes of coma have been ruled out, is sufficient for the diagnosis of brain death.

66. Protocol-driven therapy using benzodiazepines to stop seizures, followed by antiepileptic medication to prevent recurrence, is the mainstay of therapy for status epilepticus.

67. Acute ischemic stroke is a medical emergency that can be treated effectively. Time is brain!

68. The major characteristics of headache in aneurysmal rupture include the suddenness of onset, the severity, the quality, and associated symptoms.

69. Ventilatory failure and autonomic dysfunction are the major complications of Landry-Guillain-Barré syndrome. Monitoring vital capacity, inspiratory force, heart rate, and blood pressure are keys to following up with patients.

70. Close monitoring of respiratory function using measurements of vital capacity and inspiratory force is required in patients in myasthenic crises. In patients with myasthenia and respiratory failure, the distinction should be made between myasthenic crises and cholinergic crisis.

71. If you suspect a patient in the ICU has a component of alcohol withdrawal, institute benzodiazepine therapy. Beta blockers or clonidine may be useful adjuvants for patients who exhibit hypertension and tachycardia.

72. Cerebral perfusion pressure therapies have been and remain the mainstays of treatment for traumatic brain injury. Cerebral perfusion pressure therapy is designed to maintain adequate cerebral blood flow and aggressively treat elevations in intracranial pressure.

73. Early excision and grafting are the keys to optimal survival and healing for burns. Maintain a high index of suspicion for smoke inhalation and intubate early.

74. Early small bowel obstructions can be managed conservatively (with nasogastric tube decompression and IV fluids) if the patient does not have systemic indicators of inflammation or peritoneal signs.

75. Untreated tension pneumothoraces are associated with high mortality rates and therefore represent medical emergencies.

76. It is not a flail chest, but rather the underlying associated pulmonary contusion, that places patients at high risk for respiratory insufficiency.

77. In blunt chest trauma, normal physical examination, chest radiography, ECG, and transthoracic echocardiography findings identify a low-risk subgroup of patients but do not effectively rule out myocardial contusion. Due to its anterior location, the right ventricle is the most common site of contusion.

78. Extubation in the operating room can be safely performed in select patients undergoing liver transplantation.

79. Patients receiving a heart transplant via the biatrial technique will have two P waves on ECG: one for the donor and one for the recipient atria.

80. When using succinylcholine as muscle relaxant for emergent intubation in the ICU, keep in mind its potential adverse effects, such as an increase in serum potassium levels; blood pressure changes and cardiac arrhythmias; increased intracerebral, intraocular, and intragastric pressure; and trigger for rhabdomyolysis and malignant hyperthermia.

81. The most frequently used analgesic agents in the ICU are opioids; that is, morphine, fentanyl, hydromorphone, and sufentanil. Morphine has an active metabolite, morphin-6-glucuronid, which is more potent and longer-lasting and may accumulate, especially in renal insufficiency, causing anesthesia and respiratory depression for several days.

82. If a critically ill patient has fluctuating changes in mental status and seems confused, assess the patient for delirium using the Confusion Assessment Method for the Intensive Care Unit. If the patient is diagnosed with ICU delirium, assess all causes and remove all precipitating factors, if possible.

83. Tetanus as a clinical disease can be completely prevented by appropriate vaccination. It may occur after any disruption in skin integrity, including minor-appearing injuries.

84. Naloxone will reverse most opiate sedation unless the patient has already suffered hypoxic encephalopathy, in which case a partial response or no response may be seen.

85. Heated, humidified oxygen delivery is an effective and simple-to-apply therapy for patients with mild to moderate hypothermia who are hemodynamically stable.

86. The adage, "A patient is not dead until warm and dead" is contravened only by obviously lethal (nonhypothermic) injury, no code status, inability to perform chest wall compressions, discovery of clotted or frozen intravascular contents, endangerment of rescuers, or sound physician judgment.

87. If a person who comes from a hot environment or is undergoing strenuous exercise presents with an altered mental status, consider heat stroke. Heat stroke is a true medical emergency requiring immediate action; the longer it takes to lower the person's core temperature, the worse his or her condition will be.

88. In treating a patient with a severe and persistent unexplained metabolic acidosis in whom ingestion of methanol or ethylene glycol cannot be ruled out, a loading dose of 15 mg/kg of fomepizole (Antizol) will, if either of these agents is present, prevent metabolism to toxic metabolites for approximately 12 hours.

89. If a patient has a severe unexplained metabolic acidosis, consider, treat, and rule out aspirin, methanol, and ethylene glycol ingestion. Early hemodialysis after acute aspirin intoxication should be instituted for a high and rising salicylate level, mental status changes indicating early cerebral edema, pulmonary edema, or renal failure/oliguria.

90. The most important determinant of the risk of hepatotoxicity after a large acute acetaminophen overdose is the time to treatment with the first dose of N-acetylcysteine. After massive acetaminophen overdoses, metabolic acidosis, coma, renal toxicity, and pancreatitis also can occur.

91. Although the potential adverse effects on the fetus of radiologic investigations and drug therapy should always be considered, appropriate investigation and treatment of the mother are almost always in the fetus's best interest.

92. The mainstay of pharmacologic management of delirium is haloperidol. There is some evidence to support the use of risperidone, olanzapine, and quetiapine. Benzodiazepines should not be used as monotherapy for delirium except in special circumstances such as delirium due to alcohol withdrawal.

93. For patients with a history of alcohol abuse, thiamine should be given before any glucose infusion to prevent Wernicke-Korsakoff syndrome.

94. Neuroleptic malignant syndrome can occur at any age in either sex with exposure to any antipsychotic medication. Antipsychotic agents are not the only substances that can cause neuroleptic malignant syndrome; antiemetics and illicit drugs should be considered as well.

95. Although it is technically a legal definition, the competency of a patient can be determined by most health care providers. When in doubt about any moral or ethical issue, consult the institution's ethics committee.

96. Withdrawal of support is a clinical procedure, and, if possible, procedures should follow a protocol. Patients should not receive treatment that will not benefit them, but actions should not take place to hasten a patient's death.

97. The multidisciplinary critical care committee and team can play a pivotal role in the coordination of the delivery of care.

98. The incidence of ventilator-associated pneumonia can be reduced with the use of the ventilator bundle.

99. Your ICU population will not be considered as subjects of material for publication in a high-level scientific journal nor for benchmarking issues unless you provide an objective measurement of general severity at admission.

100. Unwanted variation in clinical care may be responsible for up to 50% of deaths in the ICU. The ICU intervention with the largest effect on mortality, morbidity, and costs is the use of intensivists and closed ICUs.

I. BASIC LIFE SUPPORT

GENERAL APPROACH TO THE CRITICALLY ILL PATIENT

Manuel Pardo, Jr., MD, and Michael A. Gropper, MD, PhD

This book deals with many different aspects of critical care. Each disorder has specific diagnostic and management issues. However, when initially evaluating a patient, one must have a conceptual framework for the patterns of organ system dysfunction that are common to many types of critical illness. Furthermore, in the patient with multiple organ failure, resuscitation or "stabilization" is often more important than establishing an immediate, specific diagnosis.

1. **Which organ systems are most commonly dysfunctional in critically ill patients?**
   The respiratory system, the cardiovascular system, the internal or metabolic environment, the central nervous system (CNS), and the gastrointestinal tract.

2. **What system should be evaluated first?**
   The first few minutes of evaluation should address life-threatening physiologic abnormalities, usually involving the airway, the respiratory system, and the cardiovascular system. The evaluation should then expand to include all organ systems.

3. **Which should be performed first—diagnostic maneuvers or therapeutic maneuvers?**
   The management of a critically ill patient differs from the typical sequence of history and physical examination followed by diagnostic tests and therapeutic plans. The pace of assessment and therapy is quicker, and simultaneous evaluation and treatment are necessary to prevent further physiologic deterioration. For example, if a patient has a tension pneumothorax, the immediate placement of a chest tube may be lifesaving. Extra time should not be taken to transport the patient to a monitored setting. If there are no obvious life-threatening abnormalities, it may be appropriate to transfer the patient to the intensive care unit (ICU) for further evaluation. Many patients are admitted to the ICU solely for continuous electrocardiogram monitoring and more frequent nursing care.

RESPIRATORY SYSTEM

4. **How do you evaluate the respiratory system?**
   The most important function of the lungs is to facilitate oxygenation and ventilation. Physical examination may reveal evidence of airway obstruction or respiratory failure. These signs include cyanosis, tachypnea, apnea, accessory muscle use, gasping respirations, and "paradoxic" respirations. Auscultation may reveal rales, rhonchi, wheezing, or asymmetric breath sounds.

5. **Define *paradoxic respirations* and *accessory muscle use*. What is their significance?**
   Normal breathing involves simultaneous rise and fall of the abdomen and chest wall. A patient with paradoxic respirations has asynchrony of abdominal and chest wall movement. With inspiration, the chest wall rises as the abdomen falls. The opposite occurs with exhalation. *Accessory muscle use* refers to the contraction of the sternocleidomastoid and scalene muscles

with inspiration. These patients have increased "work of breathing," which is the amount of energy the body consumes for the work of the respiratory muscles. Most patients use accessory muscles before they develop paradoxic respirations. Without support from a mechanical ventilator, patients with paradoxic respirations will eventually develop respiratory muscle fatigue, hypoxemia, and hypoventilation.

6. **What supplemental tests are useful in evaluating the respiratory system?**
   Although all tests should be individualized to the particular clinical situation, arterial blood gas (ABG) analysis, pulse oximetry, and chest radiography rapidly provide useful information at a relatively low cost-benefit ratio.

7. **What therapy should be considered immediately in a patient with obvious respiratory failure?**
   Mechanical ventilation may be an immediate life-sustaining therapy in a patient with obvious or impending respiratory failure. Mechanical ventilation can be carried out *invasively* or *noninvasively*. Invasive ventilation is carried out via endotracheal intubation or tracheotomy. Noninvasive ventilation is instituted with a nasal mask or a full face mask. Even if the patient does not have obvious respiratory distress, supplemental oxygen should be administered until the oxygen saturation is measured. The risk of developing oxygen-induced hypercarbia is rare in any patient, including those with an acute exacerbation of chronic obstructive pulmonary disease.

CARDIOVASCULAR SYSTEM

8. **How do you evaluate the cardiovascular system?**
   The most important function of the cardiovascular system is the delivery of oxygen to the body's vital organs. The determinants of oxygen delivery are cardiac output and arterial blood oxygen content. The blood oxygen content, in turn, is determined primarily by the hemoglobin concentration and the oxygen saturation. It is difficult to determine the hemoglobin concentration and the oxygen saturation by physical examination alone. Therefore, the initial evaluation of the cardiovascular system focuses on evidence of vital organ perfusion.

9. **How is vital organ perfusion assessed?**
   The measurement of heart rate and blood pressure is the first step. If the systolic blood pressure is below 80 mmHg or the mean blood pressure is below 50 mmHg, the chances of inadequate vital organ perfusion are greater. However, because blood pressure is determined by cardiac output and peripheral vascular resistance, it is not possible to estimate cardiac output from blood pressure alone. The vital organs and their method of initial evaluation are as follows:
   - **Lungs** (*see* questions 4–7)
   - **Skin:** Assess warmth and capillary refill in all extremities.
   - **CNS:** Assess level of consciousness and orientation.
   - **Heart:** Measure blood pressure and heart rate, and ask for symptoms of myocardial ischemia (e.g., chest pain).
   - **Kidneys:** Measure urine output and creatinine.

10. **What supplemental tests are useful in the initial evaluation of the cardiovascular system?**
    Electrocardiography is a potentially useful diagnostic test with a low cost-benefit ratio. Cardiac enzyme tests, such as troponin measurement, are generally available within hours and can suggest myocardial injury. Other tests, which may entail more risk and cost, should be

determined after the initial evaluation. This may include echocardiography, right heart catheterization, central venous pressure measurement, or coronary angiography.

11. **What therapies should be considered immediately in a patient with hypotension and evidence of inadequate vital organ function?**
Fluid and vasopressor therapy can rapidly restore vital organ perfusion, depending on the cause of the deterioration. In most patients, a fluid challenge is well tolerated, although it is possible to precipitate heart failure and pulmonary edema in a volume-overloaded patient. Other therapies that may be immediately lifesaving include thrombolysis or coronary angioplasty for an acute myocardial infarction. Patients with hypotension from sepsis may benefit from early therapy involving defined goals for blood pressure, central venous pressure, central venous oxygen saturation, and hematocrit.

   Rivers E, Nguyen B, Havstad S, et al: Early goal-directed therapy in the treatment of severe sepsis and septic shock. N Engl J Med 345:1368–1377, 2001.

METABOLIC ENVIRONMENT

12. **How do you evaluate the metabolic environment?**
The clinical laboratory is required for most metabolic tests. It is difficult to evaluate the metabolic environment by physical examination alone.

13. **Why are metabolic changes important to detect in a critically ill patient?**
Metabolic abnormalities such as acid-base, fluid, and electrolyte disturbances are common in critical illness. These disorders may compound the underlying illness and require specific treatment themselves. They may also reflect the severity of the underlying disease. Metabolic disorders such as hyperkalemia and hypoglycemia can be life threatening. Prompt testing and treatment may reduce morbidity and improve patient outcome.

14. **Which laboratory tests should be performed in the initial evaluation of the metabolic environment?**
The selected tests should have a rapid reporting time, be widely available, and be likely to produce a change in management. Tests that fit these criteria include measurements of glucose, white blood cell count, hemoglobin, hematocrit, electrolytes, anion gap, blood urea nitrogen, creatinine, and pH. Some of these tests may be unnecessary in a particular patient, and supplemental testing may be useful in others.

CENTRAL NERVOUS SYSTEM

15. **How do you evaluate the CNS?**
A neurologic examination is the first step in evaluating the CNS. The examination should include assessment of mental status (i.e., level of consciousness, orientation, attention, and higher cortical function). CNS disturbances in critical illness can be subtle. Common changes include fluctuations in mental status, changes in the sleep-wake cycle, or abnormal behavior. The remainder of the neurologic examination includes assessment of respiratory pattern, cranial nerves, sensation, motor function, and reflexes.

16. **What diagnostic tests and therapies should be immediately considered in a patient with altered mental status?**
Oxygen therapy may be useful in patients with altered mental status from hypoxemia. Pulse oximetry or ABG analysis should be done to evaluate this. IV dextrose may be lifesaving in patients with hypoglycemia. Additional diagnostic tests may be indicated depending on the

clinical situation. Lumbar puncture, head computed tomography (CT) or magnetic resonance imaging scan, electroencephalography, and metabolic testing may be useful in directing specific therapies.

KEY POINTS: THE GENERAL APPROACH TO CRITICALLY ILL PATIENTS

1. In the first few minutes, try to identify any life-threatening problems that require immediate treatment.

2. In patients with respiratory distress, consider whether immediate mechanical ventilation is necessary to prevent respiratory arrest.

3. Administer a fluid challenge for hypotensive patients without evidence of pulmonary edema.

4. When possible, use treatment strategies that have demonstrated benefit in clinical trials of critically ill patients.

GASTROINTESTINAL TRACT

17. **How do you evaluate the gastrointestinal tract?**
    History and abdominal and rectal examination are the first steps in an initial evaluation of the gastrointestinal tract. Abdominal catastrophes such as bowel obstruction and bowel perforation are common inciting events leading to multiple organ failure. In addition, abdominal distention can reduce the compliance of the respiratory system, leading to progressive atelectasis and hypoxemia. Further diagnostic tests such as chest radiography, plain radiography of the abdomen, or abdominal CT scan may be useful in certain patients. For example, the finding of "free air" in the abdomen may lead to surgery for correction of bowel perforation.

OTHER ISSUES

18. **Besides the information about current organ system function, what else should one learn about a patient in the initial evaluation?**
    After assessing current medical status, one should develop a sense for the "physiologic reserve" of the patient, as well as the potential for further deterioration. This information may often be gained by observing the patient's response to initial therapeutic maneuvers. It is also important to realize that patients may not desire cardiopulmonary resuscitation or other life-support therapies. If the patient has completed an advance directive, such as a durable power of attorney for health care, these guidelines should be followed or discussed further with the patient.

    Franklin C: 100 thoughts for the critical care practitioner in the new millennium. Crit Care Med 28:3050–3052, 2000.

19. **What measures can be taken to reduce patient morbidity in the ICU?**
    The prevention of complications in the ICU is an important patient safety issue. Each ICU should develop strategies to prevent complications such as venous thromboembolism, nosocomial pneumonia, and central line infections. In the last several years, a number of clinical trials have

focused on reducing morbidity and mortality among critically ill patients. Many of these studies have evaluated common ICU problems such as acute respiratory distress syndrome, sepsis, and postoperative hyperglycemia. Practices such as hand washing can have a major impact on the incidence of complications.

WEBSITE

Making Health Care Safer: A Critical Analysis of Patient Safety Practices
http://www.ahrq.gov/clinic/ptsafety/

BIBLIOGRAPHY

1. Gropper MA: Evidence-based management of critically ill patients: Analysis and implementation. Anesth Analg 99:566–572, 2004.

CHAPTER 2

CARDIOPULMONARY RESUSCITATION

David Shimabukuro, MDCM

Most of the information provided in this chapter can be reviewed in greater detail by referring to specific guidelines published by the American Heart Association (AHA), in conjunction with the International Liaison Committee on Resuscitation. Please visit the AHA's website at http://www.heart.org and follow the links to Cardiopulmonary Resuscitation and Emergency Cardiovascular Care (CPR & ECC). The 2005 CPR & ECC Guidelines can be found in Circulation 112(24 Suppl), 2005.

1. **What is meant by cardiopulmonary resuscitation (CPR)?**

   To most people, *CPR* refers to basic life support (BLS), which encompasses rescue breathing and closed-chest compressions. For health care providers, the term can be much broader and can include advanced cardiac life support (ACLS), pediatric advanced life support, and advanced trauma life support. Thus, it is very important for the physician to be specific whenever discussing resuscitation with patients and their families.

2. **Is iatrogenic cardiopulmonary arrest very common?**

   It probably occurs much more often than it really should. Without a doubt, errors of omission and commission contribute to the incidence and poor outcome of in-hospital cardiopulmonary arrests. In a study of 562 in-hospital arrests, a major unsuspected diagnosis was present (and proved by autopsy) in 14% of cases. The two most common missed diagnoses were pulmonary embolus and bowel infarction, which together accounted for 89% of all missed conditions. Retrospective reviews indicate that as many as 15% of in-hospital arrests are probably avoidable. These cases can be attributed to respiratory insufficiency and hemorrhage that are often undetected or diagnosed too late, as aberrations in patients' vital signs and their complaints (especially dyspnea) are frequently ignored.

   Direct iatrogenesis also contributes to in-hospital cardiopulmonary arrests. Almost every procedure, including esophagogastroduodenoscopy, bronchoscopy, central venous line placement, and an abdominal computed tomography scan with contrast has, on occasion, been associated with an arrest. The injudicious use of lidocaine, sedative-hypnotics, and opiates are primarily responsible for these types of arrests throughout the hospital. Careful hemodynamic monitoring, especially pulse oximetry, by a dedicated practitioner can decrease the occurrence of this easily avoidable complication.

   Bedell SE, Fulton EJ: Unexpected findings and complications at autopsy after cardiopulmonary resuscitation (CPR). Arch Intern Med 146:1725–1728, 1986.

3. **What are the ABCDs of resuscitation?**

   According to all published guidelines, the ABCDs of resuscitation are airway, breathing, circulation, and defibrillation.

4. **How is BLS performed?**

   The ABCDs should guide, streamline, and organize the resuscitation of all patients who are unconscious or in cardiopulmonary extremis.

   - **Airway:** The patient's airway is opened by performing a head tilt–chin lift or a jaw thrust. These maneuvers will thereby displace the mandible anteriorly, lifting the tongue and epiglottis away from the glottic opening. To help improve airway patency, if suction is available, the mouth and oropharynx are suctioned and a plastic oropharyngeal or nasopharyngeal airway is inserted.

- **Breathing:** Once the airway has been opened, the adequacy of respirations needs to be determined. Look at the chest to see whether it is rising; listen and feel for air movement. If necessary, assist respirations by performing mouth-to-mouth, mouth-to-mask, or bag-valve-mask breathing. For an apneic patient, give two breaths. The technique used will depend on the clinical setting, the equipment available, and the rescuer's skill and training. In addition, to avoid insufflation of the stomach with consequent emesis and aspiration, one should deliver slow even breaths, allowing for full exhalation. Furthermore, keeping peak inspiratory pressures low and using the Sellick maneuver (applying digital pressure to the cricoid cartilage) may reduce the possibility of this hazard.

- **Circulation:** After opening the airway and assessing breathing, check for a spontaneous circulation by palpating the carotid pulse. If the patient is pulseless, begin chest compressions. Place the heels of the hands, one atop the other, on the lower half of the sternum. Be careful to avoid the ribs and the xiphoid process because a fracture of either could be very deleterious. Compress the chest smoothly and forcefully, approximately 100 times per minute, allowing for full chest recoil. The force used should be enough to depress the chest by 4–5 cm. Until the airway is definitively secured, the recommended sequence is 30 chest compressions to two ventilations (one cycle of CPR). The patient should be reevaluated after every five cycles (about 2 minutes). Once there is a definitive airway, chest compressions are performed continuously and 8–10 breaths per minute are given (asynchronous).

- **Defibrillation:** As soon as an automatic external defibrillator or monitor/defibrillator becomes available, it should be attached to the patient and the cardiac rhythm analyzed. If indicated, a single high-energy shock should be delivered, followed immediately by 2 minutes of CPR and then reevaluation of the patient.

For adults, if the rescuer is alone in the community, once it is established that the patient is unconscious, the emergency medical services system should be activated, and an automatic external defibrillator should be retrieved (if one is readily available) before continuing with the ABCDs. In the hospital setting, help should always be called for immediately. Of note, CPR should ideally only be performed by those persons who have been certified by the AHA. Certification is easily obtained by attending one or two classes taught by qualified instructors. Most communities offer these classes to the general public.

5. **How does blood flow during closed-chest compressions?**
   There are two basic models derived from animal studies that explain the movement of blood during closed-chest compressions. In the cardiac pump model, the heart is squeezed between the sternum and spine. Systole occurs when the heart is compressed; the atrioventricular valves close and the pulmonary and aortic valves open, ensuring ejection of blood with unidirectional, antegrade flow. Diastole occurs with the release of the squeezed heart resulting in a fall in intracardiac pressures; the atrioventricular valves open while the pulmonary and aortic valves close. Blood is subsequently drawn into the heart from the vena cavae and lungs.

   In the thoracic pump model, the heart is considered a passive conduit. Closed-chest compression results in uniformly increased pressures throughout the thoracic cavity. Forward flow of blood occurs with each squeeze of the heart and thorax due to the relative noncompliance of the arterial system (i.e., they resist collapse) and the one-way valves preventing retrograde flow in the venous system. Both of these models probably contribute to blood flow during CPR.

Paradis NA, Martin GB, Rivers EP, et al: Coronary perfusion pressure and the return of spontaneous circulation in human cardiopulmonary resuscitation. JAMA 263:1106–1113, 1990.

6. **What is the main determinant of a successful resuscitation?**

There are two principal factors that can highly influence the outcome of resuscitation. The first factor is access to defibrillation. For most adults, the primary cause of sudden, nontraumatic cardiac arrest is ventricular tachycardia (VT) or ventricular fibrillation (VF), for which the recommended treatment is electric defibrillation. The second factor is time—or more specifically, time to defibrillation. Survival from a VF arrest decreases by 7% to 10% for each minute of delay. Defibrillation at the earliest possible moment is vital in facilitating a successful resuscitation. Interestingly, only 15% of patients who experience an out-of-hospital arrest survive to discharge; the percentage is even lower for those who have an in-hospital event.

7. **What is the role of pharmacologic therapy during ACLS?**

The immediate goals of pharmacologic therapy are to improve myocardial blood flow, increase ventricular inotropy, and terminate life-threatening arrhythmias, thereby restoring and/or maintaining spontaneous circulation. Combined α/β-adrenergic agonists, such as epinephrine, and smooth muscle V_1 agonists, such as vasopressin, augment the mean aortic-to-ventricular end-diastolic pressure gradient (coronary perfusion pressure) by increasing arterial vascular tone. Although primarily α-adrenergic agonists, phenylephrine and norepinephrine also increase arterial pressure and myocardial blood flow, but neither has been shown to be superior to epinephrine. Of note, recent data (both animal and human) have shown that vasopressin may be advantageous over epinephrine when comparing patients' survival rates to hospital discharge and residual neurologic deficits.

In addition to improving or maintaining myocardial blood flow, pharmacologic therapy during ACLS is also aimed at terminating or preventing arrhythmias, which can further damage an already severely ischemic heart. VT and VF markedly increase myocardial oxygen consumption at a time when oxygen supply is tenuous because of poor delivery. Intracellular acidosis only causes the myocardium to be more dysfunctional and irritable, which makes the heart more vulnerable to arrhythmias. Amiodarone, a class III antiarrhythmic agent, has become the drug of choice for the treatment of the majority of life-threatening arrhythmias.

8. **Is sodium bicarbonate indicated in the routine management of cardiopulmonary arrest?**

No! The primary treatment of metabolic acidosis from tissue hypoperfusion and hypoxia during a cardiac arrest is adequate chest compressions and ventilation. The metabolic acidosis is usually unimportant in the first 15–18 minutes of resuscitation. If adequate ventilation can be maintained, the arterial pH usually remains above 7.2. Some argue that during CPR, ventilation is at best suboptimal, leading to a combined metabolic and respiratory acidosis, dropping the pH well below 7.2. Studies have shown that severe acidosis leads to depression of myocardial contractile function, ventricular irritability, and a lowered threshold for VF. In addition, a markedly low pH interferes with the vascular and myocardial responses to adrenergic drugs and endogenous catecholamines, reducing cardiac chronotropy and inotropy. Although it is appealing to administer sodium bicarbonate in this situation, the clinician must keep in mind that the bicarbonate ion, after combining with a hydrogen ion, generates new carbon dioxide. Cell membranes are highly permeable to carbon dioxide (more so than bicarbonate) and, therefore, administration of sodium bicarbonate causes a paradoxic intracellular acidosis. The resultant intramyocardial hypercapnia leads to a profound decline in cardiac contractile function and failure of resuscitation. The generated carbon dioxide also needs to be eliminated to prevent worsening of an already present respiratory acidosis. Given the poor cardiac output during CPR and probable suboptimal ventilation, this may be quite difficult.

Because the optimal acid-base status for resuscitation has not been established and no buffer therapy is needed in the first 15 minutes, the routine administration of sodium bicarbonate for acidosis resulting from a cardiac arrest is not recommended. Only restoration of the spontaneous circulation with adequate tissue perfusion and oxygen delivery can reverse this ongoing process.

9. **What are the arrhythmias associated with most cardiopulmonary arrests?**
Most sudden, nontraumatic cardiopulmonary arrests in adults are caused by VF or VT from myocardial ischemia or infarct caused by coronary artery disease. Electrolyte disturbances (hypokalemia or hypomagnesemia), prolonged hypoxia, and drug toxicity can also be important inciting factors in patients with multiple medical problems. Also not uncommon are brady-asystolic arrests (as many as 50% of in-hospital arrests). One cause of this arrhythmia could be unrecognized hypoxemia or acidemia. Other causes include heightened vagal tone precipitated by medications, an inferoposterior myocardial infarction (Bezold-Jarisch reflex), or invasive procedures. A third common arrest rhythm seen is pulseless electric activity (PEA). A common etiology is prolonged arrest itself. Typically, after 8 minutes or more of VF, electrical defibrillation induces a slow, wide-complex PEA that tends to be terminal and is known as a *pulseless idioventricular rhythm*. On most occasions of an unsuccessful resuscitation, VF degrades to pulseless idioventricular rhythm before the patient becomes asystolic. The rhythm of PEA can also be narrow and fast, which accompanies other reversible life-threatening conditions, rather than just representing a terminal rhythm. Examples are cardiac tamponade, hypovolemia, pulmonary embolus, or tension pneumothorax. These are discussed later in some detail.

10. **What are the most common immediately reversible causes of cardiopulmonary arrest?**
An alert clinician should recognize at the patient's bedside the following treatable causes of cardiopulmonary arrest:
- **Hypovolemia:** This should be suspected in all cases of arrest associated with rapid blood loss. This "absolute" hypovolemia occurs in settings such as trauma (pelvic fractures), gastrointestinal hemorrhage, or rupture of an abdominal aortic aneurysm. A "relative" hypovolemia can occur with sepsis or anaphylaxis resulting from extensive capillary leak. Regardless of the type, a large amount of fluid (crystalloid, colloid, blood) should be rapidly administered and the cause of the hypovolemia corrected (e.g., by taking the patient to the operating room or administering antibiotics).
- **Hypoxia:** Hypoxia from a variety of etiologies can lead to a cardiac arrest. Tracheal intubation with the delivery of a high concentration of oxygen is the treatment of choice while the cause of the hypoxia is determined and definitive management instituted.
- **Hydrogen ions (acidosis):** These can lead to myocardial failure resulting in cardiogenic shock and arrest. The high hydrogen ion concentration also increases myocardial irritability and arrhythmia formation. A known preexisting severe acidosis can be partially compensated for by hyperventilation, but sodium bicarbonate may still need to be administered. The underlying cause of the acidosis should be diagnosed and corrected.
- **Hyperkalemia:** This condition is encountered in patients with renal insufficiency, diabetes, and profound acidosis. Peaked T waves and a widening of the QRS complex, with the electrical activity eventually deteriorating to a sinus-wave pattern, herald hyperkalemia. Treatment includes the administration of calcium chloride, sodium bicarbonate, insulin, and glucose. *Hypokalemia* and other electrolyte disturbances leading to a cardiac arrest are much less common. Treating the abnormality should help restore spontaneous circulation.
- **Hypothermia:** This condition should be easily detected on examination of the patient. The electrocardiogram (ECG) may reveal Osborne waves that are pathognomonic. All resuscitation efforts should be continued until the patient is euthermic.
- **Tablets or toxins:** Ingestion of these items should be considered in those patients with an out-of-hospital cardiac arrest. Some of the more common intoxications include carbon monoxide poisoning after prolonged exposure to smoke or exhaust fumes from incomplete combustion, cyanide poisoning during fires involving synthetic materials, and drug overdoses (intentional or unintentional). High-flow, high-concentration, and, if possible, hyperbaric oxygen, along with the management of acidosis, are the cornerstones of treatment for carbon

monoxide and cyanide poisonings. In addition, IV sodium nitrite and sodium thiosulfate can be used to help remove cyanide from the circulation. Tricyclic antidepressant drugs act as a type IA antiarrhythmic agent and cause slowing of cardiac conduction, ventricular arrhythmias, hypotension, and seizures. Aggressive alkalinization of blood and urine, in addition to seizure control, should aid in controlling toxicity. An opiate overdose causes hypoxia from hypoventilation, whereas an overdose of cocaine can lead to myocardial ischemia. Naloxone reverses the effects of opioids and should be administered immediately if an opioid overdose is suspected.

- **Cardiac tamponade:** Cardiac tamponade presents with hypotension, a narrowed pulse pressure, elevated jugular venous pressure, distant and muffled heart sounds, and low-voltage QRS complexes on the ECG. Trauma victims and patients with malignancies are at greatest risk. Pericardiocentesis or subxiphoid pericardiorrhaphy can be lifesaving.
- **Tension pneumothorax:** This condition must be recognized immediately. Most often it occurs in patients who have experienced trauma or in patients receiving positive-pressure ventilation. The signs of a tension pneumothorax are rapid-onset hypotension, hypoxia, and an increase in airway pressures. Subcutaneous emphysema and reduced breath sounds on the affected side with tracheal deviation toward the unaffected side are commonly noted. The placement of a 14- or 16-gauge IV catheter into the second intercostal space at the midclavicular line or into the fifth intercostal space at the anterior axillary line for immediate decompression is imperative for restoration of circulation. A chest tube can be placed after the tension pneumothorax is converted to a simple pneumothorax.
- **Thrombosis of a coronary artery:** This condition can lead to myocardial ischemia and infarct. Reperfusion is a vital determinant for eventual outcome. Cardiac catheterization is the primary choice if it is immediately available; thrombolysis is a good alternative.
- **Thrombosis of the pulmonary artery:** Thrombosis of the pulmonary artery can be devastating. Some patients may present with dyspnea and chest pain, similar to acute coronary syndromes, but those who present in cardiac arrest have a minimal chance of survival. Therapy would include immediate thrombolysis to unload the right ventricle while restoring pulmonary blood flow.

11. **How should VF be treated?**

Early defibrillation with a single countershock at an energy level of 360 joules for a monophasic waveform defibrillator is recommended to minimize myocardial damage and to prevent the development of post-countershock pulseless bradyarrhythmias or tachyarrhythmias. Each subsequent shock, following five cycles of CPR, should continue to be at 360 joules if the patient remains in pulseless VT or VF. If using a biphasic waveform defibrillator, the energy level equivalent to a 360-joule monophasic waveform shock, as determined by the manufacturer, should be used. If this energy level is not known and it is firmly established that one is using a biphasic waveform defibrillator, it is recommended that a single countershock of 200 joules be administered.

If the initial single countershock is not successful at terminating the VF, according to ACLS guidelines, epinephrine or vasopressin should be given while CPR continues. After five cycles or 2 minutes of CPR, the rhythm should be reevaluated. If the patient remains in VF or pulseless VT, the defibrillator should be charged appropriately while CPR continues. When ready, the patient should be cleared and the shock delivered; CPR should be immediately reinstituted and rhythm analysis delayed. After five cycles or 2 minutes of CPR, the patients should once again be reevaluated. If this process is still unsuccessful, an antiarrhythmic agent, amiodarone or lidocaine, should be administered. Venous access and a definitive airway should be obtained during periods of patient reevaluation. CPR is not to be interrupted unless absolutely necessary. The sequence should always be five cycles of CPR, patient evaluation and drug administration, charge of defibrillator with CPR in progress, defibrillation, immediate resumption of five cycles of CPR, patient evaluation and drug administration, etc.

12. **Is pulseless idioventricular rhythm treatable?**
    Delayed electrical defibrillation or prolonged VF frequently results in a pulseless idioventricular rhythm or asystole. In the majority of cases, the idioventricular rhythm is not amenable to treatment and results in death. In animal experiments, high-dose epinephrine (0.1–0.2 mg/kg) has helped to restore cardiac contractility and pacemaker activity; however, several clinical studies have shown no benefit in long-term survival or neurologic outcome. It is not recommended at this time.

    Brown CG, Martin DR, Pepe PE, et al: A comparison of standard-dose and high-dose epinephrine in cardiac arrest outside the hospital. N Engl J Med 327:1051–1055, 1992.

13. **How is asystole treated?**
    In brief:
    1. Rapidly determine whether there is any evidence that resuscitation should not be attempted.
    2. Perform CPR and confirm the absence of electrical cardiac activity (a flatline in an ECG may be due to technical mistakes). Rotate the monitoring leads 90 degrees (if using pads/paddles) and maximize the amplitude to detect fine VF (if present,defibrillation should be performed immediately). Verify the absence of pulses at the carotid or femoral artery.
    3. Every 5 minutes, administer atropine 1 mg (up to 3 mg) to counter any vagal activity and epinephrine 1 mg to increase myocardial perfusion.
    4. Always consider stopping resuscitative efforts.

14. **What are the appropriate routes of administration of drugs during resuscitation?**
    The preferred choice is by the IV route. If a central venous catheter is in place, this should be used over a peripheral venous line. Administration of drugs through a peripheral venous line will result in a slightly delayed onset of action, although the peak drug effect is similar to that achieved via the central route. Drugs administered peripherally should be followed with at least 20 mL of normal saline to ensure central delivery. Intracardiac administration should not be performed.

    The "NAVEL" drugs (i.e., naloxone, atropine, vasopressin, epinephrine, lidocaine) are absorbed systemically after endotracheal administration. Although pulmonary blood flow, and hence systemic absorption, is minimal during CPR, recent animal studies suggest that comparable hemodynamic responses can occur. At this time, standard IV doses are recommended for the endotracheal route.

    Virtually every resuscitation drug can be administered in conventional doses via the intraosseous route. This method is preferred in pediatric patients, in whom an IV line cannot be established rapidly.

KEY POINTS: CARDIOPULMONARY RESUSCITATION

1. Iatrogenic cardiopulmonary arrests can occur during procedures; extra care needs to be taken to monitor patients during procedures.

2. Remember the reversible causes of cardiac arrest: hypovolemia, hypoxia, hydrogen ions (acidosis), hypothermia, hyperkalemia, toxins, tablets, and tension pneumothorax.

3. If you do not have IV access, you can give the NAVEL drugs—naloxone, atropine, vasopressin, epinephrine, and lidocaine—down the endotracheal tube. You can give all the drugs via the intraosseous route.

4. Only 5–20% of patients will undergo CPR and survive their hospitalization. You cannot identify the survivors before CPR.

15. **What is the usual outcome of in-hospital CPR?**
Most patients who receive CPR in the hospital do not survive. In fact, only 5–20% of patients live to be discharged home. Furthermore, many patients who do survive have severe impairments of independence and cognition. Unfortunately, it is not yet possible to confidently predict the outcome of in-hospital resuscitation.

McGrath RB: In-house cardiopulmonary resuscitation—after a quarter of a century. Ann Emerg Med 16:1365–1368, 1987.

CHAPTER 3

PULSE OXIMETRY AND CAPNOGRAPHY

Philip E. Bickler, MD, PhD

1. **What is pulse oximetry?**

   Pulse oximetry is a continuous noninvasive estimation of arterial hemoglobin oxygen saturation. It is a means of routinely monitoring oxygenation in diverse clinical settings including the operating room, emergency ward, and intensive care unit (ICU). Clinical use of pulse oximeters falls into two main categories: (1) as a screening or warning system of arterial hemoglobin/ oxygen desaturation and (2) as an endpoint for titration of therapeutic interventions. Because the instruments detect pulsatile blood flow, they also serve as heart rate monitors and as an index of tissue perfusion.

2. **How does a pulse oximeter determine arterial oxygen saturation?**

   Pulse oximetry is based on the spectrophotometric measurement of the degree of oxygen binding to hemoglobin at a point in time when the signal represents that of the arterial blood. That is, saturation is determined at the moment of the peak blood pulse, when oxygen removal by the tissues has not been significant and when the contribution of unsaturated blood in the tissue to the signal is minimal. Hemoglobin-oxygen binding is measured by the degree of absorbance of red light, and the timing of the arterial pulse is detected by an infrared light. Spectrophotometry is based on the Beer-Lambert law, which holds that optical absorbance is proportional to the concentration of the substance and the thickness of the medium. Using this principle, the two wavelengths of light are used to measure both the absorption of oxyhemoglobin (O_2Hb) and reduced hemoglobin (Hb).

   Pulse oximeters function by transmitting light from two light-emitting diodes (LEDs) through tissue containing pulsatile blood flow. Light is transmitted through the tissue at two wavelengths, 660 nm (red, principally absorbed by O_2Hb) and 940 nm (infrared, primarily absorbed by Hb), thus allowing differentiation of oxyhemoglobin from reduced hemoglobin. The infrared signal serves an additional critical function—it detects the timing of the blood pulse through the tissue. The arterial saturation is related to the ratio of the 660/940 ratios at peak pulse, thus making the calculation based on a ratio of these two ratios. This approach is really the key to pulse oximetry and represents a quantum leap from previous attempts to measure blood oxygen noninvasively. The measurement of saturation based on these ratios cancels out differences in tissue geometry, tissue and skin color, venous blood content, etc. A microprocessor algorithm is used to calculate the arterial saturation and includes empiric factors necessary to produce accurate readings for a particular instrument. Several recently introduced pulse oximeter instruments include noise/artifact rejection. These refinements also aid in the determination saturation in patients with low perfusion.

   Aoyagi T, Miyasaka K: The theory and applications of pulse spectrophotometry. Anesth Analg 94(1 Suppl): S93–S95, 2002.

3. **How accurate are pulse oximeters?**

   In published reports, pulse oximetry has an accuracy within 2–3% of the true oxyhemoglobin levels as measured *in vitro* with multiwavelength oximeters. The U.S. Food and Drug Administration requires manufacturers to demonstrate that their instruments confirm to this degree of accuracy in human subjects at between 70% and 100% oxygen saturation. Because the principle of measurement is based on a ratio of absorbance ratios, no calibration of the instrument by the user is needed or possible.

4. **Where are pulse oximetry measurements taken?**
   Pulse oximeter probes can be applied to any site that allows orientation of the LED and photodetector opposite one another across a vascular bed. If the tissue is too thick, the signal is attenuated before reaching the detector and the oximeter cannot function. Oximeters can be applied to fingers, toes, earlobes, lips, cheeks, and the bridge of the nose. Esophageal and oral probes are also in development. Several manufacturers offer "reflectance" oximeter probes that can be applied to flat tissue surfaces such as the forehead. Recently introduced earlobe-mounted sensors combine a pulse oximeter and a transcutaneous CO_2 electrode.

   Kugelman A, Wasserman Y, Mor F, et al: Reflectance pulse oximetry from core body in neonates and infants: Comparison to arterial blood oxygen saturation and to transmission pulse oximetry. J Perinatol 24(6):366–371, 2004.

5. **What factors affect pulse oximetry measurements?**
   Several factors can greatly affect the accuracy and reliability of pulse oximetry. Most errors in oximetry measurement are the result of poor signal quality (i.e., hypoperfusion, vasoconstriction) or excessive noise (i.e., motion artifact). Optical interference may be introduced by extraneous lights (especially fluorescent sources). IV dyes as well as nail polishes (especially green, blue, or black) absorb at the wavelengths used by the oximeter and can produce artificially low measurements. Contamination from venous pulsations caused by dependent venous pooling or valvular insufficiency may also cause low readings. For a similar reason, the simultaneous nature of arterial and venous pulsation during cardiopulmonary resuscitation (CPR) make oximeter data unreliable in this setting. Extreme hyperbilirubinemia has been reported to have variable effects on SpO_2 values. The presence of dysfunctional hemoglobin species can alter the ability of oximetry to reflect the true oxygen saturation. Studies show that darkly pigmented skin can falsely increase saturation estimates derived by some widely used pulse oximeters by up to 7% in the range of 70–80% saturation.

   Bickler PE, Feiner JR, Severinghaus JW: Effects of skin pigmentation on pulse oximeter accuracy at low saturation. Anesthesiology 102(4):715–719, 2005.
   Robertson FA, Hoffman GM: Clinical evaluation of the effects of signal integrity and saturation on data availability and accuracy of Masimo SE and Nellcor N-395 oximeters in children. Anesth Analg 98(3):617–622, 2004.

6. **What effects does dyshemoglobinemia have on pulse oximetry?**
   Because pulse oximeters use two wavelengths of light, they are capable of differentiating only two species of hemoglobin: Hb and O_2Hb. Given that abnormal hemoglobin species such as carboxyhemoglobin (CoHb) or methemoglobin (MetHb) also absorb red and infrared light at these same wavelengths, their presence affects the SpO_2 measurement, and their quantitative contribution cannot be determined. The pulse oximeter assumes that only "functional" hemoglobin is present (O_2Hb or Hb), and the oxygen saturation is calculated based on these amounts.

$$\text{Functional oxygen saturation } SpO_2(\%) = [O_2Hb]/([O_2Hb] + [Hb])$$

A multiwavelength CO-oximeter determines SaO_2 more accurately in the presence of dysfunctional hemoglobins because it possesses wavelengths of light that can be used to detect the presence of carboxyhemoglobin and methemoglobin.

$$\text{Fractional oxygen saturation } SaO_2(\%) = [O_2Hb]/([O_2Hb] + [Hb] + [CoHb + MetHb, \text{ etc.}])$$

For example, CoHb is read by the limited wavelength analysis of a pulse oximeter as O_2Hb (carboxyhemoglobin is scarlet red), which will falsely elevate the SpO_2 reading. The absorption pattern of MetHb is interpreted by the pulse oximeter as 85% saturation; thus, progressively higher levels of methemoglobin cause the SpO_2 value to converge on 85% regardless of the actual SaO_2. When the presence of significant amounts of dysfunctional hemoglobin is suspected, a CO-oximeter should be used to determine O_2Hb saturation.

The presence of fetal hemoglobin has not been shown to significantly affect the accuracy of SpO_2 measurements because its light absorption properties are similar those of adult hemoglobin.

Ralston AC, Webb RK, Runciman WB: Potential errors in pulse oximetry. III: Effects of interferences, dyes, dyshaemoglobins and other pigments. Anaesthesia 46(4):291–295, 1991.

7. **Will pulse oximetry detect an increase in intrapulmonary shunting?**
   Pulse oximetry can only differentiate hemoglobin oxygen saturation from desaturation. At higher levels of oxygenation, it offers little resolution because the hemoglobin is already nearly 100% saturated with oxygen. An increase in shunting sufficient to cause a decrease in PaO_2 from 200 to 100 mmHg would thus not be detectable by pulse oximetry. However, shunting or any other cause of hypoxia significant enough to cause a drop in oxygenation below approximately 60 mmHg would yield a significant drop in SpO_2 because the oxyhemoglobin dissociation curve begins to have a strong association with oxygen partial pressure at these levels. Thus, the pulse oximeter is a useful monitor of changes in oxygenation and ventilation in patients breathing room air or in those whose PaO_2 is approaching the threshold requiring acute clinical intervention.

8. **What are the complications of pulse oximetry?**
   Pulse oximetry is noninvasive and relatively safe. Complications are most commonly caused by errors in data interpretation leading to inappropriate treatment. The response to decreased saturation should include verifying that the pulse amplitude signal is free of artifacts and that an electrocardiography-derived heart rate matches that of the pulse oximeter. *If the oximeter cannot detect arterial pulsations, the SaO_2 reading will not be accurate.* The sensors contain electronic circuitry that could potentially malfunction. There have been infrequent reports of thermal burns resulting from defective LED probes. Standard pulse oximeter probes cannot be used for patients undergoing MRI both because the high radiofrequency and magnetic fields can induce probe or wire heating and cause thermal burns and because the wiring may produce artifacts in the MR images. Pressure necrosis may result from prolonged placement in one position. This occurs most often with spring-loaded sensors and in patients with impaired peripheral perfusion.

KEY POINTS: PULSE OXIMETRY

1. Pulse oximeter accuracy is most strongly degraded by low perfusion states; accept only numeric estimates of saturation that are associated with clean perfusion signals.

2. Pulse oximeters may interpret dyes, skin pigment, methemoglobinemia, and dyshemoglobinemia as alterations in hemoglobin-oxygen saturation.

9. **How can pulse oximetry measurements be obtained in patients with severe vasoconstriction?**
   The cause of vasoconstriction should be addressed. The patient with hypoperfusion should receive adequate volume therapy and inotropic support if necessary. A patient with hypothermia should receive therapy that addresses both core and peripheral warming. Heating the hand with

warm blankets can often significantly increase perfusion and improve the function of the oximeter. In selected cases, a digital nerve block using 1% lidocaine without epinephrine often restores sufficient pulsatile flow to enable SpO_2 monitoring.

10. **What is capnography? How does it work?**

Capnography is the continuous measurement of exhaled carbon dioxide over time and its graphic display (Fig. 3-1). It provides a noninvasive method to monitor both ventilation and perfusion. Most commonly, infrared spectrophotometry is used to determine the CO_2 concentration of a continuous sample of airway gas. Sampling usually occurs in one of two ways. In a mainstream capnograph, CO_2 levels are measured with a sensor (light source and detector) placed directly in line with the patient's breathing circuit. Alternatively, sidestream capnographs continuously divert a sample of gas away from the patient's breathing circuit to the capnograph for analysis and display. The mainstream method has a very brief response time, but because the sensor must be placed near the patient, long-term monitoring may prove to be cumbersome. The sidestream method, because it uses a thin plastic sampling tube, is lighter and allows for greater flexibility, but because transit time is unavoidable, a slower response time (approximately 1.5 seconds) results. Due to mixing of gases in the sample stream, the absolute values of the plateau and baseline may also be slightly attenuated. The sidestream device can also be used with a modified nasal cannula to monitor CO_2 concentrations in the airway of nonintubated patients.

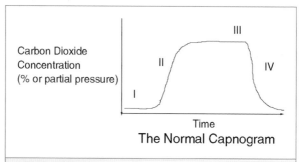

Figure 3-1. A capnogram is a plot of airway CO_2 versus time. Phase I (inspiratory baseline) refers to inspired gas devoid of CO_2. Phase II (beginning expiration) represents expiration of anatomic dead space followed by gas from respiratory bronchioles and alveoli. Phase III (alveolar plateau) corresponds with exhalation of alveolar gases. The last portion of the plateau is termed *end-tidal* (PETCO$_2$). Phase IV (inspiratory downslope) is the beginning of the next inspiration.

11. **What other methods are used to measure CO_2 in respiratory gases?**

The most commonly used method for measuring carbon dioxide in expired gases is infrared light absorbance. In addition, technologies such as Raman spectrometry and mass spectrometry are reliable, accurate, and responsive but generally more expensive. However, these options also offer detection of a variety of other gases and anesthetic vapors. Colorimetric detectors that attach to endotracheal tubes are available to help assess endotracheal tube placement. The colorimetric detector uses a pH-sensitive indicator strip to semiquantitatively detect exhaled CO_2. Although portable and convenient, these devices yield results that are often more difficult to interpret than conventional capnographs, and they can only be used once.

12. **Why is measurement of end-tidal carbon dioxide important?**

A capnograph provides a continuous display of the CO_2 concentration of gases in the airways. The CO_2 partial pressure at the end of normal exhalation (end-tidal CO_2, $PETCO_2$) is a reflection of gas leaving alveoli and is an estimate of the alveolar CO_2 partial pressure, $PACO_2$. When ventilation and perfusion are well matched, the $PACO_2$ closely approximates the $PaCO_2$, and thus $PaCO_2 \approx PACO_2 \approx PETCO_2$. The presence of cyclical exhaled CO_2 is useful in confirming airway patency, verifying endotracheal tube placement, and verifying the adequacy of pulmonary ventilation. In addition, decreases in cardiac output caused by hypovolemia or cardiac dysfunction result in decreased pulmonary perfusion. This causes an increased alveolar dead space, which dilutes $PETCO_2$. The resulting depression of end-tidal CO_2 can be observed by capnography. Animal studies show that a 20% decrease in cardiac output causes a 15% decrease in $PETCO_2$.

13. **What can a capnogram reveal about the patient's condition?**

Alterations in the shape of the capnogram in an intubated, ventilated patient often provide clues to alterations in pulmonary pathology and malfunction of ventilation equipment. For example, a staircase pattern in phase II may indicate sequential emptying of the lung, which may occur in main stem partial bronchial obstruction. An upward sloping plateau in phase III is a classic indication of late emptying of poorly ventilated alveolar spaces with elevated PCO_2, which may occur with expiratory obstruction at the level of smaller airways, as seen in chronic obstructive pulmonary disease (COPD), bronchospasm, and other forms of ventilation perfusion mismatching. A pulmonary embolus is another cause of a decrease in end-tidal CO_2.

Gravenstein N, Good ML: Noninvasive assessment of cardiopulmonary function. In Civetta JM, Taylor RW, Kirby RR (eds): Critical Care, 2nd ed. Philadelphia, J.B. Lippincott, 1992, pp 291–312.

14. **What factors affect the arterial–end-tidal CO_2 gradient?**

The normal gradient between $PaCO_2$ and $PETCO_2$, $P(a-ET)CO_2$, is <6 mmHg. The gradient between $PaCO_2$ and $PETCO_2$ increases when pulmonary perfusion is reduced or ventilation is maldistributed. This occurs with the development of high ventilation/perfusion alveolar units (increased dead space ventilation). The result is an increased $P(a-ET)CO_2$ and decreased $PETCO_2$. Examples of this state are COPD, pulmonary hypoperfusion, and pulmonary emboli. Technical failures such as accidental extubation and endotracheal tube cuff leak can also cause a decrease in $PETCO_2$.

15. **Is it possible to see an expired CO_2 waveform after esophageal intubation?**

The stomach may contain some exogenous CO_2 or carbonated solutions before intubation. Also, ineffective mask ventilation may force previously exhaled gas from the pharynx into the stomach. Initially, this may produce a normal capnogram tracing, but because CO_2 is not continuously generated, the expired concentration will fall toward zero as sequential breaths dilute the existing gases. Esophageal intubation should be suspected if the capnogram tracing begins to "fall off" after five or six breaths.

Takeda T, Tanigawa K, Tanaka H, et al: The assessment of three methods to verify tracheal tube placement in the emergency setting. Resuscitation 56(2):153–157, 2003.

16. **What physiologic parameters affect the measurement of $ETCO_2$?**

End-tidal CO_2 may be altered by changes in CO_2 production and elimination. $ETCO_2$ may be expected to increase during hypermetabolism, such as during hyperthermia or sepsis, and decrease with hypothermia or hypometabolism. More often, however, changes in the pulmonary system affect CO_2 elimination. Hypoventilation and rebreathing cause increased $ETCO_2$, whereas hyperventilation and ventilation/perfusion mismatching produce decreased $ETCO_2$. Only in circumstances that result from ventilation/perfusion mismatching (e.g., hypoperfusion, embolism, grossly impaired diffusion) will the $PETCO_2$ fail to accurately reflect the state of the arterial carbon dioxide levels ($PaCO_2$). Because this gradient between end-tidal and arterial CO_2 reflects a greater degree of inefficient ventilation, the respiratory system must make up for this inefficiency by increasing the minute ventilation (via increased tidal volume or respiratory rate) to maintain clearance of the body's CO_2 production.

KEY POINTS: CAPNOGRAPHY

1. An upsloping trace of the capnogram during expiration (alveolar plateau, phase III) occurs with airway obstruction such as in asthma or COPD.

2. Capnography is valuable in the evaluation of the effectiveness of circulatory and ventilatory support measures during CPR.

17. **How does capnography assist in CPR efforts?**
In the course of CPR, capnography not only can help verify tracheal intubation, it can also monitor the adequacy of circulatory assistance. The presence of exhaled CO_2 during CPR is useful in that it provides evidence of enough circulation to produce CO_2 transport from tissues to the lungs. Thus, assuming constant minute ventilation and CO_2 production, changes in $PETCO_2$ reflect the status of overall circulation. Some investigators have suggested that if the $PETCO_2$ is >15 mmHg at the beginning of CPR, it may predict successful resuscitation. Failure to achieve any recovery of $PETCO_2$ should prompt consideration of a diagnosis of inadequate cardiac filling. This may be caused by hypovolemia, tamponade, pneumothorax, or pulmonary embolism. Low $PETCO_2$ also may be caused by alveolar hyperventilation, or it may indicate ineffective CPR. The return of spontaneous circulation is heralded with a substantial increase in $PETCO_2$, primarily because of increased flow of hypercarbic blood to the lungs.

Callaham M, Barton C: Prediction of outcome of cardiopulmonary resuscitation from end-tidal carbon dioxide concentration. Crit Care Med 18(4):358–362, 1990.

18. **Is pulse oximetry cost-effective?**
The effectiveness of pulse oximetry in the ICU must be extrapolated from studies of its use in the operating/recovery room. These reports have suggested that the enhanced early detection of arterial oxygen desaturation afforded by pulse oximetry may lead to improved outcomes, such as a decreased incidence of perioperative myocardial ischemia. However, its benefit in terms of decreasing the incidence of respiratory complications has been difficult to demonstrate, even in large populations.

There are few published data that permit direct, outcome-based conclusions concerning either the clinical impact or cost-benefit ratio of pulse oximetry. One study has demonstrated a decrease in total cost of care associated with the introduction of pulse oximetry and capnography. The savings realized were a result of a reduced need for arterial blood gas (ABG) measurements and associated operating costs. Pulse oximetry and capnography may aid in the weaning of ventilatory support by decreasing the need for ABG sampling. In a consensus statement, the Technology Assessment Task Force of the Society of Critical Care Medicine asserted that routine use of pulse oximetry in critically ill patients results in cost savings because of the positive impact on patient outcomes, but it also acknowledged the need for more detailed study of the subject.

Ely EW, Baker AM, Evans GW, Haponik EF: The distribution of costs of care in mechanically ventilated patients with chronic obstructive pulmonary disease. Crit Care Med 28:408–413, 2000.

1. **What are the indications for placement of an arterial line?**
   Arterial catheters are used when frequent arterial blood samples are necessary or when close, accurate, real-time measurement of blood pressure is needed. Usually this need arises when a patient is profoundly hypotensive or hypertensive or when fast-acting blood pressure medications are being used.

2. **What is the Allen test?**
   In most people, the radial artery is connected by the palmar arch vessels to the ulnar artery. If the radial artery is damaged or thrombosed, the ulnar artery will keep the hand alive. The Allen test ensures that this dual blood supply and palmar arch are patent. The radial and ulnar arteries are squeezed manually until the hand blanches. Then the ulnar artery is released. If the hand turns pink, then the ulnar artery and palmar arch are patent, and the radial artery can be cannulated without fear of hand necrosis.

3. **What are the risk factors for thrombosis after arterial cannulation?**
   - Big catheter relative to the size of the vessel
   - Multiple punctures
   - Long duration of use
   - Shock
   - Vasoconstricting drugs

4. **What is overdampening? What causes it?**
   Proper measurement of pressures using catheters depends on appropriate tubing. When catheter tubing is too pliable, is kinked, or has an air bubble in it, the waveform will be overdampened. This results in artificially depressed systolic pressure and artificially elevated diastolic pressures. Mean pressures are not affected by dampening.

5. **What hemodynamic events are represented by the *a wave,* the *c wave,* and the *v wave* on a central venous/right atrial pressure waveform?**
   - **a wave:** Atrial contraction (after p wave on an electrocardiogram [ECG])
   - **c wave:** Tricuspid valve closure (at the end of the QRS complex on an ECG)
   - **v wave:** Atrial filling (after the t wave) (Fig. 4-1)

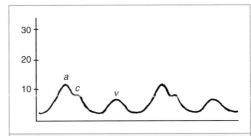

Figure 4-1. Central venous pressure/right atrial pressure tracing.

6. **Central venous pressure (CVP) tracings vary during every patient breath. At what point in the respiratory cycle should we measure CVP to avoid respiratory artifact?**
   - In a spontaneously breathing patient, a breath produces negative thoracic pressures. Therefore, to avoid artificially low measurements, the CVP should be measured just before a breath (just before the baseline starts to drop).
   - In a patient undergoing positive pressure ventilation, each breath is accompanied by positive thoracic pressure. Therefore, CVP is measured just before the baseline starts to rise.

7. **What data does the pulmonary artery catheter give us?**
   The pulmonary artery catheter gives us values for pressures, such as right atrial pressure, pulmonary capillary wedge pressure, and pulmonary artery diastolic pressure. It also measures cardiac output, and blood can be drawn from it to generate a mixed venous blood gas.

8. **Why are we interested in the mixed venous O_2 saturation (SvO_2)?**
   When tissue beds are poorly perfused (such as when a patient is in shock), they will extract more oxygen from the blood, and the venous blood returning to the heart will be more deoxygenated than in a healthy person. Therefore, a low SvO_2 can be used to diagnose hypoperfusion/shock.

9. **What is a normal value for SvO_2?**
   The normal value is 60–75%.

10. **Is a high SvO_2 always good?**
    No. Patients with septic shock are unable to properly extract and use oxygen, so venous blood returning to the heart will be very oxygen rich. Also, single-organ ischemia may not affect SvO_2.

11. **Why are we interested in the pressure in the pulmonary capillaries?**
    When the catheter tip is wedged in the pulmonary artery, the tip (theoretically) measures the pressure in a continuous column of blood that extends from the catheter tip, through the pulmonary capillaries and pulmonary veins, and into the left atrium and ventricle. Left ventricular pressure correlates with left ventricular end-diastolic volume, which in turn is related by a Starling curve to myocardial contractility. Therefore, the wedge pressure is used to help decide whether the left ventricle is being filled enough to allow it to maximally contract.

12. **Why is a pulmonary artery catheter often called a "Swan"?**
    The pulmonary artery catheter does float gracefully downstream like a swan, but in fact the flow-directed pulmonary catheter was developed in 1968 by Dr. Jeremy Swan and Dr. William Ganz at the Cedars-Sinai Medical Center.

13. **What are the characteristics of a right ventricular pressure tracing?**
    A sharp upstroke and downstroke, with a slight rise between the end of the downstroke and the beginning of the next upstroke (Fig. 4-2).

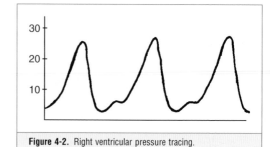

Figure 4-2. Right ventricular pressure tracing.

14. **What are the characteristics of a pulmonary artery pressure tracing?**
    - A sharp upstroke and downstroke, with a dicrotic notch (pulmonic valve closure) in the middle of the downstroke
    - Slight downward slope in the valley between diastole and systole (Fig. 4-3)

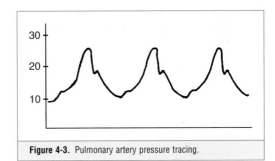

Figure 4-3. Pulmonary artery pressure tracing.

15. **What are the complications of pulmonary artery catheters?**
    Complications that can arise from central venous cannulation include arterial injury (8%), pneumothorax (2–4%), hydrothorax (2%), infection (5%), venous thrombosis (60%), injury to phrenic and laryngeal nerve, and brachial plexus injury. Complications of the pulmonary artery catheter itself include arrhythmia (13–70%), right bundle branch block (3%), cardiac injury (<1%), pulmonary artery rupture (<1%), and catheter knotting.

16. **Describe the changes in systolic and diastolic pressure values in a catheter passing from the right ventricle to the pulmonary artery.**
    - Systolic pressure stays roughly the same.
    - Diastolic pressure rises.

17. **What is the thermodilution method?**
    This describes the way that a pulmonary artery catheter is used to measure cardiac output. A small amount of cold or room temperature fluid (injectant) is injected via a proximal hole in the catheter. This injectant mixes with blood in the flowing pulmonary artery and then passes a thermometer at the catheter tip. The more warm blood flowing through the vessel, the higher the temperature at the catheter tip. This temperature, along with the volume and temperature of the injectant, is input into a bedside computer that estimates cardiac output.

18. **Do pulmonary artery catheters help or hurt patients?**
    The use of pulmonary artery catheters has been called into question in numerous studies over the last decade. There is scant literature showing that the use of these devices decreases mortality in the intensive care unit. Some studies have suggested that this lack of benefit may be due to the fact that many caregivers who use pulmonary artery catheters lack a sophisticated understanding of their use and in interpretation of the data they provide.

    Connors A, Speroff T, Dawson N, et al: The effectiveness of right heart catheterization in the initial care of critically ill patients. JAMA 276:889–897, 1996.
    Dalen J, Bone R: Is it time to pull the pulmonary artery catheter? JAMA 16:916–918, 1996.

19. **Should the catheter balloon be inflated during insertion and removal of pulmonary artery catheters?**
    The balloon should be inflated while the catheter is advanced or inserted and deflated during withdrawal. Advancing the catheter without the balloon inflated may result in improper placement, or, more importantly, rupture of a vessel wall with the catheter tip.

20. **How is systemic vascular resistance (SVR) measured?**
SVR is not measured. It is calculated from mean arterial pressure (MAP), cardiac output (CO), and CVP using the following formula:

$$SVR = [(MAP - CVP) \times 80]/CO$$

21. **What is the difference between global and local perfusion monitoring? What are some examples of global tissue perfusion monitoring?**
Global tissue monitoring measures overall changes in oxygen metabolism. Local tissue perfusion monitoring measures perfusion of specific tissue beds. Examples of global tissue perfusion monitoring include measurement of oxygen consumption and delivery, mixed venous oxygen saturation, and serum lactate.

KEY POINTS: COMMON WAYS OF MONITORING PERFUSION

1. DO_2/VO_2 measurement (global perfusion)

2. SVO_2 measurement (global perfusion)

3. Lactate levels (global perfusion)

4. Gastric or sublingual tonometry (local tissue perfusion)

22. **What is the formula for oxygen delivery (DO_2)?**

$$DO_2 = \text{cardiac output} \times \text{oxygen content}$$
$$= CO \times (1.3[\text{Hb}]O_2 \text{ saturation} + 0.002 \, PO_2)$$

23. **Which is a more important determinant of the oxygen content of blood—PO_2 or O_2 saturation?**
O_2 saturation is more important. The parenthetic part of the equation in question 22 is the formula for oxygen content, and it shows that PO_2 is multiplied by 0.002, making it clinically irrelevant.

24. **What is a "sacrificial lamb" tissue bed?**
This phrase refers to a tissue bed that is among the first to lose its blood flow when the body becomes hypoperfused. *Local* tissue perfusion monitoring is based on measurement of perfusion of these tissue beds. Because they are the first areas of the body to lose perfusion, they can be sensitive indicators of early shock.

25. **What tissue beds have been chosen for perfusion monitoring?**
Gastric mucosa, sublingual mucosa, and skin are three examples. Near infrared spectrometry has been used to measure perfusion in a number of other organs as well.

26. **What does a gastric tonometer measure?**
A gastric tonometer is a gastric catheter with a bubble at the tip that lodges against the gastric mucosa. Infrared spectrometry is used to measure the partial pressure of CO_2 in the bubble. This is used to calculate gastric mucosal pH, which is used to assess gastric mucosal perfusion.

INTERPRETATION OF ARTERIAL BLOOD GASES

E. Michael Canham, MD

CHAPTER 5

1. **What do arterial blood gas (ABG) instruments measure?**
   The current ABG instruments measure pH, PCO_2, and PO_2 using three separate electrodes. The blood gas samples are placed through an inlet into a temperature-controlled chamber (usually 37°C), where the blood is exposed to these three electrode tips. Newer ABG machines have simultaneous co-oximeter measurements as well. Consequently, using an absorption spectrophotometer, measurements of reduced hemoglobin, oxyhemoglobin, carboxyhemoglobin, and methemoglobin can also be made.

   Severinghaus JW, Astraup P, Murray JF: Blood gas analysis and critical care medicine. Am J Respir Crit Care Med 157:S114–S122, 1998.

2. **When should ABGs be analyzed?**
   Analysis of ABGs is used extensively in the critical care setting to evaluate both acid-base status and oxygen and carbon dioxide gas exchange. Analysis of ABGs is indicated in virtually all cardiopulmonary conditions.

   Raffin TA: Indications for arterial blood gas analysis. In Sox HC Jr (eds): Common Diagnostic Tests, 2nd ed. Philadelphia, American College of Physicians, 1990, pp 100–119.

3. **What are the problems associated with obtaining ABGs?**
   The arterial puncture may result in acute hyperventilation, which is often minimized by good technique, by use of a small needle, or by instillation of a local anesthetic. After the sample is obtained, all air bubbles should be expelled and the syringe capped. Air bubbles that are mixed or agitated into the sample will equilibrate with the blood, possibly altering the PO_2. The sample should be placed on ice unless the analysis is performed within 15 minutes. Plastic syringes may allow greater diffusion of gases than glass syringes and thus should also be run promptly. In the absence of extreme leukocytosis, an iced, glass ABG syringe will maintain the PO_2 value for up to 3 hours.

KEY POINTS: SITUATIONS IN WHICH AN ARTERIAL BLOOD GAS ANALYSIS IS REQUIRED

1. An ABG analysis is required if carboxyhemoglobin or methemoglobinemia is suspected.

2. Assessment of acid-base status necessitates an ABG analysis.

3. ABG analysis is required in the presence of poor oximetry signal due to hypoperfusion, hypothermia, severe anemia, or venous congestion.

4. Calculation of the alveolar gas equation involves ABG analysis.

4. **What does extreme leukocytosis ("leukocyte larceny") do to the ABG analysis?**
   The presence of large numbers of leukocytes or platelets will reduce the PO_2 value, giving a false impression of hypoxemia. This drop in PO_2 is negligible if the sample is stored in ice and analyzed within 1 hour. Presumably the ongoing metabolism of the cellular elements of

blood consume oxygen, reducing PO_2. Another mechanism of pseudohypoxemia may be explained by the interference of the oxygen electrode because of the markedly increased numbers of leukocytes or platelets. A centrifuged ABG specimen of plasma may be used to measure the PO_2.

Charan NB, Mark M, Caravalho P: Use of plasma for arterial blood gas analysis in leukemia. Chest 105:954–955, 1994.

Hess CE, Nichols AB, Hunt WB, Suratt PM: Pseudohypoxemia secondary to leukemia and thrombocytosis. N Engl J Med 301:361–363, 1979.

5. **How long after starting or stopping supplemental oxygen should one wait before ABG samples can be drawn at a point when they will reflect baseline or plateau values?**
   In patients with severe obstructive lung disease and air trapping, 25 minutes may be required; however, in the absence of significant lung disease, 5–7 minutes would be adequate.

Cugell DW: How long should you wait? [editorial]. Chest 67:253, 1975.

6. **What is the alveolar gas equation?**
   The alveolar gas equation is a formula used to approximate the partial pressure of oxygen in the alveolus (PAO_2):

$$PAO_2 = (PB - PH_2O)FiO_2 - (PaCO_2 \div R)$$

where PB is the barometric pressure, PH_2O is the water vapor pressure (usually 47 mmHg), FiO_2 is the fractional concentration of inspired oxygen, and R is the gas exchange ratio. (The rate of CO_2 production to O_2 use is usually around 0.8 at rest.) For example, at sea level:

$$PAO_2 = (760 - 47)0.21 - (40 \div 0.8) = 100 \text{ mmHg}$$

7. **What is the alveolar-arterial PO_2 difference, or "A-a gradient" (i.e., AaO_2 gradient)?**
   After calculation of the PAO_2 from the alveolar gas equation, the AaO_2 gradient can be obtained by subtracting the PaO_2 measured from the ABGs. For example, at sea level (where PCO_2 is 40, and PO_2 is 92):

$$100 \text{ mmHg} - 92 \text{ mmHg} = 8 \text{ mmHg}$$
$$PAO_2 - PaO_2 = AaO_2 \text{ gradient}$$

The normal AaO_2 gradient is dependent on age, body position, and nutritional status. The AaO_2 gradient is widened under normal conditions by age, obesity, fasting, supine position, and heavy exercise. One predictive equation for estimating PO_2 (at PB = 760 mmHg) in relation to age is as follows:

$$PO_2 = 109 - 0.43 \times \text{age (in years)}$$

Sorbini CA, Grassi V, Solinas E, Muiesan G: Arterial oxygen tension in relation to age in healthy subjects. Respiration 25:3–13, 1968.

8. **How is the AaO_2 gradient useful?**
   The AaO_2 gradient may be widened by any significant cardiopulmonary condition that results in hypoxemia and/or hypocarbia. Hypoxemia caused by simple alveolar hypoventilation will not widen the AaO_2 gradient. Most pulmonary emboli, on the other hand, will widen the AaO_2 gradient because even if hypoxemia does not occur, hypocarbia is very common.

Cvitanic O, Marino PL: Improved use of arterial blood gas analysis in suspected pulmonary emboli. Chest 95:48–51, 1989.

9. **What is the difference between a calculated versus a measured oxygen saturation?**
   The calculated oxyhemoglobin saturation is calculated from the measured values of PaO_2 and pH by the Severinghaus slide rule, a nomogram, or the blood gas instrument microprocessor. The measured oxyhemoglobin saturation is obtained with a co-oximeter (a spectrophotometer). Errors in the calculation of oxygen saturation may occur if carboxyhemoglobin is present, which is

commonly seen in cigarette smokers. Carbon monoxide does not affect oxygen tension (PaO_2) but does bind and displace oxygen from hemoglobin. Consequently, the calculated oxygen saturation is falsely elevated.

The calculated oxygen saturation may also be in error if the oxyhemoglobin dissociation curve is displaced by changes in 2,3-diphosphoglycerate (2,3-DPG). The binding of 2,3-DPG to hemoglobin reduces the affinity of hemoglobin for oxygen, facilitating the unloading of oxygen at the tissue level. The binding of 2,3-DPG to

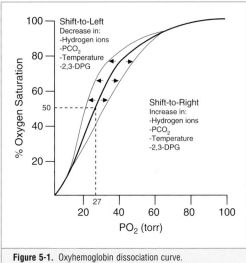

Figure 5-1. Oxyhemoglobin dissociation curve.

hemoglobin shifts the oxyhemoglobin dissociation curve to the right. A common example of 2,3-DPG depletion occurs in the storage of blood. Consequently, a patient receiving multiple units of stored blood, with a leftward shift of the oxyhemoglobin dissociation curve, will have a calculated oxygen saturation less than the measured oxygen saturation (Fig. 5-1).

Hemoglobinopathies will also cause a discrepancy between the measured and calculated oxygen saturation, depending on which way they shift the oxyhemoglobin dissociation curve.

Severinghaus JW: Blood gas calculator. J Appl Physiol 21:1108–1116, 1966.

10. **How do continuous intra-arterial blood gas monitors (CIABGMs) work?**
    Most of the CIABGMs in development or in current use utilize optical fiber sensors (i.e., optodes), which quantify photochemical reactions from light absorption, light reflection, or fluorescence. The optical fibers transmit a light signal down the fiber, where it interacts with a dye. Changes in the concentration of the measured substance (i.e., CO_2, O_2) within the dye complex causes an alteration of the light signal by absorption, reflection, or fluorescence. The CIABGM probe generally consists of three fiberoptic fibers with specific dyes for measuring pH, PCO_2, and PO_2. Additionally, a thermocouple is included for continuous temperature measurement of blood. The role of CIABGM is unclear until outcome and cost-benefit studies are completed.

Venkatesh B, Hendry SP: Continuous intra-arterial blood gas monitoring. Intensive Care Med 22:818–828, 1996.

11. **What are point-of-care (POC) ABGs?**
    Current technology allows measurement of ABGs at the bedside with handheld blood gas analysis devices that use disposable cartridges. Several commercially available devices provide different test options to measure in addition to routine ABG values. Consequently, the reliability of each measured parameter may differ from one device to another.

12. **How do POC ABGs work? What are their advantages and disadvantages?**
    The heparinized ABG specimen is placed into the POC cartridge, where the blood flows to different sites/sensors for analysis. The pH and PCO_2 are measured by direct potentiometry, and the PO_2 is measured amperometrically. The values for HCO_3, total CO_2, base excess, and oxygen saturation are calculated. POC testing can be performed by nurses, physicians, and respiratory therapists, and the ABG results are obtained more rapidly and may influence critical

decisions. The major disadvantages include cost per cartridge, lack of preanalysis calibrations to ensure accuracy, and the lack of inclusion of co-oximetry measurements.

Severinghaus JW, Astraup P, Murray JF: Blood gas analysis and critical care medicine. Am J Respir Crit Care Med 157:S114–S122, 1998.

13. **Given that oximetry is so readily available, painless, and accurate, why is ABG analysis necessary?**

Oximetry and the newer technology that made it more accessible, affordable, and accurate have decreased the need for ABG analysis in monitoring oxygen saturation. In fact, in many hospitals the number of ABG analyses performed has decreased with the influx of oximeters into virtually every department within a hospital. However, relying on oximetry alone can lead to misdiagnosis, increased cost, and potentially fatal respiratory arrest. Consider the following examples of pitfalls of using oximetry alone that have been observed in practice:

1. A patient was noted to have oxygen desaturation via oximetry during a routine check after minor orthopedic surgery. The physicians evaluated this oximetric abnormality by ordering chest radiography, pulmonary function tests, and a ventilation-perfusion lung scan, all of which yielded normal results. Finally, AGB analysis was done and revealed alveolar hypoventilation alone with a normal AaO$_2$ gradient. The oxygen desaturation was simply the result of an increased PCO$_2$ from hypoventilation in a patient receiving narcotics.

2. After an episode of smoke inhalation, a patient came to the emergency department for headache and nausea. The oxygen saturation by oximetry was normal, and the patient was nearly dismissed after symptomatic treatment alone. Fortunately, recognizing the limitation of oximetry in differentiating oxygenated hemoglobin from carboxyhemoglobin, the physician drew an ABG sample, which revealed profound carbon monoxide poisoning. The patient was treated appropriately with 100% oxygen and close monitoring.

3. A house officer was asked to see a febrile, septic patient with a respiratory rate of 40 breaths/min and a chest radiograph revealing early alveolar infiltrates bilaterally. The administration of oxygen was initiated, and with the use of oximetry, the oxygen saturation was titrated to 90%. The patient required FiO$_2$ of 100% by nonrebreather mask to achieve the 90% oxygen saturation. Unfortunately, the house officer did not draw an ABG sample and failed to realize that with marked hyperventilation and respiratory alkalosis, the oxyhemoglobin dissociation curve is shifted to the left, thereby causing a much higher oxygen saturation for a given PaO$_2$. Had ABG analysis been done at that time, it would have revealed pH of 7.58, PACO$_2$ of 22, PAO$_2$ of 50, and O$_2$ saturation of 90%—all clearly indicating intubation and assisted ventilation with positive end-expiratory pressure. Later that evening, the patient suffered a near-fatal respiratory arrest (*see* Fig. 5-1).

4. You are asked to consult on a patient who has just completed a transesophageal echocardiogram. Conscious sedation was used with a local anesthetic spray (benzocaine). Oxygen saturation as measured by oximetry drops to 75%. POC ABG reveals normal pH and PCO$_2$ and a PO$_2$ of 250 mmHg on supplemental oxygen. However, the blood specimen appears brownish! A second ABG sample sent to the lab with co-oximetry reveals a methemoglobin level of 24%. Benzocaine-induced methemoglobinemia is diagnosed and resolves with the administration of IV methylene blue.

BIBLIOGRAPHY

1. Asmussen E, Nielsen M: Alveolo-arterial gas exchange at rest and during work at different O$_2$ tensions. Acta Physiol Scand 50:153–160, 1960.
2. Cissik JH, Salustro J, Patton OL, Louden JA: The effects of sodium heparin on arterial blood gas analysis. Cardiovasc Pulm 5:17–21, 1977.
3. Hansen JE: Arterial blood gases. Clin Chest Med 5:227–237, 1989.
4. Hansen JE, Simmons DH: A systematic error in the determination of blood PCO$_2$. Am Rev Respir Dis 115:1061–1063, 1977.

FLUID THERAPY

James E. Wiedeman, MD, and Mark W. Bowyer, MD, DMCC, COL, USAF, MC

CHAPTER 6

1. **How is water distributed throughout the body?**

   Total body water comprises 60% of body weight in males and 50% of body weight in females (Fig. 6-1). The distribution of this water is 40% in intracellular space (30% in females due to larger amounts of subcutaneous tissue and smaller muscle mass) and 20% in extracellular space. The extracellular fluid is broken down into 15% interstitial and 5% plasma. Total body water deceases with age; 75–80% of a newborn's weight is water.

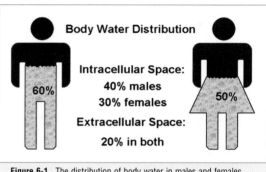

   Figure 6-1. The distribution of body water in males and females.

2. **What are sensible and insensible fluid losses? How are maintenance fluid requirements calculated?**
   - Insensible losses (nonmeasurable)
     - Skin: 600 mL
     - Lungs: 200 mL
   - Sensible losses (measurable)
     - Fecal: 200 mL
     - Urine: 800–1500 mL
     - Sweat: Variable

   These losses account for 2000–2500 mL/day, giving a 24-hour fluid requirement of 30–35 mL/kg to maintain normal fluid balance.

3. **What are fluid maintenance requirements for children?**

   Twenty-four-hour fluid requirements for children have been formulated based on weight:
   - **0–10 kg:** 100 mL/kg
   - **11–20 kg:** 1000 mL + 50 mL/kg for every kilogram above 10 kg
   - **20 kg:** 1500 mL + 20 mL/kg for every kilogram above 20 kg

4. **Describe the clinical features of volume deficit and volume excess.**
   - **Deficits:** These lead to changes in the central nervous system (e.g., decreased mentation), cardiovascular system (e.g., tachycardia, hypotension), skin (e.g., decreased turgor), and metabolism (e.g., hypothermia).

- **Excesses:** Excesses cause distended neck veins, S_3 gallop, basilar rales, and peripheral edema. It is important to note that volume deficit and excess are clinical diagnoses, independent of changes in concentration (e.g., sodium) or composition (e.g., potassium, calcium, magnesium, or bicarbonate).

5. **What are the classes of hemorrhagic shock, how do they relate to a tennis game, and what fluid should be administered in each class?**
   See Table 6-1.

6. **What is the "3:1 rule" in fluid therapy after acute blood loss?**
   Three milliliters of crystalloid is given for each milliliter of blood loss to compensate for administered fluid that is lost into the interstitial and intracellular spaces.

7. **What are the common sources, volumes, and compositions of gastrointestinal fluid losses?**
   See Table 6-2.

8. **What empiric replacement fluids can be used for fluid losses?**
   - **Sweat:** D_5 1/4 normal saline with 5 KCl/L
   - **Gastric:** D_5 1/2 normal saline with 30 KCl/L

TABLE 6-1. CLASSES OF HEMORRHAGIC SHOCK

Class of Shock	Tennis Score	% Blood Loss	Resuscitation Fluid
I	15	$\leq$15%	LR
II	30	15–30%	LR
III	40	30–40%	LR + blood
IV	Game over	>40%	LR + blood

LR = lactated Ringer's solution.

TABLE 6-2. COMMON SOURCES, VOLUMES, AND COMPOSITIONS OF GASTROINTESTINAL FLUID LOSSES

Source	Composition (mEq/L) Na	K	Cl	HCO₃	Volume
Gastric (NG tubes, vomiting)	60	10	130	—	100–400 mL
Duodenum (fistulas)	140	5	80	—	100–2000 mL
Bile (T tubes, fistulas)	145	5	100	35	50–800 mL
Pancreas (fistulas)	140	5	75	115	100–800 mL
Ileum (ileostomies, fistulas)	140	5	104	30	100–9000 mL
Colon (diarrhea)	60	30	40	20	

Na = sodium, K = potassium, Cl = chlorine, HCO_3 = bicarbonate, NG = nasogastric.

- **Bile, pancreas, small bowel:** Lactated Ringer's solution
- **Colon:** D₅ 1/2 normal saline with 30 KCl/L
- **Third space (interstitial loss):** Lactated Ringer's solution

KEY POINTS: FLUID THERAPY

1. Total body water is 60% of body weight (40% intracellular and 20% extracellular). Plasma (blood) volume is 5% of body weight.

2. Diagnose volume deficit or excess by clinical examination, not laboratory study results.

3. Avoid fluid and electrolyte abnormalities by measuring and replacing ongoing gastrointestinal losses with appropriate fluids.

4. Use lactated Ringer's solution to treat acute volume resuscitation.

9. **What is the difference between crystalloids and colloids? Give examples of each.**
   - **Crystalloid:** Crystalloids are mixtures of sodium chloride and other physiologically active solutes. The distribution of sodium will determine the distribution of the infused crystalloid. Examples are normal saline, lactated Ringer's solution, and hypertonic saline.
   - **Colloid:** High-molecular-weight substances that stay in the vascular space and exert an osmotic force are colloids. Examples are albumin, hetastarch, dextran, and blood.

10. **Describe the composition of normal saline and lactated Ringer's solution. Which should be used for acute resuscitation?**
    Table 6-3 summarizes the composition of normal saline and lactated Ringer's solution. Lactated Ringer's solution is preferable for acute volume replacement because normal saline can result in hyperchloremic metabolic acidosis.

CONTROVERSY

11. **What evidence-based data exist to support the use of various resuscitation fluids?**
    - **Lactated Ringer's solution:** This remains the least expensive and best fluid for trauma resuscitation.
    - **Albumin, Hespan, other colloids:** No evidence from randomized controlled trials exists to demonstrate that resuscitation with colloids reduces the risk of death, pulmonary edema, or hospital stay compared with resuscitation with crystalloids in patients with trauma or burns,

TABLE 6-3. COMPOSITION OF NORMAL SALINE AND RINGER'S SOLUTION					
	Na	Cl	K	Ca	Lactate
Normal saline (mEq/L)	154	154	—	—	—
Lactated Ringer's solution (mEq/L)	130	109	4	3	28

Na = sodium, Cl = chlorine, K = potassium, Ca = calcium.

or after surgery. Because colloids are more expensive, it is difficult to justify their continued use in this setting.

- **Hypertonic saline:** The only benefit is shown in patients with head trauma/cerebral edema.

BIBLIOGRAPHY

1. Alderson P, Bunn F, Lefebvre C, et al: Human albumin solution for resuscitation and volume expansion in critically ill patients. Cochrane Database Syst Rev(4):CD001208, 2004.

2. Bunn F, Alderson P, Hawkins V: Colloid solutions for fluid resuscitation. The Cochrane Database of Systemic Reviews, The Cochrane Collaboration, John Wiley & Sons, 2005: www.cochrane.org/cochrane/revabstr/AB001319.htm

3. Fan E, Stewart TE: Albumin in critical care: SAFE but worth the salt? Crit Care 8:297–299, 2004.

4. Roberts I, Alderson P, Bunn F, et al: Colloids versus crystalloids for fluid resuscitation in critically ill patients. The Cochrane Database of Systemic Reviews, The Cochrane Collaboration, John Wiley & Sons, 2005: www.cochrane.org/reviews/en/ab000567.html

CHAPTER 7

NUTRITION IN CRITICALLY ILL PATIENTS

Lee-lynn Chen, MD, and Annette Stralovich-Romani, RD, CNSD

1. **Describe the metabolic changes that occur during critical illness.**
   Critical illness is frequently accompanied by starvation and malnutrition. Metabolic changes associated with critical illness include a shift to a hypermetabolic and hypercatabolic state that is characterized by the release of catecholamines, glucocorticoids, inflammatory mediators, and cytokines. Consequences of these changes include anorexia, weight loss, loss of lean body mass, alterations in immune function, and impaired wound healing.

2. **What are the goals of nutritional support in critically ill patients?**
   The goals of nutritional support in critically ill patients include the preservation and repletion of lean body mass, prevention of macronutrient and micronutrient deficiencies, reduction in overall morbidity and mortality, improvement in patient outcomes, and avoidance of complications related to the delivery of the nutritional support. Other goals of more specialized nutritional support may be to improve immune function, to improve wound healing, or to support hepatic protein synthesis, among others.

3. **Discuss the initial nutritional assessment of a critically ill patient and the clinical indicators of malnutrition.**
   Assessment of nutritional status begins with a history and physical examination. Indicators of malnutrition include recent involuntary weight loss (which can be masked by fluid retention), changes in appetite or bowel habits, presence of persistent gastrointestinal (GI) symptoms, muscle wasting, and signs of specific micronutrient deficiencies such as glossitis or anemia.

   Many patients enter the intensive care unit (ICU) malnourished, and their nutritional status tends to decline with length of stay in the hospital. Serum hepatic protein levels are linked in clinical practice to nutritional status and severity of illness. Because the half-life of albumin is 21 days and that of prealbumin is 2–3 days, albumin is a better indicator of a patient's chronic nutritional status, and prealbumin serves as a marker of changes in the current nutritional state. Often in the ICU, albumin and prealbumin levels are both low despite apparent sufficient nutritional support. Serum levels of albumin, prealbumin, and transferrin (also known as *negative acute phase proteins*) decrease in response to infection, injury, or trauma and increase with recovery from these same conditions. Conversely, positive acute phase proteins such as C-reactive protein (CRP) increase with stresses of critical illness and decrease with health. Prealbumin and CRP should be monitored weekly as a gauge of both severity of illness and adequate nutritional support.

   Fuhrman MP, Charney P, Mueller CM: Hepatic proteins and nutrition assessment. J Am Diet Assoc 104:1258–1264, 2004.

4. **What are the daily nutritional requirements for critically ill patients?**
   A well-balanced fuel mix is advised, as follows:
   - **Glucose:** Fifty to fifty-five percent of total calories should be administered as carbohydrates. Conditions such as chronic obstructive pulmonary disease or an inability to wean the patient from mechanical ventilation might warrant decreasing the amount of carbohydrates; this decision can frequently be guided by calculation of the respiratory quotient (*see* question 6).

KEY POINTS: GOALS OF NUTRITIONAL SUPPORT IN CRITICALLY ILL PATIENTS

1. Nutritional support is useful in the preservation and repletion of lean body mass.

2. Prevention of macronutrient and micronutrient deficiencies is achieved.

3. A reduction in overall morbidity and mortality results from nutritional support.

4. Improvement in patient outcomes and avoidance of complications are related to the delivery of the nutritional support.

- **Fat:** Thirty percent of total caloric intake should be administered as fat. Most enteral formulas contain 30% of the total calories as fat. Omega-3 fatty acids may provide an anti-inflammatory effect and are used increasingly for patients with acute respiratory distress syndrome.
- **Protein:** Between 15% and 20% of total calories per day should be administered as proteins or amino acids. Therapy is generally initiated with 1.2–1.5 gm/kg/day and adjusted after measuring nitrogen retention and other clinical indicators of protein catabolism. Considerations that might warrant a decrease in protein administration include worsening hepatic encephalopathy with a rising blood ammonia level or with renal failure without dialysis (*see* question 8).

The nutritional requirements for many micronutrients such as vitamins, minerals, and other trace elements are still not well established. Electrolytes such as sodium, potassium, magnesium, and phosphate should be supplied and serum levels monitored.

Chan S, McCowen KC, Blackburn GL: Nutrition management in the ICU. Chest 115:145S–148S, 1999.

5. **How can energy requirements be estimated in a critically ill patient?**
Resting energy expenditure can be estimated by using the Harris-Benedict equation.
   - **For males:** Resting energy expenditure (REE) = 66.5 + 13.75 × (weight in kilograms) + 5 × (height in centimeters) − 6.76 × (age in years)
   - **For females:** REE = 655 + 9.56 × (weight in kilograms) + 1.86 × (height in centimeters) − 4.68 × (age in years)

   A major limitation of the Harris-Benedict equation in critically ill patients is that it was derived from indirect calorimetry data in healthy volunteers. To correct for disease states and degrees of stress, the REE is multiplied by factors to better estimate the energy expenditure of critically ill patients. These factors range from 1.2 to 2.0.

   For patients who weigh more than 30% of ideal body weight, an adjusted ideal body weight should be used—otherwise, actual body weight should be used to calculate the energy requirement.

   Indirect calorimetry provides a more accurate way to measure energy expenditure in the ICU by measurement of respiratory gas exchange. Bedside devices (a metabolic cart) measure oxygen consumption (VO_2), carbon dioxide production (VCO_2), and minute ventilation (VE) that are then used in the Weir equation to determine energy expenditure. A major limitation to the use of indirect calorimetry in the ICU is that the measurements become unreliable when the inspired oxygen concentration is greater than 60%. The Weir equation is as follows:

   $$\text{Energy expenditure} = [(VO_2) \times (3.941) + (VCO_2) \times (1.11)] \times 1440$$

6. **How is the respiratory quotient (RQ) defined? How can it be used clinically?**
The RQ is the ratio of the patient's carbon dioxide production (VCO_2) to his or her oxygen consumption (VO_2). These values are obtained by indirect calorimetry at the patient's bedside. The RQ is helpful in guiding the planning of nutritional therapy. The physiologic range for RQ

values is 0.7 to 1.2 and is influenced by the relative contribution from fat, protein, and carbohydrate. RQ values for fat, protein, and carbohydrate are 0.7, 0.8, and 1.0, respectively. Thus, an RQ of >1.0 might suggest excessive carbohydrate or calorie provision that can result in increased CO_2 production and cause difficulty weaning from mechanical ventilation. A RQ of <0.7 might suggest underfeeding and use of ketones as a fuel source.

7. **What are some of the specific nutritional considerations for patients dependent on a ventilator for respiration?**
Nutritional depletion can affect the immune system and predispose to infection, weaken the respiratory muscles, and exacerbate respiratory failure. Malnutrition also causes hypoalbuminemia, thereby potentially accelerating the formation of pulmonary edema fluid. Electrolyte abnormalities such as hypophosphatemia or hypermagnesemia can worsen the function of already weak respiratory muscles. Overfeeding with calories or carbohydrate can lead to excessive CO_2 production and can exacerbate respiratory failure.

8. **How can protein requirements be assessed in a critically ill patient?**
Protein reserves do not exist in the body and must be continually replenished. Table 7-1 provides an estimate of protein requirements. The goal of protein provision is to minimize the degree of net nitrogen loss. A nitrogen balance remains the best available marker of the effects of nutritional intervention and is defined as the nitrogen intake minus the nitrogen losses from urine, skin, and feces:

$$\text{Nitrogen balance (gm)} = (\text{protein intake}/6.25) - (\text{urinary urea nitrogen} + 2 \text{ to } 4)$$

Nitrogen balance determines the quantity of protein required to maintain equilibrium between nitrogen intake and losses. Positive nitrogen balance is associated with improved outcomes and is the best single marker of the effectiveness of nutritional support. Due to the catabolic state associated with critical illness, a positive nitrogen balance is frequently difficult to achieve. Liver failure renders nitrogen balance calculations inaccurate due to decreased urea nitrogen production, whereas excessive diarrhea, high ostomy output, serous drainage from wounds, or other fluid losses make the calculations difficult due to excessive unmeasured losses.

TABLE 7-1. ESTIMATED PROTEIN REQUIREMENTS

Condition	Requirement (gm/kg/day)
Normal renal function	
Maintenance	0.8–1.2
Moderate stress	1.3–1.5
Severe stress	1.5–2.0
Renal failure	
Nondialyzed	0.8–1.2
Hemodialyzed	1.0–1.4
CAPD	1.3–1.5
CAVHD/CVVHD	1.6–1.8
Hepatic failure	Begin at 1.0 gm of protein/kg/day and increase as tolerated to 1.5–2.0 gm of protein/kg/day
Hepatic failure with encephalopathy	0.6–0.8 (no less than 40 gm/day)

CAPD = continuous ambulatory peritoneal dialysis, CAVHD = continuous arteriovenous hemodialysis, CVVHD = continuous veno-venous hemodialysis.

A nitrogen balance cannot be interpreted in the presence of renal dysfunction (creatinine clearance <50 mL/min) or with elevated ammonia levels.

Stralovich-Romani A, Mahutte C, Luce J: Administrative, nutritional, and ethical principles for the management of critically ill patients. In George RB, Light RW, Matthay M, et al (eds): Chest Medicine: Essentials of Pulmonary and Critical Care Medicine, 5th ed. Philadelphia, Lippincott Williams and Wilkins, 2005, pp 497–516.

9. **What is the preferred modality of nutritional delivery—enteral or parenteral?**
   Enteral feeding is the preferred method. Critical illness frequently is associated with atrophy of intestinal mucosa and gut-associated lymphoid tissue (GALT), disruption of normal intestinal flora by antibiotics, ileus induced by a variety of drugs, and decreased production of gastric acid caused by proton pump inhibitors. All of these factors can lead to barrier dysfunction in the gut. The result of this breakdown in intestinal structure and barrier function can lead to malabsorption and bacterial translocation. The term *bacterial translocation* describes the migration of bacteria from the gut lumen to the lymph tissue or bloodstream and has been implicated in the pathogenesis of sepsis and the septic inflammatory response syndrome. "Trophic" or "trickle" feeds (i.e., 10 mL/h) have not been shown to achieve the desired effects in the GI tract; approximately 60% of goal feedings are required to achieve the therapeutic benefits of enteral feeding. Compared with parenteral nutrition, enteral feedings also have reduced infectious complications and expense.

   DeWitt RC, Kudsk KA: The gut's role in metabolism, mucosal barrier function, and gut immunology. Infect Dis Clin North Am 13:465–481, 1999.

10. **When should patients in the ICU be fed?**
    Early enteral nutrition (i.e., within 24 hours of admission) is associated with significantly lower incidence of infections and a reduced length of hospital stay. The presence of bowel sounds and the passage of flatus are not necessary before the institution of enteral nutrition. Potential benefits to early enteral nutrition include attenuation of the stress response, lessening of gut atrophy, and decrease in abnormal gut permeability associated with starvation.

    Marik P, Zloga GP: Early enteral nutrition in acutely ill patients: A systematic review. Crit Care Med 29:2264–2270, 2001.

11. **Describe the routes of administration and the preferred method of delivery for enteral nutrition.**
    Enteral nutrition is generally administered nasoenterically via gastric or small bowel feeding tubes:
    - **Intragastric feedings:** Intragastric feedings require adequate motility and increase the risk of aspiration but do not require the placement of a nasoenteric tube into the small bowel, which can be technically more challenging and may even require fluoroscopic guidance.
    - **Transpyloric (small bowel) feedings:** These feedings are better tolerated, have fewer complications, and can be used even in the presence of gastric and colonic ileus.
    Enteral nutrition can be delivered via bolus, intermittent, or continuous feeding:
    - **Bolus feeding:** Bolus feeding involves the delivery of a large volume of formula over a short period of time and carries a greater risk of aspiration, diarrhea, nausea, vomiting, and distention.
    - **Intermittent feeding:** Intermittent feeding delivers a defined volume of formula over 1–12 hours. Bolus and intermittent feeds must be administered in the stomach.
    - **Continuous feedings:** These feedings deliver a small amount of formula continuously over 24 hours via a mechanical pump. In the setting of critical illness, continuous feedings delivered into the small bowel are far better tolerated than the other aforementioned methods with a lower incidence of aspiration, stress ulceration, and diarrhea, and are thus the preferred method of delivery.

    Binnekade J, Tepaske R, Bruynzeel P, et al: Daily enteral feeding practice in the ICU: Attainment of goals and interfering factors. Crit Care Med 9:R218–R225, 2005.

12. **How should enteral feed tolerance be monitored?**
    Check residuals every 4 hours. If the residuals are >200 mL, hold feedings for 2 hours, and then recheck. If the residuals are <200 mL, resume tube feedings at the previous flow rate or volume of feeding (if bolus/intermittent feeding). If the residuals are still >200 mL after holding feeds for 2 hours, then check feeding tube placement with kidney, ureter, and bladder analysis. Consider promotility agents or advancing the feeding tube through the pylorus and into the duodenum or jejunum. Residuals should be minimal with small bowel feeds. In fact, studies have shown that patients fed through a jejunal feeding tube versus gastric feeding tube received a significantly higher percentage of their daily goal caloric intake and had a lower rate of pneumonia. Additionally, tube feedings postpylorically delivered only need to be held 2–4 hours before a procedure (i.e., extubation).

13. **What types of enteral nutrition solutions are available? How is the right solution selected for a patient?**
    Enteral nutrition formulas are solutions that can contain water, carbohydrate, protein, fat, vitamin, minerals, and electrolytes. There is tremendous variety in the commercially available enteral nutritional formulas. Formulas are frequently classified as polymeric (intact), oligomeric (semielemental/peptide-based), monomeric (elemental), or modular. Polymeric formulas contain intact nutrients and require a fully functional GI tract. Elemental and semielemental formulas contain partially digested nutrients and have applications in patients with compromised GI function. Modular formulas consist of different macronutrient modules that can be combined to meet specific nutritional needs of a particular patient.
    There has been a tremendous proliferation in disease-specific formulas that frequently contain specific pharmaconutrients, immunomodulatory substances, or specific combinations of macro- and micronutrients. These formulas are generally expensive with few data to support improved outcome or efficacy and should be selected with care.

KEY POINTS: OBJECTIVE CRITERIA FOR EVALUATING NUTRITIONAL STATUS

1. Prealbumin and C-reactive protein (CRP) levels should be measured weekly.

2. Nitrogen balance should be established.

3. Indirect calorimetry should be performed.

4. A calorie count must be undertaken.

14. **What are some of the clinical conditions that provide newer applications for enteral nutrition?**
    - **Acute pancreatitis:** Patients with acute pancreatitis were previously kept non per os (NPO) and fed parenterally. Jejunal feedings, which bypass the cephalic and gastric phases of digestion and thus decrease stimulation for exocrine pancreatic secretion, have come to be viewed as a safe and efficacious way to provide nutrition for these patients. In fact, jejunal feeding is considered the standard of care for patients with acute pancreatitis. Enteral nutrition is preferred to maintain the intestinal barrier. It lowers infectious complications, reduces surgical intervention, and reduces the length of hospital stays.
    - **Enterocutaneous fistula:** Enteral feedings are being used more frequently in the management of enterocutaneous fistulae. The enteral feeding must be infused 40 cm distal to the fistula to prevent reflux.

- **Short gut syndrome:** A combination of enteral and parenteral nutritional support can be used to manage short gut syndrome. The enteral nutrition is infused at a very low continuous rate to promote intestinal adaptation and to sustain the GALT.

  Cynober L, Moore FA: Nutrition and Critical Care. Basel, Switzerland, Nestec, Ltd., 2003.

15. **What are some of the potential complications associated with enteral nutrition, and how can these be minimized?**

    Complications of enteral nutrition can be classified as mechanical, GI, or metabolic.

    - **Mechanical complications:** Mechanical complications include obstruction of the tube with medications or pills, irritation of or erosion into nasal or gastric tissue with the associated risk of bleeding, infection or perforation, pulmonary injury during placement, and displacement of the tube with the associated risk of aspiration. To minimize these complications, tubes should be flushed frequently with water, tubes should be soft and well lubricated for insertion, and tube position should be verified before use.

    - **GI complications:** These complications include diarrhea, nausea, vomiting, constipation, and aspiration. Nausea and vomiting are frequently caused by large-volume gastric residuals or drugs and can sometimes be improved by postpyloric placement of the feeding tube and delivery by continuous infusion. Ileus is often associated with narcotic drug administration and can be treated with small doses of oral naloxone with little change in systemic analgesic effect of the opioid. The risk of aspiration is decreased by proper postpyloric tube placement, elevation of the head of the bed, use of smaller feeding tubes, elimination of drugs that decrease lower esophageal sphincter tone, and frequent checks of tube feeding residuals.

    - **Metabolic complications:** Complications of the metabolism are similar to those for parenteral nutrition but are usually less severe. These include hyperglycemia, electrolyte imbalances, and dehydration or overhydration. Frequent monitoring of blood glucose and urine output and judicious use of blood and urine testing can detect these and lead to appropriate alterations in the feedings to prevent or treat these complications as they arise. Tight blood glucose control to levels between 80 and 110 mg/dL with an insulin drip can decrease morbidity and mortality.

      Montejo JC: The Nutritional and Metabolic Working Group of the Spanish Society of Intensive Care Medicine and Coronary Units: Enteral nutrition-related gastrointestinal complications in critically ill patients: A multicenter study. Crit Care Med 27:1447–1453, 1999.

16. **What are the contraindications to enteral feedings?**

    Critically ill patients who do not have adequate GI function should not receive enteral feedings. Conditions that may lead to a nonfunctioning GI tract include ischemic bowel, intestinal obstruction, severe malabsorption, or high-output fistulae with effluent >500 mL/day. High-volume diarrhea or severe distention while receiving tube feedings requires an evaluation and may require discontinuation of tube feeds. As mentioned previously, pancreatitis, enterocutaneous fistulae, and recent GI surgery are not usually contraindications to enteral feeds.

17. **What are the indications for parenteral nutrition in critically ill patients?**

    Parenteral nutrition is indicated when patients demonstrate absolute gut failure or when they are unable to meet their nutritional requirements by oral or tube feedings. This includes patients who may be meeting some of their nutritional requirements by the enteral route but are not tolerating full enteral nutritional support. The majority of patients are solely receiving nourishment through tube feedings and are started on total parenteral nutrition (TPN) only if they cannot tolerate tube feedings to meet their full requirements.

    Jeejeebhoy KN: Total parenteral nutrition: Potion or poison? Am J Clin Nutr 74:160–163, 2001.

18. **What are the usual electrolytes that are added to parenteral nutrition solutions? How does acid-base status affect the choice of electrolytes and their concentration in the parenteral nutrition solution?**

Sodium chloride, potassium chloride, sodium acetate, potassium acetate, calcium gluconate, and magnesium sulfate are the usual electrolytes added to TPN solutions.

Acetate is metabolized to bicarbonate. For patients without significant acid-base abnormalities, the ratio of chloride to acetate administered is generally kept at 1:1. For patients with a metabolic alkalosis, the acetate can be minimized to decrease the amount of bicarbonate produced. For patients with a metabolic acidosis, the acetate in the parenteral nutrition solution should be maximized to increase the amount of bicarbonate produced.

19. **Describe the basic composition of TPN solutions.**

The usual concentration of carbohydrate, in the form of dextrose, is 20–30%. The usual concentration of amino acids ranges from 3% to 15%. IV fat emulsions contain soybean or safflower oil, egg yolk phospholipid, and glycerin. These are available in emulsions of 10%, 20%, or 30%. Multivitamins and certain medications are often added to parenteral nutrition formulas.

The following vitamins and minerals are suggested as supplements for parenteral nutrition: vitamin A, vitamin D, vitamin E, vitamin K, folic acid, niacin, riboflavin, thiamine, pyridoxine (vitamin B_6), vitamin B_{12}, pantothenic acid, biotin, zinc, copper, chromium, and manganese. Patients with liver failure who have a total bilirubin level >10 should exclude manganese and copper from the solution because these are excreted via the biliary system, and with liver/biliary disease, can lead to hepatic deposition of these elements. Multivitamin preparations do not contain iron due to concern about the possibility for allergic reactions. This may require additional supplementation, if indicated.

20. **What are some of the complications of parenteral nutrition?**

Complications of parenteral nutrition can be classified as mechanical, metabolic, infectious, and hepatobiliary.

- **Mechanical complications:** Mechanical complications encompass those related to the catheters used for delivery of parenteral nutrition. Among these are pneumothorax associated with placement of a central venous catheter, thrombus formation and embolization, and air embolus.
- **Metabolic complications:** The most common metabolic complication is hyperglycemia. Insulin can be added to the TPN solution or administered separately to control hyperglycemia. Other metabolic complications include refeeding syndrome, excess carbon dioxide production, and electrolyte abnormalities. Refeeding syndrome occurs in patients who have severe malnutrition and have feedings rapidly started. The syndrome is characterized by hypophosphatemia, hypokalemia, volume overload, and congestive heart failure.
- **Infectious complications:** These complications are generally related to the central venous access catheters used for the delivery of TPN and include catheter-related sepsis.
- **Hepatobiliary complications:** The hepatic oxidative capacity (HOC) of the liver is 4–6 mg of glucose per kg/min. If the HOC is exceeded, hepatobiliary complications of parenteral nutrition, including elevation in transaminases, alkaline phosphatase, and bilirubin, as well as steatosis (i.e., fatty liver) and acalculous cholecystitis may result.

Schloerb PR, Henning JF: Patterns and problems of adult total parenteral nutrition use in US academic medical centers. Arch Surg 133:7–12, 1998.

21. **How should a critically ill patient receiving parenteral nutrition be monitored?**

Baseline values of electrolytes (e.g., sodium, potassium, bicarbonate, magnesium, phosphate, and calcium), blood urea nitrogen, creatinine, glucose, albumin, triglycerides, complete blood count, and liver function tests (e.g., transaminases, alkaline phosphatase, and bilirubin) should be checked before therapy is initiated. After initiating therapy, blood glucose monitoring should be performed every 4–6 hours until the infusion is stabilized. Serum triglycerides should be checked 6 hours after completing the infusion of IV fat to ensure that the patient is able to adequately clear the lipids. Serum triglycerides should be <400 mg/dL. Electrolyte levels should be checked every day until the infusion is stabilized and then every 3–4 days along with a blood urea nitrogen and creatinine. Liver function test results and prealbumin and CRP levels should be checked once a week.

22. **How can the administration of propofol potentially influence the nutritional support provided to critically ill patients?**
Propofol is a sedative commonly used in the ICU. It is supplied as a 10% lipid emulsion and provides 1.1 kcal/mL. When propofol is being administered for long periods of time or in large doses, intravenous fat supplementation with TPN may need to be decreased or eliminated to avoid excessive administration of fat or calories. Patients receiving large doses of propofol should have serum triglyceride levels checked to prevent hypertriglyceridemia. Hypertriglyceridemia (>500 mg/dL) from propofol has been implicated as a cause of acute pancreatitis.

23. **What are pharmaconutrients? Give some examples.**
Pharmaconutrients are specific nutrients that are provided in addition to (or in larger amounts than) the usual macro- and micronutrients to produce specific effects on certain organs or metabolic functions. Examples of pharmaconutrients include the following:
- **Glutamine:** Glutamine is an abundant amino acid and a major gut fuel. Supplementation of enteral nutrition formulas with glutamine has been shown to maintain normal GALT size and function, decrease bacterial translocation, and increase the thickness of GI tract mucosa. Glutamine should be considered in burn and trauma patients—decreased mortality in burn patients and decreased infections in trauma patients have been reported. No effect for routine use has been reported in other critically ill patients.
- **Omega-3 fatty acid:** Older enteral nutrition formulas were high in omega-6 fatty acids that have been shown to be immunosuppressive. Newer formulas that are higher in omega-3 fatty acids have been shown to be less immunosuppressive and may provide an anti-inflammatory effect. Fish oils should be considered in patients with acute respiratory distress syndrome and are associated with a reduction in the number of days that patients require supplemental oxygen.
- **Arginine:** Arginine is an amino acid (and precursor to nitric oxide) that was initially thought to enhance immune function, wound healing, and nitrogen balance when supplied in enteral nutrition formulas. It is not recommended in critically ill patients because studies have shown a trend toward harm.

Many other substances including growth hormone, antioxidants, and nucleic acids are currently under investigation. Although many of the pharmaconutrients mentioned show promise, their precise role in routine clinical care and in improving outcomes remains uncertain.

Beale RJ, Bryg DJ, Bihari DJ: Immunonutrition in the critically ill: A systematic review of clinical outcome. Crit Care Med 27:2799–2805, 1999.

CHAPTER 8

NONINVASIVE VENTILATION

Manuel Pardo, Jr., MD

1. **What is noninvasive ventilation?**
   Noninvasive ventilation is mechanical ventilation without the use of an endotracheal tube or tracheotomy.

2. **What are the main types of noninvasive ventilation?**
   The two main types are positive-pressure and negative-pressure noninvasive ventilation. With the former, positive pressure is applied to the airway to inflate the lungs directly. With negative-pressure ventilation, negative pressure is applied to the abdomen and thorax to draw air into the lungs through the upper airway. This chapter deals mainly with positive-pressure ventilation, the most commonly used noninvasive ventilator mode in the intensive care unit (ICU).

3. **When did noninvasive ventilation first become widely used? For what disease?**
   Noninvasive ventilation became widely used during the poliomyelitis epidemics of the 1920s through the 1950s. The ventilators used included the rocking bed, various types of tank respirators or "iron lungs," and body-wrapping cuirass respirators. Patients with chronic respiratory failure after polio could be supported for years with these forms of negative-pressure noninvasive ventilation.

4. **Why did the use of noninvasive ventilation decrease in the 1950s and 1960s?**
   The success of the polio vaccines led to the control of the epidemic. In addition, the use of positive-pressure ventilation became more widely used. The success of this form of "invasive" positive-pressure ventilation was described during the Copenhagen polio epidemic of 1952. At the start of the epidemic, the Blegdam Hospital had only seven ventilators, yet up to 70 patients required ventilatory support simultaneously. Lassen and Ibsen developed the technique of tracheotomy and manual intermittent positive-pressure ventilation and described their success in 1953.

   Woollam CH: The development of apparatus for intermittent negative pressure respiration. (2) 1919–1976, with special reference to the development and uses of cuirass respirators. Anaesthesia 31:666–685, 1976.

5. **Why has the use of noninvasive positive-pressure ventilation (NIPPV) increased in recent years?**
   Several developments have led to its increased use. The use of continuous positive airway pressure for obstructive sleep apnea was described in the early 1980s. The development of a more comfortable nasal mask was important to the success of this therapy. These masks became widely available in the 1980s and were found to be effective in delivering NIPPV. Inexpensive portable ventilators have been developed specifically for NIPPV (Fig. 8-1). As physicians have gained experience with this mode of ventilation, it has been used in many different forms of acute and chronic respiratory failure. In the past 5–10 years, randomized clinical trials have evaluated NIPPV in a variety of patient populations in the ICU setting.

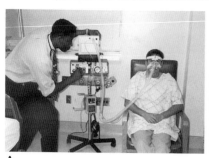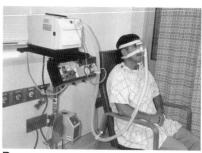

A   B

Figure 8-1. A demonstration of noninvasive positive pressure ventilation with a nasal mask. *A,* The respiratory therapist is adjusting the inspiratory pressure support level and checking for proper mask fit. *B,* The mask must be fitted properly to minimize air leak but to avoid excessive pressure on the skin.

6. **What are the advantages of NIPPV compared with conventional mechanical ventilation with an endotracheal tube?**
    In most studies of NIPPV in the ICU setting, the main outcome measure has been the need for tracheal intubation. For those patients who avoid intubation, the main advantage is the avoidance of artificial airway complications. Several studies document a lower infection rate (e.g., nosocomial pneumonia and sinusitis) with NIPPV, which may be related to the maintenance of the protective glottic barrier. Other advantages include reduced need for sedative medications. Some NIPPV trials have demonstrated reductions in ICU length of stay, ICU mortality, or in-hospital mortality.

7. **What are the disadvantages and contraindications of NIPPV?**
    Patient selection is crucial to ensuring success with noninvasive ventilation. Patients who are uncooperative, need immediate intubation, have upper airway pathology, are hemodynamically unstable, or have excessive secretions are not likely to succeed. NIPPV should be contraindicated in these patients. In practical terms, NIPPV can initially require significant attention from a respiratory therapist, ICU nurse, or both. Early generations of noninvasive ventilators had limitations on the amount of oxygen that could be delivered.

8. **Has noninvasive ventilation been used for chronic respiratory failure? For what disorders?**
    As previously described for the polio epidemics, negative-pressure ventilation has a long history of success for chronic respiratory failure. Similar benefits have also been shown in uncontrolled studies for NIPPV. The disorders for which it has been used include thoracic restrictive diseases (e.g., kyphoscoliosis, chest wall deformities), central hypoventilatory disorders, and slowly progressive neuromuscular diseases (e.g., amyotrophic lateral sclerosis, muscular dystrophy). If the patient is able to maintain only brief periods of spontaneous breathing, tracheotomy along with positive-pressure ventilation is usually a better option. Otherwise, intermittent (usually nocturnal) noninvasive ventilation may be successful in controlling hypercarbia and promoting daytime independence.

9. **Can noninvasive ventilation be used for patients with acute respiratory failure?**
    Noninvasive ventilation has been used for acute respiratory failure of diverse causes. Patient selection is important because clinical trials have not demonstrated uniform benefit for all

causes of acute respiratory failure. The earliest studies involved patients with acute exacerbations of chronic obstructive pulmonary disease (COPD).

10. **Which patients with acute respiratory failure are most likely to benefit from NIPPV?**

Patients with acute exacerbations of COPD are most likely to benefit, in terms of reduction in the need for tracheal intubation and decreased mortality. The benefits in this patient population may be limited to those with more severe exacerbations. Other populations likely to have a decreased intubation rate with NIPPV include patients with immune compromise from solid organ transplants or hematologic malignancies, cardiogenic pulmonary edema, respiratory failure after lung resection, and respiratory failure immediately after elective abdominal surgery. If NIPPV is used for patients who do not fit in these categories, consider limiting the time to 2 hours unless clear improvement is evident.

Calfee CS, Matthay MA: Recent advances in mechanical ventilation. Am J Med 118:584–591, 2005.

Squadrone V, Coha M, Cerutti E, et al: Continuous positive airway pressure for treatment of postoperative hypoxemia: A randomized controlled trial. JAMA 293:589–595, 2005.

11. **Which patients with acute respiratory failure are not likely to benefit from NIPPV?**

Patients with contraindications to NIPPV (*see* question 7) are inappropriate candidates. Unselected patients with postextubation respiratory failure are not likely to benefit and may even have a higher mortality rate. Patients with hypoxemic respiratory failure of various causes may have a reduced need for intubation with NIPPV, but there may be no survival advantage. The exception may be patients with a high risk of mortality with prolonged mechanical ventilation, such as an immunocompromised patient with multiple organ dysfunction. There are few data on NIPPV in patients with acute lung injury or acute respiratory distress syndrome.

Esteban A, Frutos-Vivar F, Ferguson ND, et al: Noninvasive positive-pressure ventilation for respiratory failure after extubation. N Engl J Med 350:2452–2460, 2004.

Keenan SP, Sinuff T, Cook DJ, et al: Does noninvasive positive pressure ventilation improve outcome in acute hypoxemic respiratory failure? A systematic review. Crit Care Med 32:2516–2523, 2004.

12. **What are the complications of noninvasive ventilation?**

The main complication of negative-pressure ventilation is development of upper airway obstruction and hypoxemia during sleep. This complication may be caused by changes in the upper airway muscle activation when exposed to ventilator breaths. Complications of NIPPV include pressure necrosis of the skin, aerophagia, and intolerance of the mask. The incidence of mask intolerance can be as high as 25%.

KEY POINTS: NONINVASIVE VENTILATION

1. For patients with acute exacerbations of COPD, noninvasive ventilation is associated with decreased need for tracheal intubation and improved survival.

2. For patients with hypoxemic acute respiratory failure, noninvasive ventilation may decrease the need for tracheal intubation but may not improve survival.

3. Do not use noninvasive ventilation for patients with an urgent need for tracheal intubation.

4. Noninvasive ventilation can be effective long-term management for some patients with chronic respiratory failure.

13. **What ventilator settings can be used for NIPPV?**

A range of ventilator settings and modes may be effective for a given patient. The most common setting is inspiratory pressure support ventilation. A typical setting for a patient with acute exacerbation of COPD is inspiratory pressure of 10–20 cm H_2O and expiratory pressure of 0–2 cm H_2O. Some ventilators incorporate a backup ventilator rate so that patients are given a mandatory breath if their respiratory rate is less than the desired rate. The pressure level is adjusted by subjective comfort or by measurement of the exhaled tidal volume. An exhaled tidal volume of 6–8 mL/kg is appropriate for most patients. The method of oxygen enrichment depends on the specific ventilator.

14. **What type of masks can be used for NIPPV?**

The most common type is a full face mask or nasal mask. Full face masks provide a better seal but are generally considered less comfortable than nasal masks. Other devices include nasal "pillows" and "helmet" masks that seal around the neck.

MECHANICAL VENTILATION

Carolyn H. Welsh, MD

CHAPTER 9

1. **What are the two major indications for mechanical ventilation?**

   Most patients requiring mechanical ventilation have ventilatory failure and are unable to exchange air and expire carbon dioxide (CO_2), resulting in a high PCO_2 and low pH. Causes of this type of respiratory failure include recovery from general anesthesia, drug overdose, neuromuscular disease, chest wall deformity, and exacerbations of chronic obstructive lung disease or asthma. In general, patients with acute ventilatory failure require ventilation support if they hypoventilate to a $PCO_2 > 50$ mmHg with pH < 7.30. Patients with acute superimposed on chronic ventilatory failure may have a much higher PCO_2, up to 80 or 90 mmHg, before requiring intubation, because they develop a compensatory metabolic alkalosis.

   Less frequently, patients require ventilation primarily for hypoxemia. Such patients are often able to ventilate well, with a low arterial PCO_2. Causes of hypoxemic respiratory failure include pneumonia, aspiration, acute respiratory distress syndrome (ARDS), and pulmonary emboli. Usually, patients with hypoxemia require mechanical ventilation for a $PO_2 < 50$ mmHg on a 100% oxygen nonrebreather mask.

2. **What are the common modes of ventilation?**

   Mechanical ventilation for adults is primarily positive pressure ventilation in contrast to normal breathing, where there is negative pressure in the thorax with inspiration. For volume-limited modes of ventilation, the delivered breath is limited by a preset volume. For pressure-limited modes, breath volume is limited by a preset pressure. Volume-limited ventilation using assist control or intermittent mandatory ventilation (IMV) and pressure-limited ventilation using pressure support ventilation are the most common modes in intensive care units (ICUs).

3. **How do assist control and synchronized intermittent mandatory ventilation (SIMV) differ?**

   Assist control (also called *continuous mandatory ventilation*) and SIMV share several common features. Both deliver a preset volume such that, if set at a tidal volume of 500 mL and a rate of 15, both will deliver at least a 7.5-L minute ventilation. To improve patient comfort, both accommodate extra patient-initiated breaths.

   Assist control and SIMV differ in that the former delivers each initiated breath to the full preset tidal volume, whereas the latter delivers each patient-initiated breath to only as much volume as pressure from the patient's muscles generates while also delivering the full preset tidal volume at the preset rate. SIMV often increases the work of breathing by the amount of work required to overcome valve pressures in the ventilator circuit. Due to this increased work of breathing, IMV may hasten fatigue and compromise weaning.

4. **What is the role of pressure support ventilation mode in ventilating patients?**

   This is a pressure-limited mode used primarily for weaning and occasionally as primary ventilator support. Airflow is limited by pressure and is patient triggered with pressure delivered only during inspiration. It is thought to improve patient ventilator synchrony and comfort and reduces the work of breathing. It is not an ideal choice when ventilatory drive is blunted from disease or sedative medications because sufficient ventilation may not be achieved.

Pressure support ventilation may be advantageous in asthmatic exacerbations to avoid high peak airway pressures and is currently a preferred weaning mode.

5. **How are ventilator settings selected?**
Ventilator settings are chosen to minimize airway pressure and optimize oxygen exchange and acid-base status. Patients start with a fraction of inspired oxygen (FiO_2) of 1.00 (100% oxygen). If the PO_2 is high on arterial blood gas (ABG) analysis, the FiO_2 is decreased to give a PO_2 of 60–90 mmHg. When possible, a fraction of inspired oxygen of 0.4–0.5 is selected to avoid oxygen toxicity. Respiratory rate is set to achieve adequate minute ventilation (product of rate multiplied by tidal volume) and roughly varies from 10 to 25 breaths/min. An initial tidal volume of 6–8 mL/kg is selected, approximately 450 mL for a 70-kg person. For decades, clinicians chose tidal volumes of 10–12 mL/kg because this easily normalized acid-base status. Tidal volume selection changed when randomized clinical trials showed improved survival rates in a subgroup of patients—those with acute lung injury or ARDS who received low (6 mL/kg) compared with higher tidal volumes (12 mL/kg). For routine postoperative care, somewhat larger tidal volumes are still used, although even in this setting, lower tidal volumes may protect the lungs from ventilator-induced lung injury.

Gajic O, Dara SI, Mendez JL, et al: Ventilator-associated lung injury in patients without acute lung injury at the onset of mechanical ventilation. Crit Care Med 32:1817–1824, 2004.

6. **How are ventilator settings monitored for adequacy and safety?**
Peak airway pressures are assessed to fine-tune tidal volumes, targeting peak pressures < 35 mmHg to avoid ventilator-induced lung injury. If peak and plateau airway pressures are high, clinicians seek explanations (i.e., bronchospasm, pulmonary edema, or auto–positive end-expiratory pressure [PEEP]). After at least 20 minutes on a setting, an ABG is obtained to assess ventilation. Limiting peak airway pressures is more important than ideal acid-base status. Ventilator management has changed from prioritizing normal acid-base status to maintaining low airway pressures. Respiratory acidosis is tolerated to achieve acceptable pressures.

7. **What are the common complications of mechanical ventilation?**
Ventilator-induced lung injury, barotrauma, hemodynamic compromise, and pneumonia. High airway pressures may damage airway epithelium, leading to ventilator-induced lung injury. In addition, high airway pressures may induce rupture of the alveolar wall at its weakest point, leaking air into the bronchovascular sheath. If air remains in the sheath, it tracks through the mediastinum, leading to pneumothorax and subcutaneous emphysema. Air entering pulmonary vessels can cause the devastating air emboli syndrome characterized by livedo reticularis, cardiac arrhythmias, and unexplained altered mental status or stroke. Other complications of positive-pressure ventilation include increased intracranial pressure, fluid retention, renal failure, hyponatremia, and tracheal damage, as well as infections such as sinusitis and pneumonia.

KEY POINTS: COMMON COMPLICATIONS OF MECHANICAL VENTILATION

1. Ventilator-induced lung injury is a frequent complication.

2. Barotrauma includes pneumothorax and air embolism.

3. Hemodynamic compromise or hypotension commonly occurs with mechanical ventilation.

4. Another danger is ventilator-associated pneumonia.

8. **What is ventilator-induced lung injury? How do we prevent it?**

Ventilator-induced lung injury is caused by alveolar overdistention leading to inflammatory mediator release, alveolar rupture, and epithelial injury in the setting of high positive airway pressure. Positive-pressure ventilation in ARDS may worsen the outcome by causing this type of damage. In a large trial involving patients with ARDS, use of low tidal volumes improved mortality rates by 22%. A pressure-protective strategy encompasses lowering of peak and plateau airway pressures, use of smaller tidal volumes, permissive hypercapnia, and changes in the contour of ventilator airway pressure waveforms. Permissive hypercapnia tolerates an elevated PCO_2 to achieve the lower airway pressures.

Acute Respiratory Distress Syndrome Network: Ventilation with lower tidal volumes as compared with traditional tidal volumes for acute lung injury and the acute respiratory distress syndrome. N Engl J Med 342:1301–1308, 2000.

9. **Do mechanical ventilators affect the cardiovascular system?**

Positive-pressure ventilation decreases cardiac output and may lead to hypotension. One mechanism is by positive pressure in the thorax diminishing venous return to the heart by compression of the inferior vena cava, thus creating a low cardiac output state. In patients with cardiogenic pulmonary edema, however, the lowering of venous return to the heart during mechanical ventilation may lessen edema and improve cardiac function (Fig. 9-1).

10. **How is ventilator-associated pneumonia prevented?**

Interest has focused on ventilator-associated pneumonia as a potentially preventable complication of mechanical ventilation, particularly as noninvasive positive airway pressure ventilation (NIPPV) is associated with lower pneumonia rates than intubation. There are several other ways that ventilator-associated pneumonia can be prevented. Elevation of the head of the bed, a simple and inexpensive maneuver, is supported overwhelmingly in evidence-based studies. Other strategies are listed in Box 9-1.

Dodek P, Keenan S, Cook D, et al, for the Canadian Critical Care Trials Group of the Canadian Critical Care Society: Evidence-based clinical practice guideline for the prevention of ventilator-associated pneumonia. Ann Intern Med 141:305–313, 2004.

11. **What is PEEP?**

PEEP is application of positive pressure to the ventilator expiration circuit. In effect, PEEP works by increasing the functional residual capacity of the lung, preventing the collapse of some alveoli while overdistending others. PEEP usually leads to improved ventilation-perfusion matching in the pulmonary circulation.

12. **What are the indications for using PEEP?**

PEEP is primarily used to improve arterial oxygenation in severely hypoxemic patients or to decrease the FiO_2 to avoid oxygen toxicity. PEEP may be a pressure-protective strategy to avoid lung injury; it may by improving ventilation-perfusion matching and oxygenation while minimizing transalveolar cycling pressures.

13. **What is auto-PEEP?**

Auto-PEEP (intrinsic PEEP) is the inadvertent development of PEEP due to the ventilator delivery of a positive-pressure breath before complete exhalation of the previous breath. Thus, it is seen in patients with high minute ventilation, as in ARDS, or in diseases of airflow limitation, such as asthma and chronic obstructive lung disease. Detection involves occlusion of the expiratory port at end exhalation, allowing equilibration of airway and circuit pressure. The complications of auto-PEEP are similar to those of applied PEEP: diminished cardiac output, hypotension, and inaccurate pulmonary artery catheter measurements leading to inappropriate fluid and pressor administration or diuresis.

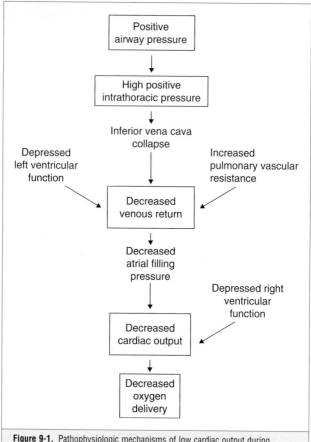

Figure 9-1. Pathophysiologic mechanisms of low cardiac output during mechanical ventilation. Decreased venous return due to compression of the inferior vena cava is key.

14. **How can auto-PEEP be remedied?**
    Primary treatment for auto-PEEP is treatment of the underlying bronchospasm. Other treatment approaches include raising inspiratory flow rates to maximize expiratory time, increasing endotracheal tube size, and lowering minute ventilation by decreasing respiratory rate or tidal volume. If this dangerous problem persists, the patient should be sedated and occasionally paralyzed. Applying PEEP in centimeters equivalent to the original auto-PEEP is helpful in the treatment of some patients with auto-PEEP.

15. **What do you do if a patient on a ventilator is agitated or the ventilator alarm sounds?**
    Agitation is a clue to machine malfunction or a change in the patient's medical status. Remove the patient from the ventilator and ventilate with a resuscitation bag while evaluating the problem. Common ventilator problems include inadvertent disconnection of the patient from the ventilator and use of inappropriate ventilator settings such as low trigger sensitivity, low flow

BOX 9-1.   STRATEGIES TO PREVENT VENTILATOR–ASSOCIATED PNEUMONIA

- Elevation of the head of the bed
- Orotracheal (not nasotracheal) intubation
- Good oral care
- Hand washing
- Heat moisture exchanger preferred to humidifier cascade to humidify airways
- Closed suctioning systems
- Earliest possible extubation
- Noninvasive positive pressure ventilation

Possibly effective strategies

- Subglottic secretion drainage
- Kinetic beds

rates, or ventilator response delay. Poor synchrony of the patient with the ventilator can lead to development of auto-PEEP (see previous discussion). Check the ventilator for problems with settings and connections, which are correctable. Changes in medical condition that may affect ventilation include both airway and neurologic problems. Box 9-2 includes a partial list of such problems.

16. **Are there other helpful treatments, in addition to mechanical ventilation itself, for acute respiratory failure?**

For patients with acute bronchospasm in whom positive-pressure ventilation poses a risk for pneumothorax, vigorous pharmacologic treatment of the underlying disease may abolish the need for mechanical ventilation. Negative-pressure ventilators may benefit adults with normally compliant lungs. For patients with respiratory failure due to an exacerbation of chronic obstructive pulmonary disease (COPD), NIPPV reduces need for intubation, lowers the frequency of complications, and shortens patient hospital stay. For patients with ARDS who remain hypoxic, inhaled nitric oxide therapy has been attempted. Placement in a prone position improves oxygenation in 70% of patients; however, in a clinical trial, prone positioning offered no survival benefit. High-frequency oscillation is again undergoing scrutiny for mechanical ventilation. Severely hypoxemic patients are occasionally treated with extracorporeal membrane oxygenation, bypassing the diseased lungs to oxygenate blood and tissue. This, however, remains unproved and may worsen survival rates.

   Gattinoni I, Tognoni G, Presenti A, et al: Effect of prone positioning on the survival of patients with acute respiratory failure. N Engl J Med 345:568–573, 2001.

17. **What is NIPPV? When should it be used?**
NIPPV is the use of a standard ventilator to deliver positive-pressure breaths by mask rather than by endotracheal tube. NIPPV reduces the need for endotracheal intubation, lowers the frequency of infectious complications, and shortens ICU or hospital stay. A mortality benefit for NIPPV compared with intubation has been shown in exacerbations of COPD. Sound data support the use of NIPPV in such patients and in selected patients with hypoxemic respiratory failure, pneumonia, and pulmonary edema.

   Masip J, Roque M, Sanchez B, et al: Noninvasive ventilation in acute cardiogenic pulmonary edema: systematic review and meta-analysis. JAMA 294:3124–3130, 2005.

18. **When should patients undergo tracheostomy?**
Standard recommendations have been to reserve tracheostomy, the insertion of a tube in the neck for attachment to the ventilator, until after a patient has spent 3 weeks on the ventilator.

BOX 9-2. REASONS FOR AGITATION DURING MECHANICAL VENTILATION

Machine malfunction

- Inadvertent disconnection of the patient from the ventilator
- Inappropriate ventilator settings
  - Low trigger sensitivity
  - Low flow rates
  - Ventilator response delay
  - Auto-PEEP

Changes in medical condition

- Mucous plugs/copious secretions
- Bronchospasm
- Pneumothorax
- Pulmonary edema
- Acidosis
- Sepsis
- Carbon dioxide retention
- Hypoxemia
- Lobar collapse
- Pulmonary emboli
- Pain
- Hallucinations
- Awakening from sedation
- Alcohol or drug withdrawal

PEEP = positive end-expiratory pressure.

Views on this are changing, and currently the timing of tracheostomy for certain patients is shorter than 1 week. Reasons to perform early tracheostomy include underlying neurologic disease, failure of extubation, and expectation of need for prolonged ventilation. Early tracheostomy leads to earlier ICU discharge in selected patients.

Griffiths J, Barber VS, Morgan L, Young JD: Systematic review and meta-analysis of studies of the timing of tracheostomy in adult patients undergoing artificial ventilation. BMJ 330:1243–1247, 2005.

WEBSITES

1. Acute Respiratory Distress Syndrome Network: The National Institutes of Health ARDS network offers information on completed and ongoing clinical trial studies and publications on patients with acute lung injury, including ventilation studies.
http://www.ardsnet.org

2. Critical Care Research Network: This is a Canadian consortium of critical care investigation including mechanical ventilation.
http://www.criticalcareresearch.net

DISCONTINUATION OF MECHANICAL VENTILATION

CHAPTER 10

Theodore W. Marcy, MD, MPH, and Katherine Habeeb, MD

1. **What proportion of patients can be readily removed from mechanical ventilation?**

   The majority of patients (75%) supported with mechanical ventilation are able to resume unsupported breathing within 7 days of intubation if the illness that resulted in respiratory failure resolves or improves. The ventilator "weaning mode" is not critical and does not determine success or failure. Instead, the clinician's primary—and challenging—task is to determine when the patient is ready for ventilator discontinuation. Continuing mechanical ventilation beyond the time that is necessary exposes the patient to risks of nosocomial infection and ventilator-induced lung injury. Conversely, removing a patient prematurely from ventilatory support can lead to severe stress from respiratory and cardiovascular decompensation and exposes the patient to the risks associated with reintubation.

   Esteban A, Anzueto A, Frutos F, et al: Characteristics and outcomes in adult patients receiving mechanical ventilation: A 28-day international study. JAMA 287:345–355, 2002.

   Tobin M: Advances in mechanical ventilation. N Engl J Med 344:1986–1996, 2001.

2. **When should patients receiving mechanical ventilation be assessed for ventilator discontinuation?**

   Every patient receiving mechanical ventilation should be assessed for ventilator discontinuation on a *daily* basis as long as his or her medical status meets the following criteria:

   - Resolution or improvement in the underlying cause of respiratory failure
   - Adequate oxygenation ($PaO_2/FiO_2 > 150–200$ on $FiO_2 = 0.50$ and positive end-expiratory pressure $= 5–8$ cm H_2O)
   - Hemodynamic stability (not requiring pressors more than dopamine $5\,\mu g/kg/min$)
   - Patient capable of initiating adequate inspiratory efforts

   Evidence indicates that systematic daily weaning assessments improve patient outcomes, reduce the number of days patients are dependent on the ventilator, and reduce the number of patients who require tracheostomies.

3. **How, exactly, should this assessment be done?**

   As of yet, no systematic weaning protocol has been agreed upon. However, most protocols have a stepwise assessment that varies in the details. For all patients who fulfill the medical criteria previously listed, there is first an initial brief trial or *readiness assessment* during which patients are closely observed for 1–5 minutes while receiving minimal or no support (continuous positive airway pressure $= 5$ cm H_2O) to assess their ability to undergo a formal spontaneous breathing trial (SBT). If the patient does well during the readiness assessment, an SBT is performed for between 30 and 120 minutes. During this time, patients are closely monitored for signs of respiratory insufficiency, hemodynamic deterioration, or patient discomfort. Full ventilatory support is promptly reinitiated if problems develop. Successfully completing an SBT is highly predictive of successful ventilator discontinuation. These steps are illustrated in Fig. 10-1.

   Ely E, Meade M, Haponik E, et al: Mechanical ventilator weaning protocols driven by nonphysician health-care professionals: Evidence-based clinical practice guidelines. Chest 120:454S–463S, 2001.

   MacIntyre N: Current issues in mechanical ventilation. Chest 128(Suppl 5):561S–567S, 2005.

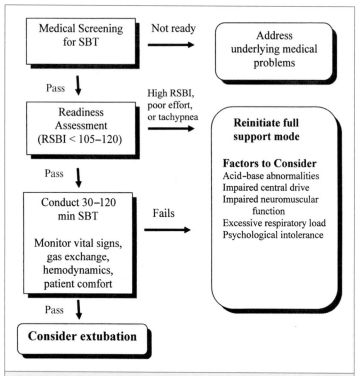

Figure 10-1. A protocol for daily assessment for extubation. SBT = spontaneous breathing trial, RSBI = rapid shallow breathing index calculated by frequency of breaths/min divided by tidal volume in liters.

4. **What is the rapid shallow breathing index (RSBI)? How is it used?**
   The RSBI is calculated using the following formula:

$$\frac{\text{Respiratory rate (breaths/min)}}{\text{Tidal volume (liters)}}$$

   Higher values for the RSBI signify a pattern of breathing often seen in patients with respiratory muscle fatigue who tend to have weak inspiratory efforts and consequently higher respiratory rates. Values greater than 105–120 predict patients who may not tolerate an SBT. The RSBI is most often measured during the readiness assessment to identify patients who should go forward with an SBT.

5. **To which mode should the ventilator be set during the SBT?**
   The specific ventilatory mode during the SBT is not critical. The choices usually include the following:
   - T-piece circuit that provides a constant flow of oxygen past the endotracheal tube with an extension downstream to prevent entrainment of room air

- Low levels of pressure support ventilation of 5–8 cm H_2O
- Continuous positive airway pressure

A disadvantage of T-piece trials is that the patient is not connected to the ventilator's alarm systems that supplement clinician monitoring for apnea or tachypnea. The choice among these options will depend on each provider's experience and preferences.

6. **What are the traditional weaning parameters, and how are they used?**
   Traditional weaning parameters include maximal inspiratory pressure, minute volume, vital capacity, maximum voluntary ventilation, thoracic compliance, and respiratory resistance. In the past, they were used to predict the likelihood of success with weaning trials. It is now known that they do not discriminate well between patients who will succeed and those who will fail after extubation. Assessment during a carefully monitored SBT appears to provide the most clinically useful information regarding ventilator discontinuation. Measurement of traditional weaning parameters is generally not necessary.

   Meade M, Guyatt G, Cook D, et al: Predicting success in weaning from mechanical ventilation. Chest 120 (Suppl 6):400S–424S, 2001.

7. **Describe what to do about sedation and analgesia with such a patient.**
   Patients are often medicated with sedatives and analgesics while on mechanical ventilation to reduce patient pain and discomfort and to limit patient movements that could lead to accidental extubation or other injuries. Continuous sedation may provide a more constant level of sedation, but this has been associated with a longer duration of mechanical ventilation, days spent in the intensive care unit (ICU), and hospitalization compared to intermittent sedation protocols. Patients randomly assigned to undergo a planned interruption of continuous sedation on a daily basis had reduced days of mechanical ventilation and days in the ICU compared with those who were randomly assigned to receive continuous sedation. There were no apparent adverse effects of interruption of sedation. The optimal method of providing sedation and analgesia for these patients is not known. However, minimizing sedatives to the level that achieves a specified sedation target and attempting to awaken the patient daily appear to be important aspects of patient management during mechanical ventilation.

   Heffner J: A wake-up call in the intensive care unit. N Engl J Med 342:1520–1522, 2000.
   Kress J, Pohlman A, O'Connor M, Hall J: Daily interruption of sedative infusions in critically ill patients undergoing mechanical ventilation. N Engl J Med 342:1471–1477, 2000.

8. **What do you do with patients who fail during the SBT?**
   Two actions are necessary:
   - Place the patient back on a full ventilatory support mode (e.g., assist/control).
   - Perform a comprehensive review of potential contributing factors to the failure.

   To sustain spontaneous ventilation successfully, patients must have an intact respiratory center drive, adequate neuromuscular function, and relief of excessive loads on the respiratory muscles. Box 10-1 provides one method of systematically reviewing possible causes of failure during an SBT. Patients often have more than one cause for failure to wean, and correction of these factors may require multiple interventions. In general, it is recommended to wait 24 hours before attempting another SBT.

   Manthous C, Schmidt G, Hall J: Liberation from mechanical ventilation: A decade of progress. Chest 114(3):886–901, 1998.

9. **What criteria are important when considering removal of an artificial airway?**
   Successful completion of an SBT does not necessarily indicate that the patient is ready for extubation. Reintubation for respiratory failure occurs in about 13–19% of patients who are extubated by this protocol. The rate is higher—about 25%—among those who have been intubated for longer than 48 hours. Other risk factors include older age, increased severity of

> ### BOX 10-1. FACTORS TO CONSIDER WHEN PATIENTS FAIL TESTS OF INSPIRATORY EFFORTS OR SPONTANEOUS BREATHING TRIALS
>
> 1. The patient has an increasing $PaCO_2$ without increases in respiratory effort or rate.
>   - (a) Inadequate respiratory center drive due to excessive narcotics, sedatives, hypothyroidism, or brain injury
>   - (b) Appropriate compensation for metabolic alkalosis due to excessive diuresis or nasogastric suctioning
>   - (c) Return to a chronic hypercapnic state after inappropriate overventilation in patients with COPD or sleep apnea
> 2. The patient has tachypnea, tachycardia, or distress.
>   - (a) Impaired neuromuscular function
>   - Fatigue due to prolonged high loads, inadequate rest, or ventilator dyssynchrony
>   - Hypothyroidism
>   - Electrolyte deficiencies (e.g., hypokalemia, hypophosphatemia, hypomagnesemia)
>   - Critical illness myopathy/polyneuropathy
>   - Steroid myopathy
>   - Effects of drugs (e.g., aminoglycosides, neuromuscular antagonists)
>   - Sepsis
>   - Diaphragmatic paresis or paralysis due to phrenic nerve injury resulting from cold cardioplegia or thoracic or neck surgery
>   - Prolonged malnutrition
>   - (b) Excessive respiratory load
>   - Increased airway resistance (e.g., asthma, COPD, excessive secretions, small endotracheal tube)
>   - Air trapping and increased threshold load due to positive residual pressures (particularly in patients with COPD)
>   - Decreased respiratory system compliance (e.g., pulmonary edema, fibrosis, pneumonia, abdominal distention, thoracic cage abnormalities, pleural effusions)
>   - High minute ventilation requirements (e.g., fever, sepsis, metabolic acidosis, high physiologic dead space, excessive caloric intake, pulmonary embolism)
>   - (c) Impaired left ventricular function
>   - (d) Psychological dependence: a diagnosis of exclusion, but not rare in patients confined to intensive care units
>
> COPD = chronic obstructive pulmonary disease.

illness, anemia, and cardiac failure. Unfortunately, reintubation is associated with a significantly increased mortality compared with patients not requiring reintubation, even when controlling for the severity of illness among these patients. Patients who have an ineffective cough, increased volume of secretions, and reduced alertness are at higher risk for respiratory failure even if they pass an SBT. Extubation should be postponed if secretions are copious, if frequent suctioning is required, or if the patient is somnolent with a poor cough. A cuff leak test, although neither sensitive nor specific, may alert clinicians to the possibility of laryngeal edema if there is no detectable leakage of air with endotracheal balloon deflation.

10. **What about using noninvasive ventilation (NIV) for patients who develop respiratory failure after extubation?**
   The initial use of NIV—ventilators that interface with the patient through a full face or nasal mask rather than an endotracheal tube—has improved outcomes in subsets of patients who

present with acute respiratory failure, including patients with COPD and cardiogenic pulmonary edema. However, the situation may be different in patients who develop respiratory failure after extubation. A randomized trial of NIV versus standard medical therapy (including reintubation) in patients with respiratory failure after extubation did not observe a decrease in reintubation rates among those randomly assigned to receive NIV. In addition, NIV was associated with an *increase* in ICU mortality, particularly among those patients who did require reintubation, suggesting that a delay in reintubation was deleterious. This suggests that the use of NIV for patients who are failing after extubation should be limited to patients with COPD and hypercapnia and, if used, should be closely monitored with a decision to reintubate the patient if there is no improvement within a short (2-hour) period of time.

Esteban A, Frutos-Vivar F, Ferguson ND, et al: Non-invasive positive-pressure ventilation for respiratory failure after extubation. N Engl J Med 350:2452–2460, 2004.

KEY POINTS: DISCONTINUATION OF MECHANICAL VENTILATION

1. Daily systematic assessments of ventilated patients for the ability to breathe spontaneously are more important than the mode of ventilation used for weaning.

2. A respiratory therapist–driven or nurse-driven protocol for this daily assessment can safely reduce the duration of mechanical ventilation and performs better than standard physician assessments.

3. Sedation and analgesia should be minimized or interrupted on a daily basis.

4. Systematic attention to medical conditions that impair spontaneous breathing, such as left ventricular dysfunction, muscle fatigue, and metabolic abnormalities, must be part of this daily assessment.

11. **Define prolonged mechanical ventilatory support (PMV).**

    A recent consensus conference defined patients receiving PMV as those who need at least 6 h/day of ventilatory support for ≥ 21 days. These patients generally require a tracheostomy for optimal care. It is estimated that about 3–7% of patients receiving mechanical ventilatory support meet this definition. One-year survival rates among these patients range from 23% to 76%, with older age and poor functional status before the acute illness predicting a worse prognosis. In patients receiving PMV, the criteria used in the weaning protocols previously described for acutely ill patients do not apply. Many of these patients are managed in long-term care units outside the ICU.

    MacIntyre N, Epstein S, Carson S, et al: Management of patients requiring prolonged mechanical ventilation: Report of a NAMDRC consensus conference. Chest 128:3937–3954, 2005.

12. **Should these patients be managed with different modes of ventilation?**

    Patients receiving PMV often require a gradual withdrawal of ventilatory support over an extended period of time. No definite evidence indicates that gradual withdrawal of support itself facilitates physiologic improvement. Nonetheless, there may be no other way of determining when the patient has recovered sufficiently to resume spontaneous ventilation 24 h/day.

    Common modes used in patients receiving PMV include pressure support ventilation, synchronized intermittent mandatory ventilation, and intermittent unsupported trials with tracheostomy collar. As in acutely ill patients, a therapist-driven protocol approach to weaning, regardless of the mode, appears to improve outcomes in comparison to clinical judgment alone.

Clinicians should continue efforts to identify and correct physiologic reasons for the patient's inability to resume spontaneous ventilation (*see* Box 10-1). Ventilatory support should be withdrawn gradually during the day, allowing rest and sleep on full support modes at night. Once the patient tolerates spontaneous ventilation throughout the day, withdrawal of nocturnal ventilation may proceed relatively quickly.

Scheinhorn D, Chao D, Stearn-Hassenpflug M, Wallace W: Outcomes in post-ICU mechanical ventilation: A therapist-implemented weaning protocol. Chest 119:236–242, 2001.

13. **Why is there such an emphasis on protocols?**
    In most recent studies, systematic weaning protocols, protocols to minimize or interrupt sedation, and raising the head of the bed have been associated with improved patient outcomes and reductions in the cost of care. One hospital that implemented a multifaceted, hospital-wide quality improvement program for weaning observed a significant decrease in mean days spent receiving mechanical ventilation, ICU days, hospital days, and cost per patient compared with the year before the program, even though patients were more ill. In the one study that did *not* demonstrate a change with a weaning protocol, there was a high physician-to-patient ratio (9.5 physician-hours per bed per day), and the physicians used a structured systems-based rounding template that prompted review of ventilator-related issues.

    In summary, clinicians should minimize the duration of mechanical ventilation by identifying and treating underlying causes of respiratory failure while systematically monitoring patients daily for evidence that ventilatory support might be successfully discontinued.

Krishan J, Moore D, Robeson C, et al: A prospective, controlled trial of a protocol-based strategy to discontinue mechanical ventilation. Am J Respir Crit Care Med 169:673–678, 2004.
Smyrnios N, Connolly A, Wilson M, et al: Effects of a multifaceted, multidisciplinary, hospital wide quality improvement program on weaning from mechanical ventilation. Crit Care Med 30:1224–1230, 2002.

WEBSITE

Institute for Healthcare Improvement: Intensive Care
http://www.ihi.org/IHI/Topics/CriticalCare/IntensiveCare

TRACHEAL INTUBATION AND AIRWAY MANAGEMENT

Manuel Pardo, Jr., MD

CHAPTER 11

1. **What is the airway?**
   The airway is the conduit through which air and oxygen must pass before reaching the lungs. It includes the anatomic structures extending from the nose and mouth to the larynx and trachea.

2. **What is airway management?**
   Airway management is making sure that the airway remains patent. It is the first step in the ABCs of basic resuscitation (B = breathing, C = circulation).

3. **Why does airway management precede management of breathing and circulation?**
   If the airway is completely obstructed, no oxygen can reach the lungs and no carbon dioxide can leave the lungs. If oxygen does not reach the lungs, the heart and circulation will have no oxygen to distribute to the body's vital organs.

4. **Describe the ways to manage the airway.**
   The airway may remain patent without any intervention and can be managed with or without tracheal intubation. Airway management without intubation can involve a variety of maneuvers. In unconscious patients, the tongue commonly obstructs the airway. Techniques to open the airway include the head tilt–chin lift maneuver and the jaw thrust maneuver. Placement of oral or nasal airways may also help to maintain a patent airway. The use of a face mask with a bag-valve device (e.g., Ambu-bag) is the usual next step in airway management. In the majority of patients, it is possible to maintain a patent airway without tracheal intubation. If tracheal intubation is required, it can be accomplished through surgical or nonsurgical techniques.

5. **What are the indications for tracheal intubation?**
   There are five main indications:
   - Upper airway obstruction
   - Inadequate oxygenation
   - Inadequate ventilation
   - Elevated work of breathing
   - Airway protection

6. **Explain upper airway obstruction as an indication for tracheal intubation.**
   If the upper airway is obstructed and cannot be opened with the previously described maneuvers, the trachea must be intubated to avoid life-threatening hypoxemia. Although intubation will bypass the anatomic area of obstruction, the cause should be determined to evaluate appropriate timing of extubation or need for further treatment.

7. **Explain how to evaluate hypoxemia as an indication for tracheal intubation.**
   If the patient's oxygen saturation is consistently less than 90% despite the use of high-flow oxygen delivered through a face mask, tracheal intubation should be considered. One hundred percent oxygen can be delivered reliably only with an endotracheal tube. Other factors to

consider are the adequacy of cardiac output, blood hemoglobin concentration, presence of chronic hypoxemia, and reason for the hypoxemia. For example, patients with hypoxemia due to intracardiac right-to-left shunts may have chronic hypoxemia. In these patients, the administration of 100% oxygen with an endotracheal tube may not be effective in raising the oxygen saturation level.

8. **Explain how to evaluate hypoventilation as an indication for tracheal intubation.**
   With hypoventilation, the blood PCO_2 progressively rises, which also lowers the blood pH level (respiratory acidosis). With increasing CO_2 levels, patients eventually become unconscious (CO_2 narcosis). Low systemic pH may be associated with abnormal myocardial irritability and contractility. The exact level of pH or PCO_2 that requires assisted ventilation must be determined for each patient. Chronic respiratory acidosis (e.g., in a patient with severe chronic obstructive pulmonary disease) is usually better tolerated than acute respiratory acidosis.

9. **Explain how to evaluate elevated work of breathing as an indication for tracheal intubation.**
   Normally, the respiratory muscles account for less than 5% of the total body oxygen consumption. In patients with respiratory failure, this can increase to as much as 40%. It can be difficult to assess the work of breathing by clinical examination. However, patients who have rapid shallow breathing, use of accessory respiratory muscles, or paradoxic respirations have a predictably high work of breathing. The results of an arterial blood gas analysis (i.e., pH, PCO_2, and PO_2) may be initially normal in such patients. Eventually, the respiratory muscles fatigue and fail, causing inadequate oxygenation and ventilation. Mechanical ventilation can sometimes be done without tracheal intubation (*see* Chapter 8, Noninvasive Ventilation) but is more reliably accomplished with intubation.

10. **Explain "airway protection" as an indication for tracheal intubation.**
    In an awake patient, protective airway reflexes normally prevent the pulmonary aspiration of gastric contents. Patients with altered mental status from a variety of causes may lose these protective reflexes, increasing the risk of aspiration pneumonia. Tracheal intubation with a cuffed tube can decrease the risk of aspiration. However, liquids can still leak around the endotracheal tube cuff, and the glottic barrier is bypassed, which plays a role in bacterial colonization of the lower airways.

11. **What are the surgical techniques for tracheal intubation?**
    Surgical techniques include cricothyroidotomy or tracheotomy, which involves placing an endotracheal tube directly into the trachea through the cricothyroid membrane or between two tracheal rings (*see* Chapter 12, Tracheotomy and Upper Airway Obstruction).

12. **What are the commonly used nonsurgical techniques for tracheal intubation?**
    Nonsurgical techniques can be divided into techniques that incorporate direct vision and "blind" techniques. The most commonly used direct vision intubation technique is direct laryngoscopy. The laryngoscope is placed in the mouth and manipulated to expose the larynx. An endotracheal tube is then placed through the larynx into the trachea. Another direct vision technique uses the flexible fiberoptic bronchoscope. An endotracheal tube is loaded onto the bronchoscope, which is advanced through the larynx via the nose or mouth. Once the bronchoscope is in the trachea, the endotracheal tube is advanced into position. Blind intubation is generally performed through the nose because the nasopharynx guides the endotracheal tube toward the larynx.

13. **Which drugs can be given to facilitate tracheal intubation?**
    Sedative or analgesic agents are given to reduce the discomfort of laryngoscopy and to blunt the hemodynamic response. Muscle relaxants can make direct laryngoscopy easier to perform.

The main risks of sedative or analgesic drugs in this setting are hypotension and respiratory depression. The muscle relaxants cause paralysis of all skeletal muscle, including the respiratory muscles. If the trachea cannot be intubated, the patient may not resume spontaneous breathing if sedatives, analgesics, or muscle relaxants have been given.

14. **What equipment should be prepared before direct laryngoscopy is attempted?**
    Before laryngoscopy is attempted, all equipment should be checked for proper function. This includes laryngoscope blades, laryngoscope handle, suction source, suction catheter, oxygen source, self-inflating bag or breathing circuit, face mask, oral airways, nasal airways, sedative agents, muscle relaxants, IV line, and patient monitors.

15. **How is direct laryngoscopy accomplished?**
    The technique varies slightly depending on the type of blade used (Figs. 11-1 and 11-2). First, the head is placed in the "sniffing" position with cervical spine in flexion and atlanto-occipital joint in extension. The blade is inserted into the right side of the mouth. Then the tongue is moved to the left. With a curved (Macintosh) blade, the tip is inserted between the base of the tongue and the superior surface of the epiglottis, an area called the

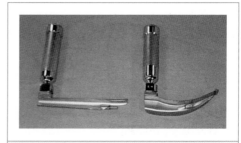

Figure 11-1. Two types of commonly used laryngoscope blades. The straight blade (left) is a size 3 Wisconsin blade. The curved blade (right) is a size 3 Macintosh blade.

vallecula. If a straight (Miller or Wisconsin) blade is used, the tip is manipulated to lift the epiglottis. With both blade types, once the tip is in position, the blade is moved forward and upward to expose the larynx. An endotracheal tube is then inserted into the trachea. Gentle downward pressure on the thyroid cartilage may help to improve the view of the larynx.

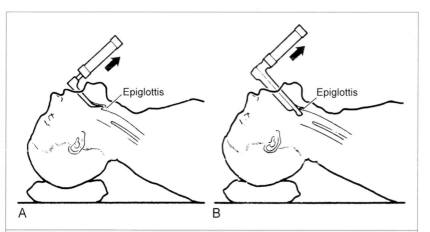

Figure 11-2. Procedure for direct laryngoscopy. *A,* A curved laryngoscope blade is placed in the vallecula. Lifting the blade forward and upward exposes the larynx. *B,* A straight blade is used to lift the epiglottis directly and expose the larynx. (From Gal TJ: Airway management. In Miller RD [ed]: Miller's Anesthesia, 6th ed. New York, Churchill-Livingstone, 2005, p 1634.)

16. **What maneuver can be performed to minimize the risk of aspiration during direct laryngoscopy?**
    Cricoid pressure consists of firm manual pressure on the cricoid cartilage. This maneuver can occlude the esophagus and reduce the chance of gastric distention from mask ventilation. It can also prevent regurgitation of gastric contents into the pharynx.

17. **What is a "difficult airway"? What is a "difficult intubation"?**
    A difficult airway is a clinical situation in which an anesthesiologist or other specially trained clinician has difficulty with mask ventilation or tracheal intubation. Difficult intubation can be defined as one requiring more than three attempts at laryngoscopy or more than 10 minutes of laryngoscopy. Although the definitions are arbitrary, the inability to maintain a patent airway (with or without intubation) may be associated with anoxic brain injury and death.
    American Society of Anesthesiologists: Practice Guidelines for Management of the Difficult Airway: www.asahq.org/publicationsAndServices/Difficult%20Airway.pdf

18. **How do you evaluate the airway for potential difficulty?**
    The history should address the ease of prior tracheal intubations. Patients who have general anesthesia for surgery frequently undergo tracheal intubation. The anesthetic record for the procedure should document the ease of intubation and the equipment used. On examination, one must evaluate four anatomic features: mouth opening, pharyngeal space, neck extension, and submandibular compliance.

19. **How do you evaluate mouth opening and pharyngeal space to predict difficult intubation?**
    In the adult, a mouth opening of 2–3 fingerbreadths is usually adequate. One measure of pharyngeal space is the Mallampati class (Fig. 11-3). The patient is asked to sit upright with the head in a neutral position. Then he or she is asked to open the mouth as widely as possible and protrude the tongue as far as possible. The classification is based on the pharyngeal structures seen.

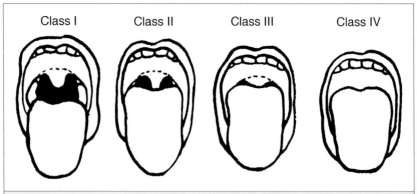

Figure 11-3. The Mallampati classification to evaluate pharyngeal space.

- **Class I:** The soft palate, fauces, entire uvula, and tonsillar pillars are visible.
- **Class II:** The soft palate, fauces, and part of the uvula are visible.
- **Class III:** The soft palate and base of the uvula are visible.
- **Class IV:** The soft palate is not visible at all.

Patients with class I airways are generally easier to intubate than patients with class IV airways. However, this test addresses only one of the four anatomic features required for easy direct laryngoscopy.

20. **How do you evaluate neck extension and submandibular compliance to predict difficult intubation?**
A normal adult has approximately 35 degrees of extension at the atlanto-occipital joint. A decrease in extension may make it impossible to view the larynx with direct laryngoscopy. It can be difficult to assess the submandibular compliance by physical examination. Assessment of the mandibular space can be attempted by measuring the distance from the chin to the thyroid cartilage, the *thyromental distance*. An adult with less than 6.5 cm of thyromental distance may have a greater chance of difficult intubation than one with greater than 6.5 cm. Combining the various physical exam tests improves the ability to predict a difficult intubation, but no combination is foolproof.

21. **How do you manage a potentially difficult intubation?**
Three types of plans must be made when managing a difficult airway. The first is the primary approach to the intubation. The second is the plan for an emergency nonsurgical airway. Finally, there should be a plan for an emergency surgical airway (cricothyroidotomy or tracheotomy). Many factors affect the management plan for a potentially difficult airway. These factors include the indication for intubation, the urgency of the intubation, the availability of skilled personnel, and the availability of special equipment. Because an awake, cooperative, spontaneously breathing patient normally has a patent airway, an awake intubation may be the safest. Topical or local anesthetics can be used to decrease airway sensation and patient discomfort.

22. **What are the ways to provide an emergency nonsurgical airway?**
If tracheal intubation and mask ventilation are not possible and the airway is not patent, an emergency airway must be provided. The options for providing an emergency nonsurgical airway include laryngeal mask ventilation, transtracheal jet ventilation, or esophageal-tracheal Combitube ventilation. The laryngeal mask is the most widely available of the three options. It is inserted into the posterior pharynx and lies opposite the larynx. In elective situations, it has a success rate of over 90%. It is less successful in emergencies, but its widespread availability makes it a valuable option in managing the difficult airway. Special versions of the laryngeal mask incorporate features designed to facilitate blind passage of an endotracheal tube into the trachea.

   LMA North America Education Center: www.lmana.com/prod/components/education_center/education_center.html

23. **How is tracheal intubation confirmed?**
Auscultation for bilateral breath sounds and absence of stomach inflation should be done after each intubation attempt. However, these signs may still be present with an esophageal intubation. Carbon dioxide capnography is one of the most reliable methods to confirm placement. The laryngoscopic view may be useful. If an experienced clinician clearly sees the tube between the vocal cords, this is definitive confirmation. The endotracheal tube itself commonly blocks sight of the vocal cords, and inexperienced clinicians may insert the tube in the esophagus despite having a good view of the larynx. Other confirmation methods include fiberoptic bronchoscopy or an esophageal detector device.

24. **What are the immediate, short-term complications of tracheal intubation?**
Immediate complications of intubation include dental injury, cervical spine injury, pharyngeal trauma, laryngeal injury, aspiration of gastric contents, and tracheal rupture. Nosebleed is a risk with nasal intubations. The most common injuries are minor lip trauma and tooth damage.

KEY POINTS: AIRWAY MANAGEMENT IN PATIENTS IN THE INTENSIVE CARE UNIT

1. In most patients, it is possible to maintain a patent airway without tracheal intubation.

2. Before managing a patient's airway, confirm the availability and function of all equipment that may be used.

3. The five main indications for tracheal intubation are upper airway obstruction, inadequate oxygenation, inadequate ventilation, elevated work of breathing, and airway protection.

4. To predict a difficult intubation, evaluate four anatomic features on physical examination: mouth opening, pharyngeal space, neck extension, and submandibular compliance.

5. Confirm endotracheal tube placement immediately with a reliable method such as carbon dioxide capnography.

WEBSITES

1. American Society of Anesthesiologists Practice Guidelines for Management of the Difficult Airway
www.asahq.org/publicationsAndServices/Difficult%20Airway.pdf

2. LMA North America Education Center
www.lmana.com/prod/components/education_center/education_center.html

BIBLIOGRAPHY

1. Gal TJ: Airway management. In Miller RD (ed): Miller's Anesthesia, 6th ed. New York, Churchill Livingstone, 2005, pp 1617–1652.

CHAPTER 12

TRACHEOTOMY AND UPPER AIRWAY OBSTRUCTION

John E. Heffner, MD

1. **What are the different techniques for obtaining tracheal access in critically ill patients?**

   A standard tracheotomy is a surgical procedure wherein a tracheostomy tube is inserted through an incisional tracheostoma. The tube enters the trachea between cartilaginous rings. The rings can be divided for passage of the tube by various surgical techniques, including incision and dilation of the inter-ring membranes, vertical incisions through rings, removal of portions of the anterior tracheal wall including ring segments, or formation of an anterior tracheal tissue flap (Björk flap). The stoma spontaneously closes after removal of the tracheostomy tube.

   The term *percutaneous tracheotomy* refers to various procedures that have in common either a modified Seldinger technique for placing a standard or modified tracheostomy tube or a forceps or dilator technique to cannulate and dilate tracheal tissue between cartilaginous rings. For the Seldinger technique, a small cutaneous incision is made over the trachea and a needle, guidewire, and introducer are placed below the first or second tracheal ring into the tracheal lumen. A single horn-shaped dilator is introduced through the tract into the trachea over the introducer. A tracheostomy tube loaded onto a stylet is then placed through the dilated tissue structures, followed by removal of the stylet. For the forceps technique, a specialized guidewire dilating forceps (GWDF) is used. The GWDF has a groove that allows loading of a guidewire onto the forceps, which are used to dilate the trachea, thread the wire, and insert a tracheostomy tube over the wire. Most intensivists in the United States use the modified Seldinger technique with a single-horned percutaneous dilator.

   A cricothyroidotomy is a surgical technique for placement of an airway into the trachea through the cricothyroid space. The superficial location of anatomic landmarks at the level of the cricothyroid membrane offers simplicity of technique, which makes cricothyroidotomy the preferred technique for placement of a surgical airway in emergency settings. Most centers do not use the cricothyroidotomy technique for placing tubes for long-term airway access because of the risks for subglottic stenosis.

   A minitracheotomy allows the percutaneous placement of a 7 Fr cannula through the tracheal rings for patients with difficulty clearing airway secretions. The minitracheotomy tube is just large enough to allow passage of a suction catheter for frequent removal of secretions.

   Bonde P, Papachristos I, McCraith A, et al: Sputum retention after lung operation: Prospective, randomized trial shows superiority of prophylactic minitracheostomy in high-risk patients. Ann Thorac Surg 74:196–203, 2002.

   deBoisblanc BP: Percutaneous dilational tracheostomy techniques. Clin Chest Med 24:399–407, 2003.

   Ernst A, Critchlow J: Percutaneous tracheostomy: Special considerations. Clin Chest Med 24:409–412, 2003.

   Goumas P, Kokkinis K, Petrocheilos J, et al: Cricothyroidotomy and the anatomy of the cricothyroid space: An autopsy study. J Laryngol Otol 111:354–356, 1997.

   Isaacs JH Jr, Pedersen AD: Emergency cricothyroidotomy. Am Surg 63:346–349, 1997.

   van Heurn LW: When and how should we do a tracheostomy? Curr Opin Crit Care 6:267–270, 2000.

   Wood DE: Tracheostomy. Chest Surg Clin North Am 6:749–764, 1996.

KEY POINTS: TYPES OF TRACHEOSTOMY PROCEDURES

1. Standard tracheotomy involves the surgical incision and dissection of the neck.

2. In a percutaneous tracheotomy, needle or dilator insertion of a guidewire occurs, allowing passage of a tracheostomy tube.

3. Emergency airway placed through the cricothyroid space is a cricothyroidotomy.

4. Minitracheotomy involves the needle insertion of a small tube that allows airway suctioning.

2. **Should all tracheotomies in critically ill patients be performed in the operating room (OR)?**
Not necessarily. Tracheotomy in intubated patients undergoing mechanical ventilation can be done efficiently and safely in the intensive care unit (ICU), thereby avoiding patient transport and OR scheduling delays. The patient's critical care room must be transformed, however, to an OR environment, with adequate instrumentation, sterile fields, personnel, lighting, and suction. At present, however, most standard surgical tracheotomies are performed in the OR. Most intensivists who perform percutaneous tracheotomies prefer the ICU setting for the procedure; the ability to perform percutaneous tracheotomies in the ICU safely and quickly is seen as one of the advantages of the procedure. Percutaneous dilational tracheotomies can be performed in the ICU at a lower cost than standard tracheotomies in the OR. This cost advantage no longer applies when both procedures are performed in the ICU.

Grover A, Robbins J, Bendick P, et al: Open versus percutaneous dilatational tracheostomy: Efficacy and cost analysis. Am Surg 67:297–301, 2001.

Massick DD, Yao S, Powell DM, et al: Bedside tracheostomy in the intensive care unit: A prospective randomized trial comparing open surgical tracheostomy with endoscopically guided percutaneous dilational tracheostomy. Laryngoscope 111:494–500, 2001.

3. **Is percutaneous dilational tracheotomy performed as a blind technique with dilator insertion directed by neck and airway palpation?**
Percutaneous dilational tracheotomy was first described as a blind technique in which the operator directed the needle and guidewire into the airway guided by careful palpation of the neck. Reports of extraluminal insertion of tracheostomy tubes and lacerations of the posterior tracheal wall by needles and guidewires promoted the performance of percutaneous dilational tracheotomy under direct bronchoscopic visualization. A bronchoscope with video imaging is inserted through the endotracheal tube, which is pulled back into the subglottic region of the airway to allow visualization of the tracheotomy site. The operator then can observe the needle and guidewire entering the trachea to ensure proper placement of the introducer and dilator. Some intensivists perform percutaneous tracheotomy with bedside ultrasonographic guidance.

Kollig E, Heydenreich U, Roteman B, et al: Ultrasound and bronchoscopic controlled percutaneous tracheostomy on trauma ICU injury. Injury 31:663–668, 2000.

Sustic A, Zupan Z, Antoncic II: Ultrasound-guided percutaneous dilatational tracheostomy with laryngeal mask airway control in a morbidly obese patient. J Clin Anesth 16:121–123, 2004.

Winkler WB, Karnik R, Seelmann O, et al: Bedside percutaneous dilational tracheostomy with endoscopic guidance: Experience with 71 ICU patients. Intens Care Med 20:476–479, 1994.

4. **Is emergency tracheotomy the surgical procedure of choice in apneic patients with acute upper airway obstruction?**
No. Tracheotomy is acceptably safe when performed electively in an OR environment under controlled clinical conditions. Risks of surgical complications increase fivefold, however, when

tracheotomy is applied in an emergency situation. An emergency cricothyroidotomy provides the greatest likelihood of successful airway placement with the lowest risks for complications in patients with acute upper airway obstruction who cannot undergo translaryngeal intubation.

Burkey B, Esclamado R, Morganroth M: The role of cricothyroidotomy in airway management. Clin Chest Med 12:561–571, 1991.

Gillespie MB, Eisele DW: Outcomes of emergency surgical airway procedures in a hospital-wide setting. Laryngoscope 109:1766–1769, 1999.

Walls RM: Cricothyroidotomy. Emerg Med Clinic North Am 6:725–736, 1988.

5. **What is the most lethal complication of tracheotomy in the perioperative period?**
Inadvertent decannulation of a tracheostomy tube during the first 3–5 days after its placement represents a potentially lethal clinical event. It may take several days for a tracheostomy incision to form a stomal tract that allows blind replacement of a decannulated tracheostomy tube. Before this time, attempts to reinsert a tracheostomy tube will most likely create a false tissue tract in the pretracheal space. Subsequent attempts to ventilate the patient with positive pressure through a misplaced tube result in profound cervical emphysema and external compression of the trachea, leading to asphyxia.

A general rule dictates that only surgeons experienced with the patient's cervical anatomy should attempt replacement of a decannulated tube within the first 5 days after surgery. In the absence of a skilled surgeon, patients who require urgent airway control can undergo translaryngeal intubation and replacement of the tracheostomy tube under a controlled setting after they stabilize. If the patient cannot be intubated through the nose or mouth because of upper airway obstruction, a narrow-caliber, cuffless endotracheal tube can be inserted through the surgical incision into the trachea with the assistance of a lighted laryngoscope blade. In some patients, the trachea may require initial intubation with a flexible endotracheal stylet ("tube changer") or nasogastric tube over which an airway can be guided into place. Other complications are listed in Box 12-1.

BOX 12-1.   COMPLICATIONS OF TRACHEOTOMY

- Aspiration and pneumonia
- Acute cardiopulmonary arrest with surgical misplacement
- Herniation of tracheal rings
- Mediastinitis
- Peristomal cellulitis
- Pneumomediastinum and pneumothorax
- Posterior tracheal wall perforation
- Stomal erosion or breakdown
- Stoma site infection
- Stomal hemorrhage
- Subglottic stenosis or atresia
- Surgical emphysema
- Tracheal dilation
- Tracheal granulomas with obstruction
- Tracheal ring rupture
- Tracheal stenosis
- Tracheoesophageal fistula
- Tracheoinnominate fistula
- Tracheomalacia

---

6. **How is a cricothyroidotomy performed?**
The cricothyroid membrane is located approximately 2–3 cm below the thyroid notch. The membrane, which is typically 1 cm in height, lies below the vocal cords but within the subglottic

larynx. A surgical scalpel is used to incise the overlying skin and stab the membrane. The resultant opening into the airway is enlarged with a spreader, allowing placement of a tracheostomy tube. Commercially available instruments designed for emergency situations allow puncture of the membrane and introduction of an airway cannula in one maneuver.

7. **Can mechanically ventilated patients with a tracheostomy speak?**
Several techniques promote speech in mechanically ventilated patients with a tracheostomy tube in place. Patients with low to moderate minute ventilation requirements can whisper intelligibly if the tracheostomy tube cuff is deflated to allow a small "cuff leak" during the ventilatory inspiratory cycle. Addition of a small amount of positive end-expiratory pressure (PEEP) creates a leak throughout inspiration and expiration and promotes more continuous and spontaneous speech. A "speaking tracheostomy tube" provides an external cannula that directs compressed gas to exit the tube below the vocal cords, allowing some patients to communicate in whispered tones. An "electrolarynx" placed against the neck near the laryngeal cartilage generates a vibratory tone that can be articulated with practice into intelligible speech. If patients have limited or no mechanical ventilatory requirements, a one-way valve can be placed in-line between a fenestrated tracheostomy tube with a deflated cuff and the ventilator tubing, allowing expiration through the native airway and promoting intelligible speech (Fig. 12-1).

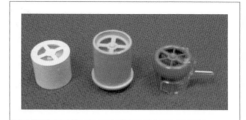

Figure 12-1. One-way tracheotomy valves that allow spontaneous speech.

Godwin JE, Heffner JE: Special critical care considerations in tracheostomy management. Clin Chest Med 12:573–583, 1991.

Hoit JD, Banzett R: Simple adjustments can improve ventilator-supported speech. Am J Speech Lang Pathol 56:87–96, 1997.

Hoit JD, Lohmeier HL: Influence of continuous speaking on ventilation. J Speech Lang Hear Res 43:1240–1251, 2000.

Leder SB: Importance of verbal communication for the ventilation dependent patient. Chest 98:792–793, 1990.

8. **What precautions should be exercised in patients with a cuffed tracheostomy tube who undergo general anesthesia?**
Some volatile anesthetics, such as nitrous oxide, diffuse more rapidly into a tracheostomy tube cuff than oxygen or nitrogen can diffuse out and thereby increase intracuff pressures. During a 2-hour operation, cuff pressures may increase from 15 mmHg to over 80 mmHg, which can cause ischemic injury to the tracheal mucosa. Appropriate precautions include frequent monitoring of cuff pressures in the OR or inflation of the tube cuff at the outset of the surgical procedure with the anesthetic gas mixture administered to the airway.

9. **What is the ideal size of tracheostomy tube for a patient?**
No one size is best for all patients because tracheal caliber and clinical situations vary. Small-caliber tubes may decrease the incidence of tracheal stenosis at the stoma site because of the smaller tracheal incision required. Unfortunately, small tubes present difficulties in airway suctioning, spontaneous ventilation, and fiberoptic bronchoscopy. Furthermore, small tubes have small cuffs that may damage the tracheal mucosa because they require high intracuff

pressures to overdistend in order to seal the airway. Overly large tubes require wide stomas and prohibit adequate cuff inflation to cushion the rigid tube from the tracheal mucosa and to effectively prevent aspiration. The best approximation of ideal size requires the surgeon to select a tube with an outer diameter two-thirds the inner caliber of the patient's trachea at the point of insertion.

10. **Should tracheostomy tube cuff pressures be checked periodically in patients undergoing mechanical ventilation?**
Frequent monitoring of cuff pressure with a pressure gauge provides the best measure to prevent tracheal injury at the cuff site. Other techniques exist to estimate in-cuff pressure. These include finger palpation of the external inflation bulb, minimal occlusive volume, and the tension felt by the operator on an inflating syringe. None of these techniques substitutes for direct measurements of intracuff pressure. Up to 45% of patients will experience overinflated cuffs if not monitored with pressure gauges. Cuff pressures in excess of mucosal capillary perfusion pressures (usually 25 mmHg) can rapidly cause mucosal ischemia and resultant tracheal stenosis. Reliance on minimal leak technique to inflate cuffs without actually measuring cuff pressures may prevent detection of patients with high cuff pressure requirements. A linear relationship exists between the intracuff pressure required to seal the airway (minimal leak cuff pressure) and the peak inspiratory pressure generated by positive pressure ventilation. Patients with peak inspiratory pressures above 48 cm H_2O will usually require cuff inflations pressures above 25 mmHg.

If a tracheotomy tube is underinflated (<15 mmHg) in a patient undergoing mechanical ventilation, the risks for aspiration and nosocomial pneumonia increase. Therefore, most experts recommend maintaining cuff pressure between 15 and 25 mmHg. Clinicians should notice the units of measurement of cuff pressures and make the appropriate conversion from centimeters of water (cm H_2O) to millimeters of mercury (mmHg) to allow adherence to cuff pressure standards (cuff pressure in millimeters of mercury = [measured cuff pressure in centimeters of water]/1.36).

Bernhard WN, Cottrell JE, Sivakumaran C, et al: Adjustment of intracuff pressure to prevent aspiration. Anesthesiology 50:363, 1979.

Norwood S, Vallina VL, Short K, et al: Incidence of tracheal stenosis and other late complications after percutaneous tracheostomy. Ann Surg 232:233–241, 2000.

Rello J, Sonora R, Jubert P, et al: Pneumonia in intubated patients: Role of respiratory airway care. Am J Respir Crit Care Med 154(1):111–115, 1996.

11. **What should the clinician consider in any patient with airway hemorrhage after the first 48 hours of insertion of a tracheostomy tube?**
Bleeding within the first 48 hours of tracheotomy is usually a result of hemorrhage from the incisional wound. Any bleeding that develops more than 48 hours after surgery should suggest the possibility of a tracheoinnominate fistula, which develops as a communication between the trachea and innominate artery from erosion of the tracheal wall as a result of pressure necrosis caused by the tracheostomy tube tip or cuff. This life-threatening complication requires immediate evaluation by a thoracic surgeon capable of performing an emergency sternotomy for ligation of the innominate artery because massive hemorrhage often develops after an initial "herald" episode of mild to moderate bleeding.

Allan JS, Wright CD: Tracheoinnominate fistula: Diagnosis and management. Chest Surg Clin North Am 13:331–341, 2003.

12. **How should you evaluate a patient who continues to have cough and shortness of breath 2 months after removal of a tracheostomy tube?**
Although these symptoms often accompany underlying lung disease, they also occasionally represent the only clinical manifestations of a tracheoesophageal fistula. Patients undergoing

positive-pressure mechanical ventilation may experience gastric distension or frequent belching. Recurrent aspiration of esophageal secretions may manifest as nosocomial pneumonia. A tracheoesophageal fistula related to pressure necrosis by the tube cuff or catheter tip occurs as a complication of tracheostomy in fewer than 1% of patients. Risk factors include excessive tube movement, high ventilator inflation pressures, overinflated cuffs, prolonged intubation, diabetes mellitus, and the presence of a nasogastric tube.

Suspicion of a tracheoesophageal fistula should be pursued with contrast imaging studies, such as a cine-esophagram. Endoscopic evaluation either by bronchoscopy or esophagoscopy may fail to identify the fistula tract.

Reed MF, Mathisen DJ: Tracheoesophageal fistula. Chest Surg Clin North Am 13:271–289, 2003.

13. **What are the indications for tracheotomy in critically ill patients?**
Common indications include removal of airway secretions, relief of upper airway obstruction, provision of airway access for long-term mechanical ventilation, and prevention of aspiration.

14. **Do ventilator-dependent patients wean faster from the ventilator if an "early" tracheotomy is performed?**
Several prospective, randomized studies that enrolled ventilator-dependent, critically ill patients have examined potential benefits of performing early tracheotomy (after 3–7 days of intubation) compared with delayed tracheotomy (8 days or longer after intubation). Some of these studies demonstrated lower rates of hospital-acquired pneumonia and shorter duration of mechanical ventilation among patients undergoing early tracheotomy. Unfortunately, design flaws in these studies prevent widespread acceptance of their findings. Evidence-based guidelines for weaning patients from ventilatory support, recently published by the American College of Chest Physicians, reported no high-grade evidence that routine performance of early tracheotomy promotes earlier weaning.

Many intensivists, however, suggest that tracheotomy probably does promote earlier weaning from mechanical ventilation more through the impact of tracheostomy on altering physician behavior than any specific physiologic effects of the tube. For instance, increased patient comfort from removal of an endotracheal tube may allow earlier discontinuation of sedative drugs and more rapid weaning. Placement of a tracheotomy for intubated patients does decrease the work of breathing, but it is not established that the degree of decreased work is clinically important.

Durbin CG Jr: Indications for and timing of tracheostomy. Respir Care 50:483–487, 2005.
Heffner JE: The role of tracheotomy in weaning. Chest 120(6 Suppl):477S–481S, 2001.
Maziak DE, Meade MO, Todd TR: The timing of tracheotomy: A systematic review. Chest 114:605–609, 1998.
Moscovici da Cruz V, Demarzo SE, Sobrinko JB, et al: Effects of tracheostomy on respiratory mechanics in spontaneously breathing patients. Eur Respir J 20:112–117, 2002.
Pierson DJ: Tracheostomy and weaning. Respir Care 50:526–533, 2005.
Rana S, Pendem S, Pogodzinski MS, et al: Tracheostomy in critically ill patients. Mayo Clin Proc 80:1632–1638, 2005.

15. **When should a tracheotomy be performed in a ventilator-dependent patient?**
No study or accumulation of data from combined investigations has determined the ideal time to perform a tracheotomy in patients who require long-term mechanical ventilation. Recent consensus, however, is that the decision should be individualized, with a tracheotomy being performed when a patient appears likely to benefit from the procedure. The potential benefits of tracheotomy over prolonged translaryngeal intubation include improved comfort, enhanced ability to communicate, greater mobility, and diminished risk for direct laryngeal injury.

Consensus further emphasizes that the decision whether to apply a tracheotomy in ventilator-dependent patients should be determined by a patient's anticipated likelihood of requiring prolonged mechanical ventilation rather than by the arbitrary duration of ventilator dependency that has already transpired. As an example, patients with respiratory failure should be evaluated within 7 days of treatment with a translaryngeal endotracheal tube for the probability of successful extubation within the first 10–14 days of intubation. Patients determined unlikely to improve rapidly on the basis of severity of disease should undergo tracheotomy at an early and convenient opportunity rather than waiting for an arbitrary and obligate 1–2 weeks of mechanical ventilation.

Durbin CG Jr: Indications for and timing of tracheostomy. Respir Care 50:483–487, 2005.
Heffner JE: Timing of tracheotomy in mechanically ventilated patients. Am Rev Resp Dis 147:768–771, 1993.
Heffner JE: Tracheotomy application and timing. Clin Chest Med 24:389–398, 2003.

16. **Describe the role of a fenestrated tracheostomy tube in the ICU.**
Newer fenestrated tracheostomy tubes with multiple small holes in their greater curvature assist speech and weaning from tracheostomy in spontaneously breathing patients without stimulating growth of granulation tissue. After removal of an inner cannula (if present) and deflation of the cuff, patients can breathe around the cuff and through the fenestrations in addition to the stoma to decrease airway resistance. Placement of a one-way valve, such as the Passy-Muir valve, on the tracheostomy tube allows patients to inhale through the tube and exhale out their native upper airways, thereby promoting speech.

Some physicians recommend placement of a fenestrated tracheostomy tube to facilitate gradual weaning toward decannulation. Others prefer to use a stomal button, arguing that placement of a fenestrated tube interferes with spontaneous clearing of secretions through the native airway and delays decannulation.

17. **What is a tracheal button?**
Tracheal buttons, such as the Olympic tracheal button and the Montgomery tracheal button, assist weaning from a tracheostomy tube (Fig. 12-2). Designed as a straight, rigid, or flexible plastic or Silastic tube, tracheal buttons fit through the stoma to maintain its patency in case patients need suctioning or reinsertion of a tracheostomy tube through the tract. The button is ideal for patients with borderline ventilatory status because the distal end abuts the anterior tracheal wall and does not protrude into the airway to impede respiration or clearance of secretions by coughing.

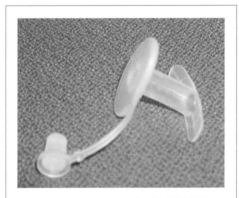

Figure 12-2. A tracheotomy stoma button. The silicone distal flange deforms to allow placement into the trachea through the stoma tract.

18. **Why do patients aspirate after removal of a tracheostomy tube?**
Scarring at the stoma site may interfere with the rostrocaudal excursion of the larynx during swallowing, which is necessary for glottic closure. In addition, prolonged diversion of ventilation away from the glottis causes attenuation of the vocal cord adductor response that is important in aspiration prevention.

19. **Can a percutaneous tracheotomy be safely performed in a ventilated patient who requires PEEP?**

Percutaneous tracheotomy can be performed successfully in patients with severe respiratory failure who require high levels of PEEP. One reported series performed the procedure under bronchoscopic guidance for patients with mean PEEP levels of 16.6 cm H_2O (range, 12–20 cm H_2O) and found no deterioration of arterial oxygen at 1 and 24 hours after the procedure compared with patients with lower PEEP levels (mean, 7.6 cm H_2O; range, 5.4–9.8 cm H_2O).

Beiderlinden M, Groeben H, Peters J: Safety of percutaneous dilational tracheostomy in patients ventilated with high positive end-expiratory pressure (PEEP). Intens Care Med 29:944–948, 2003.

WEBSITES

1. Bliznikas D, Baredes S: Percutaneous tracheostomy
www.emedicine.com/ent/topic682.htm

2. Cook Incorporated, Inc: Video clips of percutaneous tracheostomy
www.cookgroup.com/cook_critical_care/education/video/index.html

CHAPTER 13

CHEST TUBES

Mark W. Bowyer, MD, DMCC, COL, USAF, MC

1. **What is the purpose of a chest tube?**
   A chest tube is used to evacuate fluid and air from the pleural space and to reestablish a negative intrapleural pressure so that the lung can reexpand.

2. **Describe the clinical conditions in which you would place a chest tube.**
   Chest tubes are generally placed for the treatment of pneumothorax (both tension and simple) and hemothorax in trauma and in nontraumatic conditions. In addition, chest tubes are used for the drainage of large symptomatic or recurrent pleural effusions, in the treatment of empyema and chylothorax, and as drainage of the pleural space after esophageal rupture.

3. **How often is a chest tube the sole therapy needed to treat penetrating chest trauma?**
   In 85% of cases of penetrating trauma to the chest, chest tube insertion is therapeutic and potentially lifesaving.

4. **How does a chest tube work?**
   The suction design for chest tubes is based on a three-bottle system. In this system, the first bottle is connected directly to the patient's chest tube for fluid collection. The second bottle is connected to the first bottle and is used for a water seal. The third bottle connects the first two bottles to wall suction and is used to control the amount of suction applied to the system (Fig. 13-1). Modern systems have the same three compartments as the original three-bottle system, but they are contained together in one sealed plastic container.

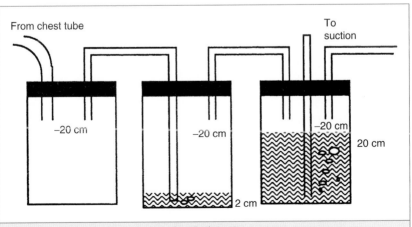

Figure 13-1. The classic three-bottle chest tube collection system.

5. **How much suction is applied to the chest tube?**
   Under most circumstances, about −20 cm H_2O is applied to the chest tube via the collection system. This is usually adequate to keep the pleural space evacuated but not so high as to damage the lung. More suction can be used if needed. The highest pressure ever routinely used is −40 cm H_2O.

6. **Where are the landmarks for chest tube placement?**
   Chest tubes are generally placed in the fourth or fifth intercostal space just anterior to the midaxillary line and directed apically in the chest cavity. The nipple line is generally used in males to estimate the fifth intercostal space and the inframammary fold or crease in women (Fig. 13-2, *A*).

   Griffiths JR, Roberts N: Do junior doctors know where to insert chest drains safely? Postgrad Med J 81:456–458, 2005.

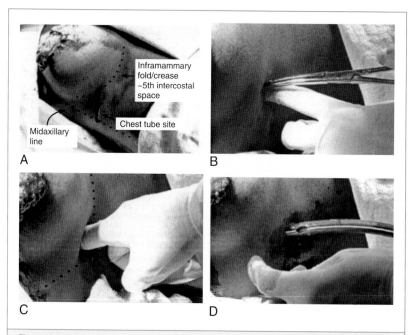

Figure 13-2. The steps for inserting a chest tube. *A,* The inframammary fold is used to estimate the site for chest tube insertion just anterior to the midaxillary line. *B,* After a skin incision is made, a clamp is advanced up and over the next rib, spreading muscle and entering the chest. *C,* A gloved finger is placed into the chest to ensure proper position and to lyse any adhesions that might prevent tube placement. *D,* The chest tube is inserted toward the apex and advanced until the last hole is in the chest.

7. **How does one select an appropriately sized chest tube?**
   The size should be tailored to the specific need. Large chest tubes (i.e., 36 Fr) should be used to drain a hemothorax. In patients with this condition, smaller tubes can become obstructed with blood clots requiring repeat tube placement. Small chest tubes (i.e., 10–14 Fr) should be used exclusively for treatment of a simple pneumothorax. In the setting of the intensive care unit, the most commonly used tube is 28 Fr. This allows for treatment of a pneumothorax as well as drainage of pleural fluid. It will continue to function even in the presence of a large pulmonary air leak in a patient receiving positive-pressure ventilation.

   Bauman MH: What size chest tube? What drainage system is ideal? And other chest tube management questions. Curr Opin Pulm Med 9:276–281, 2003.

8. **How is a chest tube placed?**
The area is prepared and draped (*see* Fig. 13-2, *A*) and local anesthesia using 1% lidocaine is administered. A small incision is made below the planned interspace, and a tract for insertion is made by bluntly spreading the muscle using either a Kelly clamp (Fig. 13-2, *B*) or Mayo scissors. After entering the pleura, a digital examination of the chest cavity should be performed to ensure proper position and to lyse any local adhesive bands that would prevent insertion of the tube (Fig. 13-2, *C*). The tube can then be inserted using a blunt-tip clamp and directed to the appropriate location in the chest (Fig. 13-2, *D*). The chest tube should be sewn in place with a single silk suture and connected to the drainage system.

9. **What are the possible complications of chest tube placement?**
Older chest tubes may include a metal trocar, which has been responsible for a large number of the perforation complications listed in Box 13-1. If a trocar comes with the chest drain set, it should be immediately discarded or only used to hold up tomato plants.

Chest Trauma: Intercostal Chest Drains: www.trauma.org/thoracic/CHESTdrain.html

---

BOX 13-1. COMPLICATIONS OF CHEST TUBE PLACEMENT

Traumatic perforation of:
- Lung
- Heart chambers
- Inferior vena cava
- Pulmonary artery
- Diaphragm
- Intra-abdominal organs
- Breast prosthesis

Intercostal neuralgia

Bleeding from intercostal vessels

Reexpansion pulmonary edema

Infection

Improper tube placement:
- Outside chest
- Not far enough into chest
- Into lung fissure

---

10. **What is reexpansion pulmonary edema? Is it treatable?**
Reexpansion pulmonary edema is a rare event resulting in unilateral pulmonary edema from rapid evacuation of a pleural effusion or rapid reexpansion of the lung in the case of a pneumothorax. Although it is rare, a mortality of up to 20% has been noted in recognized cases. Most reported cases have occurred after drainage of large collections, that is, more than 2 L that have existed for longer than 3 days. Differential lung ventilation has shown some early promise in treatment.

Cho SR, Lee JS, Kim MS: New treatment method for reexpansion pulmonary edema: Differential lung ventilation. Ann Thorac Surg 80:1933–1934, 2005.

11. **How can you decrease the likelihood of reexpansion pulmonary edema?**
    Efforts to decrease the likelihood of this occurrence include the following: (1) allowing the initial drainage of a large pleural effusion, or the initial reexpansion of a large, chronic pneumothorax using water seal only; and (2) clamping the chest tube for several hours after draining the initial 2 L of a large chronic pleural effusion.

12. **How do you monitor a patient with a chest tube?**
    The amount and character of fluid output should be monitored throughout the day. The presence or absence of an air leak should also be noted by looking for the presence of bubbles in the water seal chamber during inspiration or coughing. When a continued air leak is noted, it is important to ensure that the leak is not within the system itself. This can be checked by sequentially clamping the tube before each connection and looking for an air leak. If there is a leak from the system, it must be replaced. It is also important make sure that there is no leak where the chest tube enters the chest and to check the chest radiograph to see that the last hole in the chest tube is within the chest.

13. **How much blood draining from a hemothorax should prompt operative intervention?**
    Acutely, a drainage of 1500 mL of blood or more from the hemothorax, which represents approximately 40% of the circulating blood volume, should raise serious concerns that the hemorrhage may require operative intervention. In general, more than 800 mL in 1 hour, 400 mL/h for 2 consecutive hours, 200 mL/h for 4 consecutive hours, or 800 mL over 8 hours should also prompt consideration for operative intervention.

14. **Can blood drained from the chest tube be given back to the patient?**
    Yes, an autotransfusion container can be placed between the chest tube and the collection/drainage device. This blood can be given back to the patient without further processing.

15. **Should chest tubes be clamped when patients are being transported?**
    No! During transport, when suction is unavailable, the patient should be transported on water seal, and the water seal chamber should be kept at least 20 cm H_2O below the level of the patient to prevent reflux of fluid up the tube with any high negative intrathoracic pressures that may occur. Clamping the chest tube during transport could result in a tension pneumothorax if a significant air leak from the lung is present.

16. **What is chest tube stripping?**
    Stripping is the practice of compressing the chest tube (or the drainage tube coming from it), either with the thumb and forefingers or with a mechanical stripper, and pulling away from the chest wall while continuing to compress the tube. The objective is to generate a negative pressure to dislodge any clots within the tube and to promote pleural drainage. There is no evidence that stripping the tube actually accomplishes this goal. It is a procedure whose routine use should probably be abandoned.

17. **What is a Heimlich valve? How is it used?**
    A Heimlich valve is a simple one-way flutter valve. Air that is moving from the pleural space can exit the valve, but air cannot enter because the distal end collapses with inspiration. It is usually used in an outpatient setting or during transport of patients to prevent a pneumothorax. It is usually not used in critically ill patients.

KEY POINTS: CHEST TUBE BASICS

1. Tension pneumothorax is a clinical diagnosis, not an x-ray diagnosis.
2. Eighty-five percent of penetrating chest trauma can be treated with a chest tube alone.
3. Use large-bore (36 Fr) tubes to drain blood, and smaller tubes (10–14 Fr) to remove air.
4. An initial drainage of more than 1500 mL of blood mandates surgical exploration.
5. Chest tubes should be hooked to underwater suction at -20 cm H_2O.
6. When drainage is less than 100 mL/day, and there is no air leak on water seal for 24 hours, the chest tube can be removed.

18. **When are chest tubes removed?**
Chest tubes can be pulled when no air leak is noted on water seal for 24 hours, the drainage falls below 100 mL/day, and the chest radiograph demonstrates complete expansion of the lung. Mechanical ventilation should not be a deterrent to removal of the chest tube because the risk of recurrent pneumothorax after chest tube removal in these patients is low. One exception to the previously discussed rule is when the tube has been placed for an empyema. Pulling a chest tube that is draining an empyema cavity may result in reaccumulation of the abscess cavity.

19. **How is a chest tube removed?**
The classic teaching for removal of a chest tube is as follows: After taking down the dressing, carefully cut the sutures holding the tube is place. Place a greased gauze pad on a 4 × 4 dressing and hold it over the chest tube exit site. Instruct the patient to take a large breath and perform a Valsalva maneuver, then rapidly pull the chest tube while covering the exit site with the greased gauze dressing. If great care is not taken during this maneuver, a pneumothorax may occur, requiring replacement of the chest tube.

20. **Should a chest tube be removed at end-inspiration or end-expiration? Does it make a difference?**
As described previously, the classic teaching has been that chest tubes need to be removed at end-inspiration. This belief has been recently challenged in the literature, with a recent randomized study showing no difference in the rate of post-removal pneumothorax after removal at end-inspiration or end-expiration.

   Bell RL, Ovadia P, Abdullah F, Spector S, Rabinovici R: Chest tube removal: End-inspiration or end-expiration? J Trauma 50:674–677, 2001.

21. **Does removal of a chest tube mandate obtaining a post-removal chest radiograph?**
Once again, one of the cherished classic teachings has been challenged by recent literature. At least two recent studies have challenged this dogma and suggest that chest radiography after the removal of chest tubes should not be a routinely performed procedure but should be based on good clinical judgment.

22. **Should patients receiving a chest tube be treated with antibiotics?**
Yes, administration of prophylactic antibiotics to patients requiring chest tube for isolated chest injury reduces the incidence of pneumonitis but does not appear to influence the risk of empyema. The ideal regimen is 24 hours of a first-generation cephalosporin.

Luchette FA, Barre PS, Oswanski MF, et al: Practice Management Guidelines for Prophylactic Antibiotic use in Tube Thoracostomy for Traumatic Hemopneumothorax. Eastern Association for Trauma: www.east.org/tpg/chesttube.pdf

23. **How should the diagnosis of a tension pneumothorax be made?**
The diagnosis of tension pneumothorax is a clinical one. Classic signs are deviation of trachea, distended neck veins, and hyperexpanded chest with increased percussion. Do *not* wait for x-ray confirmation or you may have a dead patient.

CHAPTER 14

BRONCHOSCOPY

Amy E. Morris, MD, and Lynn M. Schnapp, MD

1. **What is flexible bronchoscopy?**
   Bronchoscopy literally means "to see the airways" and provides a means to visualize the upper airways, trachea, and bronchi. Flexible bronchoscopy uses a small-caliber fiberoptic scope, which is passed either through the nose or mouth or through a tracheostomy or endotracheal tube (Fig. 14-1). The bronchoscope is then directed down the trachea to the main carina and beyond to the regions of interest. In most patients, the airways can be visualized at least to the segmental bronchi.

   Wang KP, Mehta AC (eds): Flexible Bronchoscopy. Cambridge, Blackwell Scientific, 1995.

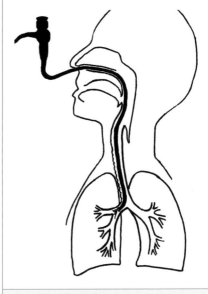

Figure 14-1. Flexible bronchoscopy.

2. **How is flexible bronchoscopy performed?**
   Flexible bronchoscopy can be performed at the bedside or in a specialized suite with the assistance of a nurse and a respiratory therapist. Preparation includes the following steps:
   1. Numb the patient's nose and pharynx with topical lidocaine.
   2. Set up suction equipment and monitoring for cardiac rhythm, blood pressure, and oxygenation saturation. Supplemental oxygen should be provided.
   3. Control cough and gag with small doses of short-acting narcotic and benzodiazepines.
   4. Lubricate the bronchoscope with topical lidocaine jelly. Anesthesia of the posterior pharynx, vocal cords, and carinas is important because advancing the bronchoscope past these areas is the least tolerated part of the procedure.

3. **How is rigid bronchoscopy different from flexible bronchoscopy?**
   Rigid bronchoscopy is performed with the patient under general anesthesia, using a rigid hollow tube that provides a large working channel, direct illumination, and an attachment to allow mechanical ventilation during the procedure. This technique is preferable to flexible bronchoscopy when more suction is required (as in the work-up of hemoptysis), during removal of foreign bodies, during surgical or laser removal of endobronchial lesions, or in the placement of endobronchial stents. Rigid bronchoscopy requires a stable cervical spine and the ability to manipulate the mandible.

4. **When should intubation be considered before bronchoscopy?**
   A spontaneously breathing patient scheduled to undergo flexible bronchoscopy without an artificial airway or mechanical ventilation should be cooperative, without violent coughing, and without risk for upper airway obstruction or hypoxic or hypercarbic respiratory failure. Patients who do not fit these criteria, but in whom bronchoscopy is considered a necessary procedure, may require intubation before the procedure. In all cases, equipment for endotracheal intubation should be easily accessible.

5. **How is bronchoscopy different for patients receiving mechanical ventilation?**
   Fiberoptic bronchoscopy can be performed through an endotracheal tube at least 7.0 mm in diameter by using a special adapter. Topical anesthesia is achieved with 1–2 mL of 2% lidocaine through the endotracheal tube. A silicone-based lubricant is applied to the bronchoscope to facilitate passage through the endotracheal tube. The bronchoscope will partially obstruct the tube, causing increased airway pressure and potentially increased air trapping. The respiratory therapist should set the ventilator on a volume mode with increased peak airway pressure limits to ensure that the patient receives adequate minute ventilation. The fractional concentration of oxygen in inspired gas (FiO_2) should be increased (usually to 1.0) because bronchoscopy and lavage may cause transient hypoxia.

   Hertz MI, Woodward ME, Gross CR, et al: Safety of bronchoalveolar lavage in the critically ill, mechanically ventilated patient. Crit Care Med 19:1526–1532, 1991.

6. **What are the indications for bronchoscopy in the intensive care unit (ICU)?**
   Bronchoscopy allows inspection of the airways, collection of samples from the lower airways, and performance of various interventions (Table 14-1). In the ICU, it is most commonly used to

TABLE 14-1.	INDICATIONS FOR BRONCHOSCOPY	
	Indication	Goal
Inspection	Hemoptysis	Localize bleeding
		Search for endobronchial lesion
	Infection	Identify evidence of inflammation or pus
	Aspiration	Look for foreign bodies
	Mass	Look for endobronchial masses
	Chest trauma	Find evidence of airway injury
	Inhalational injury	Find evidence of airway injury
Sample collection	Pulmonary infiltrates (infectious)	Obtain samples for Gram stain, silver stain, bacterial cultures, and viral and fungal studies
	Pulmonary infiltrates (noninfectious)	Identify alveolar hemorrhage
		Check for eosinophilia (analyze cell count and differential)
	Mass or adenopathy	Perform transbronchial biopsy for cytology/pathology
Interventions	Hemoptysis	Control bleeding
	Bronchial obstruction	Remove mucus or foreign bodies
		Perform laser removal of masses
		Place stent
	Alveolar proteinosis	Perform lavage
	Intubation	Visualize anatomy for tube placement

diagnose infection via bronchoalveolar lavage (BAL) or protected specimen brush. In BAL, the tip of the bronchoscope is wedged into a subsegmental bronchus while 5- to 30-mL aliquots of saline are injected and aspirated into sterile traps. Alveolar contents are collected while the bronchoscope position prevents flooding of other regions of the lung. The protected specimen brush is a sterile brush with a gelatin cap that is inserted into a potentially infected area, agitated, then withdrawn and sent for culture.

Raoof S, Mehrishi S, Prakash UB: Role of bronchoscopy in modern medical intensive care unit. Clin Chest Med 22:241–261, 2001.

7. **What other kinds of samples can be collected by bronchoscopy?**
   - **Cytology brush:** An abrasive brush is agitated against potentially malignant tissue and then sent for cytologic analysis.
   - **Transbronchial biopsy:** The bronchoscope is advanced as far as possible into subsegmental bronchi, then biopsy forceps are pushed past distal airways into the pulmonary parenchyma to obtain lung tissue. This technique may be used to diagnose infection (i.e., fungal disease), granulomatous diseases (i.e., sarcoidosis), or malignancy.
   - **Wang needle aspiration:** A technique used in diagnosis and staging of cancer. A short, rigid needle is thrust through the airway wall, usually near the main carina, into subcarinal or paratracheal lymph nodes. Suction is then applied to aspirate cells, which are sent for cytologic evaluation.

8. **List the absolute and relative contraindications for bronchoscopy.**
   - **Absolute contraindications:** These include an inability to maintain a patent airway during the procedure, such as in upper airway obstruction, laryngospasm, or intubation with a small endotracheal tube; an inability to oxygenate or ventilate adequately during bronchoscopy; active cardiac ischemia; malignant arrhythmias; and severe hemodynamic instability.
   - **Relative contraindications:** These include poor patient cooperation, elevated intracranial pressure, presence of lung abscess, and severe coagulopathy. Patients with impending respiratory failure or laryngeal edema may undergo bronchoscopy more safely if the airway is secured by elective endotracheal intubation before the procedure.

9. **What are the potential complications of bronchoscopy?**
   Flexible bronchoscopy is generally a safe procedure. However, complications do occur, with an incidence in observational studies of 0.1% for death and 2–5% for major complications (Table 14-2). Sources of complication include the bronchoscopic procedures themselves and anesthetic/sedative medications.

10. **What is the role of bronchoscopy in the diagnosis of community-acquired pneumonia (CAP)?**
    CAP in an immunocompetent host does not require microbiologic confirmation by bronchoscopy and is typically treated with empiric antibiotics. However, bronchoscopy may be indicated in patients with preexisting lung disease, immunosuppression, or critical illness because the microbiologic flora involved are less predictable. In patients whose conditions fail to respond to initial treatment for CAP, bronchoscopic sampling may provide information about bacterial resistance or atypical organisms or may reveal noninfectious etiologies.

11. **Discuss the role of bronchoscopy in an immunosuppressed patient with pulmonary infiltrates.**
    The differential diagnosis of pulmonary infiltrates in an immunocompromised host is broad and includes a long list of infectious and noninfectious etiologies. Bronchoscopy is particularly useful in these patients to guide therapy by collecting samples that are analyzed by culture, special stains, and serologies. These methods are useful in the diagnosis of infections with *Pneumocystis carinii,* atypical bacteria, viruses (e.g., cytomegalovirus, respiratory syncytial

TABLE 14-2. POTENTIAL COMPLICATIONS OF BRONCHOSCOPY

Intervention	Potential Complication	Prevention
Passing bronchoscope through nose	Epistaxis, nasal discomfort	Topical anesthesia and vasoconstriction
Passing bronchoscope through pharynx	Gagging, emesis, aspiration	Topical anesthesia, benzodiazepines
Passing bronchoscope into trachea	Laryngospasm, cough, laryngeal trauma	Topical anesthesia
	Bronchospasm	Pretreatment with beta agonists
Bronchoalveolar lavage	Postprocedure fever	Minimize lung contamination by oral secretions
	Hypoxemia	Supplemental oxygen; good wedge technique
Cytology brush	Endobronchial hemorrhage	Avoid vascular lesions
Transbronchial biopsy	Hemorrhage	Avoid vascular lesions
	Pneumothorax	Avoid distal biopsies; consider fluoroscopy
Topical lidocaine administration	Arrhythmias, seizures	Use <7 mg/kg (<25 mL) of 2% lidocaine
Conscious sedation	Hypotension	Intravenous access, prehydration in hypovolemic patients
	Respiratory depression	Avoid oversedation, stimulate patient

virus, adenovirus), fungal pathogens, and mycobacteria. In addition, bronchoscopy and cytology may reveal alveolar hemorrhage, malignancy, or other noninfectious sources that are more common in this population than in immunocompetent hosts.

Pisani RJ, Wright AJ: Clinical utility of bronchoalveolar lavage in immunocompromised hosts. Mayo Clin Proc 67:221–227, 1992.

12. **What is the role of bronchoscopy in the diagnosis of ventilator-associated pneumonia (VAP)?**
The clinical diagnosis of VAP is made when an intubated patient develops a fever or leukocytosis, a new x-ray infiltrate, and purulent tracheal secretions. However, these findings are not specific for pneumonia. Recent studies show that patients who undergo invasive (i.e., bronchoscopic) diagnosis of VAP have less antibiotic use and a lower 14-day mortality rate than patients diagnosed using a noninvasive, empiric approach. Thus, bronchoscopic diagnosis of VAP and subsequent adjustment of antibiotics (or search for nonpulmonary source of infection) is becoming standard of care in many ICUs. Protected brush specimens or BAL samples are sent for quantitative cultures; $\geq 10^3$ and $>10^4$ colonies of bacteria, respectively, are generally considered diagnostic for VAP.

Fagon JY, Chastre J, Wolff M, et al: Invasive and noninvasive strategies for management of suspected ventilator-associated pneumonia: A randomized trial. Ann Intern Med 132:621–630, 2000.

13. **What are the alternatives to bronchoscopy for sample collection in the diagnosis of VAP?**

In patients for whom bronchoscopy is unavailable or contraindicated, blind protected brush sampling or nonbronchoscopic ("mini") BALs may be viable and less expensive alternatives. In both techniques, a catheter is inserted into the airways without bronchoscopic guidance until resistance is encountered. Then the protected brush is extended or saline is injected to obtain the sample, and the apparatus is withdrawn. Some studies comparing the quality of samples obtained by these methods to standard bronchoscopic techniques have demonstrated similar sensitivity and specificity, although neither is currently a standard approach in most adult ICUs.

14. **Are transbronchial biopsies safe in patients receiving mechanical ventilation?**

Several studies have demonstrated higher complication rates in mechanically ventilated patients. The largest case series showed a pneumothorax rate of 14%, compared with a previously reported 5% rate in spontaneously breathing patients. Other studies identified higher rates of bleeding and pneumothorax in mechanically ventilated patients who undergo biopsies. However, no study has identified increased mortality, and valuable diagnostic information is obtained in the majority of patients. Mechanical ventilation is therefore not an absolute contraindication to transbronchial biopsy, which may provide a less morbid alternative to surgical lung biopsy in selected cases.

O'Brien JD, Ettinger NA, Shevlin D, Kollef MH: Safety and yield of transbronchial biopsy in mechanically ventilated patients. Crit Care Med 25:440–446, 1997.

15. **Can BAL be safely performed in patients with the acute respiratory distress syndrome?**

Yes—if the partial arterial oxygen tension (PaO_2) is at least 80 mmHg (with an FiO_2 as high as 1.0) and if the patient has no absolute contraindications for bronchoscopy. A study of 110 patients with acute respiratory distress syndrome who met these criteria found no significant morbidity or mortality associated with bronchoscopy and BAL. The protocol included sedation to improve patient cooperation and to minimize coughing during the procedure. The investigators found a nonsustained decrease in oxygen saturation (to <90%) in 4.5% of patients. Mild, self-limited bleeding followed the procedure in 34% of patients.

Steinberg KP, Mitchell DR, Maunder RJ, et al: Safety of bronchoalveolar lavage in patients with adult respiratory distress syndrome. Am Rev Respir Dis 148:556–561, 1993.

16. **How is bronchoscopy used in the evaluation and management of hemoptysis in the ICU?**

Bronchoscopy can play a role in localization of the site of bleeding, cessation of hemoptysis, and interventions to prevent compromise of the unaffected lung. Initial management of hemoptysis includes airway protection because the danger of hemoptysis is suffocation rather than exsanguination. Then, if the site of bleeding is identified by bronchoscopy, local injection of cold saline, epinephrine, vasopressin, or fibrin as well as laser or electrocautery can be performed via the bronchoscope. Bronchoscopy can be used to tamponade bleeding, either using the tip of the bronchoscope or a Fogarty balloon placed through the suction channel.

17. **What are the limitations of bronchoscopy in hemoptysis?**

When bleeding is brisk, the small suction channel of the flexible bronchoscope may be overwhelmed; in such cases, rigid bronchoscopy may be preferable. For patients unable to expectorate the blood adequately, endotracheal intubation and mechanical ventilation may be needed before bronchoscopy. In patients with persistent bleeding despite bronchoscopic maneuvers, interventional radiology may be required to localize the bleed, followed by interventional radiology embolization or surgical resection.

KEY POINTS: BRONCHOSCOPY

1. Flexible bronchoscopy is most commonly used in the ICU to diagnose and guide antibiotic choices for ventilator-associated pneumonia.

2. Complications of bronchoscopy may occur due to topical anesthesia, sedation, or the procedure itself and include hypoxia, pneumothorax, and hypotension.

3. Bronchoscopy samples can be obtained via bronchoalveolar lavage, protected brush specimen, cytology brush, or biopsy.

4. Chest physiotherapy appears to be as effective as bronchoscopy in treating atelectasis, although bronchoscopy has a role in retained, inspissated secretions or foreign bodies.

5. Bronchoscopy can be safely performed in mechanically ventilated patients, including those with acute respiratory distress syndrome.

18. **What is the role of bronchoscopy in potential lung donors?**
Bronchoscopy is routinely performed on potential lung donors before the decision is made to perform lung explantation. The purpose of this examination is threefold. First, the anatomy of the airways is assessed. Second, the operator searches for evidence of airway trauma, infection, or previous aspiration; it is likely that the lungs will be rejected if any of these is found. Third, samples are taken and sent for culture so that the microbiologic flora (if present) can be known before transplantation and covered in the recipient, who will soon be heavily immunosuppressed.

19. **Is bronchoscopy indicated for management of patients with acute lobar atelectasis?**
Probably not. Bronchoscopy can be effective in improving atelectasis; however, studies have shown no added benefit of bronchoscopy over vigorous respiratory therapy alone, in either intubated or spontaneously breathing patients. However, bronchoscopic intervention may be beneficial in some cases for the removal of retained, inspissated secretions or foreign bodies.

Marini JJ, Pierson DJ, Hudson LD: Acute lobar atelectasis: A prospective comparison of fiberoptic bronchoscopy and respiratory therapy. Am Rev Respir Dis 119:971–978, 1979.

20. **How is bronchoscopy used in performing tracheostomy in the ICU?**
Bronchoscopy is often performed during percutaneous tracheostomy in the ICU to confirm tracheal puncture, to avoid injury to the posterior tracheal wall, and to ensure appropriate tracheostomy tube placement. Several studies suggest bronchoscopic guidance reduces complications from percutaneous tracheostomy.

Mallick A, Venkatanath D, Elliot SC, et al: A prospective randomised controlled trial of capnography vs. bronchoscopy for Blue Rhino percutaneous tracheostomy. Anaesthesia 58:864–868, 2003.

CHAPTER 15

PACEMAKERS AND DEFIBRILLATORS

Noah E. Gordon, MD, and Linda L. Liu, MD

1. **Describe the evolution of the modern implantable pacemaker.**
   Paul Zoll was the first to report successful transcutaneous cardiac pacing in 1952. The 1960s and 1970s brought about temporary transvenous pacing, transtelephonic monitoring, and a movement from asynchronous pacing to an "inhibited" response. Atrioventricular (AV) sequential pacing (DVI) became popular in the mid 1970s, but was later replaced by the dual-chamber pacemaker capable of pacing, sensing, and responding in both chambers (DDD).

2. **What are some other milestones in pacemaker development?**
   Advances in technology over the decades have led to optimization of many aspects of the evolving pacemaker:
   - Pacer leads (presently are polyurethane-insulated, bipolar design, small surface electrodes)
   - Miniaturization
   - Battery longevity
   - Programmability (a magnetic switch can be closed within the pulse generator to allow it to receive radiofrequency signals transmitted from the programmer)
   - Rate-adaptive pacing (activity sensors for detection of minute ventilation)
   - Bidirectional telemetry
   - Autoprogrammability (ability to optimize a parameter based on preprogrammed criteria or logic)

3. **What is the deal with the crazy pacing code?**
   The discipline of pacing required a nomenclature that would allow clinicians to have an abbreviated yet specific "code" that could describe devices. The first position of the code reflects the chamber(s) in which stimulation occurs, and the second position refers to the chamber(s) in which sensing occurs. The third position refers to the mode of setting (or how the pacemaker responds to a sensed event). The fourth position reflects rate modulation, and the fifth position of the code is now used to indicate whether multisite pacing is present. Inclusion of nomenclature to designate multisite pacing is owed to the growing use of cardiac resynchronization therapy (CRT) and the use of dual-site atrial pacing (Table 15-1).

4. **Practice with the generic pacemaker code: explain the AOO, VVI, and DDD modes.**
   - **AOO:** Asynchronous atrial-only pacing. The pacing device emits a pacing pulse regardless of the underlying cardiac rhythm.
   - **VVI:** Ventricular-only antibradycardia pacing. Failure of the ventricle to produce an intrinsic event within the appropriate time window results in ventricular pacing. With no atrial sensing, there can be no AV synchrony in a patient with any intrinsic atrial activity.
   - **DDD:** Dual-chamber antibradycardia pacing. In the absence of intrinsic activity in the atrium, it will be paced. After any sensed or paced atrial event, an intrinsic ventricular event must occur before the expiration of the AV timer or the ventricle will be paced.

TABLE 15-1. THE GENERIC PACEMAKER CODE

Position 1: Pacing Chamber(s)	Position 2: Sensing Chamber(s)	Position 3: Response to Sensing	Position 4: Programmability	Position 5: Multisite Pacing
0 = none	**0** = none	**0** = none	**0** = none	**0** = none
A = atrium	**A** = atrium	**I** = inhibited	**R** = rate modulation	**A** = atrium
V = ventricle	**V** = ventricle	**T** = triggered		**V** = ventricle
D = dual (A+V)	**D** = dual (A+V)	**D** = dual (T+I)		**D** = dual (A+V)

5. **What is rate-adaptive pacing?**
   The normal heart rate response to increased physiologic demand is linearly related to oxygen demand/consumption. Circumstances requiring heart rate variation include exercise, emotion, anxiety, baroreflexes, vagal maneuvers, hypovolemia, fever, and anemia. The ideal sensor and response algorithm for rate-adaptive pacing would mimic this with physiologic detectors. Optimal sensors would detect primary determinants of sinoatrial node function (e.g., such as circulating catecholamine levels or autonomic nervous system activity), whereas less sophisticated sensors would detect external changes in response to exercise (e.g., accelerometers to sense body movement).

6. **What pacing mode is best?**
   A number of retrospective studies performed in the 1980s and 1990s consistently demonstrated the superiority of dual-chamber devices (DDD or DDDR) in terms of morbidity and mortality. In recent years, prospective trials showed no difference in mortality between the DDD/DDDR and VVI/VVIR groups. Despite this, clinical bias is toward dual-chamber pacing in the United States, likely due to the greater clinical programming flexibility and a perception that quality-of-life improvements in specific subsets of patients (age > 65 years) warrants continued use in the majority of patients.

7. **What is neurocardiogenic syncope? Is pacing indicated for neurocardiogenic syncope?**
   Neurocardiogenic syncope encompasses vasovagal syncope and carotid sinus hypersensitivity. Despite several prospective clinical trials of pacing for these disorders, considerable controversy exists regarding which patients to pace and clinical criteria to use to choose pacing candidates. The guidelines of the American College of Cardiology (ACC)/American Heart Association (AHA)/National Association for Sport and Physical Education (NASPE) outline specific indications for pacemaker use; in general, there is a tendency to use a dual-chamber pacemaker with rate-drop response for patients with documented significant cardioinhibition and recurrent syncope.

8. **Does pacing alter a patient's risk of sudden cardiac death (SCD) with hypertrophic cardiomyopathy?**
   Observational studies had demonstrated an improvement in patients with hypertrophic cardiomyopathy and symptoms refractory to medical treatment. However, several randomized control trials that followed showed a clinical improvement in only some patients without definitive evidence that pacing altered the risk of SCD. Practically, most cardiologists institute pacing in many of these patients as part of an implantable cardiac defibrillator (ICD) system being used for primary or secondary prevention of SCD.

9. **What are the latest ACC/AHA/NASPE class I guidelines for implantations of cardiac pacemakers?**

ACC/AHA class I guidelines refer to "conditions for which there is evidence and/or general agreement that a given procedure or treatment is useful and effective." Table 15-2 lists class I guidelines for pacemaker insertion.

TABLE 15-2. CLASS I GUIDELINES FOR PACEMAKER INSERTION

Major Indication	Class I Recommendation for Pacemaker
Acquired AV block in adults	Third-degree and advanced second-degree AV block at any anatomic level, associated with bradycardia with symptoms, arrhythmias requiring drugs that result in symptomatic bradycardia, documented periods of asystole >3 seconds, after catheter ablation of AV junction, postoperative AV block not expected to resolve, neuromuscular diseases with AV block
Chronic bifascicular and trifascicular block	Intermittent third-degree AV block, type II second-degree AV block, alternating bundle-branch block
Sinus node dysfunction	Sinus node dysfunction with documented symptomatic bradycardia, including frequent sinus pauses that produce symptoms
Prevention and termination of tachyarrhythmias	Symptomatic recurrent SVT after drugs and catheter ablation fail, symptomatic recurrent sustained VT as part of an automatic defibrillator system
Hypersensitive carotid sinus and neurocardiogenic syncope	Recurrent syncope caused by carotid sinus stimulation, minimal carotid sinus pressure induces ventricular asystole >3 seconds
Congenital heart disease	Advanced second- or third-degree AV block associated with symptomatic bradycardia/ventricular dysfunction/low CO, sinus node dysfunction with correlation of symptoms during age-inappropriate bradycardia, postoperative AV block not expected to improve with 1 week, congenital third-degree AV block with a wide QRS escape rhythm/complex ventricular ectopy/ventricular dysfunction, congenital third-degree AV block in an infant with a ventricular rate <50 or congenital heart disease with a rate <70 bpm, sustained pause-dependent VT
Cardiomyopathies (hypertrophic obstructive and idiopathic dilated)	Same as recommendations for sinus node dysfunction or AV block
Cardiac transplantation	Symptomatic bradyarrhythmias/chronotropic incompetence not expected to resolve

AV = atrioventricular, SVT = supraventricular tachycardia, VT = ventricular tachycardia.

10. **What is CRT?**
    Cardiac resynchronization therapy is the term applied to reestablishing synchronous contraction between the left ventricular free wall and the ventricular septum in an attempt to improve left ventricular efficiency and subsequently improve functional class. CRT has generally been used to describe biventricular or multisite ventricular pacing, but cardiac resynchronization can also be achieved by left ventricular pacing alone in some patients.

11. **Is cardiac resynchronization effective?**
    It seems so. A number of randomized clinical trials demonstrating the safety and efficacy of CRT have been completed. In the most recent ACC/AHA/NASPE guidelines for pacing, biventricular pacing in medically refractory, symptomatic New York Heart Association class III/IV patients with idiopathic dilated or ischemic cardiomyopathy, prolonged QRS interval (>130 ms), left ventricular end-diastolic diameter >55 mm, and left ventricular ejection fraction < 0.35 is included as a class IIa indication.

12. **Is there a role for CRT in the management of atrial fibrillation?**
    Randomized clinical data are now available assessing CRT in patients with chronic atrial fibrillation. These trials have consistently demonstrated functional improvement in this group of patients; consequently, more and more cardiologists are using CRT in this population.

13. **What is "high-voltage CRT"?**
    These are devices combining CRT and ICD capabilities. The indications for high-voltage CRT are in evolution; however, given the widespread acceptance of CRT, as well as the high incidence of ventricular tachyarrhythmias in patients with left ventricular dysfunction, it is likely that this unit will become the device of choice for these patients in the future.

14. **Summarize the pacing strategies for the prevention of atrial fibrillation.**
    Dual-site and alternate-site pacing, specifically atrial septal pacing, have been explored to reduce the burden of atrial fibrillation. As yet, no approach has emerged as singularly superior. Examples of available algorithms include those that respond to premature atrial contractions (PACs) (atrial pacing rate increases in presence of a PAC), atrial overdrive pacing to consistently maintain the atrial pacing rate above the intrinsic atrial rate, and postmode switching algorithm to pace at a faster atrial rate until the pathologic atrial rhythm is terminated and the original dual-chamber pacing mode is resumed.

15. **Describe the proposed mechanism of defibrillation.**
    Spontaneous reentry arrhythmias can be initiated by the interaction between a propagating wavefront and an obstacle in its path or triggered by a spontaneous premature beat (e.g., premature ventricular contraction). Defibrillation aims to bring an abrupt halt to this process and to rapidly restore normal cardiac rhythm and cardiac output, thus preventing cardiac death. To achieve successful defibrillation, a critical electric stimulus must be applied to fibrillating tissue to reset the myocardial cells. This stimulus must produce a sufficient potential gradient to alter the transmembrane potential in an adequate portion of the fibrillating myocardium; and yet, the stimulus must not lead to the development of more fibrillation.

16. **Discuss the pertinent parameters for defibrillators and how these are optimized.**
    Parameters for defibrillation include waveforms (direct versus alternating, monophasic versus biphasic, dampened sine wave versus truncated exponential waveform), circuit design (capacitors with or without inductors), electrode positioning (anteroposterior versus anteroapical configurations), energy selections, and role of transthoracic impedance. Modern defibrillators are direct current, impedance compensated biphasic waveform devices, using straightforward capacitor discharge circuits (so they can be small enough for internal implantation), with electrodes positioned anteroposterior. Biphasic waveforms may offer efficacy at lower energy and peak voltages than monophasic waveforms.

17. **What is an ICD? What is the generic defibrillator code?**

ICDs defibrillate life-threatening ventricular tachycardia or ventricular fibrillation. The NASPE/ British Pacing and Electrophysiology Group generic defibrillator code is similar to the generic pacemaker code, with four positions referring to shock chamber, antitachycardia pacing chamber, tachycardia detection, and antibradycardia pacing chamber. For robust information, the fourth position is expanded into its complete generic pacemaker code (Table 15-3).

TABLE 15-3. THE GENERIC DEFIBRILLATOR CODE			
Position 1: Shock Chamber(s)	**Position 2: Antitachycardia Pacing Chamber(s)**	**Position 3: Tachycardia Detection**	**Position 4: Antibradycardia Pacing Chamber(s)**
0 = none	**0** = none	**E** = electrogram	**0** = none
A = atrium	**A** = atrium	**H** = hemodynamic	**A** = atrium
V = ventricle	**V** = ventricle		**V** = ventricle
D = dual (A+V)	**D** = dual (A+V)		**D** = dual (A+V)

18. **Practice with the generic defibrillator code: explain the VVE-DDDRV mode.**

To decipher the first three positions of the defibrillator code, first look at Table 15-3. For the final "position" (which is actually five letters), use Table 15-1 to decode the pacemaker. This is a biventricular pacing defibrillator possessing ventricular shock and antitachycardia pacing, with a dual-chamber, rate-adaptive, antibradycardia programmed pacer.

19. **What are the latest ACC/AHA/NASPE class I guidelines for ICD therapy?**

Box 15-1 lists the 2002 recommended guidelines for ICD therapy.

BOX 15-1. GUIDELINES FOR ICD PLACEMENT

Cardiac arrest due to VF or VT not due to a transient or reversible cause

Spontaneous sustained VT in association with structural heart disease

Syncope of undetermined origin with clinically relevant, hemodynamically significant sustained VT or VF induced at EP study when drug therapy is ineffective, not tolerated, or not preferred

Nonsustained VT in patients with coronary disease, prior MI, LV dysfunction, inducible VF, or sustained VT at EP study that is not suppressible by a class I antiarrhythmic drug

Spontaneous sustained VT in patients who do not have structural heart disease that is not amenable to other treatments

ICD = implantable cardiac defibrillator, VF = ventricular fibrillation, VT = ventricular tachycardia, EP = electrophysiology, MI = myocardial infarction, LV = left ventricular.

20. **What is an "R on T" phenomenon?**

If a pacemaker stimulus (R) fires during the vulnerable phase of a ventricular extrasystole (T), ventricular tachycardia or ventricular fibrillation may occur. Theoretically, this phenomenon may result when the magnet-induced asynchronous pacing competes with the patient's own heart rhythm. This "competitive pacing" was a concern with older-generation pacers. In modern pacemakers, the switch to asynchronous pacing is coupled to the next cardiac event to avoid competition at the outset.

21. **Discuss how a temporary pacemaker may fail.**

The most common cause of temporary transvenous pacemaker failure is the loss of contact between an electrode wire and the heart. In this case, pacemaker spikes appear on the monitor without QRS complexes. To restore cardiac pacing, the pacing electrode must be advanced until it comes into contact with the myocardium to "capture" or pace the heart. The absence of pacemaker spikes means one of two things—there is no energy left in the battery, or one of the electrode wires is disconnected from the generator.

22. **What is electromagnetic interference (EMI), and what is its relevance to pacemakers?**

EMI refers to any electromagnetic radiation with the potential to affect implantable devices (pacemakers). Some hospital sources of EMI are electrocautery, diathermy, external cardioversion/defibrillators, and magnetic resonance imaging. Possible responses to interference include inappropriate inhibition or triggering of a paced output, asynchronous pacing, reprogramming, damage to device circuitry, and triggering of a defibrillator discharge. Strategies to minimize these responses involve use of bipolar leads, noise protection algorithms that filter out unwanted signals, using magnets to decrease inappropriate pacemaker triggering, and avoiding/minimizing exposure to EMI.

23. **What do magnets do when applied to a pacemaker?**

Magnets can be used to protect a pacemaker-dependent patient and can be applied over the pacemaker to avoid inhibition by potential sources of interference. However, not all pacemakers will switch to a continuous asynchronous mode when a magnet is applied. Depending on the manufacturer and model, possible magnet responses include no apparent change in rate or rhythm, brief asynchronous pacing, continuous or transient loss of pacing, and asynchronous pacing without rate response. It is advisable to confirm magnet behavior before magnet use (such information can be obtained from the manufacturer directly or from the patient's pacing clinic).

KEY POINTS: POSSIBLE EFFECTS OF A MAGNET ON A PACEMAKER

1. Possible effects of a magnet on a pacemaker include no apparent change in rate or rhythm.

2. A magnet may elicit brief asynchronous pacing (10–64 beats).

3. Continuous or transient loss of pacing is another possible effect.

4. Application of a magnet can also cause asynchronous pacing without rate response.

24. **What is an automated external defibrillator (AED)?**

AEDs are computerized, portable devices that allow lay rescuers to provide defibrillation during cardiac arrest with minimal training. AEDs are placed in airports, airplanes, casinos, office buildings, and other public locations. They analyze multiple features of the electrocardiogram and advise shock for ventricular fibrillation and monomorphic or polymorphic ventricular tachycardia only. The user must clear the area and the patient before pressing the "shock" button to prevent harming bystanders.

WEBSITES

1. AHA information for patients with an implantable cardioverter defibrillator or a pacemaker
   www.americanheart.org

2. Guidant website
   www.guidant.com

3. Medtronic website
   www.medtronic.com

4. St. Jude Medical website
   www.sjm.com

CHAPTER 16

CIRCULATORY ASSIST DEVICES

Lundy J. Campbell, MD

1. **What types of circulatory assist devices are available?**
   There are several types of circulatory assist devices currently available, and each type is designed to achieve different patient care goals. These will each be discussed in detail in this chapter. However, there has been a renewed interest in the use of long-term circulatory assist devices, and there have been many recent advances made in this field. The major types of circulatory assist devices can be categorized as:
   - Intra-aortic balloon pumps (IABPs)
   - Left ventricular assist devices (LVADs)
   - Right ventricular assist devices (RVADs)
   - Biventricular assist devices
   - Total artificial hearts

KEY POINTS: MAIN TYPES OF CIRCULATORY ASSIST DEVICES

1. The main types of circulatory assist devices include the intra-aortic balloon pump.

2. The LVAD is another types of circulatory assist device.

3. Circulatory assist devices can be RVADs.

4. The biventricular assist device assists both ventricles.

5. Another option for circulatory assistance is the total artificial heart.

2. **What is an IABP?**
   An IABP consists of a large control module (i.e., monitors, software, pump, gas cylinder) attached to a catheter that has an externally mounted balloon. The balloon catheter is placed into the patient while the control module remains outside. Via the control module, the balloon is set to inflate just after the closure of the aortic valve, at the onset of diastole, and to actively deflate just before the opening of the aortic valve (systole). The balloon is normally inflated with 40 mL of helium (low viscosity) or carbon dioxide (high blood solubility).

3. **How is an IABP placed into a patient?**
   In most patients, the balloon catheter is percutaneously introduced into the femoral or iliac artery through a sheath. The catheter is advanced until the tip is just distal to the take-off of the left subclavian artery while also ensuring that the balloon remains above the level of the renal arteries (Fig. 16-1). Fluoroscopic guidance is most often used to achieve proper placement. The catheter can also be properly positioned under direct visualization intraoperatively when a sternotomy or thoracotomy has already been performed. If the femoral and iliac arteries are severely diseased, the IABP catheter can be placed via a transthoracic route by a cardiovascular surgeon.

4. **What are the goals of intra-aortic balloon counterpulsation?**
   The primary goal of an IABP is to improve myocardial function by increasing myocardial oxygen supply and decreasing myocardial oxygen demand. Secondary gains include an increase in cardiac output, ejection fraction, and increased coronary perfusion pressure, resulting in an improvement in systemic perfusion with a decrease in heart rate, pulmonary capillary wedge pressure, and systemic vascular resistance.

5. **How does an IABP accomplish these goals?**
   Coronary blood flow and myocardial oxygen supply are improved by balloon inflation that leads to augmentation of diastolic pressure and blood flow to the failing heart. The balloon on the catheter is set to inflate at the onset of diastole (at closure of the aortic valve or at the dicrotic notch on an arterial waveform). The inflation of the balloon causes retrograde blood flow and an increase in pressure toward the aortic root, thereby increasing coronary perfusion pressure. This increase in perfusion pressure improves oxygen delivery and can improve

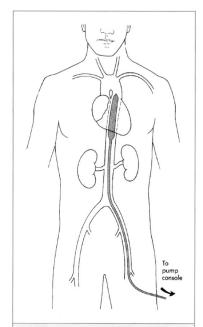

Figure 16-1. Intra-aortic balloon pump (IABP) placement: balloon tip is distal to the left subclavian artery, and the balloon end is proximal to the renal arteries. (From Flynn J, Bruch N: Introduction to Critical Care Skills. St. Louis, Mosby, 1993.)

cardiac performance in an ischemic myocardium. When an IABP is properly functioning, the augmented diastolic pressure should be greater than the patient's unassisted systolic pressure.

Balloon deflation causes unloading during systole, thus decreasing the workload of the left ventricle and decreasing myocardial oxygen demand. Specifically, at the end of diastole and just at the start of systole, the balloon is set to deflate rapidly, leaving an area of markedly decreased volume and pressure. The low pressure in this region decreases the afterload of the left ventricle, resulting in an improvement in cardiac output and end-organ perfusion. This decrease in afterload should be represented as a balloon-assisted end-diastolic pressure that is less than the patient's unassisted end-diastolic pressure (Figs. 16-2 and 16-3).

Ryan EW, Foster E: Augmentation of coronary blood flow with intra-aortic balloon pump counter-pulsation. Circulation 102:364–365, 2000.

Takeuchi M, Nohtomi Y, Yoshitani H, et al: Enhanced coronary flow velocity during intra-aortic balloon pumping assessed by transthoracic Doppler echocardiography. JACC 42:368–376, 2004.

6. **What are the indications for placement of an IABP?**
   The most common indications for the use of an IABP are left ventricular failure, cardiogenic shock, or unstable angina refractory to medical therapy. Other applications include use as a bridge to coronary artery bypass grafting after failed percutaneous transluminal coronary angioplasty or a bridge to cardiac transplant in end-stage heart failure. It is also placed in patients who are initially unable to wean from cardiopulmonary bypass during cardiac surgery.

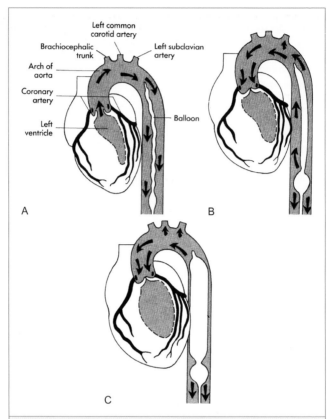

Figure 16-2. *A,* Balloon deflation decreases left ventricular afterload. *B* and *C,* Balloon inflation increases coronary perfusion pressure. (From Flynn J, Bruch N: Introduction to Critical Care Skills. St. Louis, Mosby, 1993.)

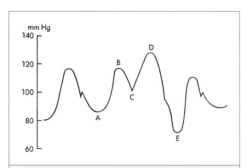

Figure 16-3. Intra-aortic balloon pump (IABP) waveform. *A,* End-diastolic pressure. *B,* Systolic pressure. *C,* Dicrotic notch (balloon inflates). *D,* Augmented diastolic pressure. *E,* Assisted end-diastolic pressure. (From Flynn J, Bruch N: Introduction to Critical Care Skills. St. Louis, Mosby, 1993.)

KEY POINTS: INDICATIONS FOR PLACEMENT OF A CIRCULATORY ASSIST DEVICE

1. Indications for placement of a circulatory assist device include cardiogenic shock.

2. Unstable angina is another indication for placement of a circulatory assist device.

3. Placement of a circulatory assist device should be considered in the presence of ventricular failure.

4. When a patient is experiencing acute, severe mitral valve regurgitation, placement of a circulatory assist device is indicated.

5. Circulatory assist device placement is indicated as a bridge to revascularization or transplant.

6. Bridge to recovery is an indication for placement of a circulatory assist device.

7. **What are the contraindications to the use of an IABP?**
   The major absolute contraindications are structural aortic problems, such as dissection or aneurysm, in which IABP use could lead to a worsening of the aortic injury or even rupture. In addition, aortic valvular insufficiency negates the effectiveness of the device and may even worsen cardiac output by increasing the regurgitant fraction. Although severe peripheral vascular disease is not an absolute contraindication to IABP placement, one needs to consider that the catheter can more readily cause lower limb ischemia or infarct. Finally, its use in patients with no hope of recovery should be very carefully evaluated and the benefits clearly defined.

KEY POINTS: MAJOR CONTRAINDICATIONS TO THE USE OF AN INTRA-AORTIC BALLOON PUMP

1. Aortic dissection is a major contraindication to the use of an IABP.

2. Another contraindication to IABP is aortic aneurysm.

3. IABP should not be used in the presence of aortic valvular insufficiency.

4. If there is no chance for recovery or transplantation, IABP should not be used.

8. **How is the IABP controlled?**
   Proper use of the IABP consists of setting the augmentation frequency ratio as well as adjusting the timing of the start of balloon inflation and deflation. The *augmentation frequency ratio* refers to how often the balloon inflates with respect to the cardiac cycle. Maximal support occurs when the balloon inflates with each cardiac cycle, also known as a 1:1 ratio. Less support can be obtained by sequentially decreasing the augmentation ratio to 1:2 or 1:3 (i.e., the balloon inflates once every second or third cardiac cycle). As the augmentation ratio is decreased, the risk of forming a thrombus on the balloon significantly increases; thus, a ratio of 1:3 should not be used for a prolonged period.

The triggering of balloon inflation and active deflation can be accomplished by several means: (1) the R wave on the electrocardiogram (ECG); (2) the arterial waveform; (3) ventricular pacemaker spikes; or (4) a preset rate. Of these, the most common method is the ECG R wave. Triggering from the R wave causes balloon inflation to begin in the middle of the T wave and active balloon deflation to occur just before the start of the QRS complex. Newer IABP devices can trigger appropriately even if the patient is in atrial fibrillation. The exact timing of balloon inflation and deflation can be manually adjusted. If the ECG cannot be used for any reason (e.g., too much artifact during patient transport), most clinicians use the arterial waveform as a second choice.

Overwalder P: Intra aortic balloon pump (IABP) counterpulsation. Internet J Thorac Cardiovasc Surg 2(2):1999: www.ispub.com/ostia/index.php?xmlPrinter=true&xmlFilePath&=journals/ijpf/vol1n1/iabp.xml

9. **What are the potential complications with IABP use?**
   Although complications can arise from anywhere within the IABP device as a result of mechanical failure, the most common complications are related to the presence of the intra-aortic balloon catheter itself and the technique used for insertion. The rapid inflation/deflation cycling of the balloon causes trauma to the formed elements of blood, leading to anemia and thrombocytopenia. There may also be platelet dysfunction or activation of clotting factors, which may result in disseminated intravascular coagulation, arterial thrombosis, and embolization. Because of the risk of thrombus formation and the possibility of an embolus, patients with an IABP are systemically anticoagulated. Thus, bleeding at the insertion site tends to occur quite frequently. In addition, other complications that may occur at the site of insertion include infection or pseudoaneurysm formation. Furthermore, improper technique with device insertion can result in incorrect positioning with loss of effective diastolic augmentation, possible limb or visceral ischemia, or aortic dissection or perforation, leading to massive hemorrhage. Finally, the balloon can perforate or rupture, causing a gas embolus and device ineffectiveness.

10. **How are patients weaned from IABP support?**
    To be successfully weaned from IABP support, patients must not be in cardiogenic shock. They should have an adequate blood pressure and cardiac output on little or no vasopressor or inotropic support. A mean arterial pressure ≥ 65 mmHg and a cardiac index > 2 L/min/m^2 are the usual criteria. Weaning is generally accomplished by decreasing the augmentation ratio every 1–6 hours, as tolerated, until a ratio of 1:3 is achieved. The balloon catheter can then be removed when the patient is no longer anticoagulated. An alternative strategy for IABP weaning is to decrease the balloon filling volume by 10 mL every 1–6 hours until a final filling volume of 20 mL is reached.

11. **What's new in IABPs?**
    A permanent implantable IABP (the Kantrowitz Cardio VAD) has been developed and has undergone limited human testing. This device provides the same hemodynamic and physiologic effects as all other IABPs, but it is surgically implanted into the wall of the descending thoracic aorta. The device has a 60-mL balloon that is electrically powered and pneumatically driven by a wearable harness similar to an implantable ventricular assist device (VAD). This device has the possible advantage of not requiring systemic anticoagulation and does not pose a significant risk of cerebrovascular accidents. Additional testing needs to be done to assess the long-term efficacy and safety of this device.

Jeevanandam V, Jayakar D, Anderson AS, et al: Circulatory assistance with a permanent implantable IABP: Initial human experience. Circulation 106:183–188, 2002.

12. **What are the major types of VADs?**
    - **Extracorporal nonpulsatile VADs:** Two types of extracorporal nonpulsatile VADs are currently in use. Of the two, the more common is the centrifugal pump. Continuous flow is generated

via centrifugal forces created at the base of the pump using a spinning impeller. Roller pumps, although much more familiar, are not frequently used due to their increased deleterious effects on the formed elements of blood. Roller pumps generally provide a more consistent cardiac output, but they tend to cause greater shearing forces, which results in thrombocytopenia, anemia, and formation of microemboli.

- **Extracorporal pulsatile pumps:** These are either pneumatic or electric. In pneumatic pumps, compressed gas is "driven" during systole into a pneumatic chamber adjacent to the blood sac, which is then squeezed with resultant ejection of blood. During diastole, the gas is actively removed, causing a vacuum effect that draws blood into the blood sac. Electric pumps operate on the same basic principle but use a piston and plate to compress the blood sac for ejection during systole. Whether the pumps are nonpulsatile or pulsatile, the term *extracorporal* implies that the device chambers and/or pump mechanism remain external.

- **Implantable pulsatile VADs:** Presently, the totally implantable pulsatile type is the most commonly used VAD as a bridge to transplant and as an aid to cardiac recovery. Of these, the most widely used portable left ventricular assist systems are the Thoratec Heartmate and Baxter's Novacor. Both devices can operate in either a fixed mode or, more frequently, an automatic mode that mimics normal physiology. In the automatic mode, the device ejects when the pump is 90% full; it detects a reduction in the rate of filling or senses an increase in native heart rate. Thus, as the patient's workload increases, the pump fills faster and cardiac output correspondingly increases to meet the demand. The cannulas are typically placed through the diaphragm, with the device chambers implanted in the abdomen and the control module with power source remaining external (normally on a belt or shoulder strap carried by the patient).

- **Axial-flow pumps:** This is a new type of implantable VAD that uses a continuous axial-flow pump rather than a pulsatile centrifugal pump. These pumps flow continuously throughout the cardiac cycle and may have the additional advantages of improved ventricular unloading, as well as lack of stasis, which may minimize thrombus formation and bacterial adhesion.

- **Total artificial heart:** Because of the scarcity of suitable donor hearts, there has been renewed interest in the use of total artificial hearts as a bridge to cardiac transplantation. These devices continue to have problems with long-term use, but results to date appear promising when used for a relatively short period in patients in whom a VAD is contraindicated.

Copeland JG, Smith RG, Arabia FA, et al: Cardiac replacement with a total artificial heart as a bridge to transplantation. N Engl J Med 351:859–867, 2004.

Goldstein DJ, Oz MC, Rose EA: Implantable left ventricular assist devices. N Engl J Med 339:1522–1532, 1998.

13. **How does a VAD work?**

VADs can be used to assist the right (RVAD), left (LVAD), or both ventricles (BiVAD). When placed temporarily, the cannulas are normally inserted into the atria with blood returned to the pulmonary artery or aorta. If the device is to be used as a bridge to cardiac transplantation, the cannulas are inserted into the apices of the heart. Regardless of the exact device used, its placement, and its components, VADs are capable of supporting up to 100% of the cardiac output, thereby bypassing the need for any ventricular work or activity.

14. **What are the indications for the placement of a VAD?**

VADs are used in patients as a bridge to cardiac transplantation or as an aid in cardiac recovery. Possible transplant patients include those with chronic heart failure or acute decompensation of chronic heart failure, postcardiotomy failure, or acute myocardial infarction in an already failing heart. Patients who may benefit from VAD support as an aid in recovery include those with severe myocarditis, severe ventricular arrhythmias unresponsive to pharmacologic therapy, postcardiotomy failure, or acute myocardial infarction with resulting heart failure.

15. **How are patients selected for VAD support?**

Once maximal pharmacologic and IABP therapy prove unsuccessful, most clinicians use the following parameters to consider initiation of VAD support:

- Cardiac index < 2 L/min/m^2
- Systolic blood pressure < 80 mmHg
- Mean arterial pressure < 65 mmHg
- Systemic vascular resistance > 2100 dynes/sec/cm^5
- Urine output < 20 mL/h
- Pulmonary capillary wedge pressure > 20 mmHg

16. **What are the contraindications for VAD use?**

Contraindications for VAD placement include severe multiorgan system disease or failure from which the patient is not expected to recover. In addition, disease states that cause patients to be too unstable to undergo surgical placement of the device with significant risk of death can be considered as contraindications. Specific examples include (but are not limited to) the following:

- Severe obstructive or restrictive pulmonary disease
- Severe pulmonary hypertension
- Underlying coagulopathy from liver failure or disseminated intravascular coagulation
- Dialysis-dependent renal failure
- Sepsis or current infection
- Irreversible severe cerebral injury

Although not considered a contraindication, structural heart defects should be repaired before or at the time of VAD placement. Intracardiac septal defects need to be repaired to avoid right-to-left shunting from sudden left ventricular unloading after initiation of VAD support. Preexisting mitral stenosis, mitral regurgitation, or aortic insufficiency may require correction before or during VAD implantation, as both significantly reduce cardiac output even with the device.

17. **What are the possible complications of VAD placement?**

- **Bleeding:** Hemorrhage remains the most prevalent complication associated with VAD placement. Causes of major bleeding include preoperative coagulopathy due to hepatic dysfunction, poor nutritional status, use of anticoagulants, and device-induced thrombocytopenia and platelet dysfunction. The risk of major hemorrhage has steadily declined with the continued use of these devices, but it still remains significant. In a recent large trial, the frequency of bleeding within 6 months was 42%.
- **Infection:** Postoperative patients are prone to nosocomial and device-related infections. Infection occurs most commonly at the cannula and pocket sites. Such infections are managed primarily with antibiotics and local wound care. Clinically important infections continue to occur in approximately 25–30% of patients and are caused by both gram-positive cocci (e.g., *Staphylococcus aureus, Staphylococcus epidermidis*) and gram-negative rods (e.g., *Pseudomonas aeruginosa*). On rare occasions, the entire VAD must be replaced because of significant infection or sepsis. Prophylactic antimicrobial therapy is initiated at the time of placement but discontinued if there are no signs of infection. Because of the location of the device in the chest cavity, patients are also prone to atelectasis with subsequent development of pneumonia. Therefore, aggressive respiratory therapy is vital.
- **Thromboembolism:** At the beginning of VAD use, approximately 20% of patients suffered a thromboembolic event. The current rate of major embolic events is reported to be as low as 0.01 per patient-month. This significant decrease is attributed to the use of textured blood-contacting surfaces within the VAD itself, which prevent thrombus formation. Although major embolic events have decreased, asymptomatic cerebral microemboli continue to occur in 34–67% of recipients. Systemic anticoagulation remains controversial at present.
- **Right ventricular failure:** Historically, severe right heart failure, which required the implantation of an RVAD, occurred in 20% of patients in whom an LVAD was placed. Fortunately, improved perioperative management and use of inhaled nitric oxide have

decreased the need for RVAD placement over the past several years. The major risk factor for right heart failure is perioperative hemorrhage necessitating multiple blood transfusions. As a result of severe bleeding, the cytokines interleukin (IL)-1b, IL-6, IL-10, and tumor necrosis factor alpha are released into the circulation. These cytokines, in turn, mediate the release of platelet-activating factor, which causes vasoconstriction of the pulmonary vasculature, thus inducing pulmonary hypertension and subsequent right heart failure.

- **Device malfunction:** In a long-term study of VAD use in patients with end-stage heart failure, the probability of device failure was 35% at 24 months. When a VAD is used for a shorter period (up to 12 months), then the likelihood of device failure is exceedingly small.
- **Other end-organ failure:** Patients who receive VADs are at very high risk for sepsis, acute lung injury, acute respiratory distress syndrome, acute renal failure, or hepatic dysfunction. Some of these complications are directly related to the device itself (infection), but most are due to the underlying disease severity in patients in whom a VAD is placed.

Rose EA, Gilijns AC, Moskowitz AJ, et al: Long-term use of left ventricular assist device for end-stage heart failure. N Engl J Med 345:1435–1443, 2001.

18. **How is weaning from a VAD accomplished?**
Weaning is attempted only in patients in whom a VAD was placed as a bridge to recovery or the heart has undergone sufficient remodeling so that a transplant is no longer necessary. The patient must be adequately assessed to ensure sufficient recovery of myocardium before weaning can be attempted. Methods to determine recovery include echocardiography, radionucleotide scans, and exercise testing. If the patient is hemodynamically stable, has demonstrated adequate myocardial recovery, and no longer meets the criteria for device placement, weaning trials can begin. Weaning is generally accomplished by sequentially reducing VAD flow rates while cardiac performance (e.g., ejection fraction, cardiac output) is closely monitored. If the patient is able to tolerate a VAD support of only 1–1.5 L/min, the device can usually be discontinued.

CHAPTER 17

ACUTE PNEUMONIA

Rachel H. Dotson, MD, and Jeanine Wiener-Kronish, MD

1. **Define severe community-acquired pneumonia (CAP).**
   Severe community-acquired pneumonia refers to CAP that requires management in the intensive care unit (ICU). The mortality rate for patients with severe CAP is high, and the empiric antimicrobial regimen for this subgroup differs from antibiotic coverage recommended for less severe cases of pneumonia. Ultimately, the decision to admit a patient to the ICU must be based on clinical judgment; however, various indices have been validated to predict the need for ICU admission and can supplement clinical decision-making. The modified American Thoracic Society (ATS) rules define severe CAP by the presence of either one of two major criteria (septic shock or need for mechanical ventilation) *or* two of three minor criteria (systolic blood pressure [SBP] $\leq$ 90 mmHg, multilobar pneumonia, and $PaO_2/FiO_2 < 250$). The British Thoracic Society guidelines recommend that patients with two or more of the following be considered for ICU admission: altered mental status, blood urea nitrogen > 19.1 mg/dL, respiratory rate ≥ 30 breaths/min, and either DBP ≤ 60 mmHg or SBP < 90 mmHg (CURB = confusion, urea, respiratory rate, blood pressure).

2. **Which pathogens most commonly cause severe CAP?**
   Table 17-1 lists the most common culprits. *Streptococcus pneumoniae* is the most frequently identified causative organism. Pathogens are identified in fewer than 50% of cases. Culturing the blood or pleural fluid in addition to respiratory tract specimens may increase the diagnostic yield. Furthermore, *Legionella pneumophila* can often result in severe illness; therefore, urinary antigen for *L. pneumophila* serogroup 1 should be measured. Whether or not a specific organism is identified does not appear to affect mortality; however, microbiologic data can be used to tailor therapy.

3. **Is the sputum Gram's stain and culture helpful diagnostically for CAP?**
   Sputum Gram's stain and culture can be performed noninvasively and are inexpensive diagnostic tests. A sputum Gram's stain specimen is considered satisfactory for interpretation when the neutrophil count is >25 per low-power field and <10 epithelial cells. There is some controversy regarding how the results of a sputum Gram's stain should influence clinical practice. The ATS recommends that this test be used to broaden antibiotic therapy to treat unsuspected organisms not covered by the usual empiric regimen. Conversely, the Infectious Diseases Society of America (IDSA) guidelines suggest that empiric antimicrobial therapy be narrowed based on sputum Gram's stain findings. Keep in mind the diagnostic limitations of sputum Gram's stain and culture, including the inability to visualize atypical organisms, contamination by oral flora, and the difficulty encountered by some patients to provide adequate specimens.

4. **What determines the selection of empiric antimicrobial therapy for patients with severe CAP?**
   The initial empiric antibiotic regimen depends on the presence of risk factors for *Pseudomonas aeruginosa*. These include malnutrition, underlying structural pulmonary disease such as bronchiectasis, >7 days of broad-spectrum antibiotic therapy within the past month, leukopenic

immunosuppression, and steroid use (>10 mg prednisone per day). Recommended antibiotics according to the most recent ATS guidelines are listed in Table 17-1. The current IDSA guidelines also note that exposure to an antibiotic within the preceding 3 months predicts resistance to that antibiotic class. Prompt administration (within 4 hours of presentation) of appropriate empiric antibiotics is strongly encouraged because studies suggest that delays in treatment are associated with worse outcomes.

5. **Who is at risk for penicillin-resistant *S. pneumoniae* pneumonia, and does this affect treatment?**
   Risk factors for infection due to penicillin-resistant *S. pneumoniae* include age older than 65 years, recent beta-lactam therapy, multiple comorbidities, alcoholism, immunosuppression, noninvasive disease, and contact with a child who attends day care. Several investigations indicate that penicillin-resistant *S. pneumoniae* pneumonia (in the absence of meningitis) can be successfully treated with beta-lactam antibiotics without adversely affecting mortality *unless* the minimal inhibitory concentration is ≥4 mg/L.

   S. pneumoniae resistance against macrolides and fluoroquinolones is increasing. Clinical failures with macrolides are rare despite macrolide resistance; however, fluoroquinolones with less potency against *S. pneumoniae* are likely to be ineffective against resistant strains.

   Campbell GD Jr, Silberman R: Drug-resistant *Streptococcus pneumoniae*. Clin Infect Dis 26:1188–1195, 1998.

   Clavo-Sanchez AJ, Giron-Gonzalez JA, Lopez-Prieto D, et al: Multivariate analysis of risk factors for infection due to penicillin-resistant and multidrug-resistant *Streptococcus pneumoniae*: A multicenter study. Clin Infect Dis 24:1052–1059, 1997.

KEY POINTS: INITIAL MANAGEMENT OF ACUTE PNEUMONIA

1. Treat empirically if pneumonia is clinically suspected.

2. Select the initial empiric therapy based on the current bacteriology and resistance patterns at each institution. Alternatively, published evidence-based practice guidelines may be used.

3. Obtain cultures of respiratory tract specimens to identify pathogen(s), preferably before the initiation of antibiotics. However, the administration of antibiotic therapy should not be delayed for diagnostic testing.

4. Narrow the initial antibiotic regimen based on quantitative culture results and clinical response (i.e., de-escalation).

5. Avoid excessive antibiotic use by de-escalating therapy when appropriate and prescribing the minimal duration of therapy required for efficacy.

---

6. **What is meant by "de-escalation" of antibiotic therapy?**
   Antibiotic use promotes the development of antibiotic resistance; therefore, restricted use of antimicrobial drugs should be encouraged. If the patient is responding favorably, the initial empiric antibiotic regimen should be de-escalated, or narrowed to the most specific antibiotic based on the results of respiratory tract cultures and sensitivities.

7. **When is it safe to switch a patient to oral therapy?**
   Conversion to oral therapy may be considered in a clinically stable patient who demonstrates the following: improvement in cough and shortness of breath, defervescence (<100°F) on two

TABLE 17-1. COMMON PATHOGENS THAT CAUSE SEVERE COMMUNITY–ACQUIRED PNEUMONIA AND EMPIRIC ANTIBIOTIC THERAPY*†

Organisms	Therapy‡ǁ

a. No risks for *Pseudomonas aeruginosa*

Organisms	Therapy
Streptococcus pneumoniae (including DRSP)	Intravenous β-lactam (cefotaxime, ceftriaxone)§
Legionella spp.	*plus either*
Hemophilus influenzae	Intravenous macrolide (azithromycin)
Enteric gram-negative bacilli	*or*
Staphylococcus aureus	Intravenous fluoroquinolone
Mycoplasma pneumoniae	
Respiratory viruses	
Miscellaneous	
Chlamydia pneumonlae,	
Mycobacterium tuberculosis, endemic fungi	

b. Risks for *Pseudomonas aeruginosa*ǁ

Organisms	Therapy
All of the above pathogens plus *P. aeruginosa*	Selected intrevenous antipseudomonal β-lactam (cefepime, imipenem, meropenem, piperacillin/tazobactam)¶ *plus* intravenous antipseudomonal quinolone (ciprofloxacin)
	or
	Selected intravenous antipseudomonal β-lactam (cefepime, imipenem, meropenem, piperacillin/tazobactam)¶ *plus* intravenous aminoglycoside
	plus either
	Intravenous macrolide (azithromycin)
	or
	Intravenous nonpseudomonal fluoroquinolone

*Excludes patients at risk for HIV.
†In roughly one-third to one-half of the cases no etilogy was identified.
‡In no particular order.
§Antipseudomonal agents such as cefepime, piperacillin/tazobactam, imipenem, and meropenem are generally active against DRSP and other likely pathogens in this population, but not recommended for routine use unless the patient has risk factors for *P. aeruginosa.*
ǁCombination therapy required.
¶If β-lactam allergic, replace the listed β-lactam with aztreonam and combine with an aminoglycoside and an antipneumococcal fluoroquinolone as listed.
Data from Niederman MS, Mandell LA, Anzueto A, et al; American Thoracic Society: Guidelines for the management of adults with community-acquired pneumonia. Diagnosis, assessment of severity, antimicrobial therapy, and prevention. Am J Respir Crit Care Med 163:1730–1754, 2001, with permission.

separate measurements 8 hours apart, white blood cell count trending toward normal, and satisfactory oral intake and gastrointestinal tract absorption.

8. **What defines a treatment failure?**
   The majority of patients receiving appropriate therapy show a favorable clinical response within 72 hours. Therefore, initial antibiotic therapy should not be changed within 72 hours of initiation unless indicated by significant clinical worsening or microbiologic data. Remember that certain host factors, such as advanced age, alcoholism, and chronic obstructive pulmonary disease (COPD), have been associated with delayed resolution despite appropriate treatment. Radiographic resolution of pneumonia lags behind clinical improvement and in some cases may take up to 8–10 weeks to clear completely.

9. **Discuss the potential reasons why a patient may not respond favorably to empiric therapy.**
   Clinical deterioration or a lack of response to empiric antimicrobial therapy within 3 days often indicates treatment failure, warranting thorough reassessment and additional investigation. The following should be considered:
   1. Inappropriate antimicrobial therapy
      - Is the dosing adequate?
      - Are all potential bacterial pathogens covered by the empiric regimen?
      - Are the organisms resistant, or has a previously sensitive pathogen developed resistance?
      - Is the pathogen bacterial? Consider other pathogens, including viruses, endemic fungi, and mycobacteria.
      - Is the host immunocompromised and at risk for opportunistic infections such as *Pneumocystis jiroveci?*
      - Is the disease infectious? Has the patient been misdiagnosed (*see* question 11)?
   2. Complications of lung infection or hospitalization
      - Has the patient developed a lung abscess or empyema?
      - Does the patient have acute respiratory distress syndrome (ARDS)?
      - Have the bacteria seeded extrapulmonary sites (e.g., endocarditis, septic arthritis, meningitis)?
      - Has the patient acquired a new nosocomial infection (e.g., urinary tract infection, central line infection, sinusitis)?

10. **How should a patient with nonresolving pneumonia be evaluated?**
    The clinician should review initial culture results and sensitivities and collect additional lower respiratory tract and blood cultures. Broadening empiric therapy may be indicated while awaiting the results of additional testing. All patients should have a repeat chest radiograph at this time. Additional history taking may reveal human immunodeficiency virus risk factors, tick exposure, travel history, or other diagnostic clues. Further testing, such as chest computed tomography scan or ultrasound, should be directed at the likely cause of treatment failure. If the procedure can be performed safely, a thoracentesis of a pleural effusion can exclude a complicated effusion or empyema. Bronchoscopy has good diagnostic utility, and specimens should be sent for quantitative bacterial cultures and sensitivities, as well as for stains and cultures of unusual organisms (e.g., mycobacteria, viruses, endemic fungi, and *P. jiroveci*). If the diagnosis remains elusive, a trial of corticosteroids or a thoracoscopic or open lung biopsy may be considered in the appropriate clinical setting.

   Ioanas M, Ferrer M, Cavalcanti M, et al: Causes and predictors of nonresponse to treatment of intensive care unit–acquired pneumonia. Crit Care Med 32:938–945, 2004.

11. **Which noninfectious processes can present with signs and symptoms of acute pneumonia?**
    Noninfectious conditions that can mimic acute pneumonia include ARDS, traumatic pulmonary contusion, pneumonitis resulting from connective tissue disease (e.g., systemic lupus

erythematosus), acute hypersensitivity pneumonitis, drug-induced pneumonitis, diffuse alveolar hemorrhage (e.g., Goodpasture's syndrome), Wegener's granulomatosis, bronchiolitis obliterans organizing pneumonia, acute interstitial pneumonia (Hamman-Rich syndrome), acute eosinophilic pneumonia, pulmonary embolism with infarction, atelectasis, chemical pneumonitis (aspiration), and malignancy (e.g., bronchoalveolar carcinoma, lymphangitic carcinomatosis, Kaposi sarcoma).

12. **What about viral pneumonia?**
Viral pneumonia can be severe, particularly in elderly or immunocompromised patients or when complicated by a secondary bacterial infection, such as *S. pneumoniae, Staphylococcus aureus,* or *Haemophilus influenzae*. When suspected, the influenza virus can be detected using a rapid antigen detection assay, which can distinguish influenza A from B. Antiviral therapy against influenza A (e.g., amantadine, rimantadine, oseltamivir, or zanamivir) or influenza B (e.g., oseltamivir or zanamivir) is recommended if started within 48 hours of symptom onset. Specific antiviral therapy does not exist against parainfluenza, respiratory syncytial virus, adenovirus, metapneumovirus, coronavirus (severe acute respiratory syndrome agent), or hantavirus. Management of these infections involves supportive care and vigilant infection control measures.

13. **Which patients with severe CAP and acute respiratory failure benefit from noninvasive positive pressure ventilation (NPPV)?**
Clinical trials have demonstrated that the use of NPPV for acute respiratory failure from severe CAP can reduce the need for intubation and decrease mortality in patients with COPD or immunocompromised states. Patients must be suitable candidates for NPPV based on current practice guidelines. There is no evidence to support the use of NPPV in immunocompetent patients who do not have COPD but do have severe CAP.

14. **What is health care–associated pneumonia (HCAP)?**
The term *HCAP* refers to pneumonia that develops in a patient who lives in a nursing home or long-term care facility; undergoes hemodialysis; has received IV antimicrobial therapy, chemotherapy, or wound care within the preceding 30 days; or has been hospitalized for at least 2 days within the preceding 90 days. The causative pathogens in these patients are similar to those responsible for hospital-acquired pneumonia and ventilator-associated pneumonia (VAP) and are often multidrug resistant.

15. **Summarize the pathogenesis of VAP.**
The majority of cases are due to microaspiration of pathogens colonizing the oropharynx. Endotracheal intubation interferes with normal host defenses by impairing the patient's ability to cough and disrupting the protective barrier between the oropharynx and trachea. Bacteria-laden oropharyngeal secretions pool and leak around the cuff of the endotracheal tube and infect the lower respiratory tract. This is facilitated when the patient is supine. It has been hypothesized that the endotracheal tube is colonized with bacteria encased in biofilm and that tube manipulation or suctioning results in embolization of bacteria into the lower respiratory tract. Other less common sources of bacteria include the paranasal sinuses, dental plaque, gastrointestinal tract, and rarely hematogenous spread from another site of infection.

Chastre J: Conference Summary: Ventilator-associated pneumonia. Respir Care 50:975–983, 2005.

16. **List the most common pathogens responsible for VAP.**
The most common causative organisms are listed in Table 17-2. The relative frequency of these pathogens and their respective resistance patterns vary depending on the institution, prior exposure to antibiotics, host factors, and the duration of mechanical ventilation. Clinicians should be familiar with their institution's spectrum of common nosocomial pathogens and current resistance patterns.

TABLE 17-2. ETIOLOGIC PATHOGENS THAT CAUSE VENTILATOR-ASSOCIATED PNEUMONIA

Pseudomonas aeruginosa
Staphylococcus aureus
Enterobacteriaceae
- *Klebsiella* species
- *Escherichia coli*
- *Proteus* species
- *Enterobacter* species
- *Serratia* species
- *Citrobacter* species

Acinetobacter spp.
Stenotrophomonas maltophilia
Haemophilus influenzae
Legionella pneumophila
Streptococcus species
Coagulase-negative staphylococci
Neisseria species
Anaerobes

Polymicrobial infection (particularly common in ARDS).
ARDS = acute respiratory distress syndrome.

---

17. **What are the diagnostic criteria for VAP?**
Universally agreed-upon diagnostic criteria for VAP do not exist; however, commonly used criteria include the presence of *all* of the following:
1. Mechanical ventilation for >48 hours
2. A new and persistent infiltrate on chest radiograph or ARDS (in the setting of ARDS, it may be impossible to visualize a new infiltrate on chest radiograph)
3. Two of the following three findings:
   - Fever (temperature > 38°C)
   - Leukocytosis or leukopenia
   - Purulent tracheal secretions
4. Quantitative bacterial cultures of a lower respiratory tract specimen at or above the threshold defined as consistent with lung infection
   The use of clinical criteria alone without microbiologic data tends to lead to overdiagnosis of lung infection.

18. **Discuss the differences between qualitative and quantitative bacterial cultures of endotracheal aspirates from patients suspected of VAP.**
Colonization of the endotracheal tube occurs within 5 days of mechanical ventilation and, thus, qualitative cultures of endotracheal aspirates rarely yield negative results. Qualitative cultures are sufficiently sensitive (82%) to identify the infecting pathogen but lack specificity (27%). Therefore, quantitative cultures are necessary to distinguish oropharyngeal contaminants from infection. The recommended threshold for quantitative cultures of endotracheal aspirates ranges from 10^5 to 10^6 colony-forming units (CFU)/mL. Unless antibiotic therapy has been started or adjusted within the preceding 72 hours, *sterile* cultures from endotracheal aspirates have a strong negative predictive value (94%).

Chastre J, Fagon JY: Ventilator-associated pneumonia. Am J Respir Crit Care Med 165:867–903, 2002.

19. **What are the various invasive methods for obtaining lower respiratory tract specimens for quantitative cultures?**
    Bronchoscopic methods include bronchoalveolar lavage and protected specimen brush. Nonbronchoscopic methods can be performed in intubated patients by respiratory therapists and include minibronchoalveolar lavage and protected telescoping catheter. Bronchoscopic and nonbronchoscopic methods have similar performance characteristics; however, the diagnostic threshold for each procedure varies. Although nonbronchoscopic procedures are performed blindly and most frequently sample the right lower lobe, studies have shown that VAP is a diffuse process that typically involves every pulmonary lobe, particularly the posterior lower lobes.

20. **What are the advantages of quantitative cultures of lower respiratory tract specimens over a clinical approach for the diagnosis of VAP?**
    A microbiologic diagnosis using quantitative cultures of lower respiratory tract specimens not only establishes the presence of lung infection, but also identifies the etiologic organism. Several studies have shown that unless antibiotic therapy was initiated or changed within 72 hours preceding sampling, antibiotics can be safely discontinued when quantitative cultures of lavage specimens are below the diagnostic threshold. Qualitative or semiquantitative cultures of the trachea rarely yield negative results due to tracheal colonization even in the absence of lung infection.

    A multicenter, randomized, controlled trial of over 400 patients meeting clinical criteria for VAP showed that a diagnostic strategy involving bronchoscopic sampling and quantitative cultures resulted in significantly less antibiotic use and decreased 14-day mortality when compared with a clinical diagnostic strategy using qualitative cultures of endotracheal aspirates.

    Fagon JY, Chastre J, Wolff M, et al: Invasive and noninvasive strategies for management of suspected ventilator-associated pneumonia: A randomized trial. Ann Intern Med 132:621–630, 2000.

21. **Are there factors that predispose patients to nosocomial lung infection with drug-resistant organisms?**
    Hospital-acquired pneumonia (HAP) or VAP that develops within the first 4 hospital days is described as *early-onset*. A patient is at risk for infection with drug-resistant pathogens when HAP or VAP develops ≥5 days of hospitalization (i.e., *late-onset*) or if, within the preceding 3 months, the patient was hospitalized or received antibiotics. Additional risk factors for multidrug-resistant pathogens are listed in Table 17-3 and should be considered when prescribing empiric therapy for nosocomial pneumonia.

22. **What determines the selection of the initial empiric antibiotic therapy for HAP, HCAP, and VAP?**
    Investigations have shown that early, appropriate (meaning, effective against the etiologic pathogen) antimicrobial therapy for VAP improves outcomes. The ATS guidelines recommend empiric therapy. The initial selection of antibiotics depends on whether the patient has risk factors for drug-resistant nosocomial pathogens and whether the pneumonia is classified as early- or late-onset. Individual institutions differ in patterns of antimicrobial resistance; therefore, many hospitals have antibiotic guidelines or antibiograms for empiric therapy based on likely pathogens and local antimicrobial resistance patterns. If the patient has received antibiotics recently, empiric therapy should include antimicrobials from a different class than the patient received (Tables 17-4 and 17-5).

23. **What is the duration of antimicrobial therapy for HAP, HCAP, and VAP?**
    In a prospective, randomized clinical trial, an 8-day treatment strategy for culture-proven VAP resulted in a significant decrease in multidrug-resistant bacteria and more antibiotic-free days with no differences in mortality, ICU length of stay, or mechanical ventilator–free days compared with a 15-day regimen. A higher rate of recurrence was documented with the 8-day regimen when

---

TABLE 17-3. RISK FACTORS FOR MULTIDRUG-RESISTANT PATHOGENS CAUSING HOSPITAL-ACQUIRED PNEUMONIA, HEALTHCARE-ASSOCIATED PNEUMONIA, AND VENTILATOR-ASSOCIATED PNEUMONIA

- Antimicrobial therapy in preceding 90 days
- Current hospitalization of 5 days or more
- High frequency of antibiotic resistance in the community or in the specific hospital unit
- Presence of risk factors for HCAP:
    □ Hospitalization for 2 days or more in the preceding 90 days
    □ Residence in a nursing home or extended care facility
    □ Home infusion therapy (including antibiotics)
    □ Chronic dialysis within 30 days
    □ Home wound care
    □ Family member with multidrug-resistant pathogen
- Immunosuppressive disease and/or therapy

Data from American Thoracic Society; Infections Diseases Society of America. Guidelines for the management of adults with hospital-acquired, ventilator-associated, and health care–associated pneumonia. Am J Respir Crit Care Med 171:388–416, 2005, with permission.

TABLE 17-4. INITIAL EMPIRIC ANTIBIOTIC THERAPY FOR HOSPITAL-ACQUIRED PNEUMONIA OR VENTILATOR-ASSOCIATED PNEUMONIA IN PATIENTS WITH NO KNOWN RISK FACTORS FOR MULTIDRUG-RESISTANT PATHOGENS, EARLY ONSET, AND ANY DISEASE SEVERITY

Potential Pathogen	Recommended Antibiotic
*Streptococcus pneumoniae**	Ceftriaxone
Haemophilus Influenzae	*or*
Methicillin-sensitive *Staphylococcus aureus*	Levofloxacin, moxifloxacin, or ciprofloxacin
Antibiotic-sensitive enteric gram-negative bacilli	*or*
Escherichia coli	Ampicillin/sulbactam
Klebsiella pneumoniae	*or*
Enterobacter species	Ertapenem
Proteus species	
Serratia marcescens	

*The frequency of penicillin-resistant *S. pneumoniae* and multidrug-resistant *S. pneumoniae* is increasing; levofloxacin or moxiflox-acin are preferred to ciprofloxacin and the role of other new quinolones, such as gatifloxacin, has not been established.
Data from American Thoracic Society; Infections Diseases Society of America. Guidelines for the management of adults with hospital-acquired, ventilator-associated, and health care–associated pneumonia. Am J Respir Crit Care Med 171:388–416, 2005, with permission.

TABLE 17-5. INITIAL EMPIRIC THERAPY FOR HOSPITAL-ACQUIRED PNEUMONIA, VENTILATOR-ASSOCIATED PNEUMONIA, AND HEALTH CARE–ASSOCIATED PNEUMONIA IN PATIENTS WITH LATE-ONSET DISEASE OR RISK FACTORS FOR MULTIDRUG-RESISTANT PATHOGENS AND ALL DISEASE SEVERITY

Potential Pathogens	Combination Antibiotic Therapy*
Pathogens listed in Table 17-4 and MDR pathogens	Antipseudomonal cephalosporin (cefepime, ceftazidime)
Pseudomonas aeruginosa	*or*
Klebsiella pneumoniae (ESBL +)[†]	Antipseudomonal carbepenem (imipenem or meropenem)
Acinetobacter species[†]	
	or
	β-Lactam/β-lactamase inhibitor (piperacillin–tazobactam)
	plus
	Antipseudomonal fluoroquinolone[†] (ciprofloxacin or levofloxacin)
	or
	Aminoglycoside (amikacin, gentamicin, or tobramycin)
	plus
Methicillin-resistant *Staphylococcus aureus* (MRSA)	Linezolid or vancomycin[‡]
Legionella pneumophila[†]	

*Initial antibiotic therapy should be adjusted or streamlined on the basis of microbiologic data and clinical response to therapy.
[†]If an ESBL+ strain, such as *K. pneumoniae*, or an *Acinetobacter* species is suspected, a carbepenem is a reliable choice. If *L. pneumophila* is suspected, the combination antibiotic regimen should include a macolide (e.g., azithromycin) or a fluoroquinolone (e.g., ciprofloxacin or levofloxacin) should be used rather than an aminoglycoside.
[‡]If MRSA risk factors are present or there is a high incidence locally.

the infection was due to *Acinetobacter* or *Pseudomonas* species; therefore, VAP due to these organisms should be treated for 15 days. Because the infecting pathogens are similar, HAP and HCAP can be treated similarly. Extended therapy (14–21 days) may be indicated in the setting of multilobar disease, cavitation, malnutrition, or necrotizing gram-negative infection.

Chastre J, Wolff M, Fagon J-Y, et al: Comparison of 8 to 15 days of antibiotic therapy for ventilator-associated pneumonia in adults. JAMA 290:2588–2598, 2003.

24. **Describe measures that can decrease the risk of VAP.**
    1. Avoid intubation when possible, and apply NPPV when appropriate.
    2. Consider orotracheal tubes preferentially over nasotracheal tubes.
    3. Minimize the duration of mechanical ventilation with the aid of weaning protocols.
    4. Apply continuous aspiration of subglottic secretions.

5. Maintain an endotracheal tube cuff pressure >20 cm H_2O to prevent leakage of oropharyngeal secretions containing bacteria into the lungs.
6. Avoid unnecessary manipulation of the ventilator circuit.
7. Carefully discard contaminated condensate from the ventilator circuit.
8. Keep the head of the bed elevated 30 degrees.
9. Avoid heavy sedation and paralytics because they impair the patient's ability to cough.
10. It does not appear that sucralfate or therapies that decrease gastric acid increase the incidence of nosocomial pneumonia.

Cook D, Guyatt G, Marsahall J, et al: A comparison of sucralfate and ranitidine for the prevention of upper gastrointestinal bleeding in patients requiring mechanical ventilation. N Engl J Med 338:791–797, 1998.

Mallow S, Rebuck JA, Osler T, et al: Do proton pump inhibitors increase the incidence of nosocomial pneumonia and related infectious complications when compared with histamine-2 receptor antagonists in critically ill trauma patients? Curr Surg 61:452–458, 2004.

Messori A, Trippoli S, Vaiani M, et al: Bleeding and pneumonia in intensive care patients given ranitidine and sucralfate for prevention of stress ulcer: Meta-analysis of randomized controlled trials. BMJ 321:1–7, 2000.

25. **Under what circumstances is a thoracentesis indicated for a parapneumonic effusion?**

If the patient is clinically stable and a thoracentesis can be performed safely, then significant (>10 mm on lateral decubitus film) or loculated pleural effusions should be sampled whenever a complicated parapneumonic effusion (persistent bacterial invasion of the pleural space) or an empyema (frank pus in the pleural space) is suspected. Thoracentesis is also indicated when the diagnosis is elusive and the patient's condition is not responding favorably to empiric antibiotic therapy. Pleural fluid should be analyzed for cell count and differential, protein, glucose, lactate dehydrogenase (LDH), Gram's stain, acid-fast stain, and cultures for bacteria, fungi, and mycobacteria. Drainage is required for complicated parapneumonic effusions and empyemas.

WEBSITES

1. American Thoracic Society
www.thoracic.org

2. Infectious Diseases Society of America
www.idsociety.org

CHAPTER 18

ASTHMA

Gil Allen, MD, and David A. Kaminsky, MD

1. **What are important factors to address when taking the history of patients with acute severe asthma?**

    Box 18-1 summarizes the important historical points in a patient with acute severe asthma. If the clinician is able to obtain a history from the patient, it is important to first exclude other possible causes of the patient's presentation. A prior history of heart failure may suggest wheezing and shortness of breath resulting from left ventricular failure and pulmonary edema. A history of allergies or prior anaphylactic reactions, along with a recent exposure to certain foods, new medications, or other known triggers, could be an important warning of potentially imminent upper airway inflammation and closure. A history of recent-onset cough, wheezing, and hemoptysis with unilateral inspiratory and expiratory wheezes could be clues to an intrabronchial tumor, such as a carcinoid or carcinoma. Pulmonary embolism can also mimic asthma and should especially be considered in the patient with dyspnea, anxiety, and hypoxemia, but clear breath sounds. In this case, it would be important to elicit any history of prior deep venous thrombosis or embolism and pertinent risk factors. In a patient with dyspnea, anxiety, and inspiratory stridor, vocal cord dysfunction should be considered. A history of anxiety, voice changes, or sudden truncation of vocalizations can be a clue to this disorder. Spirometry can be an especially useful tool in the emergency department (ED) when evaluating these patients, and flow-volume loops often yield the characteristic truncated or flattened inspiratory loops. It is important to remember that the majority of these patients also have true asthma, but they often appear more flow limited than they actually are. If their peak expiratory flow rate (PEFR) is at baseline and there are no signs of fatigue, low doses of benzodiazepines can often break the cycle of paradoxical vocal cord closure.

    Rodrigo GJ, Rodrigo C, Hall JB: Acute asthma in adults: A review. Chest 125:1081–1102, 2004.

BOX 18-1. IMPORTANT HISTORICAL POINTS IN ACUTE ASTHMA

- History of asthma (i.e., when diagnosed, type of treatment, common triggers)
- Factors related to asthma control (e.g., frequency of use of medications, nocturnal symptoms, history of hospitalization, intubation, use of oral steroids)
- Timing of onset of symptoms (i.e., gradual versus sudden)
- Nature of symptoms (e.g., wheezing, chest pain, intermittent versus continuous, associated cough, sputum production, fever)
- Exclude other causes of shortness of breath (e.g., heart failure, pulmonary embolus)
- Exclude other causes of wheezing (e.g., bronchospasm from allergic reaction, endobronchial tumor)
- Consider paradoxical vocal cord closure on inspiration (i.e., vocal cord dysfunction)

2. **List some important indicators of a severe asthma attack.**
   - Use of accessory muscles
   - Inability to speak in full sentences
   - Heart rate > 130 beats/min
   - Pulsus paradoxus > 15 mmHg
   - Respiratory rate > 30 breaths/min
   - Inability to lie down
   - A silent chest
   - Somnolence
   - Advancing fatigue
   - Normal or elevated $PaCO_2$

3. **Which patients are at greatest risk of near-fatal or fatal asthma?**
   A recent survey of North American adult asthmatics presenting to the ED identified a number of factors associated with a high number of ED visits, including nonwhite race, Medicaid or other public (or no) insurance, and markers of chronic asthma severity, such as history of hospitalization, intubation, or recent inhaled corticosteroid use. Although it is difficult to identify such patients prospectively, other risk factors have been identified retrospectively. Patients with a high degree of bronchial reactivity, a history of poor compliance with therapy and follow-up, and those judged to be poor at perceiving the severity of their own attack, as demonstrated by a poor correlation between reported symptoms and PEFR values, are also at increased risk of near-fatal asthma. These are patients for whom home monitoring of PEFR is strongly indicated.

   Patients who develop sudden, severe attacks or those who have severe, slowly progressive disease are both typically at risk. A history of marked diurnal variation in FEV_1 is also believed to be a risk factor, but this could simply be related to its being a marker for increased bronchial responsiveness. There are historical data indicating that female gender, endotracheal intubation, and prolonged neuromuscular blockade are associated with more prolonged hospital stay, whereas elevated arterial CO_2 and lower arterial pH within 24 hours of admission are associated with increased mortality.

   Although not widely identified as a true marker of increased risk, the use of inhaled heroin is also frequently associated with near-fatal or fatal attacks of asthma. It is not known whether this is due to a direct effect of the inhaled drug (or its diluents), the degree of airflow limitation, or simply the impaired judgment of the user that delays arrival to the ED for the initiation of appropriate care. However, opioids have long been known to cause bronchoconstriction via mast cell degranulation and histamine release. Although most reports of severe asthma attacks after inhalation of narcotics have been in known asthmatics, they have also been reported in patients without any prior history of asthma.

   Afessa B, Morales I, Cury JD: Clinical course and outcome of patients admitted to an ICU for status asthmaticus. Chest 120:1616–1621, 2001.

   Griswold SK, Nordstrom CR, Clark S, et al: Asthma exacerbations in North American adults: Who are the "frequent fliers" in the emergency department? Chest 127:1579–1586, 2005.

   Molfino NA, Nannini LJ, Rebuck AS, Slutsky AS: The fatality-prone asthmatic patient: Follow-up study after near-fatal attacks. Chest 101:621–623, 1992.

4. **How should one treat a severe asthma attack?**
   - **Beta agonists:** These are the first-line therapy in an acute asthma attack. It is now widely accepted that the inhaled forms of these drugs are superior to the subcutaneous or IV route, with fewer adverse affects. The subcutaneous route is still reserved for patients who are so dyspneic that they are unable to take deep-enough breaths, but these are usually the patients who are later intubated. It is also accepted that metered-dose inhalers are equally as effective as aerosolized delivery, provided good technique is used with a spacer device. Nebulized or aerosolized delivery is still used frequently in the ED, in part from convention and in part because less instruction and observation are needed to ensure good delivery.

- **Corticosteroids:** These drugs also play a key role in treatment, and typical dosage is 60–125 mg of IV Solu-Medrol every 6 hours for the first 24 hours. This must be delivered as soon as possible because peak onset of action can take several hours. Therapy is typically administered every 6 hours until the attack appears to be subsiding, and then gradually tapered over days to weeks.
- **Anticholinergics:** Many studies have shown marginal benefits of adding inhaled ipratropium to beta-agonist therapy (versus beta agonists alone) in the treatment regimen of acute asthma. A recent meta-analysis showed a significant 10% increase in forced expiratory volume in 1 second (FEV_1) or PEFR and a significant reduction in hospital admissions from the ED when ipratropium was added to standard therapy regimens.
- **Aminophylline:** Oral theophylline is again becoming a popular secondary agent in chronic management of asthma. This is in part due to the recognition of its intrinsic anti-inflammatory properties, even at serum levels lower than those once thought necessary to achieve significant benefit. However, the use of IV aminophylline in the treatment of acute asthma remains controversial. Many consensus statements do not recommend its use as first-line therapy in the acute setting, and several studies have failed to show any benefit when aminophylline is added to other conventional therapies. However, there are other studies showing that with more aggressively targeted serum levels (15–20 µg/mL), the use of aminophylline can improve measures of PEFR, FEV_1, and reduce hospital admission rates. There is also limited evidence that theophylline may be beneficial adjunctive therapy in critically ill children with severe asthma whose conditions are failing to fully respond to aggressive first-line therapy. The treating physician must weigh these benefits against the higher level of undesired adverse effects that can potentially occur at such higher serum levels.
- **Inhaled anesthetic agents:** In mechanically ventilated patients with ongoing severe bronchospasm despite aggressive conventional treatment, inhaled anesthetic agents can be used for their intrinsic properties of bronchodilation. Because their delivery requires a special apparatus and conventional management is usually more effective, their use is often considered a last resort. Halothane often depresses cardiac function at doses needed for bronchodilation, and for this reason, isoflurane is the agent of choice.

Table 18-1 summarizes medications used to treat severe acute asthma.

Chien JW, Ciufo R, Novak R, et al: Uncontrolled oxygen administration and respiratory failure in acute asthma. Chest 117:728–733, 2000.

Early use of inhaled corticosteroids in the emergency department treatment of acute asthma (Cochrane Review). Cochrane Database Syst Rev 1:CD002308, 2001.

Gallagher EJ: Randomized clinical trial of intramuscular vs. oral methylprednisolone in the treatment of asthma exacerbations following discharge from an emergency department. Chest 126:362–368, 2004.

Ralston ME, Euwema MS, Knecht KR, et al: Comparison of levalbuterol and racemic albuterol combined with ipratropium bromide in acute pediatric asthma: A randomized controlled trial. J Emerg Med 29:29–35, 2005.

Rodrigo GJ, Rodrigo C: Elevated plasma lactate level associated with high dose inhaled albuterol therapy in acute severe asthma. Emerg Med J 22:404–408, 2005.

5. **Does magnesium sulfate offer any benefit in the treatment of status asthmaticus?**

Although a small number of controlled trials have yielded mixed results, one controlled study suggests that severe asthmatics ($FEV_1 < 25\%$ predicted) treated with IV magnesium sulfate in the ED had significantly reduced admission rates compared with those treated with placebo. The overall admission rate for all combined asthmatics was lower in the magnesium sulfate treatment group (25.4% versus 35.3%), but not significantly so. A more recent meta-analysis did not support these findings. Proposed mechanisms of possible benefit are:

- Blockage of calcium channels and reduced calcium entry into smooth muscle cells, leading to bronchodilation
- Possible inhibition of mast cell degranulation
- Improving respiratory muscle function by correction of lower baseline serum levels

TABLE 18-1.   PRIMARY PHARMACOLOGIC TREATMENT OF ACUTE ASTHMA*

Agent	Dose	Comments
Beta agonists	▪ 4 puffs (400 μg) by MDI + spacer every 10 minutes or ▪ 2.5 mg every 20 minutes by nebulizer	▪ Inhaled better than subcutaneous or IV ▪ MDI + spacer works as well as nebulized ▪ Levalbuterol similar to racemic albuterol, but with less tachycardia ▪ Elevated lactate levels seen after high doses
Corticosteroids	▪ 60–125 IV Solu-Medrol every 6 hours for first 24 hours, *then* ▪ Taper over 7–14 days, converting to oral therapy	▪ Single 160-mg intramuscular depot injection of methylprednisolone has been found to be as effective as an 8-day tapering course of the same dose of oral methylprednisolone once patients discharged
Anticholinergics	▪ 4 puffs (80 μg) ipratropium bromide by MDI + spacer every 10 minutes, or ▪ 500 μg every 20 minutes by nebulizer	▪ Improves lung function and reduces rate of hospitalization when added to standard care ▪ Combined use with inhaled beta agonists is beneficial
Aminophylline	▪ 6 mg/kg IV load, then 0.5 mg/kg/h	▪ Target levels = 8–12 μg/mL ▪ Use is controversial; weigh risk versus benefit
Oxygen	▪ Titrate to $SaO_2 > 92\%$	▪ Avoid excessive oxygenation, which can result in CO_2 retention ▪ Use humidified oxygen
Inhaled anesthetic agents	▪ Isoflurane the agent of choice	▪ Intrinsic bronchodilating properties ▪ Avoid halothane due to depression of cardiac function at doses necessary for bronchodilation

MDI = metered dose inhaler, SaO_2 = oxygen saturation.
*Other agents (magnesium sulfate, heliox, leukotriene antagonists) discussed in text.

Since the only reported untoward side effects from a single dose are flushing, mild fatigue, or burning at the IV site, its use in the treatment of persons with severe asthma may be warranted by its potential for lowering admission rates, but this still remains a controversial topic. Magnesium sulfate is generally delivered as 2 gm in 50 mL of normal saline given intravenously over 20 minutes. Interestingly, inhaled magnesium sulfate administered with inhaled beta agonist has also been shown to improve lung function and may reduce the rate of hospital admission.

Bloch H, Silverman R, Mancherje N, et al: Intravenous magnesium sulfate as an adjunct in the treatment of acute asthma. Chest 107:1576–1581, 1995.

6. **How can one best decide when to admit a patient and when to discharge a patient home from the ED?**

   All patients who have a poor response to treatment—defined as persistent wheezing, dyspnea, and accessory muscle use at rest despite 3 hours of treatment in the ED—should be admitted to the hospital. One study suggests that in persons with severe asthma (PEFR and $FEV_1 < 35\%$ of predicted), changes in PEFR measured 30 minutes after initiation of therapy may be a good early predictor of response to treatment after 3 hours. Any patient with worsening PEFR, rising $PaCO_2$, or advancing fatigue should, at the very least, be monitored in the intensive care unit and possibly intubated.

   Mountain RD, Sahn SA: Clinical features and outcome in patients with acute asthma presenting with hypercapnea. Am Rev Respir Dis 138:535–539, 1988.

   Rodrigo G, Rodrigo C: Early prediction of poor response in acute asthma patients in the emergency department. Chest 114:1016–1021, 1998.

7. **Which patients need to be intubated?**

   Any patient with apnea, near apnea, or cardiopulmonary arrest should be intubated. Any patient with progressive lethargy, somnolence, or near exhaustion should be intubated. An elevated $PaCO_2$ level on admission, although shown to be associated with increased mortality, may not necessarily warrant immediate endotracheal intubation. Any patient with a progressive rise in $PaCO_2$ despite therapy and increasing fatigue most likely will require intubation. Other relative indications are coexistent medical conditions that can increase minute ventilation requirements or compromise oxygen delivery, such as sepsis, myocardial infarction, metabolic acidosis, or life-threatening arrhythmias.

8. **Is normocapnia or hypercapnia an absolute indication for intubation in a person with asthma?**

   Most persons with severe asthma present with hypocapnia due to the hyperventilation associated with dyspnea and hypoxemia. A normal or elevated $PaCO_2$ is usually a sign of fatigue but can also be due to a high dead space to tidal volume ratio resulting from air trapping and ineffective ventilation of noncommunicating segments of the lung. In either case, it should be taken seriously and can be a sign of impending respiratory failure. Studies indicate, however, that most patients with normal or elevated $PaCO_2$ on blood gas analysis at initial evaluation improve before requiring mechanical ventilation. In most patients, ventilation improves with time in response to conventional therapy. Because mechanical ventilation in severe asthma can be complicated by increased air trapping and barotrauma, it is advisable not to begin mechanical ventilation in a patient with acute asthma merely because of an elevated $PaCO_2$, unless it is associated with somnolence, progressive fatigue, or significant acidosis.

9. **Can noninvasive mechanical ventilation be used safely to avoid intubation in a person with asthma?**

   Noninvasive positive pressure ventilation (NIPPV) via face mask has been shown to be safe and effective when applied to a patient with severe asthma and hypercapnia whose condition fails to improve with conventional therapy. It can be effective in unloading respiratory muscles, improving dyspnea, lowering respiratory rate, and improving gas exchange. NIPPV has been shown to be an effective potential means of avoiding endotracheal intubation and may also help avoid the need for reintubation after extubation. However, it is also critical to determine early in a patient's course whether he or she is responding appropriately to NIPPV, since delays in endotracheal intubation may be associated with worse outcomes. It should not be used in persons with asthma who have life-threatening hypoxemia, somnolence, or hemodynamic instability, and it should be aborted in patients whose conditions fail to improve or who cannot tolerate the mask. At the present time, the use of NIPPV in the treatment of acute asthma remains controversial.

Gehlbach B, Kress JP, Kahn J, et al: Correlates of prolonged hospitalization in inner-city ICU patients receiving noninvasive and invasive positive pressure ventilation for status asthmaticus. Chest 122:1709–1714, 2002.

Ram FS, Wellington S, Rowe BH, Wedzicha JA: Non-invasive positive pressure ventilation for treatment of respiratory failure due to severe acute exacerbations of asthma. Cochrane Database Syst Rev CD004360, 2005.

10. **Are helium admixtures of any proven benefit in treating severe asthma?**
When helium is blended with oxygen in an 20% O_2, 80% He mixture, the gas density becomes approximately one-third that of room air, but viscosity is increased, leading to increased laminar flow and a reduction in airway resistance in areas of greatest turbulent flow. This can result in a reduction in the work of breathing required to meet the same minute ventilation requirement when breathing room air. Because work of breathing is reduced, it would seem likely that respiratory fatigue might be delayed until conventional therapy has had time to take effect. Despite numerous trials and two recent meta-analyses, there is still no evidence that helium-oxygen (heliox) admixtures can prevent the need for endotracheal intubation. However, heliox has been shown to improve PEFR and reduce the degree of pulsus-paradoxus in acute asthma attacks. This is presumably due to the decrease in airway resistance and lower generated negative pleural pressures, but also possibly caused by improved expiratory flow and less dynamic hyperinflation (DHI). Because mixtures typically include only 20–30% oxygen, hypoxemia is a barrier to its use. However, when the patient is not hypoxemic, it is safe and worthwhile to use, particularly in patients with fatigue and hypercapnia who are at risk for progressing to the point of requiring mechanical ventilation.

Rodrigo G, Rodrigo C, Pollack CV, et al: Use of helium-oxygen mixtures in the treatment of acute asthma: A systematic review. Chest 123:891–896, 2003.

KEY POINTS: ASSESSMENT AND TREATMENT OF ACUTE ASTHMA

1. Risk factors for acute asthma include poor perception of symptoms, poor compliance with therapy, lack of medical insurance, and previous hospitalization or intubation.

2. Examination findings suggesting impending respiratory failure in acute asthma include use of accessory muscles, inability to speak full sentences, inability to lie down, and a silent chest.

3. Patients with acute asthma should be admitted to the hospital when they have failed to respond to treatment in the ED within 3 hours or when they have a normal or rising PCO_2.

4. Ventilator settings that minimize dynamic hyperinflation and its complications include low minute ventilation (preferably via both reduced tidal volume and respiratory rate), high inspiratory flow rate to minimize inspiratory time, and no external positive end-expiratory pressure.

11. **Once a patient requires intubation, what is the best management strategy?**
    1. **Intubation:** Blind nasoendotracheal intubation is often better tolerated by an awake patient, but oral endotracheal intubation is the preferred method of intubation because it permits the use of an endotracheal tube (ETT) with a larger internal diameter. This will lead to lower resistance within the respiratory circuit and allow easier deep suctioning of secretions and mucous plugs. It is important to remember that the resistance of a tube is indirectly

proportional to its internal radius (to the fourth power), and the resistance of an 8-mm ETT is roughly one-half that of a 7-mm ETT. Oral intubation is indicated for apneic, cyanotic patients. Because intubation in a person with asthma is often difficult and may induce laryngospasm or lead to increased bronchospasm, it should be performed by the most experienced person available. Sedation is usually necessary and, although sometimes warranted, paralysis should be avoided if possible. Barbiturates such as thiopental should not be used due to their association with histamine release and potential worsening of bronchoconstriction. Although narcotics such as fentanyl are often useful, one should be aware of their potential to trigger bronchoconstriction and laryngospasm.

2. **Avoiding potential complications**
   - **DHI:** When airflow limitation is severe, the next ventilated breath can be initiated before the lungs can fully empty to a normal functional residual capacity, resulting in progressive air trapping. This leads to DHI and elevated end-expiratory alveolar pressures, referred to as *intrinsic positive end-expiratory pressure* ($PEEP_i$). Measuring $PEEP_i$ can be problematic, and it is often underestimated by the brief end-expiratory pause used to estimate it on the ventilator. This is due to the often heterogeneous distribution of early airway closure that can prevent many hyperinflated segments from communicating their alveolar pressures to the transducer at the airway opening. Ideally, $PEEP_i$ should be kept below 15 cm H_2O. The key determinants of DHI are minute ventilation, tidal volume, exhalation time, and severity of airflow limitation. DHI can often be predicted by elevated plateau pressures and failure to achieve zero expiratory flow before the next delivered breath. DHI can lead to less effective respiratory muscle contraction and added work due to less optimal curvature of the diaphragm, which in turn can lead to less effective triggering of the ventilator. DHI can also lead to decreased venous return and right ventricular preload, increased right ventricular afterload (via extrinsic compression of the pulmonary vasculature), and decreased left ventricular compliance, which can all lead to diminished cardiac output and hypotension. When strongly suspected, the best immediate solution (and test) is to briefly disconnect the ETT from the ventilator circuit to allow for more complete exhalation. The other concern with DHI is that the high degree of associated $PEEP_i$ can ultimately lead to barotrauma.
   - **Barotrauma:** High airway pressures can potentially lead to pulmonary interstitial emphysema, subcutaneous emphysema, pneumomediastinum, pneumothorax, and even pneumoperitoneum. Barotrauma correlates directly with the degree of DHI. Plateau pressures are traditionally thought to be a good indicator of the degree of DHI, and a level below 35 cm H_2O is still a widely recommended target for minimizing barotrauma. However, one study has shown that end-inspiratory lung volume (the exhaled volume measured from end-inspiration to functional residual capacity (FRC) during and a period of apnea) may be a more reliable predictor of barotrauma than airway pressures. The most feared consequence of barotrauma is tension pneumothorax, typically characterized by a precipitous rise in airway pressures (peak and plateau), a drop in oxygen saturation, hypotension, tachycardia, unilaterally absent breath sounds and chest excursions, and possibly tracheal deviation. Tension pneumothorax is a clinical diagnosis, and if strongly suspected in an unstable patient, should be treated immediately with needle thoracotomy followed by chest tube placement.

3. **Ventilator settings in acute asthma (Box 18-2):** The best mode of ventilation is one that minimizes minute ventilation and allows for sufficient exhalation time to minimize DHI. This can generally be achieved with low tidal volumes of 6–8 mL/kg, a respiratory rate of 8–10 breaths/min, minimal added PEEP, and moderate inspiratory flow rates of 80–90 L/min. Decelerating flow waveforms may improve overall flow distribution and hence optimize gas exchange. Higher inspiratory flow rates with square waveforms allow for a shorter inspiratory time and hence, at the same respiratory rate, a longer expiratory time. It is the longer expiratory time, and not just the inspiratory to expiratory (I:E) ratio, that is critical. Lowering total minute ventilation is the most crucial goal, because a longer expiratory time and smaller

> **BOX 18-2. PRINCIPLES OF MANAGEMENT OF MECHANICAL VENTILATION IN ACUTE ASTHMA**
>
> The goal is to minimize DHI through the use of:
> - Minimal minute ventilation (low tidal volumes [e.g., 6–8 mL/kg]), low respiratory rate (8–10 beats/min)
> - Minimal (or zero) PEEP
> - Relatively high inspiratory flow rate (80–100 L/min), to reduce inspiratory time
> - Maintenance of plateau pressures $\leq$35 cm H_2O, and $PEEP_i$ $\leq$15 cm H_2O
> - Permissive hypercapnia up to 80 mmHg (contraindicated in patients with intracranial bleeding, cerebral edema, or a space-occupying lesion), while trying to maintain pH $\geq$7.20
>
> DHI = dynamic hyperinflation, PEEP = positive end-expiratory pressure.

burden of volume to be exhaled are what minimize DHI. Intentional hypoventilation with low minute volumes can significantly reduce the risk of DHI and barotrauma, and allowing for a maximum $PaCO_2$ of 80 mmHg or a minimum pH of 7.20 is a safe and acceptable practice when ventilating patients with severe airflow limitation. However, because an elevated $PaCO_2$ can increase cerebral perfusion, permissive hypercapnia should be avoided in patients with intracranial bleeding, edema, or a space-occupying lesion.

4. **Sedation:** Agitation can lead to hyperventilation and asynchrony with the mechanical ventilator and hence DHI and unacceptably high airway pressures. Deep anesthesia with benzodiazepines or propofol is often necessary to achieve optimal control, especially when using intentional hypoventilation and permissive hypercapnia. Paralytics should and often can be avoided if sufficient levels of sedatives are used. It is important to remember that patients are suspected to be at a higher risk of prolonged weakness when paralytics are administered in combination with corticosteroids.

Jain S, Hanania NA, Guntupalli KK: Ventilation of patients with asthma and obstructive lung disease. Crit Care Clin 14:685–705, 1998.

Williams TJ, Tuxen DV, Scheinkestel CD, et al: Risk factors for morbidity in mechanically ventilated patients with acute severe asthma. Am Rev Respir Dis 146:607–615, 1992.

12. **Can added PEEP help reduce air trapping in mechanically ventilated patients with asthma?**
Some argue that added PEEP can help minimize air trapping by "stenting" open peripheral airways. Although this may be true to some effect in patients with emphysema and easily collapsible central airways, it is unlikely to be of much benefit in persons with severe asthma. In the classic model of airflow limitation, airway collapse occurs when the extraluminal pressure overcomes intraluminal pressures (and any architectural properties of the airway itself). In patients who already have significant $PEEP_i$, and in whom distal alveolar pressures already exceed extraluminal pressures at end expiration, added PEEP will likely only increase distal alveolar pressures and worsen hyperinflation. It is important to remember that DHI can occur even in the absence of airflow limitation if the respiratory rate is high enough, so the previously mentioned strategies are still best for minimizing DHI.

13. **What are some new pharmacologic strategies for treating acute asthma?**
A recent Cochrane review found that the use of inhaled steroids in the ED reduces admission rates in patients with acute asthma, but this seems only to benefit those patients not already receiving systemic corticosteroids. Inhaled budesonide has been shown to improve markers of airway inflammation and hyper-responsiveness as early as 6 hours after dosing. Another study demonstrated that inhaled fluticasone (3000 μg/h), administered as two puffs every 10 minutes

for 3 hours, can improve lung function and reduce hospitalization rate more than treating with 500 mg of IV hydrocortisone. The rapidity of the response suggests a noninflammatory mechanism of action that may involve topical vasoconstriction. Another potential therapy for acute asthma is leukotriene blockade. One study has found that IV delivery of montelukast improved FEV_1 faster than placebo when given with standard therapy. In another study, oral administration of zafirlukast together with standard therapy resulted in a lower rate of extended care in the ED and a lower relapse rate at 28 days compared with placebo. The use of leukotriene inhibitors for acute asthma still warrants further investigation.

Comargo CA, Smithline HA, Malice MP, et al: A randomized controlled trial of intravenous montelukast in acute asthma. Am J Respir Crit Care Med 167:528–533, 2003.

Rodrigo GJ: Comparison of inhaled fluticasone with intravenous hydrocortisone in the treatment of adult acute asthma. Am J Respir Crit Care Med 171:1231–1236, 2005.

Silverman RA, Nowak RM, Korenblat PE, et al: Zafirlukast treatment in acute asthma: Evaluation in a randomized, double-blind, multicenter trial. Chest 126:1480–1489, 2004.

WEBSITE

National Institutes of Health
www.nhlbi.nih.gov/guidelines/asthma/asthgdln.htm

CHAPTER 19

CHRONIC OBSTRUCTIVE PULMONARY DISEASE

Enrique Fernandez, MD, and Anne Dixon, MD

1. **What is chronic obstructive pulmonary disease (COPD)?**

   COPD is characterized by airflow limitation that is not fully reversible. Chronic airflow limitation results from a combination of small airway disease and parenchymal destruction due to inflammatory processes. These inflammatory processes are often caused by exposure to noxious particles or gases.

2. **How many people are affected by COPD?**

   COPD is the fourth leading cause of mortality and morbidity in the United States. The number of people affected by COPD worldwide continues to increase because of exposure to tobacco smoke and aging of the population. Historically there was a higher prevalence of disease in men, but with changing patterns of exposure to tobacco, women are now affected as frequently as men. Worldwide, exposure to indoor pollution from heating and cooking fuels substantially contributes to COPD in women.

   The Global Initiative for Chronic Obstructive Lung Disease. Available at http://www.goldcopd.org.

3. **What processes are involved in the pathogenesis of COPD?**

   COPD is characterized by chronic inflammation throughout the lung, with increased neutrophils, macrophages, and CD8+ T lymphocytes. An imbalance between proteinase–antiproteinase activity and oxidative stress also contributes to the pathogenesis of this disease. Oxidative stress and proteinase–antiproteinase imbalance can be related to a combination of factors, including the inflammation itself, environmental exposures (e.g., oxidative substances in cigarette smoke), and genetics (e.g., alpha$_1$ antitrypsin deficiency).

4. **What are the major pathologic changes in COPD?**

   All structures of the lung are subjected to pathologic changes in COPD. In the central airways, inflammatory cells infiltrate the surface epithelium, edema is present, mucus-secreting glands are enlarged, and the number of goblet cells increases with mucus hypersecretion. In the peripheral airways (small bronchi and bronchioles with an internal diameter < 2 mm), chronic inflammation leads to repeated injury and repair of the airway wall. In emphysema, destruction of alveolar septa leads to confluence of adjacent alveoli and enlarged terminal air spaces. Vascular changes include thickening of the vessel wall with increased smooth muscle, proteoglycans, and collagen deposition.

5. **How do these pathologic changes produce airflow limitation?**

   Chronic inflammation causes remodeling and narrowing of the airway. The airway is also narrowed by mucus hypersecretion. Parenchymal destruction and loss of alveolar attachment to the small airways causes reduced elastic recoil of the lung and a tendency for the airways to collapse during expiration. Consequently, airflow becomes limited on expiration. This can be detected most simply with spirometry as a decrease in the ratio of forced expiratory volume in 1 second to forced vital capacity ($FEV_1/FVC < 70\%$).

6. **How is severity graded in COPD?**

   The staging system should be regarded as an educational tool and a guide to management (Table 19-1).

TABLE 19-1. CLASSIFICATION OF CHRONIC OBSTRUCTIVE LUNG DISEASE (COPD) BY SEVERITY

Stage	Severity
0: At risk	Normal spirometry
	Chronic symptoms (e.g., cough, sputum production)
I. Mild COPD	$FEV_1/FVC < 70\%$
	$FEV_1 \geq 80\%$ predicted
	With or without chronic symptoms (e.g., cough, sputum production)
II. Moderate COPD	$FEV_1/FVC < 70\%$
	$50\% \leq FEV_1 < 80\%$ predicted
	With or without chronic symptoms (e.g., cough, sputum production)
III. Severe COPD	$FEV_1/FVC < 70\%$
	$FEV_1 < 30\%$ predicted or $FEV_1 < 50\%$ predicted plus chronic respiratory failure

FEV_1 = forced expiratory volume in 1 second, FVC = forced vital capacity. From the Global Initiative for Chronic Obstrucive Lung Disease.

7. **What are the benefits of smoking cessation for a patient with COPD?**
   Smoking cessation is the most important intervention. No other intervention has been shown to decelerate the decline in lung function characteristic of this disease. In addition to the modest improvement in FEV_1 seen with smoking cessation, the rate of decline in FEV_1 may be reduced, in some cases even to the rate found in healthy nonsmokers ($\pm$30 mL/year).

8. **Why are bronchodilators used in the treatment of COPD?**
   Bronchodilators treat airway obstruction in patients with COPD. By reducing bronchomotor tone, they decrease airway resistance, which can improve airflow. This will improve emptying of the lungs and tends to reduce dynamic hyperinflation during rest and exercise and thus improve exercise performance. Spirometric changes after bronchodilator therapy may be minimal, despite significant clinical benefit, as quantified by changes in quality-of-life measures and exercise tolerance (e.g., 6-minute walk).

9. **Which bronchodilators should be used in the treatment of COPD?**
   - **Anticholinergic agents:** These agents block cholinergic transmission. Ipratropium has a duration of action of 6–8 hours. Tiotropium bromide is more potent and has a longer duration of action, allowing once-daily administration. It is more convenient but more expensive.
   - **β_2-adrenergic agents:** β_2-adrenergic agents act on airway smooth muscle. Inhaled, short-acting β_2-adrenergic agents are readily absorbed systemically and can lead to numerous systemic adverse effects, such as tachycardia, tremor, and arrhythmias. Long-acting inhaled β_2-adrenergic agents are more effective and convenient but more expensive.
   - **Methylxanthines:** These are weak bronchodilators but have multiple other effects that might be important: an inotropic effect on diaphragmatic muscle, reduced muscle fatigue, increased mucociliary clearance and central respiratory drive, and some anti-inflammatory effects. Due to the potential for toxicity with theophylline, other bronchodilators are preferred when available.

10. **Are inhaled corticosteroids beneficial in COPD?**

    Although regular use of inhaled corticosteroids do not prevent loss of lung function in patients with COPD, inhaled corticosteroids are recommended for patients with severe disease (FEV_1 < 50% predicted) and recurrent exacerbations because mounting data indicate that inhaled corticosteroids decrease the risk of exacerbations in patients with COPD.

    Sin DD, Wu L, Anderson JA, et al: Inhaled corticosteroids and mortality in chronic obstructive pulmonary disease. Thorax 60:992–997, 2005.

11. **What other pharmacologic treatments may benefit patients with COPD?**
    - **Alpha$_1$-antitrypsin replacement:** This is recommended for patients with emphysema related to deficiency of alpha$_1$-antitrypsin.
    - **Vaccines:** Patients with COPD are at risk for increased morbidity and mortality from respiratory tract infections. Pneumococcal and influenza vaccination, both alone and in combination, have been shown to reduce hospitalizations and mortality rates.
    - **Antioxidant agents:** N-acetylcysteine may reduce the frequency of exacerbations, but further studies are needed.
    - **Mucolytic therapy:** The benefit seems to be small, and widespread use cannot be recommended on the basis of current evidence.

    Immune regulators, vasodilators, respiratory stimulants, antitussives, and narcotics are not currently recommended for routine therapy.

12. **Who should get pulmonary rehabilitation?**

    Patients with all levels of COPD can benefit from exercise training programs. Pulmonary rehabilitation has been shown to improve functional status, decrease dyspnea, and reduce health care use. Pulmonary rehabilitation is currently recommended as part of the treatment plan for patients with moderate, severe, and very severe COPD.

13. **What are the indications for long-term oxygen therapy in patients with COPD?**

    For a patient at rest on room air in a stable condition:

    Arterial oxygen (PaO_2) < 55 mmHg or arterial oxygen saturation (SaO_2) < 85%

    or

    $$PaO_2 = 56-59 \, mmHg/SaO_2 = 86-89\%$$

    and one of the following:
    - Right heart failure or polycythemia
    - Desaturation during sleep
    - Desaturation during exercise

14. **What level of oxygen should be prescribed for patients with the indications listed in question 13?**

    Oxygen should be prescribed in a dose sufficient to raise the PaO_2 to 65–80 mmHg at rest during wakefulness. This PaO_2 usually is achieved with a 1- to 4-L/min oxygen flow through nasal prongs. The dose of O_2 should be increased by 1 L/min during sleep or exercise to prevent hypoxemic episodes. Oxygen should be given continuously at least 19 h/day.

15. **Is lung volume reduction surgery effective in the treatment of COPD?**

    In lung volume reduction surgery, part of the lungs are resected to reduce hyperinflation. This has beneficial effects on the mechanical action of the respiratory muscles and improves elastic recoil, which facilitates emptying of the lungs. Lung volume reduction surgery does not improve long-term survival in COPD but does improve exercise capacity in a select group of patients. Patients that benefit from lung volume reduction surgery are those with predominantly upper lobe emphysema and a low exercise capacity.

    Fishman A, Martinez F, Naunheim K, et al: A randomized trial comparing lung-volume-reduction surgery with medical therapy for severe emphysema. N Engl J Med 348:2059–2073, 2003.

16. **What factors predict death in patients with COPD?**
Long-term prognosis is hard to predict in patients with COPD. Factors that have been shown to predict mortality include low body mass index, degree of airflow obstruction, dyspnea, and exercise capacity as measured by the 6-minute walk test.

Celli BR, Cote CG, Marin JM, et al: The body-mass index, airflow obstruction, dyspnea, and exercise capacity index in chronic obstructive pulmonary disease. N Engl J Med 350:1005–1012, 2004.

17. **Are antibiotics useful in treating COPD exacerbations?**
Giving antibiotics for COPD exacerbations is associated with beneficial effects on lung function. For patients mechanically ventilated for a COPD exacerbation, withholding antibiotics has been associated with increased mortality and hospital-acquired pneumonia.

Nouira S, Marghli S, Belghith M, et al: Once daily oral ofloxacin in chronic obstructive pulmonary disease exacerbation requiring mechanical ventilation: A randomised placebo-controlled trial. Lancet 358(9298): 2020–2025, 2001.

18. **What is the role of steroids in the treatment of COPD exacerbations?**
Systemic glucocorticoids shorten the duration of the exacerbation and lead to faster improvements in lung function. A recent study suggested that nebulized budesonide may be an alternative to oral glucocorticoids in nonacidotic exacerbations.

Niewoehner DE, Erbland ML, Deupree RH, et al: Effect of systemic glucocorticoids on exacerbations of chronic obstructive pulmonary disease. Department of Veterans Affairs Cooperative Study Group. N Engl J Med 340:1941–1947, 1999.

19. **What are the causes of acute respiratory failure in patients with COPD?**
Causes include bronchial infection, pulmonary emboli, cardiac failure, pneumonia, pneumothorax, respiratory depression (usually by the injudicious use of sedatives or narcotic analgesic drugs), surgery (especially of chest and upper abdomen), stopping of medications, or occasionally malnutrition. In general, the criteria for the diagnosis of acute respiratory failure in patients with COPD include hypoxemia ($PaO_2 < 60$ mmHg), hypercapnia ($PaCO_2 > 50$–70 mmHg), and respiratory acidosis ($pH < 7.35$) associated with worsening of the patient's respiratory symptoms compared with baseline.

KEY POINTS: CHRONIC OBSTRUCTIVE PULMONARY DISEASE (COPD)

1. COPD is the fourth leading cause of morbidity and mortality in the United States.

2. Spirometry is required to grade the severity and make a diagnosis of COPD.

3. Systemic glucocorticoids are indicated only in acute exacerbations.

4. Noninvasive ventilation improves outcomes in patients with impending respiratory failure.

20. **What is the initial treatment of a severe COPD exacerbation?**
Assess the patient in terms of symptoms and signs, and obtain a chest radiograph and arterial blood gas analysis. Administer adequate oxygen: death or irreversible brain damage results within minutes when severe hypoxemia is present, whereas hypercapnia may be well tolerated.

The appropriate amount of oxygen is that which satisfies tissue oxygen needs: usually a $PaO_2 >$ 60 mmHg, without worsening the respiratory acidosis and/or further depressing sensorium. Administer beta$_2$ agonist and anticholinergic bronchodilators. Add glucocorticoids and antibiotics. Consider noninvasive ventilation.

21. **What is the role of noninvasive ventilation in the treatment of COPD exacerbations?**
Noninvasive ventilation has been used for patients with moderate to severe dyspnea and moderate to severe acidosis from a COPD exacerbation. A number of trials report improvements in acid–base balance, reduced $PaCO_2$, and decreased length of stay. Intubation rates are also reduced by noninvasive ventilation. Box 19-1 summarizes the indications and contraindications for noninvasive ventilation in COPD exacerbations; Box 19-2 summarizes indications for intubation and invasive mechanical ventilation in COPD exacerbation.

BOX 19-1. INDICATIONS AND CONTRAINDICATIONS FOR NONINVASIVE VENTILATION IN CHRONIC OBSTRUCTIVE LUNG DISEASE EXACERBATION

Indications
- Severe dyspnea
- Moderate to severe acidosis and hypercapnia
- Respiratory rate > 25

Contraindications
- Somnolence or altered mental status
- Severe hypoxemia
- Hemodynamic instability
- Craniofacial abnormalities
- High aspiration risk

BOX 19-2. INDICATIONS FOR INTUBATION AND INVASIVE MECHANICAL VENTILATION IN CHRONIC OBSTRUCTIVE LUNG DISEASE EXACERBATION

- Severe dyspnea
- Severe acidosis or hypercapnia
- Respiratory rate > 35
- Severe hypoxemia
- Failure of noninvasive ventilation
- Hemodynamic instability

---

22. **What is the prognosis for a patient requiring mechanical ventilation?**
Many studies report reasonable short-term mortality rates (25–30%) for patients intubated for a COPD exacerbation rate but high mortality rates in the long term.

23. **What is the role of positive end expiratory pressure in mechanical ventilation during a COPD exacerbation?**
The presence of positive alveolar pressure at the end of exhalation (intrinsic PEEP) may prevent the patient from triggering the ventilator. The level of external PEEP should be set just below the level of intrinsic PEEP to allow the patient to trigger the ventilator with minimal effort.

24. **What is the preferred mode of mechanical ventilation in a COPD exacerbation?**
No mode of mechanical ventilation has been shown to be superior to another during a COPD exacerbation. In general, the principles of ventilation are to minimize hyperinflation by allowing adequate expiratory time and avoiding high tidal volumes. Oxygen should be titrated to maintain an arterial partial pressure of approximately 60 mmHg. Overventilation should be avoided: these patients frequently have hypercapnia and a compensatory metabolic alkalosis at baseline.

CHAPTER 20

COR PULMONALE

John M. Taylor, MD

1. **What is cor pulmonale?**

   Literally translated from Latin, *cor pulmonale* means "pulmonary heart." The term was coined by Paul D. White, MD, in 1931. The World Health Organization in 1963 adopted the following definition of cor pulmonale: "hypertrophy of the right ventricle resulting from diseases affecting the function and/or structure of the lungs, except when these pulmonary alterations are the result of diseases that primarily affect the left side of the heart, as in congenital heart diseases." Cor pulmonale is a disease of the right ventricle characterized by hypertrophy and dilation that results from disease directly affecting the lung parenchyma or lung vasculature. Of note, right heart failure need not be present in cor pulmonale.

   Simonneau G, Gahe N, Rubin LJ, et al: Clinical classification of pulmonary hypertension. J Am Coll Cardiol 43:5S–12S, 2004.
   World Health Organization: Chronic cor pulmonale: A report of the expert committee. Circulation 27:594–615, 1963.

2. **What are the subtypes of cor pulmonale?**

   Cor pulmonale can be either acute or chronic in development. Acute cor pulmonale is the result of a sudden increase in right ventricular pressure, as seen in massive pulmonary embolism or acute respiratory distress syndrome. Chronic cor pulmonale can be further characterized by hypoxic or vascular obliterans pathophysiology. The most common disease process associated with hypoxic subtype is chronic obstructive pulmonary disease (COPD). The most common process associated with obliterans subtype is pulmonary thromboembolic disease.

3. **What is the pathophysiology of right ventricular failure?**

   Under normal physiologic conditions, the right ventricle pumps against a low-resistance circuit. Normal pulmonary vascular resistance is approximately one-tenth the resistance of the systemic arteries. The right ventricle is thin walled and able to accommodate considerable changes in volume without large changes in pressure. Increased cardiac output leads to recruitment of underperfused pulmonary vessels and distention of other pulmonary vessels. The initial pathophysiologic event in the production of cor pulmonale is elevation of the pulmonary vascular resistance. As the resistance increases, the pulmonary arterial pressure rises, and right ventricular work increases. As a response to increased right ventricular work, right ventricular hypertrophy (i.e., thickening, dilation, or both) develops. Right ventricular failure occurs when compensation through dilation and hypertrophy are exhausted. Figure 20-1 shows events that contribute to right ventricular failure.

4. **What are the causes of cor pulmonale?**

   Any process that results in pulmonary hypertension can cause cor pulmonale. *Pulmonary hypertension* is defined as mean pulmonary artery pressures > 20 mmHg at rest or > 30 mmHg with exercise. See Table 20-1 for disease processes that cause cor pulmonale.

5. **What is the pathophysiology of pulmonary hypertension?**

   Hypoxic pulmonary vasoconstriction and arterial occlusion are the major causes of pulmonary hypertension; both produce reduced blood flow with increased vascular resistance.

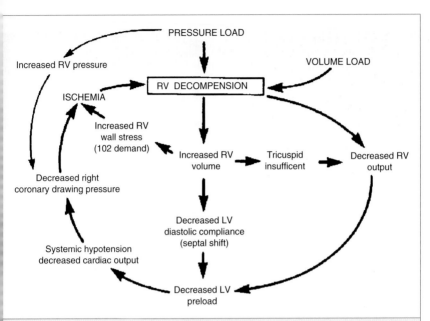

Figure 20-1. Events that contribute to right ventricular (RV) failure. LV = left ventricular. (From Wiedemann HP, Matthay RA: Management of cor pulmonale. In Scharf SM [ed]: Heart-Lung Interactions in Health and Disease. New York, Marcel Dekker, 1989, pp 920–926, with permission.)

Acute hypoxic pulmonary vasoconstriction optimizes ventilation-perfusion relationships when regional ventilation demands in the lung are not met. However, chronic hypoxemia leading to chronic vasoconstriction produces smooth muscle proliferation in the small pulmonary arteries. Decreased luminal cross-sectional diameter leads to increased resistance and increased pulmonary artery pressure. These architectural changes in the pulmonary arteries may promote platelet aggregation and activation, leading to thrombi formation that further increases pulmonary vascular resistance and pulmonary hypertension. Hypoxemia produces changes in vascular mediators such as nitric oxide, endothelin 1 (ET1), and platelet-derived growth factors (PDGF). Nitric oxide is a vasodilator; hypoxemia reduces endothelial cell production of nitric oxide and results in impaired smooth muscle relaxation. Hypoxemia increases ET1 production and PDGF-A and -B. ET1 is a potent vasoconstrictor, and PDGF-A and -B result in pulmonary vascular remodeling. Pulmonary arterial pressure increases at rest are evident when 60% or more of the lung parenchyma is affected.

Dinh-Xuan AT, Higenbottam TW, Clelland CA, et al: Impairment of endothelium dependent pulmonary artery relaxation in chronic obstructive lung disease. N Engl J Med 324:1539–1547, 1991.

Perros F, Dorfmuller P, Humbert M: Current insights on the pathogenesis of pulmonary arterial hypertension. Semin Respir Crit Care Med 26:355–364, 2005.

6. **Discuss the prevalence and incidence of right ventricular hypertrophy and edema in COPD.**
Cor pulmonale is estimated to be responsible for 7–10% of all diagnoses of heart disease. The prevalence of cor pulmonale increases with worsened airflow limitation in COPD. In fact, any disease state that worsens hypercarbia, hypoxemia, and acidemia can contribute to the further development of cor pulmonale. In the United States, 10–30% of all admissions for congestive

TABLE 20-1. CLASSIFICATION OF COR PULMONALE ACCORDING TO CAUSATIVE FACTOR

Category	Example
Diseases affecting the air passages of the lung and alveoli	Chronic obstructive pulmonary disease
	Cystic fibrosis
	Infiltrative or granulomatous defects
	Idiopathic pulmonary fibrosis
	Sarcoidosis
	Pneumoconiosis
	Scleroderma
	Mixed connective tissue disease
	Systemic lupus erythematosus
	Rheumatoid arthritis
	Polymyositis
	Eosinophilic granulomatosis
	Radiation
	Malignant infiltration
Diseases affecting thoracic cage movement	Kyphoscoliosis
	Thoracoplasty
	Neuromuscular weakness
	Sleep apnea syndrome
	Idiopathic hypoventilation
Diseases affecting the pulmonary vasculature	Primary disease of the arterial wall
	Primary pulmonary hypertension
	Pulmonary arteritis
	Toxin-induced pulmonary hypertension
	Chronic liver disease
	Peripheral pulmonary stenosis
Thrombotic disorders	Sickle cell diseases
	Pulmonary microthrombi
Embolic disorders	Thromboembolism
	Tumor embolism
	Other embolic processes (e.g., amniotic fluid, air, fat)
	Schistosomiasis and other parasitic infections
Pressure on pulmonary arteries	Mediastinal tumors
	Aneurysms
	Granulomata
	Fibrosis

Adapted from Rubin LJ (ed): Pulmonary Heart Disease. Boston, Martinus Nijhoff, 1984.

heart failure are due to right ventricular hypertrophy and failure. The prevalence of cor pulmonale in advanced COPD has been estimated to be as high as 66%.

Scharf SM, Iqbal M, Keller C, et al: Hemodynamic characterization of patients with severe emphysema. Am J Respir Crit Care Med 166:314–322, 2002.

7. **What are the symptoms and signs of cor pulmonale?**
The signs and symptoms of cor pulmonale are often subtle unless the disease process becomes far advanced. In addition, clinicians tend to focus on the disease giving rise to cor pulmonale rather than on the cor pulmonale itself. Manifestations of cor pulmonale are similar to those of right heart failure.
Symptoms of cor pulmonale
- Fatigability
- Dyspnea on exertion
- Syncope
- Chest pains
- Palpitations
- Abdominal edema or distention
- Lower extremity edema

Clinical signs of cor pulmonale
- Accentuated A wave of the jugular venous pulsations
- Prominent jugular V wave, indicating the presence of tricuspid regurgitation
- Palpable left parasternal lift
- Accentuated pulmonic component of the second heart sound
- Right-sided S_4 heart sound
- Murmurs of tricuspid and pulmonic insufficiency
- Dependent peripheral edema and hepatomegaly

Auger WA: Pulmonary hypertension and cor pulmonale. Curr Opin Pulmonol Med 4:269–295, 1983.

8. **What is the mortality associated with cor pulmonale?**
Patients with COPD have a 62% 5-year survival rate, whereas patients with COPD and pulmonary artery pressures in excess of 25 mmHg have a 5-year survival of only 36%.
The 5-year survival rate for patients with COPD who develop peripheral edema is approximately 30%. It is unclear whether pulmonary artery hypertension is the cause of death or whether it is a marker of increased mortality.

MacNee W: Pathophysiology of cor pulmonale in chronic obstructive pulmonary disease: Part two. Am J Respir Crit Care Med 150:1158–1168, 1994.
Oswald-Mammosser M, Weitzenblum E, Quoix E, et al: Prognostic factors in COPD patients receiving long-term oxygen therapy: Importance of pulmonary artery pressure. Chest 107:1193–1198, 1995.

9. **What are the electrocardiography (ECG) criteria of right ventricular hypertrophy?**
Cor pulmonale may result in loss of R waves in leads V_{1-3} and/or inferior Q waves with right axis deviation. The following are ECG findings that mimic myocardial infarction either by simulating pathologic Q or QS waves or mimicking the typical ST-T changes of acute myocardial infarction:
- Right axis deviation or rightward shift in axis
- Right atrial enlargement: An increase in the R atrial potential typically translates into a large P wave, P pulmonale, in the inferior and anterior leads. P pulmonale is present in about 20% of patients with clinical evidence of cor pulmonale. COPD can give rise to P pulmonale without evidence of right ventricular hypertrophy.
- Right ventricular hypertrophy: The sensitivity of the ECG in diagnosing right ventricular hypertrophy in patients with chronic cor pulmonale is 60–70% when assessed at autopsy.
- Right bundle-branch block
- Right precordial T-wave inversions

- Delayed intrinsicoid deflection of right precordial leads
- $S_1Q_3T_3$ pattern
- QR pattern in lead V_1 or V_3R
- An R wave in V_1 or V_3R
- An R/S ratio > 1 in V_1 or < 1 in V_5 or V_6
- An R′ in V_1 or $V_3R > 6$ mm or an R′ in $V_1 > 1.0$ (QRS duration < 0.10 second)

    Yanowitz FG: Ventricular hypertrophy. The Alan E. Lindsay ECG Learning Center in Cyberspace: http://library.med.utah.edu/kw/ecg/ecg_outline/Lesson8/index.html

10. **What tests can help determine the diagnosis of cor pulmonale?**
    - **Chest radiograph:** Radiographic signs include an enlarged pulmonary artery and/or right ventricle, a distended azygous or other central vein, oligemia of a lung lobe or entire lung (Westermark sign), and a wedge-shaped opacity (Hampton's hump). In addition, the common findings associated with COPD may be seen, including increased anterior-posterior diameter, flattening of the diaphragms, honeycombing, and hyperlucency.
    - **Computed tomography:** Main pulmonary artery diameter measurements ≥ 29 mm have a sensitivity of 84% and a specificity of 75% for diagnosis of pulmonary hypertension. There are data to suggest that an enlarged main pulmonary artery diameter and a ratio of segmental pulmonary artery diameter to corresponding bronchus diameter > 1 increases the specificity of a pulmonary hypertension diagnosis.
    - **Echocardiography:** An adequate examination is reported in up to 65–80% of patients with COPD because of the technical difficulty associated with hyperinflation. A better examination can be obtained with transesophageal echocardiography. Doppler echocardiography has aided in the assessment of pulmonary artery pressures by measuring the flow of regurgitant blood across the tricuspid valve or by measuring right ventricular ejection flow.
    - **Right heart cardiac catheterization:** This is the gold standard for thorough evaluation and diagnosis of pulmonary hypertension.
    - **Radionuclide angiography (gated blood pool scan):** This test is most useful for measuring right and left ventricular ejection fraction.
    - **Magnetic resonance imaging:** This noninvasive technique yields highly accurate dimensions of the right ventricle.

        American College of Cardiology/American Heart Association Guidelines for the Clinical Application of Echocardiography—IX. Pulmonary Disease. 95:1686–1744, 1997: www.americanheart.org/presenter.jhtml?identifier=8459
        Falaschi F, Palla A, Formichi B, et al: CT evaluation of chronic thromboembolic pulmonary hypertension. J Comput Assist Tomogr 16:897–903, 1992.

11. **What are the indications for the use of echocardiography in the evaluation of cor pulmonale?**
    See Box 20-1.

12. **Discuss nonpharmacologic treatment options for patients with cor pulmonale.**
    - **Oxygen therapy:** This is considered a mainstay of treatment for patients with COPD. Large controlled trials demonstrate that long-term administration of oxygen improves survival in hypoxemic patients with COPD. Oxygen therapy decreases pulmonary vascular resistance by diminishing pulmonary vasoconstriction and improves right ventricular stroke volume and cardiac output.
    - **Phlebotomy:** In patients with pronounced polycythemia (hematocrit $> 60\%$), phlebotomy may provide symptomatic relief. In resting patients, phlebotomy can affect a mild decrease in pulmonary artery pressure and pulmonary vascular resistance. In general, blood viscosity has less effect than blood volume on pulmonary arterial pressure. Phlebotomy, with a goal hematocrit of 50%, may improve exercise tolerance in patients with polycythemic COPD.

BOX 20-1. RECOMMENDATIONS FOR ECHOCARDIOGRAPHY IN PULMONARY AND PULMONARY VASCULAR DISEASE

Class I

1. Suspected pulmonary hypertension
2. For distinguishing cardiac versus noncardiac etiology of dyspnea in patients in whom all clinical and laboratory clues are ambiguous*
3. Follow-up of pulmonary artery pressures in patients with pulmonary hypertension to evaluate response to treatment
4. Lung disease with clinical suspicion of cardiac involvement (suspected cor pulmonale)

Class IIa

1. Pulmonary emboli and suspected clots in the right atrium or ventricle or main pulmonary artery branches*
2. Measurement of exercise pulmonary artery pressure
3. Patients being considered for lung transplantation or other surgical procedure for advanced lung disease*

Class III

1. Lung disease without any clinical suspicion of cardiac involvement
2. Reevaluation studies of right ventricular function in patients with chronic obstructive lung disease without a change in clinical status

*Transesophageal echocardiography is indicated when transthoracic echocardiographic studies are not diagnostic.
From American College of Cardiology: ACC/AHA/ASE 2003 guideline update for the clinical application of echocardiography: A report of the American College of Cardiology/American Heart Association Task Force on Practice Guidelines. American College of Cardiology Foundation, 2003: www.acc.org/clinical/guidelines/echo/index.pdf

---

Phlebotomy is not an optimal single therapy but can be considered in polycythemic patients with acute decompensation.

- **Noninvasive positive pressure ventilation (NIPPV):** For patients with acute COPD exacerbations, NIPPV has been shown to improve outcomes in acute hospitalization. No such data exist for long-term treatment of COPD or sleep-disordered breathing with NIPPV. There is evidence that oxygenation is improved in these patients, but reduction in pulmonary artery pressure is only anecdotal.

  Criner GJ: Effects of long-term oxygen therapy on mortality and morbidity. Respir Care 45:105–118, 2000.

13. **What are the pharmacologic therapies for patients with cor pulmonale?**
    - **Diuretics:** Diuretic therapy, in conjunction with a salt-restricted diet, may be needed in congestive cardiac failure to take care of the excessive water that the lungs share and to improve alveolar ventilation and gas exchange. However, the use of diuretics may produce hemodynamic adverse effects, such as volume depletion, decreased venous return to the right ventricle, and decreased cardiac output. Another complication is the production of hypokalemic metabolic alkalosis, which diminishes the CO_2 stimulus to the respiratory center, decreasing ventilatory drive.

- **Anticoagulation:** Chronic anticoagulation with warfarin may provide benefit for those patients with cor pulmonale resulting from thrombo-occlusive pulmonary disease.
- **Vasodilators:** Vasodilators improve cardiac output in many patients with cor pulmonale. However, treatment with vasodilators may be associated with adverse effects, including systemic hypotension that compromises coronary perfusion pressure, blunting of hypoxic pulmonary vasoconstriction, and circulatory collapse.

14. **Discuss the different classes of vasodilators used in the treatment of cor pulmonale.**
    Nonspecific vasodilators
    - Hydralazine increases cardiac output in patients with COPD; however, its ability to decrease pulmonary artery pressure is unpredictable.
    - Nitroprusside may provide benefit but also runs the risk of systemic hypotension and compromise of adequate coronary perfusion pressure.
    - Calcium channel blockers such as nifedipine reduce pulmonary vascular resistance and increase cardiac output only for the short term. Verapamil and diltiazem have not proved effective in dilating pulmonary vasculature.

    Pulmonary vasodilators
    - Prostaglandins decrease pulmonary artery pressure and increase right ventricular ejection fraction and cardiac output. Aerosolized prostacyclin causes pulmonary artery vasodilation and improves cardiac output and arterial oxyhemoglobin saturation in patients with chronic pulmonary hypertension.
    - Nitric oxide provides the ideal clinical scenario. It reliably decreases pulmonary vascular resistance without causing systemic hypotension and preserves or improves optimal ventilation–perfusion match. Its drawbacks are difficult administration, high cost, and a well-documented tachyphylactic effect. Multiple studies have shown that its benefits are most significant for only 1–3 days, especially in patients with acute respiratory distress syndrome.

    Inotropes with vasodilatory properties
    - Dobutamine is an inotropic agent with vasodilatory properties. Dobutamine improves right ventricular function and cardiac output, but its effect on systemic blood pressure is unpredictable. Repeat echocardiography after the institution of therapy can help to guide management. However, the effects of dobutamine (and other beta agonists, including isoproterenol and epinephrine) on pulmonary arterial pressure may be minimal and unsustained.
    - Although few data are available about its action in right heart syndrome, amrinone lowers pulmonary arterial pressure and raises cardiac output and systemic blood pressure.

    Endothelin receptor antagonist
    - Bosentan is an endothelin receptor antagonist that produces pulmonary vasodilation and attenuates ventricular remodeling when used as a chronic treatment. Studies have shown improved survival with chronic treatment.

    Lehrman S, Romano P, Frishman W, et al: Primary pulmonary hypertension and cor pulmonale. Cardiol Rev 10:265–278, 2002.
    Pulmonary Hypertension Association: Treatments. 2006: www.phassociation.org/Learn/treatment/index.asp
    Romano PM, Peterson S: The management of cor pulmonale. Heart Dis 2:431–437, 2000.

15. **Is left ventricular function impaired in chronic cor pulmonale?**
    Left ventricular dysfunction has been documented in patients with cor pulmonale. Approximately 20% of patients with severe pulmonary disease have been shown to have left ventricular dysfunction. The proposed mechanism is bulging of the ventricular septum toward the left ventricle as a result of right ventricular overload. Bowing of the ventricular septum decreases left ventricular compliance and reduces cardiac output. This interplay between right and left

ventricles is perhaps best supported by the recovery of left ventricular as well as right ventricular function in patients who have undergone lung transplantation.

Vizza CD, Lynch JP, Ochoa LL, et al: Right and left ventricular dysfunction in patients with severe pulmonary disease. Chest 113:576–583, 1998.

16. **Should digoxin be used in the treatment of COPD?**
Cardiac output improves in about 10% of patients with primary pulmonary hypertension who receive digoxin. This rate is similar to that in patients with left ventricular dysfunction. Patients who receive digoxin also show a modest increase in pulmonary pressure, perhaps due to increased cardiac output. Clinical studies show improvement in right ventricular function only in those patients who have reduced left ventricular ejection fraction. Recently, digoxin has fallen out of favor in the setting of left ventricular dysfunction; the trend in clinical medicine has been its continued use in rate control.

Mathur PN, Powles AC, Pugsley SO, et al: Effect of long-term administration of digoxin on exercise performance in chronic airflow limitation. Eur J Respir Dis 66:273–283, 1985.

17. **Discuss the considerations for ventilator management of patients with cor pulmonale.**
Hypercarbia and acidemia as well as hypoxemia increase pulmonary artery pressure. Therefore, adequate ventilation and oxygenation are critical in the management of patients with cor pulmonale. The effect of positive end-expiratory pressure (PEEP) on right ventricular function is complex and varies from patient to patient; it also depends on the level of PEEP. Clearly, higher levels of PEEP are more likely to impair right ventricular function. It is believed that PEEP used for recruiting atelectatic areas of lung, thereby improving the compliance curve, should have no deleterious effects on right ventricular function. However, if normal areas of the lung are overdistended, right ventricular function may be compromised.

KEY POINTS: COR PULMONALE

1. Right heart failure is not necessary to make the diagnosis of cor pulmonale.

2. Any process that results in pulmonary hypertension can cause cor pulmonale.

3. Chronic obstructive lung disease is the most common cause of chronic cor pulmonale.

4. Cor pulmonale is common in advanced obstructive lung disease and has a poor 5-year survival rate.

5. Ventricular interdependence can develop in late stages of cor pulmonale.

CHAPTER 21

ACUTE RESPIRATORY FAILURE

Dan Burkhardt, MD, and Martin R. Zamora, MD

1. **What is meant by *acute respiratory failure* (ARF)?**

   ARF occurs when the respiratory system is unable to either adequately absorb oxygen (i.e., hypoxemia) or excrete carbon dioxide (i.e., hypercarbia). Although both hypoxemia and hypercarbia can occur together, one process frequently predominates. ARF may occur suddenly or as a gradual process. It can occur in both healthy patients and those with chronic pulmonary disease.

2. **How is ARF defined by arterial blood gas (ABG) analysis?**

   Although no rigid criteria apply for all patients, it is generally accepted that hypoxemic respiratory failure is present when the arterial PO_2 is less than 50 mmHg when breathing room air. Hypercarbic ARF is present when PCO_2 is greater than 50 mmHg and the arterial pH is acidotic (pH < 7.30). Hypercarbia in the presence of a normal or alkalotic arterial (pH ≥ 7.40) is a normal compensatory reaction and does not constitute ARF.

3. **How can ventilation (i.e., carbon dioxide excretion) be assessed noninvasively?**

   There is no widely available noninvasive test that can accurately assess the adequacy of carbon dioxide excretion. Transcutaneous or end-tidal carbon dioxide analyzers are available, but their accuracy can be poor in certain circumstances. An abnormally low or high respiratory rate can suggest that hypercarbic respiratory failure is present, but a normal or high respiratory rate cannot exclude the diagnosis. ABG analysis remains the gold standard for the diagnosis of hypercarbic ARF.

   Gattas D, Ayer R, Suntharalingam G, Chapman M: Carbon dioxide monitoring and evidence-based practice—now you see it, now you don't. Crit Care 8:219–221, 2004.

   Soubani AO: Noninvasive monitoring of oxygen and carbon dioxide. Am J Emerg Med 19:141–146, 2001.

4. **What are the physiologic mechanisms of hypoxemic ARF? Which are reversible with supplemental oxygen?**

   - Low mixed venous oxygen
   - Alveolar hypoventilation
   - Ventilation perfusion mismatch
   - Right-to-left shunt
   - Diffusion limitation
   - Low inspired oxygen fraction (e.g., high altitude)

   Most of these physiologic mechanisms are reversible with supplemental oxygen, with the exception of shunt. Because shunting occurs when blood travels from the venous to systemic arterial circulation without passing through ventilated lung, changes in inspired oxygen concentration will not affect the shunted blood.

   Greene KE, Peters JI: Pathophysiology of acute respiratory failure. Clin Chest Med 15:1–12, 1994.

   Levy MM: Pathophysiology of oxygen delivery in respiratory failure. Chest 128(5 Suppl 2): 547S–553S, 2005.

5. **What physiologic processes can cause hypercapnic ARF?**
    Hypercapnia is the result of alveolar hypoventilation. Mechanisms responsible may be:
    - Central-decreased respiratory drive
    - Neuromuscular-decreased neural transmission or muscular translation of the drive signal
    - Abnormalities of the chest wall
    - Abnormalities of the lungs and airways

    Greene KE, Peters JI: Pathophysiology of acute respiratory failure. Clin Chest Med 15:1–12, 1994.

6. **Which disease processes are associated with each type of ARF? Which are reversible?**
    The differential diagnosis of hypoxemic ARF can be delineated based on whether there is concomitant hypercapnia and whether infiltrates are seen on the chest radiograph. If the patient is normocapnic and the chest x-ray result is normal (i.e., "clear"), pulmonary embolus, circulatory collapse, or right-to-left shunt is likely. If the chest radiograph displays diffuse infiltrates, acute respiratory distress syndrome (ARDS), cardiogenic pulmonary edema, or pulmonary fibrosis is possible. If focal infiltrates are present, the patient may have pneumonia, atelectasis, or pulmonary infarction. If the chest radiograph is clear in patients with hypercapnia, then status asthmaticus, chronic obstructive pulmonary disease (COPD), or alveolar hypoventilation resulting from drug overdose, neuromuscular weakness, paralysis, or sleep apnea syndrome is likely. If the chest radiograph shows diffuse infiltrates, end-stage pulmonary fibrosis or severe ARDS is possible, whereas if the findings are localized, the patient could have pneumonia with underlying COPD or respiratory depression resulting from drugs or oxygen therapy. In general, most of the previously mentioned disease processes are reversible. However, severe COPD, sleep apnea syndrome, diseases of the respiratory muscles, cervical fracture leading to paralysis, and kyphoscoliosis may lead to chronic carbon dioxide retention and chronic respiratory failure. In patients with these underlying disorders, ARF due to other etiologies may occur and should be investigated.

    Bartter TC, Irwin RS: Respiratory failure. Part I: A physiologic approach to managing respiratory failure. In Irwin RS, Rippe JM (eds): Irwin & Rippe's Intensive Care Medicine, ed 5. Philadelphia, Lippincott Williams & Wilkins, 2003, pp 485–488.

7. **What empiric therapy should be used emergently in patients with hypoxemic ARF?**
    Raising the PO_2 to greater than 50 mmHg is the first goal of therapy. If the patient is alert and cooperative, supplemental oxygen and close observation in the intensive care unit may be adequate. Pulse oximetry or repeat arterial blood gas analysis should be monitored frequently to assess the adequacy of therapy. If the patient is stuporous or comatose or has a decreased gag reflex, then control of the airway by endotracheal intubation is warranted. In the case of suspected opiate overdose (e.g., respiratory depression, pinpoint pupils, and coma), naloxone should be administered.

    Bartter TC, Irwin RS: Respiratory failure. Part I: A physiologic approach to managing respiratory failure. In Irwin RS, Rippe JM (eds): Irwin & Rippe's Intensive Care Medicine, ed 5. Philadelphia, Lippincott Williams & Wilkins, 2003, pp 485–488.

8. **What are the indications for endotracheal intubation?**
    - Cardiopulmonary resuscitation with the need for complete control of the airway
    - Airway protection from aspiration of gastric contents
    - Need for mechanical ventilation
    - Control of copious airway secretions
    - Complete upper airway obstruction

9. **What are the indications for mechanical ventilation?**
   Mechanical ventilation is required whenever the patient is unable to maintain adequate alveolar oxygenation or ventilation. Even in the setting of a normal PO_2 and PCO_2, excessive work of breathing may eventually lead to respiratory muscle fatigue and failure, thus necessitating mechanical ventilation. The decision for intubation and mechanical ventilation should be based on the clinical appearance of the patient and blood gas analysis results. Mechanical ventilation can also be used to provide hyperventilation to patients with head trauma to reduce intracranial pressure for the first 24–48 hours. An alternative to endotracheal intubation in patients with sufficient mental status to protect their airways is noninvasive positive pressure ventilation.

   Caples SM, Gay PC: Noninvasive positive pressure ventilation in the intensive care unit: A concise review. Crit Care Med 33:2651–2658, 2005.

   Fan E, Needham DM, Stewart TE: Ventilatory management of acute lung injury and acute respiratory distress syndrome. JAMA 294:2889–2896, 2005.

10. **What is positive end-expiratory pressure (PEEP)? When should it be used?**
    PEEP is a technique used to mechanically correct hypoxemia by increasing lung volume. PEEP increases the expiratory threshold pressure, which prevents the patient's airway pressure from falling below a preset level during the respiratory cycle. This increases the volume of gas in the patient's chest at end-expiration (i.e., functional residual capacity). The treatment would therefore be expected to be beneficial in patients with restrictive lung diseases such as ARDS because the hypoxemia in this disorder may be due to alveolar collapse, filling, or both.

11. **What is the significance of the patient who is "fighting the ventilator"?**
    The sudden onset of agitation and distress in a patient who previously was tolerating mechanical ventilation is a medical emergency and may signify acute deterioration in the underlying disease, malfunction of the ventilator, obstruction of the airway or endotracheal tube, or inadequate sedation. The patient should be disconnected from the ventilator and manually ventilated. Vital signs should be obtained, the chest examined, the airway suctioned, and ABG analysis and chest x-ray performed. If no etiology is found after these measures are taken, the ventilator setup may be incorrect for the patient's needs. Changes in the ventilator settings are appropriate so as to more closely match the machine to the patient's requirements. Increased sedation should usually only be used if other measures have failed.

12. **When can patients be weaned from mechanical ventilation?**
    Patients' health should be clinically improved with stabilization and correction of any underlying conditions that may interfere with weaning (e.g., electrolyte disturbances, fluid overload, severe anemia, or severe pain requiring analgesics or sedatives). Patients should be alert with stable vital signs and should have an intact gag reflex. Some physiologic guidelines that can be used include the following: $PO_2 > 60$ mmHg with the $FiO_2 < 50\%$ and PEEP = 0–5 cm H_2O, respiratory rate < 20, vital capacity > 10–15 mL/kg, tidal volume > 5 mL/kg, minute ventilation (VE) < 10 L/min, and negative inspiratory force of > -25 cm H_2O. No single physiologic variable can completely predict the success of a trial of ventilator liberation. Some clinicians advocate the use of frequent protocol-driven spontaneous breathing trials. A composite variable such as the rapid shallow breathing index (i.e., respiratory rate/tidal volume < 100–130 breaths/min/L) can be used to assess the adequacy of pulmonary function during these trials.

    Ely EW, Meade MO, Haponik EF, et al: Mechanical ventilator weaning protocols driven by nonphysician health-care professionals: Evidence-based clinical practice guidelines. Chest 120(6 Suppl):454S–463S, 2001.

13. **What are some postextubation complications?**
    - Hoarseness
    - Difficulty swallowing and risk of aspiration
    - Severe glottic edema leading to airway obstruction (may be treated with racemic epinephrine 0.5 mL/3 mL saline via nebulized aerosol)

KEY POINTS: ACUTE RESPIRATORY FAILURE

1. The mechanisms involved in acute hypercapnic respiratory failure include decreased central drive to breathe, weakness of respiratory muscles, abnormalities of the chest wall, and abnormalities of the lung and airways.

2. Mechanical ventilation needs to be initiated when the patient is too weak to breathe or the work of breathing is too excessive.

3. Hoarseness, difficulty swallowing, and glottic edema can occur after the endotracheal tube is removed.

BIBLIOGRAPHY

1. Acute Respiratory Distress Syndrome Network: Ventilation with lower tidal volumes as compared with traditional tidal volumes for acute lung injury and the acute respiratory distress syndrome. N Engl J Med 342:1301–1308, 2000.

2. Bartter TC, Irwin RS: Respiratory failure. Part I: A physiologic approach to managing respiratory failure. In Irwin RS, Rippe JM (eds): Irwin & Rippe's Intensive Care Medicine, ed 5. Philadelphia, Lippincott Williams & Wilkins, 2003, pp 485–488.

3. Caples SM, Gay PC: Noninvasive positive pressure ventilation in the intensive care unit: A concise review. Crit Care Med 33:2651–2658, 2005.

4. Ely EW, Meade MO, Haponik EF, et al: Mechanical ventilator weaning protocols driven by nonphysician health-care professionals: Evidence-based clinical practice guidelines. Chest 120(6 Suppl):454S–463S, 2001.

5. Fan E, Needham DM, Stewart TE: Ventilatory management of acute lung injury and acute respiratory distress syndrome. JAMA 294:2889–2896, 2005.

6. Gattas D, Ayer R, Suntharalingam G, Chapman M: Carbon dioxide monitoring and evidence-based practice—now you see it, now you don't. Crit Care 8:219–221, 2004.

7. Greene KE, Peters JI: Pathophysiology of acute respiratory failure. Clin Chest Med 15:1–12, 1994.

8. Levy MM: Pathophysiology of oxygen delivery in respiratory failure. Chest 128(5 Suppl 2):547S–553S, 2005.

9. MacIntyre NR: Current issues in mechanical ventilation for respiratory failure. Chest 128(5 Suppl 2):561S–567S, 2005.

10. MacIntyre NR, Cook DJ, Ely EW, et al: Evidence-based guidelines for weaning and discontinuing ventilatory support: A collective task force facilitated by the American College of Chest Physicians; the American Association for Respiratory Care; and the American College of Critical Care Medicine. Chest 120(6 Suppl):375S–395S, 2001.

11. Mellies U, Dohna-Schwake C, Voit T: Respiratory function assessment and intervention in neuromuscular disorders. Curr Opin Neurol 18:543–547, 2005.

12. Shneerson JM, Simonds AK: Noninvasive ventilation for chest wall and neuromuscular disorders. Eur Respir J 20:480–487, 2002.

13. Soubani AO: Noninvasive monitoring of oxygen and carbon dioxide. Am J Emerg Med 19:141–146, 2001.

14. Ware LB, Matthay MA: The acute respiratory distress syndrome. N Engl J Med 342:1334–1349, 2000.

CHAPTER 22

ACUTE RESPIRATORY DISTRESS SYNDROME

Kapilkumar Patel, MD, and Polly E. Parsons, MD

1. What is acute respiratory distress syndrome (ARDS)?

ARDS is a noncardiogenic pulmonary capillary leak syndrome characterized clinically by the development of rapidly progressive hypoxemia, diffuse alveolar infiltrates on chest x-ray, and decreased lung compliance after a known predisposing insult. Pathologically, the syndrome is characterized acutely by alveolar and interstitial edema and flooding of the alveoli with a proteinaceous exudate and inflammatory cells, including neutrophils and macrophages, followed by the development of pulmonary fibrosis.

2. How is the diagnosis of ARDS made?

The diagnostic criteria for ARDS continue to be refined. Although the pathologic findings are objective and can be agreed on, most patients do not undergo lung biopsy. The diagnosis is made clinically. The following criteria developed by the American-European Consensus Conference are currently used:

- Bilateral infiltrates identified on chest radiograph
- $PaO_2/FiO_2 < 200$
- No evidence of left atrial hypertension (or, if measured, pulmonary artery wedge pressure [PCWP] < 18 mmHg)

These criteria should be applied only to patients with a defined risk factor for ARDS and without evidence of severe chronic pulmonary disease.

Bernard GR, Artigas A, Brigham K, et al: The American European consensus conference on ARDS: Definitions, mechanisms, relevant outcomes and clinical trial coordination. Am J Respir Crit Care Med 149:818–824, 1994.

3. What is acute lung injury (ALI)?

Traditional definitions of ARDS do not include patients with mild or early evidence of ALI. Accordingly, the following criteria have been established to identify such patients:

- Bilateral infiltrates identified on chest radiograph
- $PaO_2/FiO_2 < 300$
- No evidence of left atrial hypertension (or, if measured, PCWP < 18 mmHg)

Again, these patients should have a defined risk factor for ALI and not have severe chronic pulmonary disease.

KEY POINTS: AMERICAN-EUROPEAN CONSENSUS DEFINITION OF ARDS

1. Patient experiences acute onset of disease.

2. PaO_2 divided by FiO_2 is less than 200.

3. Bilateral pulmonary infiltrates are consistent with pulmonary edema on chest x-ray.

4. No evidence of left atrial hypertension is present.

4. **What is the role of pulmonary artery catheters in the diagnosis and management of ALI/ARDS?**
   Pulmonary artery catheters are no longer necessary to make the diagnosis of ALI/ARDS. The consensus definition previously discussed indicates that, if the PCWP is measured, it should be < 18 mmHg in ALI/ARDS. Of note, however, recent studies have suggested that in patients who clinically otherwise meet criteria for ALI/ARDS, a significant percentage of them will have PCPW of 18–25 mmHg. There is ongoing discussion about how to classify this group of patients.

   The role of the pulmonary artery catheter in the management of ALI/ARDS remains under investigation. Recent trials in critically ill patients have shown no improvement in mortality with the use of pulmonary artery catheters.

   Richard C, Warszawski J, Anguel N, et al: Early use of the pulmonary artery catheter and outcomes in patients with shock and acute respiratory distress syndrome: A randomized controlled trial. JAMA 290:2713–2720, 2003.
   Shah MR, Hasselblad V, Stevenson LW, et al: Impact of the pulmonary artery catheter in critically ill patients: Meta-analysis of randomized clinical trials. JAMA 13:1664–1670, 2005.
   Ware LB, Matthay MA: Acute pulmonary edema. N Engl J Med 353:2788–2796, 2005.

5. **What is multiple-organ dysfunction syndrome?**
   The cascade of inflammatory events that results in ALI can also injure other organs, resulting in multiple-organ dysfunction syndrome. The other organs commonly involved include the kidney, central nervous system, liver, cardiovascular system, and hematologic system.

6. **How does ALI/ARDS appear radiographically?**
   See Fig. 22-1.

7. **What conditions predispose a patient to ARDS?**
   Several clinical syndromes, including sepsis, aspiration of gastric contents, trauma, pancreatitis, massive transfusions (within 24 hours), inhalation injury, drug overdose, and near drowning, have been identified as predisposing risk factors for ALI/ARDS. Sepsis is the most common, with an incidence of ALI/ARDS of approximately 40%. In addition, comorbid conditions can affect the development of ALI/ARDS. For example, alcohol abuse increases the incidence of

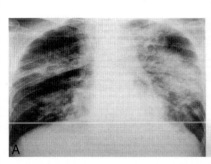
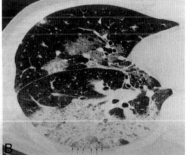

Figure 22-1. *A,* Chest radiograph shows extensive air space consolidation and ground glass opacities. ***B,*** High-resolution computed tomography image of the right lung demonstrates ground glass opacities and air space consolidation mainly in the dorsal lung regions. Also noted is a reticular pattern superimposed on the ground glass opacities (i.e., a "crazy paving" appearance). (From Muller NL, Fraser RS, Lee KS, Johkoh T: Disease of the Lung: Radiologic and Pathologic Correlations. Philadelphia, Lippincott Williams & Wilkins, 2003, with permission.)

ARDS in patients at risk, whereas diabetes mellitus decreases the incidence of ARDS in patients with sepsis. The mechanism for this observation is under investigation.

Moss M, Burnham EL: Chronic alcohol abuse, acute respiratory distress syndrome, and multiple organ dysfunction. Crit Care Med 31:S207–S212, 2003.

8. **Explain the pathogenesis of ARDS.**
   The pathogenesis of ARDS is complex, and understanding of the process continues to evolve. ARDS is initiated by the systemic release of mediators (e.g., complement fragments [specifically, C5a], endotoxin, tumor necrosis factor) that activate/stimulate neutrophils, macrophages, and platelets (and perhaps other cell types) to become sequestered within the pulmonary capillaries and release toxic products such as oxygen metabolites, proteases, and leukotrienes. This inflammatory process results in injury manifested as the loss of integrity of the components of the alveolar capillary barrier, the microvascular endothelium, and the alveolar epithelium and the development of microthrombi. As a result, edema fluid, rich in protein, accumulates with in the interstitial and alveolar spaces. In many patients, as the inflammation subsides the lung is able to repair itself. Other patients, however, have a prolonged course with the development of fibrosis. This is often referred to as *fibroproliferation.*

Bernard GR: Acute respiratory distress syndrome. Am J Respir Crit Care Med 172:798–806, 2005.
Pittet JF, Mackersie RC, Martin TR, Matthay MA: Biological markers of acute lung injury: Prognostic and pathologic significance. Am J Respir Crit Care Med 155:1187–1205, 1997.
Ware BL, Matthay MA: The acute respiratory distress syndrome. N Engl J Med 342:1334–1348, 2000.

9. **Why do patients with ARDS die?**
   Less than 10% of deaths in patients with ARDS are due to hypoxic respiratory failure. The majority of deaths that occur within 72 hours result from the original precipitating insult, whereas after 72 hours mortality is often related to infection.

10. **What is the mortality rate associated with ARDS?**
    When ARDS was first described in 1967, the mortality rate was 58%. In the past decade, the mortality rate has decreased to approximately 25–30% (28-day mortality). Survival has been shown to vary with risk factors (sepsis > trauma) and comorbid and preexisting conditions, such as age and alcohol consumption.

Milberg JA, Davis DA, Steinberg KP, et al: Improved survival of patients with acute respiratory distress syndrome (ARDS): 1983–1993. JAMA 273:306–309, 1995.
Rubenfeld GD, Cladwell E, Peabody E, Weaver J, et al: Incidence and outcomes of acute lung injury. N Engl J Med 353:1685–1693, 2005.

11. **How quickly does ARDS develop?**
    ARDS develops in approximately 80% of patients within 24 hours of onset of a predisposing condition and in 95% within 72 hours.

12. **Can ARDS be prevented?**
    No. The precipitating clinical disorder must be prevented.

13. **What therapy is available for the treatment of ARDS?**
    Currently no specific therapy is effective for ARDS, although several agents, including steroids, prostaglandin E_1, *N*-acetylcysteine, surfactant replacement, antiendotoxin antibodies, antitumor necrosis factor antibodies, ketoconazole, lisofylline, antithrombin, heparin, tissue factor pathway inhibitor, factor VIIa, and nitric oxide have been tried. However, new therapeutic modalities with significant potential continue to be developed.

Artigas A, Bernard GR, et al: The American-European consensus conference on ARDS. Part 2: Ventilatory, pharmacologic, supportive therapy, study design strategies, and issues related to recovery and remodeling. Am J Respir Crit Care Med 157:818–824, 1998.
McIntyre RC Jr, Pulido EJ, et al: Thirty years of clinical trials in acute respiratory distress syndrome. Crit Care Med 28:3314–3330, 2000.

14. **How can pneumonia be diagnosed in patients with ARDS?**
This is an area of intense discussion. The clinical diagnosis is generally based on the development of new infiltrates on chest radiograph, purulent sputum, fever, and peripheral leukocytosis. However, an autopsy study of patients with ARDS demonstrated that 80% of patients without pneumonia had fever and leukocytosis and 70% had purulent sputum. Thus, clinical parameters alone do not appear to be adequate. The other tools available include bronchoscopy with lavage, protected brush sampling, transbronchial biopsy, and open lung biopsy. The sensitivity and specificity of these procedures in patients with ARDS are not well defined. The keys to diagnosis are constant surveillance and a low threshold for evaluating and treating the patient.

15. **What are the sequelae in survivors of ARDS?**
Surprisingly, some survivors are virtually unimpaired 1 year after an episode of ARDS despite evidence of pulmonary fibrosis early in the disease course and prolonged mechanical ventilation with high positive end-expiratory pressure (PEEP) and FiO_2. However, a select few have persistent physical functional disability. The limitation is not only related to pulmonary dysfunction, but to extrapulmonary involvement (especially musculoskeletal) as well. Also, the quality of life following ARDS may be related to the preexisting comorbidities. As the number of survivors continues to increase, more research is focused on determining the long-term sequelae, and support groups have developed for patients and their families.

   Acute Respiratory Distress Syndrome Support Center: www.ards.org
   Herridge MS, Cheung AM, Tansey CM, et al: One year outcomes in survivors of the acute respiratory distress syndrome. N Engl J Med 348:683–693, 2003.
   Heyland DK, Groll D, Caeser M: Survivors of acute respiratory distress syndrome: Relationship between pulmonary dysfunction and long-term health-related quality of life. Crit Care Med 33:1549–1556, 2005.

16. **Describe the appropriate fluid management for a patient with ARDS.**
At present, there is no definitive approach to fluid management. Although improvement in oxygenation has been demonstrated with net-negative fluid balance, there has been no clear benefit in mortality. Currently, the U.S. National Institutes of Health ARDS Network is conducting a randomized, prospective, multicenter trial assessing fluid management strategies in patients with ALI/ARDS.

   ARDSNet, National Institutes of Health Acute Respiratory Distress Syndrome Clinical Network: www.ardsnet.org
   Martin GS, Moss M, Wheeler AP, et al: A randomized, controlled trial of furosemide with or without albumin in hypoproteinemic patients with acute lung injury. Crit Care Med 33:1681–1687, 2005.

17. **How should patients with ARDS be ventilated?**
The lung injury in ARDS is not homogeneous. Some areas of apparently normal lung are evident on computed tomographic scan even when the lungs appear to be diffusely involved on chest radiography. In animal models, overdistention of normal lung has been associated with the development of inflammation and alveolar flooding. These and other data suggest that patients should be ventilated with low tidal volumes. This approach was recently confirmed by a study performed by the ARDS Network, which compared tidal volumes of 12 mL/kg versus 6 mL/kg predicted body weight. The mortality rate was 39.8% for the 12-mL group and 31% for the 6-mL group. This study strongly suggests that patients with ALI/ARDS should be ventilated with low tidal volumes. In addition, PEEP has been known to improve oxygenation and lung compliance and aid in recruitment maneuvers. Although PEEP is used universally to support patients with ALI/ARDS, the optimal pressures needed to have an impact on survival have not been proved.

   Acute Respiratory Distress Syndrome Network: Ventilation with lower tidal volumes as compared with traditional tidal volumes for acute lung injury and the acute respiratory distress syndrome. N Engl J Med 342:1301–1307, 2000.

Brower RG, Lanken PN, MacIntyre N, et al, for the National Heart, Lung, and Blood Institute ARDS Clinical Trials Network: Higher versus lower positive end-expiratory pressures in patients with the acute respiratory distress syndrome. N Engl J Med 351:327–336, 2004.

18. **What is the effect of prone positioning on the survival of patients with ALI/ARDS?**
To date, results of multicenter trials are inconclusive with regard to the role of prone positioning in ALI/ARDS. In recently completed large clinical trials comparing patients ventilated in a prone versus supine position, prone positioning was associated with an improvement in oxygenation but no improvement in mortality rates.

Gattinoni L, Tognoni G, Pesenti A, et al: Effects of prone positioning on the survival patients with acute respiratory failure. N Engl J Med 345:568–573, 2001.

Guerin C, Gaillard S, Lemasson S, et al: Effects of systematic prone positioning in hypoxemic acute respiratory failure: A randomized controlled trial. JAMA 292:2379–2387, 2004.

19. **Is there a role for steroids in ARDS?**
Steroids clearly do not prevent the development of ARDS when administered to at-risk patients and do not improve mortality rates in patients with early ARDS. The use of steroids to treat persistent ARDS is currently debated.

Patients with persistent ARDS, also known as the *fibroproliferative phase of ARDS*, have ongoing inflammation that is potentially responsive to steroid therapy. The existence of the fibroproliferative phase of ARDS is relatively well accepted, and clinical studies suggest that the phase is characterized by a persistent inflammatory response (both systemic and pulmonary) and a corresponding fibroproliferative response in the lung. Several small, uncontrolled patient series suggest that the administration of steroids during this fibroproliferative phase improves mortality. A large randomized trial of steroids in late ARDS was recently completed by the ARDS Network. Preliminary results presented indicate no difference in mortality; however, other variables are being assessed.

Jantz MA, Sahn SA: Corticosteroids in acute respiratory failure. Am J Respir Crit Care Med 160:1079–1100, 1999.

CHAPTER 23

ASPIRATION

Derek Haerle, MD, and Thomas J. Donnelly, MD

1. **What is aspiration?**
   Aspiration is the inhalation of material into the airway past the level of the true vocal cords.

2. **Describe the normal host defense mechanisms against aspiration.**
   Coordination of volitional swallowing is primarily a brain stem function with modification by higher cortical centers. It is composed of oral, pharyngeal, and esophageal phases that serve to prepare the bolus, close the nasopharynx and larynx, relax the upper esophageal sphincter, and move the bolus from the upper esophagus to the stomach. Additional airway protective mechanisms are referred to as *basal mechanisms* and *response mechanisms*. Basal mechanisms include the lower (LES) and upper esophageal sphincters, whereas response mechanisms involve a series of reflexes that protect the airway in response to mechanical stretch of the esophagus or stimulation of the pharynx. Respiratory tract defenses include cilia, mucus production, lymphoid tissue, and cough. Esophageal defenses include the integrity of the LES, baseline tone, and peristalsis. Gastric defenses involve the emptying of liquids and include fundic tone, antral contractions, and pyloric tone.

   McClave SA, DeMeo MT, DeLegge MH, et al: North American Summit on Aspiration in the Critically Ill Patient: Consensus statement. J Parenter Enteral Nutr 26:S80–S85, 2002.

3. **Which patients are at risk for aspiration?**
   The risk factors for aspiration can be divided into five categories:
   - **Altered level of consciousness:** Alcohol or drug use, cerebrovascular accident, central nervous system infections or tumors, general anesthesia, hypoxia, and metabolic disturbances such as liver failure, sepsis, and uremia
   - **Gastrointestinal diseases:** Ascites, esophageal disorders, gastrointestinal bleeding, malignancy, intestinal obstruction
   - **Mechanical factors:** Endotracheal tubes, tracheostomies, nasoenteric tubes, upper airway tumors
   - **Neuromuscular diseases:** Amyotrophic lateral sclerosis, botulism, Guillain-Barré syndrome, multiple sclerosis, myasthenia gravis, Parkinson's disease, poliomyelitis, polymyositis, vocal cord paralysis
   - **Miscellaneous factors:** Obesity, pregnancy, diabetes, supine patient position

   DeLegge MH: Aspiration pneumonia: Incidence, mortality, and at-risk populations. J Parenter Enteral Nutr 26:S19–S24, 2002.

4. **What mechanisms increase the incidence of aspiration in the setting of the intensive care unit (ICU)?**
   Depression of mental status interferes with swallowing mechanisms and airway protective reflexes through disruption of coordination. The presence of endotracheal intubation or tracheostomy impedes laryngeal elevation and the inflated cuff may impinge on the esophagus, causing partial obstruction. A nasoenteric tube may compromise the integrity of the LES or increase the incidence of transient LES relaxations. Constant stimulation of the trachea in intubated patients may cause mechanical and chemoreceptor desensitization and suppress the cough reflex. Various drugs, sepsis, and pain may slow gastric emptying. Distention of the

proximal stomach, hyperglycemia, sepsis, and many drugs increase the frequency of transient LES relaxations and depress esophageal contractions, leading to increased gastroesophageal reflux.

McClave SA, DeMeo MT, DeLegge MH, et al: North American Summit on Aspiration in the Critically Ill Patient: Consensus statement. J Parenter Enteral Nutr 26:S80–S85, 2002.

5. **What are the major consequences of aspiration?**
   Aspiration can be asymptomatic or cause a variety of syndromes. The consequences of an event depend on the nature and volume of aspirated material and the host response. Large volumes of sterile, nonirritating fluid can be introduced into the airways with minor sequelae. Small volumes of oral secretions are universally aspirated during sleep in healthy persons. Clinically significant aspirations include acidic gastric contents, oropharyngeal bacteria, and particulate matter. Aspiration syndromes include pneumonitis, pneumonia, airway obstruction, atelectasis, bronchospasm, bronchitis, bronchiectasis, hoarseness, lung abscess, pulmonary hemorrhage, interstitial fibrosis, and acute lung injury (ALI)/acute respiratory distress syndrome (ARDS).

6. **What are the results of aspiration of gastric acid?**
   Aspiration of gastric acid may cause immediate and intense injury to the airway and alveolar epithelium. Bronchospasm, pulmonary edema, alveolar collapse due to loss of surfactant, and loss of intravascular fluid volume all occur. ALI/ARDS may occur. Although treatment by neutralization of airway fluids has been attempted, acid instilled into the airways is rapidly absorbed and neutralized, rendering these therapies futile.

7. **Which organisms commonly produce infectious complications in aspiration?**
   The majority of pneumonias result from aspiration of organisms that have colonized the mucosal surfaces of the oropharyngeal airways. The bacteriology of aspiration pneumonia differs based on whether it is community acquired or hospital acquired. During the first week in the ICU, the oropharynx and the stomach become increasingly colonized with more virulent organisms. Normal oral flora (e.g., *Streptococcus pneumoniae, Haemophilus influenzae,* and *Staphylococcus aureus*) are replaced by hospital-acquired resistant gram-negative organisms (e.g., *Pseudomonas aeruginosa, Acinetobacter* species, *Enterobacter* species) and methicillin-resistant *S. aureus*.

Moore FA: Treatment of aspiration in intensive care unit patients. J Parenter Enteral Nutr 26:S69–S74, 2002.

8. **What is lipoid pneumonia?**
   The aspiration of animal fats, mineral oil, or other lipid substances causes an inflammatory response in the lung that is independent of infection. The term *lipoid pneumonia* refers to persistent, alveolar infiltrates that occur after the aspiration of oil. All patients with persistent pulmonary infiltrates should be questioned about the use of oral or nasal lubricants (often oily nose drops). Patients who require a nasal emollient (i.e., patients receiving chronic oxygen therapy by nasal cannula) should be instructed to use only water-based products.

9. **How is aspiration diagnosed?**
   - By a witnessed regurgitation/aspiration event with coughing, choking, and/or expectoration of material
   - By visualization in the larynx, below the true vocal cords, of oropharyngeal secretions, gastric contents, feeding material, or marker by laryngoscopy, barium (videofluoroscopy), or radioisotope (scintigraphy)
   - By finding gastric contents or food particles in tracheal secretions

10. **How should aspiration be treated?**
The treatment of aspiration consists of confirming the diagnosis, providing supportive care, monitoring for clinical consequences, and instituting secondary prevention. Most patients do not need to be intubated. Continuing enteric feeds is not contraindicated, although measures should be taken to reduce further aspiration.

11. **How does one differentiate between aspiration pneumonitis and infectious pneumonia caused by aspiration?**
These two entities are not always clinically distinct. Because the inflammatory response and radiographic consequences (e.g., fever, leukocytosis, leukopenia, left shift, changes in sputum production, hypoxemia, new or worsening infiltrate exhibited on chest radiograph) can be identical in the first hours after an aspiration event, diagnosis has to based on respiratory cultures and clinical course.

McClave SA, DeMeo MT, DeLegge MH, et al: North American Summit on Aspiration in the Critically Ill Patient: Consensus statement. J Parenter Enteral Nutr 26:S80–S85, 2002.

12. **Is this differentiation important (*see* question 11)?**
Yes. Although all patients known to aspirate should receive aggressive pulmonary care to increase lung volumes and clear secretions, early presumptive antibiotics are not always indicated and can result in the selection of resistant organisms. On the other hand, it must be understood that critically ill patients in the ICU are at increased risk of more frequent aspiration for a variety of reasons (see previous discussion). These patients are more likely to have aspiration proceed through the stages of airway contamination to colonization, bronchiolitis, focal pneumonia, and confluent pneumonia.

Moore FA: Treatment of aspiration in intensive care unit patients. J Parenter Enteral Nutr 26:S69–S74, 2002.

13. **When should antibiotic therapy be started?**
Treatment decisions are based on three factors:
- Clinical diagnostic certainty (i.e., definite versus probable)
- Time of onset (i.e., <5 days versus >5 days)
- Whether the patient can tolerate the wrong diagnosis

There is no ideal regimen of antibiotics. When the diagnosis is uncertain, a bronchoscopy with bronchoalveolar lavage or covered brush technique can be performed. Intracellular organisms on Gram stain is diagnostic for pneumonia and should, along with local sensitivity data, guide empiric treatment. Patients who are hypotensive or appear septic may warrant empiric antibiotic therapy. The data from the quantitative cultures will be reliable only if patients have not been taking antibiotics or have been taking antibiotics for 72 hours without changes.

Guidelines for the Management of Adults with Hospital-Acquired, Ventilator-Associated and Healthcare-associated Pneumonia. Am J Respir Crit Care Med 171:388–416, 2005.
Jackson WL, Shorr AF: Update in ventilator-associated pneumonia. Curr Opin Anaesthesiol 19:117–121, 2006.
Moore FA: Treatment of aspiration in intensive care unit patients. J Parenter Enteral Nutr 26:S69–S74, 2002.

14. **What strategies can be used to prevent aspiration?**
It is important to frequently reassess the need, level, and choice of agents for analgesia and sedation. The head of the bed should be elevated to at least 30 degrees, and oral care should be optimized.

15. **Does positioning of the feeding tube in the small bowel versus the stomach affect the incidence of aspiration of enteral tube feedings?**
Studies in which infused formula has been labeled with a marker have shown that small bowel feeding can reduce the incidence of gastrointestinal reflux. Whether this leads to a decreased

incidence of pneumonia is not clear. Although studies designed to evaluate the effect of level of feeding on aspiration and pneumonia have been small and underpowered, no significant difference has been demonstrated between patients fed in the small bowel versus the stomach. Regardless, some experts recommend placing feeding tubes in the small bowel to reduce the risk of aspiration pneumonia.

Heyland DK, DeMeo MT, Drover JW, et al: Optimizing the benefits and minimizing the risks of enteral nutrition in the critically ill: Role of small bowel feeding. J Parenter Enteral Nutr 26:S51–S55, 2002.

KEY POINTS: ASPIRATION

1. Critically ill patients in the ICU are at risk for more frequent aspiration and more grave consequences after aspiration.

2. The consequences of aspiration depend on the volume and nature of aspirated material as well as the host response to the insult.

3. The bacteriology of pneumonia after aspiration depends on the flora in the oropharynx and in the gastrointestinal tract. The bacterial flora changes over time.

4. Although data are lacking, some experts recommend placing feeding tubes in the small bowel to reduce the risk of aspiration pneumonia.

16. **What clinical monitors are used to detect aspiration in patients who are enterally fed?**
    Along with clinical impression, early detection of aspiration has relied on coloring enteral feeding with dyes and the detection of elevated glucose in tracheal aspirates. Use of blue food coloring has low sensitivity and has been implicated in deaths of critically ill patients, presumably as a result of a toxic effect on mitochondria. The specificity of the glucose oxidase method for detection of glucose-containing formula is very low. Both methods should be abandoned. Gastric residual volumes are often used to assess risk of aspiration. This is not a reliable method, however, because gastric residual volumes correlate poorly with incidence of regurgitation or aspiration. Clearly, new bedside methods to detect early aspiration are needed to supplement preventative strategies.

    Maloney JP, Ryan TA: Detection of aspiration in enterally fed patients: A requiem for bedside monitors of aspiration. J Parenter Enteral Nutr 26:S34–S41, 2002.

17. **Does intubation or tracheostomy prevent aspiration?**
    No. Both intubation and tracheostomy actually breach some of the normal upper airway defenses. Balloon insufflation does not totally protect against fluid entering the airway. In patients with depressed consciousness or neuromuscular disease, however, intubation or tracheostomy may be indicated to decrease the volume of aspiration and to allow suctioning of airway contents.

18. **What preventive measures can be used during endotracheal intubation?**
    Aspiration of gastric contents during intubation can be catastrophic. Several precautions can be taken:
    - Awake intubation, without sedation, can be performed.
    - Fiberoptic intubation may be helpful, if available.
    - Pressure on the cricoid cartilage (i.e., Sellick's maneuver) occludes the esophagus and can prevent aspiration.
    - Excessive positive pressure applied before intubation often dilates the stomach and predisposes the patient to emesis.

- Ascertainment of correct placement of the endotracheal tube (ideally, by sustained end-tidal carbon dioxide and the presence of breath sounds with the absence of gastric sounds during ventilation) should be accomplished rapidly.
- Maneuvers designed to decrease gastric pH, increase LES tone, and decrease gastric volume (using H_2 blockers, metoclopramide) can be considered in high-risk persons with intubations planned several hours in advance.
- Particulate antacids can produce pulmonary damage if aspirated and should be avoided.

CHAPTER 24

HEMOPTYSIS

Michael E. Hanley, MD

1. **What is hemoptysis?**

   Hemoptysis is the expectoration of blood originating from the lower respiratory tract. It is classified based on the rate of hemorrhage. *Massive hemoptysis* is inconsistently defined but generally describes expectoration of greater than 600 mL of blood within a 24- to 48-hour period. *Frank* or *gross hemoptysis* is expectoration of less than 600 mL of blood in 24–48 hours but more than blood streaking.

2. **How are hemoptysis and pseudohemoptysis different?**

   Pseudohemoptysis is expectoration of blood originating from a source other than the lower respiratory tract. It results from either aspiration of blood from the gastrointestinal tract or blood draining into the larynx and trachea from bleeding sites in the oral cavity, nasopharynx, or larynx.

3. **Describe the differential diagnosis of hemoptysis.**

   Hemoptysis results in general from either focal or diffuse pulmonary parenchymal processes or tracheobronchial, cardiovascular, or hematologic disorders (Box 24-1). The frequency with which hemoptysis is associated with these conditions is determined by the age of the patient, the population being studied (e.g., surgical versus medical, veterans hospital versus city/county indigent hospital), and the amount of expectorated blood.

   Corder R: Hemoptysis. Emerg Med Clin North Am 21:421–435, 2003.

4. **What are the common causes of massive hemoptysis?**

   The most common cause of massive hemoptysis in patients who are not intubated when hemoptysis begins is inflammatory lung disease. This category includes tuberculosis (40%), bronchiectasis (30%), necrotizing pneumonitis (10%), lung abscess (5%), and fungal infection (5%). Pulmonary neoplasm and arteriovenous malformation account for only about 10% of cases.

   Johnston H, Reisz G: Changing spectrum of hemoptysis: Underlying causes in 148 patients undergoing diagnostic flexible fiber-optic bronchoscopy. Arch Intern Med 149:1666–1668, 1989.

5. **Name the common iatrogenic causes of hemoptysis that occur in critically ill patients.**

   When hemoptysis begins after endotracheal intubation, upper airway trauma caused by the intubation procedure, endotracheal tube, or endotracheal suction catheters must be considered. If hemoptysis begins after a latent period of 1 or more weeks after intubation, a tracheo-artery fistula may be the source of hemorrhage. This possibility is increased if a

BOX 24-1. CAUSES OF HEMOPTYSIS

Tracheobronchial disorders

Acute tracheobronchitis
Amyloidosis
Gastric aspiration
Bronchial adenoma
Bronchial endometriosis
Bronchial telangiectasia
Bronchogenic carcinoma
Broncholithiasis
Chronic bronchitis
Cystic fibrosis
Endobronchial metastasis
Endobronchial tuberculosis
Foreign body aspiration
Bronchial mucoid impaction
Tracheobronchial trauma
Tracheoesophageal fistula

Localized parenchymal diseases

Nontuberculous pneumonia
Actinomycosis
Amebiasis
Ascariasis
Aspergilloma
Bronchopulmonary sequestration
Coccidioidomycosis
Congenital and acquired cyst
Cryptococcosis
Histoplasmosis
Hydatid mole
Lung abscess
Lipoid pneumonia
Lung contusion
Metastatic cancer
Mucormycosis
Nocardiosis
Paragonimiasis
Pulmonary endometriosis
Pulmonary tuberculosis
Sporotrichosis

Cardiovascular disorders

Aortic aneurysm
Congenital heart disease
Congestive heart failure
Fat embolism
Mitral stenosis
Postmyocardial infarction syndrome
Pulmonary arteriovenous malformation
Pulmonary artery aneurysm
Pulmonary embolus
Pulmonary venous varix
Schistosomiasis
Superior vena cava syndrome
Tumor embolization

Hematologic disorders

Anticoagulant therapy
Disseminated intravascular coagulation
Leukemia
Thrombocytopenia

Diffuse parenchymal diseases

Disseminated angiosarcoma
Farmer's lung
Goodpasture's syndrome
Idiopathic pulmonary hemosiderosis
Mixed IgA nephropathy
Legionnaires' disease
Mixed connective tissue disease
Mixed cryoglobulinemia
Polyarteritis nodosa
Scleroderma
Systemic lupus erythematosus
Viral pneumonitis
Wegener's granulomatosis

Other

Idiopathic
Iatrogenic

IgA = immunoglobulin A.
Adapted from Irwin RS, Hubmayr R: Hemoptysis. In Rippe JM, Irwin RS, Alpert JS, Dalen JE (eds): Intensive Care Medicine. Boston, Little, Brown, 1985.

tracheostomy tube is present. Pulmonary artery rupture and pulmonary infarction should be considered when hemoptysis occurs in a patient with a pulmonary artery catheter. Pulmonary infarction should be suspected if a wedge-shaped infiltrate is present distal to the catheter on the chest roentgenogram.

Abreu, AR, Campos MA, Krieger BP: Pulmonary artery rupture induced by a pulmonary artery catheter: Case report and a review of the literature. J Intensive Care Med 19:291–296, 2004.

6. **Explain the significance of massive hemoptysis.**
Massive hemoptysis is generally due to hemorrhaging from the bronchial artery (systemic pressure) circulation as opposed to the low-pressure pulmonary artery circuit and therefore is more capable of generating life-threatening hemorrhage. Mortality from massive hemoptysis in some studies is 75–100%.

7. **List the tests that should be included in a routine evaluation of patients with hemoptysis.**
History, physical examination, complete blood counts including platelet count, coagulation studies, urinalysis, chest roentgenogram, and electrocardiogram.

Lordan JL, Gascoigne A, Corris PA: The pulmonary physician in critical care: Illustrative case 7: Assessment and management of massive haemoptysis. Thorax 58:814–819, 2003.

8. **What is the initial approach to the evaluation of a patient with hemoptysis in the intensive care unit (ICU)?**
Evaluation should begin with the routine tests previously described. After the patient has been hemodynamically stabilized, the site, etiology, and extent of bleeding should be determined. Identifying the site of bleeding requires visualization of the airways, including the nasopharanx and oropharynx, and examination of the chest roentgenogram. Pernasal fiberoptic bronchoscopy allows examination of the nasopharynx, larynx, and major airways and may reveal whether hemorrhaging is focal or diffuse. The presence of an endotracheal tube may compromise this examination. In this instance, upper airway bleeding may be detected by aspirating the trachea free of blood with a bronchoscope while the endotracheal balloon is expanded, and then observing fresh blood flow down from above the balloon when it is decompressed. Rigid bronchoscopy may be required if hemorrhaging is massive, such that blood cannot be adequately removed with a flexible bronchoscope.

Jean-Baptiste E: Clinical assessment and management of massive hemoptysis. Crit Care Med 28:1642–1647, 2000.

9. **How does the chest roentgenogram assist in the evaluation of hemoptysis?**
Examination of the chest roentgenogram often gives clues to both the site and etiology of hemoptysis. The presence of an infiltrate suggests the existence of a pulmonary parenchymal process. However, occasionally an infiltrate may occur after aspiration of blood coming from the upper airway. Similarly, the presence of diffuse infiltrates suggests diffuse parenchymal disease, although this roentgenographic pattern may also occur with localized bleeding associated with severe coughing, which diffusely disperses blood throughout the lungs.

KEY POINTS: MANAGEMENT GOALS IN MASSIVE HEMOPTYSIS

1. Maintain airway patency.

2. Protect the healthy lung.

3. Stop hemorrhage.

4. Prevent repeat hemorrhage.

10. **Do all patients with hemoptysis require bronchoscopy?**
    No. Bronchoscopy may not be indicated if the initial evaluation strongly suggests that hemoptysis is due to a cardiovascular etiology, a lower respiratory tract infection, or a single episode of frank hemoptysis due to acute or chronic bronchitis. However, bronchoscopy should be reconsidered in these clinical settings if the patient's hemoptysis does not improve or resolve after 24 hours of empiric therapy. Bronchoscopy is not indicated to make the specific diagnosis of a tracheo-artery fistula.

11. **Describe the immediate management of massive hemoptysis.**
    The goals of immediate management of patients with massive hemoptysis include maintaining airway patency, stopping ongoing hemorrhage, and preventing rebleeding. Maintenance of airway patency is of paramount importance because death from massive hemoptysis more commonly results from asphyxiation due to major airway obstruction than from exsanguination. Several approaches have been advocated to maintain airway patency. If hemorrhage is occurring from a focal site and the site of hemorrhage is known, the patient should be positioned with the bleeding side dependent to prevent contamination of noninvolved airways. If the site of hemorrhage is unknown or diffuse, the patient should be placed in the Trendelenburg position. Other approaches to protect uninvolved airways include bronchoscopically guided selective intubation of the nonbleeding mainstem bronchus or placement of a double-lumen endotracheal tube.

    Johnson JL: Manifestations of hemoptysis: How to manage minor, moderate, and massive bleeding. Postgrad Med 112:101–113, 2002.

12. **What specific therapies may be useful to stop ongoing hemorrhage?**
    If the cause of hemorrhage is known, specific therapy (such as antibiotics for bronchiectasis or corticosteroids for pulmonary vasculitis) should be instituted to stop ongoing hemorrhage. Coagulopathies should be corrected with administration of appropriate blood products. Life-threatening hemorrhage from a focal site may require more aggressive strategies. Surgical resection should be considered in patients with adequate underlying lung function; however, the mortality associated with this approach is high. Focal hemoptysis in patients with severe underlying respiratory disease has been successfully treated by tamponade with Fogarty catheters placed under bronchoscopic guidance, cautery with bronchoscopic laser photocoagulation, occlusion of the involved pulmonary artery with a Swan-Ganz catheter, iced normal saline lavage of hemorrhaging lung segments, topical administration of epinephrine,

and administration of IV vasopressin. Most patients, however, require bronchial artery embolization (*see* question 14).

Haponiks EF: Managing life-threatening hemoptysis: Has anything really changed? Chest 118:1431–1435, 2000.

Valipour A, Kreuzer A, Koller H, et al: Bronchoscopy-guided topical hemostatic tamponade therapy for the management of life-threatening hemoptysis. Chest 127:2113–2118, 2005.

13. **Describe the management of a tracheo-artery fistula.**
The goals of immediate management are to control bleeding and to maintain a patent airway while preparing the patient for primary surgical correction. Bleeding from a tracheo-artery fistula complicating a tracheostomy usually occurs at one of three sites: the tracheostomy tube stoma, the tracheostomy tube balloon, or the intratracheal cannula tip. Bleeding at the tracheostomy stoma can sometimes be tamponaded by applying forward and downward pressure on the top of the tracheostomy tube. Bleeding at the site of the balloon can be tamponaded by overinflating the balloon. These maneuvers should be performed immediately. However, they will not be helpful if bleeding is occurring at the cannula tip. If the bleeding stops or slows either spontaneously or subsequent to these efforts, an endotracheal tube should be placed distal to the bleeding site. However, the initial tracheostomy tube should not be removed without a surgeon present because a sudden increase in the rate of hemorrhage may necessitate blunt dissection down the anterior tracheal wall posterior to the sternum to attempt direct finger tamponade of the bleeding site.

Schaefer OP, Irwin RS: Tracheo-artery fistula. Intensive Care Med 10:64–75, 1995.

14. **What is the role of bronchial artery embolization in the management of massive hemoptysis?**
Bronchial artery embolization is important in the management of both surgical and nonsurgical causes of massive hemoptysis. It is a temporary measure for surgical lesions, facilitating the stabilization of patients while they undergo evaluation and preparation for surgery. It allows surgery to be performed in a more controlled setting. Bronchial artery embolization has become the primary mode of therapy for patients whose conditions are considered inoperable because of either diffuse lung disease or poor pulmonary function. Such patients may undergo multiple episodes of embolization over many years if hemoptysis recurs.

15. **What is the success rate of bronchial artery embolization?**
Some studies indicate success rates of 98% in the initial 24-hour period. However, 16–30% of patients rebleed in the first year after embolization. Rebleeding tends to be bimodal in occurrence, with peaks in the first month (generally due to inadequate initial embolization) and at 1–2 years (due to progression of underlying disease).

Mal H, Rullon I, Mellot F, et al: Immediate and long-term results of bronchial artery embolization for life-threatening hemoptysis. Chest 115:996–1001, 1999.

Mossi F, Maroldi R, Battaglia G, et al: Indicators predictive of success of embolisation: Analysis of 88 patients with haemoptysis. Radiol Med (Torino) 105:48–55, 2003.

16. **What complications are associated with bronchial artery embolization?**
Bronchial artery embolization is associated with low morbidity rates. The most common complications include pleuritic chest pain, fever, leukocytosis, and dysphagia. These symptoms may last for 5–7 days. Other complications are quite rare and are related to the vascular compromise of organs supplied from vessels that arise downstream from the site of catheter placement. Examples include spinal cord infarction, transverse myelitis, bronchial stenosis, bronchial-esophageal fistula, transient cortical blindness, and cerebrovascular accidents.

Saluja S, Henderson KJ, White RI: Embolotherapy in the bronchial and pulmonary circulation. Radiol Clin North Am 38:425–448, 2000.

17. **When should surgery be considered in the management of massive hemoptysis?**

Bronchial artery embolization has largely replaced surgical resection as the initial therapy in massive hemoptysis. Embolization is associated with much lower morbidity and early mortality rates than emergent surgery. However, because of high rates of recurrence after embolization, surgery should be considered for patients who have hemoptysis due to focal lung lesions and good pulmonary reserve after their conditions have been stabilized with embolization. Surgery is contraindicated in patients with advanced lung disease that results in limited pulmonary reserve, significant comorbidity (especially advanced heart disease), or lung malignancies invading the trachea, mediastinum, heart, great vessels, and parietal pleura. In contrast, it remains the treatment of choice for patients with hemoptysis related to trauma, aortic aneurysm, and bronchial adenomas.

Jougon J, Ballester M, Delcambre F, et al: Massive hemoptysis: What place for medical and surgical treatment. Eur J Cardiothorac Surg 22:345–351, 2002.

CONTROVERSIES

18. **Does the evaluation of massive hemoptysis require rigid bronchoscopy?**

For:

1. The higher suctioning capacity of rigid bronchoscopy allows superior clearing of blood from the tracheobronchial tree, permitting better evaluation of airways.
2. Rigid bronchoscopy permits superior maintenance of an adequate airway and alveolar ventilation.

Against:

1. Rigid bronchoscopy is poorly tolerated both subjectively and physiologically in acutely ill patients and allows only limited evaluation of the bronchial tree because only proximal portions of the tree are visualized. This results in insufficient time and maneuverability to permit effective lavage and evaluation of individual lung segments.
2. The increased range of flexible fiberoptic bronchoscopy permits evaluation at the level of segmental and subsegmental bronchi, resulting in increased diagnostic accuracy in both localization and visualization of bleeding site (especially the upper lobes).
3. Flexible fiberoptic bronchoscopy permits selective lavage and selective placement of Fogerty catheters in segmental and subsegmental bronchi.

19. **Should fiberoptic bronchoscopy be performed before bronchial artery embolization in patients with massive hemoptysis?**

For:

1. Fiberoptic bronchoscopy is important in guiding bronchial artery embolization by identifying the site of bleeding.
2. Fiberoptic bronchoscopy is complementary to chest computed tomography in identifying the cause of hemoptysis, allowing the institution of specific therapy aimed at the underlying lung pathology.
3. Fiberoptic bronchoscopy facilitates the introduction of balloon catheters into the airway to control hemorrhage and protect uninvolved lung parenchyma by isolating actively hemorrhaging segments.

Against:

1. A study of 29 patients who underwent bronchial artery embolization to control massive hemoptysis revealed that the site of bleeding could be identified in 80% of patients by chest radiograph alone. Bronchoscopy was essential to localizing the site of hemorrhage in only 10% of patients.

2. The site of embolization is generally identified by angiography at the time of bronchial catheterization.
3. Emergent bronchoscopy results in unnecessary delays before performance of bronchial artery embolization.
4. Endobronchial tamponade with balloon catheters is inferior to embolization as a temporary measure to control hemorrhage before the institution of more specific therapy and should be reserved for patients with contraindications to embolization.

Hsiao EI, Kirsch CM, Kagawaa FT, et al: Utility of fiberoptic bronchoscopy before bronchial artery embolization for massive hemoptysis. Am J Roentgenol 177:861–867, 2001.

Karmy-Jones, Cuschieri J, Vallieres E: Role of bronchoscopy in massive hemoptysis. Chest Surg Clin North Am 11:873–906, 2001.

CHAPTER 25

VENOUS THROMBOEMBOLISM AND FAT EMBOLISM

Pajman A. Danai, MD, and Marc Moss, MD

1. **What are the sources of pulmonary embolism (PE)?**
   The majority of PEs arise from clots in the deep veins of the legs, particularly the iliac, femoral, and popliteal veins. Clots can also originate on central venous catheters and from the pelvic veins in women with a history of obstetric difficulties or recent gynecologic surgery. Other nonhematologic sources of PE include fat particles, amniotic fluid as a complication of pregnancy, air during the placement of central venous catheters, and foreign bodies such as talc and cotton fibers in IV drug users.

2. **What are some of the risk factors for PE and deep venous thrombosis (DVT)?**
   Three general conditions that increase the risk of venous thrombosis are called *Virchow's triad:* venous stasis, hypercoagulability, and injury to the venous walls. Specific risk factors are listed in Table 25-1.

   Anderson FA, Spencer FA: Risk factors for venous thromboembolism. Circulation 107:I9–I16, 2003.

3. **How common is venous thromboembolism in critically ill patients?**
   DVT and PE are common and often underdiagnosed problems in critically ill patients. In prospective studies, 33% of medical patients in the intensive care unit (ICU) had DVTs on routine clinical screening, and 18% of trauma patients had proximal DVTs. In a retrospective series of respiratory ICU patients, 27% had PE on autopsy.

   Goldhaber SZ: Pulmonary embolism. Lancet 363:1295–1305, 2004.

TABLE 25-1. RISK FACTORS FOR VENOUS THROMBOEMBOLISM		
Hypercoagulability	**Venous Stasis**	**Vessel Wall Injury**
Antithrombin III deficiency	Prolonged bed rest	Trauma
Protein C deficiency	Congestive heart failure	
Protein S deficiency	Obesity	
Factor V Leiden mutation	Major surgical procedures	
Cancer	Pregnancy	
Hyperhomocystinemia	Limited mobility	
Antiphospholipid antibodies		
Oral contraceptives		
Hormone replacement therapy		
Nephrotic syndrome		
High levels of factor VIII		

4. **How reliable is the physical examination for diagnosing DVT?**
   You might as well flip a coin. The classic signs of DVT are leg swelling, pain to deep pressure over the calf, pain in the calf when the foot is dorsiflexed (i.e., Homans' sign), or palpable deep thrombi. Unfortunately, fewer than 50% of patients with a documented DVT have the classic findings on clinical examination.

   Miniati M, Prediletto R, Formichi B, et al: Accuracy of clinical assessment in the diagnosis of pulmonary embolism. Am J Resp Crit Care Med 159:864–871, 1999.

5. **How do patients with PE present?**
   The symptoms of PE can depend on the severity of the emboli. When there is an acute massive occlusion, patients can present with systemic hypotension, syncope, and severe refractory hypoxemia. In patients with underlying cardiac or pulmonary disease, there may be significant hemodynamic compromise with less occlusion of the pulmonary vasculature. Common signs and symptoms of PE are listed in Box 25-1.

BOX 25-1.   SIGNS AND SYMPTOMS OF ACUTE PULMONARY EMBOLISM

Pleuritic chest pain
Tachypnea
Hemoptysis
Pleural friction rub
Acute onset of tachypnea
Tachycardia
Unexplained agitation
Hypotension
Unexplained hypoxia
Asymmetric leg swelling
Unilateral leg pain
Increased difference between pulmonary artery diastolic and wedge
   pressure

---

6. **What are some specific findings of PE visible on chest radiography?**
   For most patients with PE, chest radiography yields normal results or depicts subtle abnormalities that are rarely diagnostic. Some classic radiographic findings include: Fleischner lines (i.e., linear streaks that run parallel above an elevated hemidiaphragm), Westermark sign (i.e., an area of lung lacks vascular markings), and Hampton's hump (i.e., pleural-based, wedge-shaped parenchymal density indicative of infarcted lung).

7. **What are the electrocardiographic (ECG) findings associated with PE?**
   ECG findings are also variable and relatively nonspecific. Sinus tachycardia and nonspecific ST-segment and T-wave changes occur frequently. The classic ECG findings of S1, Q3, T3, or right bundle branch block occur in fewer than 15% of patients. The development of ECG findings of acute right ventricular strain (i.e., rightward shift of the QRS axis or peaked P waves in the inferior leads) in a critically ill patient should raise concern about potential PE.

8. **Are any laboratory test result abnormalities helpful in diagnosing PE or DVT?**
   Routine laboratory studies are not helpful in the diagnostic evaluation of a patient in whom PE is suspected. Importantly, no arterial blood gas analysis findings have adequate specificity to exclude PE. Similarly, an elevated serum D-dimer level is a nonspecific finding in a patient in the ICU. However, a level below 500 ng/mL may be more useful in its negative predictive value for eliminating the diagnosis of venous thromboembolism.

   Rodger MA, Carrier M, Jones GN, et al: Diagnostic value of arterial blood gas measurements in suspected pulmonary embolism. Am J Respir Crit Care Med 162:2105–2108, 2000.

9. **When should a ventilation/perfusion (V/Q) scan be ordered in the diagnostic work-up of PE?**
    Most patients with a high-probability V/Q scan (87%) have documented PEs. If the scan has normal results, the diagnosis of PE can be reasonably excluded. Unfortunately, more than 50% of scans are nondiagnostic (i.e., intermediate or low probability), and further testing is needed. In addition, V/Q scans are difficult to interpret if the patient is mechanically ventilated or has preexisting chronic lung disease.

    Roy PM, Colombet I, Durieux P, et al: Systematic review and meta-analysis of strategies for the diagnosis of suspected pulmonary embolism. BMJ 331:1–9, 2005.

10. **What about chest computed tomography (CT) in PE?**
    The sensitivity and specificity of spiral CT approach 90%, exceeding those of V/Q scanning for the diagnosis of segmental or larger clots. Less certain is the ability of spiral CT to diagnose smaller or subsegmental emboli, for which its sensitivity is lower. However, several studies have demonstrated that fewer than 1% of patients with a negative CT scan for the diagnosis of PE will develop subsequent DVT over the next 3 months. Among the additional advantages of spiral CT is the ability to obtain diagnostic information from concurrent scanning of the mediastinum, chest wall, and lung parenchyma, which may result in an alternative diagnosis. Utility of spiral CT in the ICU is limited by patients with impaired renal function or an inability to lie flat or be safely transported to the scanner.

    Quiroz R, Kucher N, Zou KH, et al: Clinical validity of a negative computed tomography scan in patients with suspected pulmonary embolism: A systematic review. JAMA 293:2012–2017, 2005.

11. **What is the role of echocardiography in the evaluation of PE?**
    As many as 40% of patients with PE exhibit abnormalities of the right ventricle (RV), including RV dysfunction and thrombus formation (rare). Findings of RV volume and pressure overload include abnormal motion of the intraventricular septum, RV dilation, and RV hypokinesis. Patients with signs of RV dysfunction by echocardiography may be at increased risk of death from PE. Echocardiography also may diagnose conditions that simulate PE, such as aortic aneurysm, myocardial infarction, and pericardial tamponade.

    Goldhaber SZ: Echocardiography in the management of pulmonary embolism. Ann Intern Med 136:691–700, 2002.

12. **What is the recommended algorithm for the diagnosis of PE in the ICU for a patient who is hemodynamically stable?**
    Anticoagulation should be started (if not contraindicated) once PE is suspected. Although there is no consensus algorithm, the initial diagnostic test should be a V/Q scan or a spiral CT. If these tests are nondiagnostic, a Doppler ultrasound scan of the legs should be performed. If the diagnosis is still not confirmed and the clinical suspicion for PE is high, pulmonary angiography should be performed.

    Fedullo PF, Tapson VF: The evaluation of suspected pulmonary embolism. N Engl J Med 349:1247–1256, 2003.

13. **What is the recommended algorithm for the diagnosis of PE in the ICU for a patient who is hemodynamically unstable?**
    Again, anticoagulation should be started (if not contraindicated) as soon as PE is suspected. Because moving an unstable patient is difficult and potentially unsafe, the initial test should be a Doppler ultrasound scan of the legs. If nondiagnostic, echocardiography can be performed to look for signs of right ventricular dilatation, dysfunction, or possibly evidence of clot.

    Rocha AT, Tapson VF: Venous thromboembolism in intensive care patients. Clin Chest Med 24:103–122, 2003.

14. **What are the goals of treatment for PE/DVT, and how are they achieved?**
The major goals of PE and DVT therapy are to prevent further clot formation, promote resolution of existing clot, and prevent recurrence. Acutely, IV heparin should be administered. Warfarin therapy can then be started with a target level measured by the international normalized ratio of 2.0–3.0. It is important to continue the heparin until the international normalized ratio has been therapeutic for at least 2 days. The benefits of anticoagulation therapy need to be weighed against its risks. The most important complications include bleeding and thrombocytopenia. An often discussed but rare complication of warfarin therapy is skin necrosis caused by preexisting protein C or protein S deficiency.

Merli G: Anticoagulants in the treatment of deep vein thrombosis. Am J Med 118(8A):13S–20S, 2005.

15. **How long should a patient with PE/DVT be treated with anticoagulation?**
Patients with PE/DVT due to a major transient risk factor such as recent hospitalization, bed rest, or leg fracture should be anticoagulated for 3–6 months. Patients with PE/DVT not associated with a transient risk factor should be treated for at least 6 months and possibly even longer if there is a chronic hypercoagulable condition such as cancer, protein C or protein S deficiency, factor V Leiden, or antiphospholipid antibodies.

Kearon C: Duration of therapy for acute venous thromboembolism. Clin Chest Med 24:63–72, 2004.

16. **When should low-molecular-weight (LMW) heparin be used?**
LMW heparin has been found to be safe and effective in the treatment of PE and DVT, but its use in the ICU is presently under investigation. The advantages of LMW heparin include increased bioavailability with a more predictable anticoagulant response, lack of need for phlebotomy to monitor the partial thromboplastin time, infrequent daily dosing, and subcutaneous administration. In the ICU, the long half-life may complicate plans for invasive procedures, and patients receiving vasopressors have inconsistent absorption of subcutaneous medication.

Weitz JI, Hirsh J, Samama MM: New anticoagulant drugs. Chest 126:265S–286S, 2004.

17. **Which patients with PE should be treated with thrombolytic therapy?**
Classic teaching states that thrombolytic therapy should be used in patients with a massive PE causing cardiogenic shock. The use of thrombolytics has been reported to achieve faster clot lysis and improvement in right ventricular function and may lower the rate of recurrence when compared with heparin therapy alone. In patients with "submassive" PE, defined as right ventricular dysfunction without systemic hypotension, thrombolytic therapy with heparin prevents the need for escalation of therapy due to clinical deterioration, usually meaning worsening respiratory failure.

Konstantinides S, Geibel A, Heusel G, et al: Heparin plus alteplase compared with heparin alone in patients with submassive pulmonary embolism. N Engl J Med 347:1143–1150, 2002.

18. **When should the placement of an IV filter be considered?**
The most common indications are when a patient has a recurrent embolism on "adequate" anticoagulation therapy or when a patient cannot be anticoagulated due to bleeding or other contraindications.

Streiff MB: Vena caval filters. J Intens Care Med 18(2):59–79, 2003.

19. **Are there important long-term sequelae of a PE?**
Symptomatic pulmonary hypertension occurs in approximately 4% of patients within 2 years after their first episode of PE.

Pengo V, Lensing AWA, Prins MH, et al: Incidence of chronic thromboembolic pulmonary hypertension after pulmonary embolism. N Engl J Med 350:2257–2264, 2004.

20. **What is the recommended prophylactic therapy for patients at risk for the development of DVT/PE?**
Prophylaxis is recommended in all high-risk patients and has been reported to decrease the incidence of DVT by 67%. However, not all ICU patients who should be taking DVT prophylaxis actually receive this important therapy. The use of computerized electronic alert programs increased the use of prophylactic therapy and reduced the rate of DVT and PE in hospitalized patients. The most commonly used regimen is low-dose heparin, 5000 units given subcutaneously every 8 hours. LMW heparins are also efficacious as prophylaxis. Other therapies, including intermittent pneumatic compression stockings and graded elastic stockings, can be used in patients who cannot tolerate anticoagulation.

Kucher N, Koo S, Quiroz R, et al: Electronic alerts to prevent venous thromboembolism among hospitalized patients. N Engl J Med 352:969–977, 2005.

Weitz JI, Hirsh J, Samama MM: New anticoagulant drugs. Chest 126:265S–286S, 2004.

KEY POINTS: VENOUS THROMBOEMBOLISM AND FAT EMBOLISM IN THE INTENSIVE CARE UNIT

1. All high-risk patients in the ICU should receive prophylactic therapy for pulmonary embolism (PE)/deep venous thromboembolism.

2. Patients can have a PE without a significant increase in the A-a gradient.

3. There are no specific clinical, radiographic, or laboratory findings for PE. Therefore, PE should be considered in any critically ill patient with deterioration of cardiopulmonary status.

4. Symptomatic pulmonary hypertension occurs in approximately 4% of patients within 2 years after the first episode of PE.

5. Thrombolytic therapy should be used in patients with massive PE associated with cardiogenic shock.

6. Fat embolism syndrome occurs in patients with traumatic bone fractures, pancreatitis, and sickle cell crises and during orthopedic procedures or liposuction.

21. **What is the fat embolism syndrome (FES)? Who is at risk for developing it?**
Embolism of fat occurs in nearly all patients with traumatic bone fractures and during orthopedic procedures. It can also occur in patients with pancreatitis or sickle cell crises and during liposuction. Most cases are asymptomatic. FES occurs in the minority of these patients who develop signs and symptoms, usually affecting the respiratory, neurologic, and hematologic systems and the skin. Symptoms typically occur 12–72 hours after the initial injury. The presentation may be catastrophic with RV failure and cardiovascular collapse.

Bulger EM, Smith DG, Maier RV, et al: Fat embolism syndrome: A 10-year review. Arch Surg 132:435–439, 1997.

22. **How is FES diagnosed?**
Fat embolism is a clinical diagnosis. The use of bronchoscopy or pulmonary artery catheterization to detect fat particles in alveolar macrophages or blood from the pulmonary artery lack both sensitivity and specificity for the diagnosis of FES. The Gurd criteria are the most widely used method of diagnosis (Box 25-2).

Mellor A, Soni N: Fat embolism. Anaesthesia 56:145–154, 2001.

> **BOX 25-2.   GURD DIAGNOSTIC CRITERIA FOR FAT EMBOLISM SYNDROME**
>
> **Major criteria**
> *(One necessary for diagnosis)*
> Petechial rash
> Respiratory failure
> Cerebral involvement
>
> **Minor criteria**
> *(Four necessary for diagnosis)*
> Tachycardia (heart rate > 120 beats/min)
> Fever (temperature > 39°C)
> Retinal involvement
> Jaundice
> Renal insufficiency
>
> **Additional laboratory criteria**
> *(One necessary for diagnosis)*
> Thrombocytopenia
> Anemia
> Elevated erythrocyte sedimentation rate
> Fat macroglobulinemia

23. **What is the recommended treatment for FES?**
    Treatment of FES is primarily supportive. Although studied extensively, there is no compelling evidence that the use of corticosteroids is indicated for FES. Some studies have suggested that early stabilization of long bone fractures can minimize bone marrow embolization into the venous system.

WEBSITES

1. American Thoracic Society Clinical Practice Guideline: Diagnostic Approach to Acute Venous Thromboembolism
   www.thoracic.org/sections/publications/statements/pages/respiratory-disease-adults/venous1-24.htm

2. E-Medicine: Fat embolism
   www.emedicine.com/med/topic652.htm

3. Seventh American College of Chest Physicians Consensus Conference on Antithrombotic and Thrombolytic Therapy: Evidence-Based Guidelines
   www.chestjournal.org/content/vol126/3_suppl

CHEST PAIN

Jacob T. Gutsche, MD, Benjamin A. Kohl, MD, and
Clifford S. Deutschman, MS, MD

CHAPTER 26

1. **What is the differential diagnosis of chest pain?**
   Chest pain is divided into pain derived from cardiac and noncardiac causes. Cardiac causes include myocardial ischemia/infarction, aortic stenosis or dissection, hypertrophic cardiomyopathy, and myocarditis. The most common noncardiac causes are as follows:
   - **Musculoskeletal:** Chest wall trauma, arthritis, costochondritis, etc.
   - **Gastrointestinal:** Esophageal spasm, peptic ulcer, cholecystitis, pancreatitis
   - **Psychiatric:** Anxiety, somatoform disorders
   - **Pulmonary:** Pleuritis, pneumonia, pulmonary embolus
   - **Other:** Pericarditis, aortic dissection, herpes zoster

2. **How does one evaluate chest pain?**
   Immediately life-threatening causes of chest pain must be ruled out first. These include myocardial ischemia/infarction, aortic dissection, pulmonary embolism, and tension pneumothorax. After taking a history of the patient's pain and risk factors, a physical examination will direct the clinician to further diagnostic tests. Aortic dissection is classically characterized by severe ripping or tearing pain that radiates to the back. Pulmonary embolism may present with nonspecific sharp, pleuritic chest pain associated with dyspnea. A tension pneumothorax presents with sharp chest pain associated with severe dyspnea and loss of breath sounds on the affected side.

3. **What is angina?**
   Angina is the clinical manifestation of myocardial ischemia; that is, myocardial oxygen demand that exceeds oxygen availability. It is characterized by discomfort (rather than pain):
   - **Quality:** Squeezing, heaviness, fullness, tightness
   - **Severity:** Not helpful in diagnosing or ruling out coronary heart disease (CHD)
   - **Location:** Diffuse, center of the chest
   - **Radiation:** Jaw, teeth, arm, or even fingers
   - **Temporal:** Usually minutes; longer with infarction
   - **Exacerbation:** Cold, exertion, pain, stress, sexual intercourse
   - **Alleviation:** Rest, nitroglycerin

   Symptoms that may be associated with CHD-type pain include diaphoresis, dyspnea, nausea/vomiting, palpitations, and syncope. The classic sign is Levine's sign, in which the patient will hold a closed fist on the chest over the heart.

   Chronic stable angina includes predictable and reproducible chest discomfort after physical activity or emotional stress. Symptoms are typically relieved by rest or sublingual nitroglycerin. The presence of obstruction in major coronary arteries is likely, and the severity of stenosis is usually greater than 70%. Patients with severe aortic valve disease or hypertrophic cardiomyopathy may have angina-like chest pain in the absence of coronary disease.

4. **What are anginal equivalents?**
   Anginal equivalents are symptoms of myocardial ischemia other than classic angina. These include dizziness, nausea, diaphoresis, dyspnea, and pain in locations other than the chest. These usually are exacerbated and alleviated in ways similar to classic angina.

5. **What are the symptoms of atypical chest pain (noncardiac cause)?**
   - Pleuritic pain, increased with inspiration, sharp or pulsating
   - Pain in the musculoskeletal wall with varying radiation
   - Variable duration from seconds to days/weeks
   - Response to sublingual nitroglycerin possible but not guaranteed
   - Random onset and cessation

6. **What radiologic studies are helpful in the work-up of chest pain?**
   A chest x-ray is an inexpensive test that is of value in diagnosing several noncardiac causes for chest pain. These include pneumonia, pneumothorax, and rib fractures. A widened mediastinum with loss of the aortic knob may indicate aortic dissection. Cardiac ischemia may result in pulmonary edema. If either pulmonary embolus or aortic dissection is suspected, a computed tomography examination may be helpful.

7. **Is the electrocardiogram (ECG) useful in diagnosing the cause of chest pain?**
   Completely normal ECG results reduce the likelihood that chest pain is due to CHD but do not eliminate it as a possible etiology. Patients with unstable angina may have normal ECG results. Findings that are consistent with ischemia or infarction include the following:
   - ST segment elevation ≥ 0.1 mV in two contiguous leads
   - ST segment depression ≥ 0.1 mV at 80 msec from the J point
   - New-onset left bundle branch block or other conduction defect
   - T-wave inversion
   - New Q waves

   The initial ECG results may be negative in a patient with acute coronary syndrome. In cases with a high index of suspicion, the ECG should be repeated at 10-minute intervals. Patients should also have continuous two- to three-lead monitoring.

   Antman EM, Anbe DT, Armstrong PW, et al: ACC/AHA guidelines for the management of patients with ST-elevation myocardial infarction—executive summary: A report of the American College of Cardiology/American Heart Association Task Force on Practice Guidelines (Writing Committee to Revise the 1999 Guidelines for the Management of Patients with Acute Myocardial Infarction). Circulation 110:588, 2004.

8. **Is two-lead ECG monitoring sufficient to diagnose ischemia or an acute myocardial infarction?**
   ECG monitoring has become the standard of care in the operating room and in the intensive care unit (ICU). It is used to detect arrhythmias and ischemia and to assess the function of a pacemaker/automatic implantable cardioverter-defibrillator. Intraoperative studies demonstrate that continuous lead II and V_5 monitoring is 80% sensitive for ischemia detection. Adding lead V_4 will increase sensitivity to $>90\%$.

   London MJ, Hollenberg M, Wong MG, et al: Intraoperative myocardial ischemia: Localization by continuous 12-lead electrocardiography. Anesthesiology 69:232–241, 1988.

9. **How is echocardiography useful in a chest pain work-up?**
   An ECG and chest radiograph are usually sufficient to guide the chest pain work-up. Echocardiography will be able to show areas of wall motion abnormality (WMA) suggesting ischemia or infarction. This is more helpful in patients with a recent baseline echocardiograph because it demonstrates that the WMA is new. In the setting of the emergency department, absence of new WMA has been shown to have a 94–98% negative predictive value. Echocardiography may reveal right ventricular strain or a clot in the pulmonary artery in patients with pulmonary embolism but cannot be used to exclude pulmonary embolism as a diagnosis.

   Gibler WB, Runyon JP, Levy RC, et al: A rapid diagnostic and treatment center for patients with chest pain in the emergency department. Ann Emerg Med 25:1–8, 1995.

10. **What are some atypical symptoms of acute coronary syndrome?**
    Note: This differs from atypical chest pain. Up to one-third of patients suffering from an acute myocardial infarction will not present with chest pain. These patients often present with other symptoms including dyspnea, nausea/vomiting, palpitations, syncopal events, or cardiac arrest. This patient population tends to be older, diabetic, and female.

KEY POINTS: CHEST PAIN

1. There are noncardiac causes of chest pain, including musculoskeletal problems, gastrointestinal causes, pulmonary problems, psychiatric problems, and miscellaneous others.

2. Treat angina with beta blockers, angiotensin-converting enzyme inhibitors, nitroglycerin, aspirin, statins, and oxygen.

3. Patients with persistent ST-segment elevation need to be treated before obtaining cardiac isoenzymes; the goal is to achieve reperfusion within 90 minutes.

4. Characteristics of noncardiac chest pain include a pleuritic nature of pain, pain that radiates in the distribution of muscles, sharp pain, and a duration that is prolonged and random in onset and cessation.

5. Electrocardiographic characteristics of ischemia and infarction include ST-segment elevation in two contiguous leads, ST-segment depression, new-onset left bundle branch block, new Q waves, and T-wave inversions.

11. **How does one treat chronic stable angina in the ICU?**
    In critically ill patients with chronic stable angina, multiple factors may lead to myocardial oxygen demand that exceeds oxygen availability. These include pain, fever, anxiety, hypoxemia, and a host of other stressors. The treatment is directed at correcting the imbalance by treating the stressor, pharmacologically reducing myocardial oxygen demand, and increasing the oxygen supply.
    - **Beta blockers:** Beta blockers are the gold standard of treatment for reducing anginal symptoms. These agents lower heart rate, contractility, and myocardial wall tension. They have not been shown to prolong survival in patients with stable angina.
    - **Nitroglycerin and morphine:** These can lower preload to both the right and left ventricles, dilate the coronary and pulmonary arteries (reduced right ventricular afterload), and treat anginal symptoms, but they do not affect survival.
    - **Angiotensin-converting enzyme inhibitors:** Angiotensin-converting enzyme inhibitors can help manage hypertension and lower afterload and myocardial wall tension.
    Ideally, chronically used medications should be administered. These include aspirin and statins. Each have been shown to reduce cardiac events in high-risk patients. Oxygen therapy can be added.

Heart Protection Study Collaborative Group: MRC/BHF Heart Protection Study of cholesterol lowering with simvastatin in 20,536 high-risk individuals: A randomised placebo-controlled trial. Lancet 360:7–22, 2002.

Thrombosis Prevention Trial: Randomised trial of low-intensity oral anticoagulation with warfarin and low-dose aspirin in the primary prevention of ischaemic heart disease in men at increased risk. The Medical Research Council's General Practice Research Framework. Lancet 351:233, 1998.

12. **Should I wait for the cardiac enzymes to elevate in a patient with persistent ST elevation?**

No. Acute ST-segment elevation in the setting of myocardial infarction indicates thrombotic occlusion of a coronary vessel. The gold standard of treatment is reperfusion by percutaneous coronary intervention (coronary catheterization) within 90 minutes. In areas where this is not available, IV fibrinolytics should be administered. If these are not available, acetylsalicylic acid and clopidogrel (and perhaps beta blockers) should be administered.

Antman EM, Anbe DT, Armstrong PW, et al: ACC/AHA guidelines for the management of patients with ST-elevation myocardial infarction—executive summary: A report of the American College of Cardiology/American Heart Association Task Force on Practice Guidelines (Writing Committee to Revise the 1999 Guidelines for the Management of Patients With Acute Myocardial Infarction). Circulation 110:588–636, 2004.

COMMIT Collaborative Group: Addition of clopidogrel to aspirin in 45,852 patients with acute myocardial infarction: Randomized placebo-controlled trial. Lancet 366:1607–1621, 2005.

13. **What is variant angina?**

Variant angina is characterized by acute episodes of chest pain with associated ST-segment elevation on ECG. It is caused by coronary artery vasospasm, usually within 1 cm of an atherosclerotic plaque. Provocative tests with ergonovine or acetylcholine may be used to rule in patients with multiple episodes of variant angina who have negative results on coronary angiography. Tobacco and cocaine use increase the incidence of variant angina.

14. **What is mitral valve prolapse syndrome?**

Mitral valve prolapse has been associated with a constellation of symptoms including recurrent chest pain, palpitations, dyspnea, dizziness, syncope, and anxiety disorders. The chest pain is usually atypical and easily distinguishable from angina. Patients with mitral valve prolapse syndrome have been found to have elevated plasma catecholamine levels. These patients may have low serum magnesium levels and may benefit from magnesium replacement.

CHAPTER 27

ACUTE MYOCARDIAL INFARCTION AND PRESSORS

Benjamin A. Kohl, MD, and Clifford S. Deutschman, MS, MD

1. How is acute myocardial infarction (AMI) defined?

Myocardial infarction (MI) is defined as myocardial cell (myocyte) death due to ischemia. When describing the entity of MI, it is helpful to precede with words such as "acute," "healing," or "healed." AMI is classically a histologic diagnosis characterized by the presence of polymorphonuclear leukocytes in the affected region. As the myocardium begins to heal, infiltration of mononuclear cells and fibroblasts can be seen. A healed infarction is characterized by fibrous scar tissue with an absence of cellular infiltration. More commonly, however, infarcts are classified based on temporal signs and symptoms, with AMI occurring within 6 hours to 7 days, healing within 7–28 days, and healed after 28 days.

2. What are the known risk factors for coronary artery disease?

Modifiable risk factors

- Dyslipidemia
  - □ Low-density lipoprotein > 160 mg/dL
  - □ High-density lipoprotein < 35 mg/dL
- Smoking
- Cocaine abuse
- Hypertension
- Diabetes mellitus
- Obesity
- Stress
- Elevated lipoprotein a
- Decreased vitamin E
- Elevated homocysteine levels

Nonmodifiable risk factors

- Family history
- Age
- Gender (M > F)

Other potential risk factors (not as well established)

- Alcohol consumption
- Elevated fibrinogen
- *Chlamydia* infection
- Type A personality

3. What is acute coronary syndrome (ACS)? How does it differ from AMI?

ACS describes a spectrum of disorders all resulting from a common pathologic process. The clinical manifestations of ACS depend not only on the volume of myocardium affected but also on the duration of ischemia. Most commonly, ACS is precipitated by rupture or erosion of a "vulnerable" atheromatous plaque within a coronary artery. A "vulnerable" plaque is one that has a substantial lipid core and a thin fibrous cap separating thrombogenic macrophages from the blood. In contrast, more stable plaques are characterized by a relatively thick fibrous cap that protects the thrombogenic lipid core from contact with the blood. Disruption of a plaque results in a massive inflammatory and thrombogenic response, both locally and systemically. Locally plaque and thrombus propagate, narrowing the vessel lumen with potential embolization into the distal coronary circulation. There often are systemic changes in vascular tone. The dynamic process of plaque rupture may evolve with partial or complete occlusion of the vessel with thrombus. This produces ST-segment elevation on the electrocardiogram (ECG) and ultimately leads to necrosis involving full or partial ventricular myocardium in a zone supplied by the affected coronary artery. ACS may or may not culminate in AMI.

4. **What are the different ACSs? What is the difference between myocardial ischemia, MI, myocardial hibernation, and myocardial stunning?**
   ACS represents a constellation of symptoms such as unstable angina, non–Q-wave infarction, and Q-wave infarction. Symptoms include, but are not limited to, chest pain, referred pain, nausea, vomiting, dyspnea, diaphoresis, and lightheadedness. Although chest pain is thought of as the *sine qua non* of ACS, it is frequently absent in presenting patients.

   Myocardial ischemia is a general term used to describe the results of a diminution in oxygen supply relative to tissue oxygen demand. In the mid 1980s, investigators observed that subsets of patients with coronary artery disease had "reversible ischemia" or "chronic ischemia." They postulated that the reduced contractile function was an adaptation to a *chronically* insufficient oxygen supply and termed this response *myocardial hibernation.* This theory has since been substantiated, and it is well accepted that myocardial hibernation has four essential features: perfusion–contraction matching, metabolic and energetic recovery, persistent inotropic reserve, and lack of necrosis on histologic examination. Thus, restoration of normal coronary flow (e.g., coronary bypass surgery) will restore normal function to the affected myocardium. Acute coronary occlusion causes a much more rapid decrement in myocardial performance. Once flow is reestablished, however, ventricular function may slowly return to normal. The duration of this decreased function, termed *myocardial stunning,* is proportional to the duration of the preceding ischemia. Similar to hibernating myocardium, stunned myocardium is completely reversible. *Stunned,* as opposed to *hibernating* myocardium, does not have normal inotropic reserve, and thus cardiogenic shock may follow interventions such as coronary angioplasty and thrombolysis.

   Braunwald E, Rutherford JD: Reversible ischemic left ventricular dysfunction: Evidence for the "hibernating myocardium." J Am Coll Cardiol 8:1467–1470, 1986.

   Cohen M, Charney R, Hershman R, et al: Reversal of chronic ischemic myocardial dysfunction after transluminal coronary angioplasty. J Am Coll Cardiol 12:1193–1198, 1988.

   McCarthy BD, Wong JB, Selker HP: Detecting acute cardiac ischemia in the emergency department: A review of the literature. J Gen Intern Med 5:365–373, 1990.

5. **What are nonatherosclerotic causes of AMI?**
   - **Coronary artery disease other than atherosclerosis:** Spasm of coronary arteries, dissection of the coronary arteries, and a variety of coronary arteritides associated with systemic diseases including coronary mural thickening resulting from metabolic diseases and trauma to coronary arteries, including radiation therapy
   - **Embolism to the coronary arteries:** Infective endocarditis, nonbacterial thrombotic endocarditis, prosthetic valve emboli, cardiac myxoma, mural thrombus from the left atrium or the left ventricle, conditions associated with coronary bypass surgery, and angiography
   - **Myocardial supply:** Demand disproportion, aortic stenosis, aortic insufficiency, and prolonged hypotension
   - ***In situ* thrombosis:** Polycythemia vera, thrombocytosis, disseminated intravascular coagulation, thrombotic thrombocytopenic purpura (TTP), and hypercoagulable states
   - **Congenital coronary anomalies:** Anomalous origin of the left coronary artery from pulmonary artery, coronary arteriovenous fistula, and aneurysms
   - **Miscellaneous:** Cocaine abuse, myocardial contusion, and complications of cardiac catheterization

6. **How is the diagnosis of AMI made?**
   As established by the World Health Organization, the diagnosis of AMI requires at least two of the following:
   - History of angina
   - Typical ECG changes
   - Elevation of biochemical markers consistent with cardiac injury

   More recently, however, the Joint European Society of Cardiology/American College of Cardiology (ESC/ACC) committee on redefinition of MI suggested "one plus one out of two" criteria for a clinical definition of AMI. Elevation of a specific biomarker is now considered a prerequisite for the clinical diagnosis of AMI.

   Alpert JS, Thygesen K, Antman E, Bassand JP: Myocardial infarction redefined—A consensus document of The Joint European Society of Cardiology/American College of Cardiology Committee for the redefinition of myocardial infarction. J Am Coll Cardiol 36:959–969, 2000.

7. **What are the different biochemical markers used to diagnose MI?**
   The most commonly used markers are elevated plasma levels of:
   - Creatinine phosphokinase (CK) and CK, myocardial bound (CKMB)
   - Cardiac troponins
   - Myoglobin

   The plasma levels of CK enzyme increase 3–6 hours after AMI and remain elevated for 24–36 hours. CK by itself, however, is neither specific nor sensitive for the diagnosis of AMI. Thus, a consensus of experts has recommended that the diagnosis of AMI requires elevated plasma levels of CK along within increase in levels of either the MB isoform (CKMB) or troponin. CKMB is a large protein that rises about 4–8 hours after myocardial necrosis and remains elevated for 48–72 hours. Although it is more sensitive than CK for myocardial injury, its specificity is hampered by its presence in skeletal muscle.

   There are three isoforms of troponin: troponin C, troponin I, and troponin T. Only the I and T isoforms are useful in the diagnosis of myocardial injury. Whereas troponin is found in both skeletal and myocardial muscle, the cardiac isoforms are unique to cardiac muscle, and thus their sensitivity and specificity in the diagnosis of myocardial necrosis are much higher than with CK and CKMB. The specificity of troponin I is particularly high because normally it cannot be detected in healthy persons. Using this assay, about 30% of patients who were once classified as having unstable angina are now diagnosed with non–ST-segment elevation myocardial infarction (NSTEMI). In addition, both troponin T (TnT) and troponin I (TnI) may be used prognostically in patients with ACS. Patients with a negative troponin have a 30-day mortality of 5%, whereas those whose troponin is positive have a 30-day mortality of 13%. Not all troponin assays are as sensitive/specific as others. A recent study suggested that the AccuTnI (Beckman Coulter, Fullerton, CA) has the greatest sensitivity/specificity, particularly at low TnI concentrations. In the Global Utilization of Streptokinase and TPA for Occluded Coronary Arteries trial (GUSTO-II), cardiac TnT (cTnT) > 0.1 ng/mL was a better prognostic indicator for the 30-day mortality in patients with acute myocardial ischemia than abnormal ECG changes and elevated CKMB levels. The prognostic value of cTnI in patients with unstable angina or non–Q-wave MI has been demonstrated in a multicenter study. cTnI levels > 0.4 ng/mL were associated with significantly increased mortalities at 42 days, and each increase of 1 ng/mL of cTnI was associated with an increased risk of death.

   Among all the biomarkers, myoglobin rises earliest (within 2–3 hours of myocardial injury). Thus, it has a very high negative predictive value for excluding AMI if the patient presents within 4 hours from the onset of symptoms. Similar to CKMB, myoglobin is present in skeletal muscle and is not specific for myocardial injury when other muscle injury is present.

   Adams JE III, Bodor GS, Davila-Roman VG, et al: Cardiac troponin I: A marker with high specificity for cardiac injury. Circulation 88:101–106, 1993.

Antman EM, Tanasijevic MJ, Thompson B, et al: Cardiac-specific troponin I levels to predict the risk of mortality in patients with acute coronary syndromes. N Engl J Med 335:1342–1349, 1996.

Bodor GS, Porterfield D, Voss EM, et al: Cardiac troponin-I is not expressed in fetal and healthy or diseased adult human skeletal muscle tissue. Clin Chem 41:1710–1715, 1995.

McCord J, Nowak RM, McCullough PA, et al: Ninety-minute exclusion of acute myocardial infarction by use of quantitative point-of-care testing of myoglobin and troponin I. Circulation 104:1483–1488, 2001.

Ohman EM, Armstrong PW, Christenson RH, et al: Cardiac troponin T levels for risk stratification in acute myocardial ischemia. GUSTO IIA Investigators. N Engl J Med 335:1333–1341, 1996.

Panteghini M, Pagani F, Yeo KT, et al: Evaluation of imprecision for cardiac troponin assays at low-range concentrations. Clin Chem 50:327–332, 2004.

8. **What are the differences between Q-wave and non–Q-wave MIS?**
Q-wave infarctions (previously called *transmural infarctions*) account for 60–70% of all AMIs, whereas non–Q-wave MI (previously referred to as *subendocardial infarctions*) represents 30–40% of all MIs. The presence of Q waves on the ECG does not reliably document transmural versus subendocardial infarction (by autopsy data). Typical features of both are listed in Table 27-1.

9. **What is the recommended management of patients with acute MI with >0.1 mV ST-segment elevation in more than two contiguous leads?**
The immediate goal during AMI is to reestablish blood flow to the affected myocardium. This can be achieved by percutaneous coronary intervention or by pharmacologic thrombolysis. A growing body of literature has led to the consensus that percutaneous coronary intervention, if performed rapidly in a center that has significant experience with the procedure, is superior to thrombolytic therapy.

Antman EM, Anbe DT, Armstrong PW, et al: ACC/AHA guidelines for the management of patients with ST-elevation myocardial infarction—executive summary: A report of the American College of Cardiology/ American Heart Association Task Force on Practice Guidelines (Writing Committee to Revise the 1999 Guidelines for the Management of Patients with Acute Myocardial Infarction). J Am Coll Cardiol 44:671–719, 2004.

Keeley EC, Boura JA, Grines CL: Primary angioplasty versus intravenous thrombolytic therapy for acute myocardial infarction: A quantitative review of 23 randomised trials. Lancet 361:13–20, 2003.

Keeley EC, Grines CL: Primary percutaneous coronary intervention for every patient with ST-segment elevation myocardial infarction: What stands in the way?. Ann Intern Med 141:298–304, 2004.

TABLE 27-1. Q-WAVE AND NON–Q-WAVE MYOCARDIAL INFARCTIONS

Q-Wave Infarction	Non–Q-Wave Infarction
ST-segment elevation	Nonspecific ST changes or ST depression
>90% total occlusion	10–25% total occlusion of infarct-related artery
Higher CK peaks	Lower CK peaks
Predominantly systolic dysfunction	Predominantly diastolic dysfunction
Higher in-hospital mortality	Lower in-hospital mortality

CK = creatinine phosphokinase.

10. **When is thrombolytic therapy indicated?**
Thrombolytic therapy is recommended in all patients with suspected acute MI and ST-segment elevation (>0.1 mV, more than two contiguous leads) or new left bundle branch block if the patient presents within 12 hours of the onset of his or her chest pain. Even though there is an increased risk of intracranial bleeding in patients older than 75 years, thrombolytic therapy should be considered after careful screening. This reflects the fact that thrombolysis is associated with an absolute reduction in mortality (10 lives saved per 1000 patients treated). The choice of thrombolytic agents is controversial. GUSTO-I data suggested a 14% reduction in mortality with accelerated recombinant tissue plasminogen activator (rtPA) together with IV heparin compared with IV streptokinase (6.3% versus. 7.4% in 30-day mortality). However, there was a slight increase in the rate of intracranial hemorrhage with tissue plasminogen activator (tPA), especially in elderly patients. Front-loaded tPA is preferable in younger patients with anterior wall MI who present within 4 hours after onset of their chest pain. The dosing is as follows:

- Streptokinase: 1.5 million U given intravenously over 1 hour
- Accelerated tPA: 15-mg IV bolus, 0.75 mg/kg over 30 minutes up to 50 mg, then 0.5 mg/kg up to 35 mg over the next 1 hour with IV heparin (5000-U bolus), followed by an IV infusion of 1000 U/h (1200 U/h in patients weighing > 80 kg)

  Califf RM, White HD, Van de Werf F, et al: One-year results from the Global Utilization of Streptokinase and TPA for Occluded Coronary Arteries (GUSTO-I) trial. GUSTO-I Investigators. Circulation 94:1233–1238, 1996.

11. **What is the recommended management of patients with unstable angina or suspected acute MI who do not have ST elevation (NSTEMI)?**
Most patients with NSTEMI will require a coronary angiography at some point. There is accumulating evidence from clinical trials (e.g., Randomized Intervention Trial of Unstable Angina–2 [RITA-2], Fragmin and Revascularization During Instability in Coronary Artery Disease–II [FRISC-II], Intracoronary Stenting with Antithrombotic Regimen Cooling-Off [ISAR-COOL], Treat Angina with Aggrasat and Determine Cost of Theray with an Invasive or Conservative Strategy—Thrombosis in Myocardial Infarction 18 [TACTICS-TIMI 18]) that earlier angiography and intervention improve outcome. Additionally, coronary stents are more efficacious than balloon angioplasty because the newer drug-eluting stents markedly decrease in-stent restenosis.

  Cannon CP, Weintraub WS, Demopoulos LA, et al: Comparison of early invasive and conservative strategies in patients with unstable coronary syndromes treated with the glycoprotein IIb/IIIa inhibitor tirofiban. N Engl J Med 344:1879–1887, 2001.
  Henderson RA, Pocock SJ, Clayton TC, et al: Seven-year outcome in the RITA-2 trial: Coronary angioplasty versus medical therapy. J Am Coll Cardiol 42:1161–1170, 2003.
  Lemos PA, Saia F, Hofma SH, et al: Short- and long-term clinical benefit of sirolimus-eluting stents compared to conventional bare stents for patients with acute myocardial infarction. J Am Coll Cardiol 43:704–708, 2004.
  Neumann FJ, Kastrati A, Pogatsa-Murray G, et al: Evaluation of prolonged antithrombotic pretreatment ("cooling-off" strategy) before intervention in patients with unstable coronary syndromes: A randomized controlled trial. JAMA 290:1593–1599, 2003.
  Stone GW, Grines CL, Cox DA, et al: Comparison of angioplasty with stenting, with or without abciximab, in acute myocardial infarction. N Engl J Med 346:957–966, 2002.
  Wallentin L: Low-molecular-weight heparin as a bridge to timely revascularization in unstable coronary artery disease—An update of the Fragmin during Instability in Coronary Artery Disease II Trial. Haemostasis 30(Suppl 2):108–113; discussion 106–107, 2000.

12. **What is the role of beta blockade in ACS?**
Several studies have evaluated the benefit of beta blockade in patients with ST-segment elevation myocardial infarction (STEMI). The International Studies of Infarct Survival-1 (ISIS-1) compared treatment with atenolol versus placebo within 12 hours of presentation. The

administration of atenolol was associated with a 15% relative reduction in mortality over 7 days ($P = 0.05$). Similarly, the Metoprolol in Acute Myocardial Infarction (MIAMI) trial found decreased 15-day mortality in patients receiving beta blockade compared with placebo. Both of these trials consisted of patients who did not receive acute reperfusion therapy. The Thrombolysis in Myocardial Infarction Phase II (TIMI-II) compared early versus late beta blockade in patients who received thrombolytic therapy and showed lower reinfarction rates in the early group. Based on trials such as these, the most recent ACC/American Heart Association (AHA) guidelines provide the highest recommendation (class I) to prompt beta blocker administration regardless of whether reperfusion therapy is provided. Most recently, however, the Clopidogrel and Metoprolol in Myocardial Infarction Trial (COMMIT) study (a large Chinese trial of more than 45,000 patients with STEMI) showed an increased risk (by 11 cases per 1000; $P \leq 0.00001$) of cardiogenic shock in those patients already in heart failure (Killip Class II and III) who were treated with metoprolol. The data for patients with NSTEMI and unstable angina are less well established than for those with STEMI. Recent guidelines, however, provide the highest recommendation to beta blockade if there is continuous chest pain and no contraindications. Relative contraindications include bradycardia, hypotension, second- or third-degree heart block, reactive airway disease, and severe left ventricular dysfunction.

Antman EM, Anbe DT, Armstrong PW, et al: ACC/AHA guidelines for the management of patients with ST-elevation myocardial infarction—executive summary: A report of the American College of Cardiology/American Heart Association Task Force on Practice Guidelines (Writing Committee to Revise the 1999 Guidelines for the Management of Patients with Acute Myocardial Infarction). J Am Coll Cardiol 44:671–719, 2004.

Braunwald E, Antman EM, Beasley JW, et al: ACC/AHA guideline update for the management of patients with unstable angina and non–ST-segment elevation myocardial infarction—2002: Summary article. A report of the American College of Cardiology/American Heart Association Task Force on Practice Guidelines (Committee on the Management of Patients with Unstable Angina). Circulation 106:1893–1900, 2002.

Chen ZM, Pan HC, Chen YP, et al: Early intravenous then oral metoprolol in 45,852 patients with acute myocardial infarction: Randomised placebo-controlled trial. Lancet 366:1622–1632, 2005.

First International Study of Infarct Survival Collaborative Group (ISIS-1): Randomised trial of intravenous atenolol among 16,027 cases of suspected acute myocardial infarction. Lancet 2:57–66, 1986.

MIAMI Trial Research Group: Metoprolol in acute myocardial infarction patient population. Am J Cardiol 56:10G–14G, 1985.

TIMI Study Group: Comparison of invasive and conservative strategies after treatment with intravenous tissue plasminogen activator in acute myocardial infarction: Results of the thrombolysis in myocardial infarction (TIMI) phase II trial. N Engl J Med 320:618–627, 1989.

13. **What are Killip classes?**

In 1967, Killip proposed a prognostic classification of AMI based on the presence and severity of rales:

- **Class I:** No rales; no S_3
- **Class II:** Rales $< 50\%$ of lung fields, may or may not have S_3
- **Class III:** Rales $> 50\%$ of lung fields, with S_3 and pulmonary edema present
- **Class IV:** Cardiogenic shock

Despite an overall improvement in the mortality of each class compared with the patients in Killip's original report, the classification remains useful today in comparing data for treatment of patients with MI.

Killip T III, Kimball JT: Treatment of myocardial infarction in a coronary care unit: A two year experience with 250 patients. Am J Cardiol 20:457–464, 1967.

14. **What is the role of antiplatelet agents in ACS?**

The benefit of aspirin in patients with cardiac ischemia is unequivocal. More recently, multiple agents that inhibit platelets via distinct mechanisms have been added to aspirin and shown to be beneficial. A 2002 meta-analysis evaluating the efficacy of glycoprotein IIb/IIIa inhibitors in patients with ACS found significant reductions in mortality and MI at 5 days, particularly in patients who had elevated troponin levels and had subsequent revascularization. Most recently, the Clopidogrel as Adjunctive Refusion Therapy (CLARITY)-TIMI 28 trial evaluated the combined administration of aspirin, clopidogrel (300-mg load, followed by 75 mg/day), and fibrinolysis for the treatment of STEMI and found a 36% relative risk reduction of death or recurrent MI in the clopidogrel-treated group. COMMIT also showed improved outcome in patients receiving clopidogrel.

Boersma E, Harrington RA, Moliterno DJ, et al: Platelet glycoprotein IIb/IIIa inhibitors in acute coronary syndromes: A meta-analysis of all major randomised clinical trials. Lancet 359:189–198, 2002.

Chen ZM, Jiang LX, Chen YP, et al: Addition of clopidogrel to aspirin in 45,852 patients with acute myocardial infarction: Randomised placebo-controlled trial. Lancet 366:1607–1621, 2005.

Sabatine MS, Cannon CP, Gibson CM, et al: Addition of clopidogrel to aspirin and fibrinolytic therapy for myocardial infarction with ST-segment elevation. N Engl J Med 352:1179–1189, 2005.

Tendera M, Wojakowski W: Role of antiplatelet drugs in the prevention of cardiovascular events. Thromb Res 110:355–359, 2003.

15. **What is the role of 3-hydroxy-3-methylglutaryl coenzyme A (HMG-CoA) reductase inhibitors in ACS?**

Two clinical trials demonstrated that the addition of an HMG-CoA reductase inhibitor soon after presentation with ACS was of benefit. This now is considered a standard of care. The Pravastin or Atorvastin Evaluation and Infection Therapy (PROVE-IT) TIMI-22 trial randomly assigned 4162 patients to receive high-dose (atorvastatin 80 mg daily) versus moderate-dose (pravastatin 40 mg daily) statin therapy in patients with ACS. High-dose statins not only had a greater effect on low-density lipoprotein C reduction but also were associated with a statistically significant reduction in all primary composite endpoints (22.4% atorvastatin; 26.3% pravastatin; $P = 0.005$).

Cannon CP, Braunwald E, McCabe CH, et al: Intensive versus moderate lipid lowering with statins after acute coronary syndromes. N Engl J Med 350:1495–1504, 2004.

Long-Term Intervention with Pravastatin in Ischaemic Disease (LIPID) Study Group: Prevention of cardiovascular events and death with pravastatin in patients with coronary heart disease and a broad range of initial cholesterol levels. N Engl J Med 339:1349–1357, 1998.

Schwartz GG, Olsson AG, Ezekowitz MD, et al: Effects of atorvastatin on early recurrent ischemic events in acute coronary syndromes: the MIRACL study: A randomized controlled trial. JAMA 285:1711–1718, 2001.

16. **What is the role of anticoagulation in ACS?**

Unfractionated heparin (UFH) is a mainstay of treatment for unstable coronary syndrome. When added to aspirin, the combination has been shown to reduce mortality and subsequent MI. Because the anticoagulant effect of UFH is frequently unpredictable, low-molecular-weight heparins have been evaluated for efficacy. Numerous trials have shown equivalence with UFH, and one trial (Superior Yield of the New Strategy of Enoxaparin, Revascularization, and Glycoprotein IIb/IIa Inhibitors [SYNERGY]) suggested superior results with low-molecular-weight heparins.

Antman EM, McCabe CH, Gurfinkel EP, et al: Enoxaparin prevents death and cardiac ischemic events in unstable angina/non–Q-wave myocardial infarction: Results of the Thrombolysis in Myocardial Infarction (TIMI) 11B trial. Circulation 100:1593–1601, 1999.

Ferguson JJ, Califf RM, Antman EM, et al: Enoxaparin vs unfractionated heparin in high-risk patients with non–ST-segment elevation acute coronary syndromes managed with an intended early invasive strategy: Primary results of the SYNERGY randomized trial. JAMA 292:45–54, 2004.

Goodman SG, Cohen M, Bigonzi F, et al: Randomized trial of low molecular weight heparin (enoxaparin) versus unfractionated heparin for unstable coronary artery disease: One-year results of the ESSENCE Study. Efficacy and Safety of Subcutaneous Enoxaparin in Non–Q-Wave Coronary Events. J Am Coll Cardiol 36: 693–698, 2000.

17. **What is the role of aldosterone inhibition and/or angiotensin-converting enzyme (ACE) inhibition in ACS?**

In 1999, a landmark study suggested that aldosterone has deleterious effects on ventricular remodeling and that these effects could be reversed in persons experiencing heart failure by the administration of combined aldosterone blockade and ACE inhibition. The recent Eplerenone Post-AMI Heart Failure Efficacy and Survival Study (EPHESUS) investigated the effect of eplerenone, a highly selective aldosterone receptor antagonist, on mortality in patients with heart failure due to systolic dysfunction after AMI. In those patients randomly assigned to receive eplerenone, there were significant decreases in death at 16 months, hospital deaths (due to cardiovascular causes), and sudden death relative to the placebo group. This has led the ACC/ AHA to make the addition of selective aldosterone blockade to ACE inhibitors a class I recommendation.

Antman EM, Anbe DT, Armstrong PW, et al: ACC/AHA guidelines for the management of patients with ST-elevation myocardial infarction—executive summary: A report of the American College of Cardiology/American Heart Association Task Force on Practice Guidelines (Writing Committee to Revise the 1999 Guidelines for the Management of Patients with Acute Myocardial Infarction). J Am Coll Cardiol 44:671–719, 2004.

Pitt B, Remme W, Zannad F, et al: Eplerenone, a selective aldosterone blocker, in patients with left ventricular dysfunction after myocardial infarction. N Engl J Med 348:1309–1321, 2003.

Pitt B, Zannad F, Remme WJ, et al: The effect of spironolactone on morbidity and mortality in patients with severe heart failure. Randomized Aldactone Evaluation Study Investigators. N Engl J Med 341:709–717, 1999.

KEY POINTS: ACUTE MYOCARDIAL INFARCTION

1. A class I recommendation by the ACC/AHA is that a selective aldosterone blocker and an angiotensin-converting enzyme inhibitor should be given to patients with heart failure.

2. Patients with acute coronary syndrome should be anticoagulated and should receive 3-hydroxy-3-methylglutaryl coenzyme A reductase inhibitors, aspirin and clopidogrel, and a beta blocker if there is no contraindication.

3. Patients with acute ST-segment elevation myocardial infarction should receive all the drugs given for acute coronary syndrome and undergo percutaneous coronary intervention, if possible.

DYSRHYTHMIAS AND TACHYARRHYTHMIAS

Noah E. Gordon, MD, and Linda L. Liu, MD

CHAPTER 28

1. How are the tachyarrhythmias classified?

Tachyarrhythmias are usually classified according to anatomic origin, as supraventricular or ventricular. They can also be grouped using the criteria of whether or not they traverse the atrioventricular (AV) node. Atrial flutter, atrial fibrillation, atrial tachycardia, and AV nodal reentrant tachycardia (AVNRT) traverse the AV node, whereas preexcited atrial arrhythmias, ventricular tachycardia (VT), and ventricular fibrillation (VF) do not. The importance of this latter classification is that nodal blocking drugs (e.g., beta blockers, calcium channel blockers, cardiac glycosides, or adenosine) can only control the ventricular response to tachycardias that traverse the AV node.

2. What are the supraventricular tachycardias (SVTs)?

Any tachyarrhythmia arising from the atria (atrial tachycardias) or the AV junction (junctional tachycardias) is an SVT. SVTs arising from the atria include sinus tachycardia, atrial fibrillation, atrial flutter, and atrial tachycardia. The most common junctional tachycardias are AVNRT and atrioventricular reentrant tachycardia (AVRT).

3. What are the ventricular tachycardias (VTs)?

VTs can be subdivided according to their morphology (monomorphic versus polymorphic) and their duration (sustained versus nonsustained). Nonsustained VT is defined as three or more premature ventricular contractions that occur at a rate exceeding 100 beats/min and last 30 seconds or less without hemodynamic compromise.

4. What is the normal conduction pathway?

Normally, the cardiac impulse originates in the sinus node and is conducted via the internodal pathways in the atrium, through the AV node, and down the His-Purkinje system, ultimately resulting in activation of the ventricular myocardium (first at the interventricular septum, then the apex, followed by the free walls). Once conducted down through the AV node, each sinus impulse cannot return to activate the atria because of the fibrous annulus (nonconductive tissue separating atria from ventricles at all points except the AV node). This structure protects the normal heart from reentrant arrhythmias.

5. Define *preexcitation* and describe its clinical significance.

Preexcitation exists when all or part of the ventricular muscle is activated by the atrial impulse sooner than would be expected if the impulse reached the ventricles only by way of the normal AV conduction system. Clinically, the presence of preexcitation (1) is associated with a high frequency of arrhythmias; (2) results in bizarre electrocardiography (ECG) patterns that make additional ECG analysis difficult/impossible; and (3) is associated with cardiac anomalies. For example, Wolff-Parkinson-White (WPW) is often associated with Ebstein's anomaly—abnormal morphogenesis of the tricuspid valve.

6. **How can you differentiate between tachyarrhythmias of ventricular or supraventricular origin?**
First, the safest option is to regard a broad complex tachycardia of uncertain origin as VT unless good evidence suggests otherwise. If a VT is wrongly treated as an SVT, the consequences may be extremely serious. Adenosine or vagal stimulation would be better diagnostic challenges owing to their transient nature. On the ECG, independent P wave activity, QRS duration >140 msec, concordance throughout the chest leads, and fusion waves all indicate VT.

KEY POINTS: WIDE COMPLEX SUPRAVENTRICULAR TACHYCARDIAS (SVTS) FREQUENTLY MISTAKEN FOR VENTRICULAR TACHYCARDIA (VT)

1. SVT with preexisting bundle branch block can be mistaken for VT.

2. SVT with aberrant conduction includes functional block or atrial impulse too rapid for normal bundle branch conduction and can lead to mistaken diagnosis.

3. Another SVT that may be mistaken for VT is Wolff-Parkinson-White (WPW) syndrome with antidromic atrioventricular reentrant tachycardia.

4. WPW syndrome with atrial fibrillation/flutter is yet another SVT that may masquerade as VT.

---

7. **Describe the mechanism and clinical presentation of AVNRT.**
The most common cause of paroxysmal regular narrow complex tachycardias, AVNRT involves two functionally and anatomically distinct pathways in the AV node, with different conduction velocities and refractory periods. With this substrate, a premature atrial contraction (PAC) may incite a "circus movement" in the node, which gives rise to slow–fast AVNRT. Most patients with AVNRT have only mild symptoms, whereas more severe symptoms (e.g., dizziness, dyspnea, weakness, neck pulsations, and chest pain) are common in patients with very rapid ventricular rates and preexisting heart disease.

8. **Define *AVRT*. What is the most common type of AVRT?**
AVRT occurs as a result of an anatomically distinct AV connection outside of the AV node. This accessory conduction pathway allows the atrial impulse to bypass the AV node and activate the ventricles prematurely, leading to a reentry circuit and paroxysmal AVRT. The most common type of AVRT occurs as part of WPW syndrome. In WPW syndrome, an accessory pathway (bundle of Kent) connects the atria directly to the ventricles, which can lead to the formation of reentry circuits resulting in either a narrow or broad complex tachycardia.

9. **What is the characteristic ECG appearance for WPW syndrome? How is it classified?**
In sinus rhythm, the atrial impulse conducts over the accessory pathway without the delay encountered with AV nodal conduction. Because it is transmitted rapidly to the ventricular myocardium, the PR interval is short; moreover, by passing through nonspecialized myocardium via an accessory pathway, it distorts the early part of the R wave, yielding the characteristic delta wave. This slow depolarization is then rapidly overtaken by depolarization through the normal conduction system, making the remainder of the QRS complex normal in appearance.

10. **What are mechanisms of tachycardia formation in WPW syndrome?**
    In orthodromic AVRT, a PAC is conducted down the AV node to the ventricles and then back to the atria via the accessory pathway. The depolarization circles repeatedly between the atria and ventricles, producing a narrow-complex tachycardia. P waves follow the QRS, there is no delta wave, and the QRS is of normal duration. In antidromic AVRT, which only occurs in 10% of patients with WPW syndrome, the accessory pathway allows antegrade conduction with retrograde conduction through the AV node. On the ECG, a delta wave is present and the QRS can be wide and bizarre.

11. **Why is atrial fibrillation a particular problem in WPW syndrome?**
    In patients without an accessory pathway, the AV node protects the ventricle from the rapid atrial activity that occurs during atrial fibrillation. In some patients, the accessory pathway allows very rapid conduction, and the ventricular rates in atrial fibrillation can exceed 300 beats/ min, with ensuing hemodynamic compromise. Drugs that block the AV node may decrease the refractoriness of accessory connections, resulting in an increased conduction and even more rapid ventricular response. Drugs that block the accessory pathway, including procainamide and amiodarone, are safer choices in these patients.

12. **Describe the acute management of tachycardia associated with WPW syndrome.**
    If there is a narrow QRS, try vagal maneuvers first, then beta blockers, calcium channel blockers, or adenosine to interrupt the tachycardia by creating transient AV nodal conduction block. If there is a wide-complex QRS, AV nodal blocking drugs should be avoided because they may enhance antegrade accessory pathway conduction and result in degeneration to VF. Instead, drugs that block the accessory pathway, such as procainamide and amiodarone, are the drugs of choice. DC cardioversion should be used if the patient's condition is unstable or pharmacologic therapy has been unsuccessful.

13. **What are ECG characteristics of the atrial arrhythmias?**
    Sinus tachycardia has P waves of normal morphology, a regular atrial and ventricular rate greater than 100 beats/min, and one P wave preceding every QRS complex. Atrial flutter is characterized by undulating saw-toothed baseline flutter waves, atrial rates of 250–350 beats/ min, regular ventricular rhythm, and slower ventricular rates of 150 beats/min (because 2:1 AV block is common). In atrial fibrillation, P waves are replaced by oscillating baseline fibrillation waves; the atrial rate is 350–600 beats/min, and the ventricular rhythm is irregular at 100–180 beats/min.

14. **Describe the pathophysiology of atrial fibrillation, and list some of its causes.**
    Atrial fibrillation is caused by multiple reentrant circuits or "wavelets" of activation sweeping around the atrial myocardium. This low-amplitude atrial activity exhibits variability in polarity, amplitude, and cycle length. Because each contraction and subsequent stroke volume depends on the amount of time for ventricular filling between heartbeats, there is variability in both ventricular rate and blood pressure. Known causes include heart disease (ischemic, hypertensive, and valvular), thyrotoxicosis, alcohol abuse (acute/chronic), sick sinus syndrome, postcardiac surgery, pulmonary disease (acute/chronic), endogenous/exogenous catecholamine release, and idiopathic (lone).

15. **What is torsades de pointes tachycardia?**
    Torsades de pointes ("twisting of the points") is a type of polymorphic VT in which the cardiac axis rotates over a sequence of 5–20 beats, changing from one direction to another and back again. If sustained, torsades de pointes may deteriorate into VF with corresponding hemodynamic collapse. Because torsades de pointes is treated differently, it must be differentiated from atrial fibrillation with preexcitation, which may have a similar appearance on ECG.

16. **List some causes of torsades de pointes and describe the management of this arrhythmia.**
Table 28-1 lists some causes of torsades de pointes tachycardia. Management of this arrhythmia would include asynchronous DC cardioversion if the patient is hemodynamically unstable (unless precipitated by a class IC agent); identification and withdrawal of any drug associated with QT prolongation; repletion of potassium and magnesium; and increasing ventricular rate with atropine, isoproterenol, or temporary pacing.

TABLE 28-1. CAUSES OF TORSADES DE POINTES TACHYCARDIA	
Category	**Examples**
Drugs	Antiarrhythmic drugs (class IA, IC, III)
	Antimicrobial drugs (erythromycin)
	Antimalarial drugs (chloroquine)
	Calcium channel blockers (bepridil)
	Psychiatric drugs (thioridazine, haloperidol, TCAs)
	Antihistamines (terfenadine)
	Serotonin agonists/antagonists (cisapride)
	Immunosuppressants (tacrolimus)
	Antidiuretic hormone (vasopressin)
Electrolyte disturbances	Hypokalemia
	Hypomagnesemia
Congential syndromes	Jervell and Lange-Nielsen syndrome
	Romano-Ward syndrome
Other causes	Myocardial ischemia
	Myxedema
	Bradycardia due to sick sinus syndrome or 3-degree AV block
	Subarachnoid hemorrhage
	Hepatic impairment

TCA = tricyclic antidepressant, AV = atrioventricular.

17. **What are some ECG abnormalities resulting from conditions other than cardiac disease?**
Abnormalities of electrolyte concentrations, acid–base status, serum glucose, thyroid hormones, and body temperature may lead to profound changes in the electrical activity of each myocardial cell, which is manifested on the ECG. Examples are listed in Table 28-2.

18. **What are some reversible causes of both SVT and VT in the intensive care unit (ICU)?**
Box 28-1 lists some of the most common conditions in the ICU that predispose patients to arrhythmias. These conditions are reversible and should be treated before use of pharmacologic antiarrhythmic therapies is considered.

TABLE 28-2. SOME CAUSES OF ECG ABNORMALITIES OTHER THAN MYOCARDIAL ISCHEMIA

Physiologic Derangement	ECG Change
Hyperkalemia	Tall peaked T waves→loss of P waves→widened QRS→sine wave, ventricular arrhythmias, asystole
Hypokalemia	Broad, flat T waves, ST-segment depression, QT prolongation, ventricular arrhythmias (e.g., PVCs, VT, PMVT, VF)
Hypothermia	Tremor artifact from shivering, atrial fibrillation with slow ventricular rate, J waves (Osborne waves), bradycardias (especially junctional), prolonged PR/QRS/QT intervals, ventricular arrhythmias, asystole
Thyrotoxicosis	Sinus tachycardia, increased QRS voltage, atrial fibrillation, PVCs, SVTs (e.g., PACs, MAT, atrial flutter), nonspecific ST-segment and T wave changes
Hypothyroidism	Sinus bradycardia, prolonged QT interval, flat/inverted T waves, heart block, low QRS voltage, IVCDs, PVCs
Hypercalcemia	Short QT interval
Hypoglycemia	Flat T waves, prolonged QT interval
SAH	ST depression/elevation, T wave inversion

ECG = electrocardiogram, PVC = Premature ventricular contractions, VT = ventricular tachycardia, PMVT = polymorphic ventricular tachycardia, VF = ventricular fibrillation, SVT = supraventricular tachycardia, MAT = multifocal atrial tachycardia, IVCD = idioventricular conduction delay, SAH = subarachnoid hemorrhage.

BOX 28-1. POSSIBLE CAUSES OF ARRHYTHMIAS IN PATIENTS IN THE INTENSIVE CARE UNIT

Hypoxemia

Hypotension

Acidosis

Cardiac ischemia

Mechanical irritation (e.g., from central lines, chest tubes)

Proarrhythmic drugs

Electrolyte imbalances

Hypercarbia

Hypothermia

Micro/macro shock

Adrenergic stimulation (light sedation)

19. What are the two classification systems important in understanding arrhythmogenesis and pharmacologic management of arrhythmias?
    - **Sicilian gambit:** This classification underscores the critical mechanisms responsible for arrhythmogenesis to identify an arrhythmia's "Achilles heel" or vulnerable parameter.

Classifications include automaticity (enhanced normal or abnormal), triggering (early afterdepolarizations or delayed afterdepolarizations), reentry (sodium or calcium dependent), reflection, and parasystole.

- **Modified Vaughan Williams:** This classification divides antiarrhythmic agents into one of four groups: class I (block sodium channels), class II (block sympathetic activity), class III (block potassium channels/prolong action potential), and class IV (block calcium channels).

20. **List the classes of antiarrhythmic drugs according to the modified Vaughan Williams classification system, including examples, mechanisms, sites of action, and clinical uses.**
See Table 28-3.

TABLE 28-3. ANTIARRHYTHMIC DRUGS ACCORDING TO THE MODIFIED VAUGHAN WILLIAMS CLASSIFICATION SYSTEM

Class of Drug	Examples	Primary Sites of Action	Mechanisms	Uses
IA	Procainamide	HP, A, V	Slows upstroke of phase 0, moderately prolongs repolarization and PR interval and QRS duration	SVT and VT
IB	Lidocaine	V	Has limited effect on dV/dt; shortens repolarization/QT interval	VT, VF
IC	Flecainide	HP, V	Slows dV/dt; has little effect on repolarization; markedly prolongs PR and QRS intervals	SVT and VT
II	Esmolol	SAN, AVN	Slows rate of rise of phase 4/discharge of SAN and AVN; suppresses catecholamine-induced increase in pacemaker current	Tachyarrhythmias
III	Amiodarone	A, V, AVN, SAN, HP, AcP	Increases AP duration by blocking delayed rectifier current/generally reduces automaticity; slightly suppresses SAN and AVN rates	AF, Af, SVT, nodal tachycardias, VT, VF
IV	Verapamil	AVN	Depresses phase 2 and 3 of AP by blocking slow Ca current	Atrial tachyarrhythmias

HP = His-Purkinje system, A = atrium, V = ventricle, SVT = supraventricular tachycardia, VT = ventricular tachycardia, dV/dt = rate of cardiac myocyte depolarization (phase 0 of action potential), VF = ventricular fibrillation, SAN = sinoatrial node, AVN = atrioventricular node, AcP = accessory pathways, AF = atrial fibrillation, Af = atrial flutter; AP = action potential, Ca = calcium.

21. **What is a good approach to chemical cardioversion of SVTs in the ICU?**
Efforts to chemically convert SVT to sinus rhythm using antiarrhythmic agents in the ICU should be directed toward those patients who cannot tolerate or do not respond to rate control therapy or who fail to respond to DC cardioversion and remain hemodynamically unstable. Most of the antiarrhythmic agents (e.g., ibutilide, amiodarone, and procainamide) with long-term activity against atrial arrhythmias have limited efficacy when used for rapid chemical cardioversion.

22. **How should you approach chemical cardioversion of VTs in the ICU?**
The conditions of unstable patients with marginal perfusion may deteriorate with recurrent episodes of nonsustained VT and may benefit from suppression with lidocaine, beta blockade, or treatment for hypomagnesemia. Monomorphic VT can be treated with amiodarone or procainamide. Polymorphic VT, even in the setting of a normal QT interval, is usually empirically treated with magnesium and sodium channel blocking agents.

23. **Is there a role for therapeutic hypothermia after resuscitation from VF/VT arrest?**
Possibly. Much of the morbidity and mortality in VF/VT cardiac arrest stems from the resultant widespread cerebral ischemia leading to severe neurologic impairment. A recent large blinded multicenter trial examined the possible benefit of mild systemic hypothermia (32–34°C) maintained for 24 hours after resuscitation from VF cardiac arrest. At 6 months, the hypothermia group had improved cerebral performance outcomes (55% versus 39%) and lower mortality (41% versus 55%) compared with the control group.

24. **Are there subgroups of patients with a better chance of survival after out-of-hospital cardiac arrest?**
Among patients who have an out-of-hospital cardiac arrest, the overall chance of survival is low. Although various factors associated with survival have been identified, the most important factor is the initial rhythm detected by the on-site ambulance crew. VF has a much higher survival rate than a nonshockable rhythm such as asystole. Factors associated with a lower chance of survival after cardiac arrest are as follows: no bystander cardiopulmonary resuscitation, nonwitnessed arrest, arrest at home, longer time to ambulance arrival, and increased age.

WEBSITES

1. Advanced Cardiac Life Support, Updated 2005 Guidelines, Algorithms, Simulators, and Links
   www.acls.net/aclsalg.htm

2. Alan E. Lindsay ECG Learning Center in Cyberspace: ECG examples
   http://library.med.utah.edu/kw/ecg/image_index/

3. Cleveland Clinic Guide to Arrhythmias for Patients
   www.clevelandclinic.org/heartcenter/pub/guide/disease/electric/arrhythmia.htm

4. University of Arizona Health Sciences Center, Center for Education and Research on Therapeutics: Updated list of drugs implicated in QT prolongation
   www.torsades.org

CHAPTER 29

AORTIC DISSECTION

Peter M. Schulman, MD, and Rondall Lane, MD

1. **What is an aortic dissection?**
   An aortic dissection is a tearing of the layers within the aortic wall. It is classically associated with sudden onset of chest or back pain, a pulse deficit, and mediastinal widening exhibited on chest x-ray. It often results in marked hemodynamic instability and may be rapidly fatal. Prompt diagnosis and appropriate treatment are critical to maximize the possibility of survival.

2. **In which layer of the aorta (i.e., intima, media, or adventitia) does the tear usually originate?**
   The tear usually originates in the intima. It then propagates into the media, creating a false channel for blood to flow and hematoma to form. The dissection process may alternatively originate with hemorrhage in the media that secondarily causes disruption of the intima.

   Khan IA, Nair CK: Clinical, diagnostic, and management perspectives of aortic dissection. Chest 122: 311–328, 2002.

3. **In which section of the aorta (i.e., ascending, arch, descending thoracic, or descending abdominal) does the dissection most often originate?**
   In approximately 70% of patients, the intimal tear, which is the beginning of the dissection, occurs in the ascending aorta. In 20% of patients it occurs in the descending thoracic aorta, and in 10% of patients it occurs in the aortic arch. Only rarely is an intimal tear identified in the abdominal aorta.

4. **Identify and describe the two most common classification systems.**
   1. **The DeBakey classification:** This system subdivides the dissection process into three types:
      - **Type I:** Involves the entire aorta (from aortic root extending beyond ascending aorta)
      - **Type II:** Confined to the ascending aorta
      - **Type III:** Begins distal to the takeoff of the left subclavian artery (spares the ascending aorta and arch). Type IIIA is limited to the thoracic aorta, whereas type IIIB extends below the diaphragm
   2. **The Stanford or Dailey classification:** This system divides the dissection process into two types:
      - **Type A:** Involves the ascending aorta
      - **Type B:** Distal to the left subclavian artery

   Nienaber CA, Eagle KA: Aortic dissection: New frontiers in diagnosis and management. Part I: From etiology to diagnostic strategies. Circulation 108:628–635, 2003. Available online at http://circ.ahajournals.org/cgi/content/full/108/5/628.

5. **What is the incidence of aortic dissection? Compare the mortality rates of type A versus type B dissection.**
   - Aortic dissection is a relatively rare but highly lethal disease. The estimated incidence is 5–30 cases per million people per year.
   - For untreated acute dissection of the ascending aorta, the mortality rate is 1–2% per hour early after symptom onset. For type A dissection treated medically, it is approximately 20% within the first 24 hours and 50% by 1 month after presentation. Even with surgery, the

mortality rate for type A dissection may be as high as 10% after 24 hours and nearly 20% 1 month after repair.

- Although type B dissection is less dangerous then type A, it is still associated with an extremely high degree of mortality. The 30-day mortality rate for uncomplicated type B dissection is 10%. However, patients with type B dissection who develop complications such as ischemic leg, renal failure, or visceral ischemia have a 2-day mortality of 20%.

Hagan PG, Nienaber CA, Isselbacher EM: The International Registry of Acute Aortic Dissection (IRAD): New insights into an old disease. JAMA 283:897–903, 2000.

Khan IA, Nair CK: Clinical, diagnostic, and management perspectives of aortic dissection. Chest 122:311–328, 2002.

6. **What are the most important risk factors and associated conditions?**
   - **Hypertension:** Hypertension is present in 70–90% of patients with acute dissection.
   - **Advanced age:** The mean age of all patients with acute dissection in the International Registry of Acute Aortic Dissection (IRAD) was 63 years.
   - **Male gender:** Sixty-six percent of patients in the IRAD were male.
   - **Marfan syndrome and other congenital disorders:** Marfan syndrome was present in almost 5% of patients in the IRAD. Other associated congenital disorders include Ehlers-Danlos syndrome, bicuspid aortic valve, aortic coarctation, Turner's syndrome, giant-cell aortitis, and relapsing polychondritis.
   - **Pregnancy:** Fifty percent of dissections in women younger than 40 years of age occur during pregnancy, most frequently in the third trimester.
   - **Circadian and seasonal variations:** Aortic dissection occurs more frequently in the morning hours and in the winter months.
   - **Iatrogenic complications:** Iatrogenic illness can be a consequence of invasive procedures or surgery, especially when the aorta has been entered or its main branches have been cannulated.

Hagan PG, Nienaber CA, Isselbacher EM: The International Registry of Acute Aortic Dissection (IRAD): New insights into an old disease. JAMA 283:897–903, 2000.

7. **What are the most common clinical features of aortic dissection?**
   - **Pain:** The most common presenting symptom is chest pain, occurring in up to 90% of patients with acute dissection. Classically, there is sudden onset of severe anterior chest pain with extension to the back that is described as ripping or tearing in nature. However, in the IRAD, pain was more often described as sharp rather than ripping or tearing. The pain is usually of maximal intensity from its inception and is frequently unremitting. It may migrate along the path of the dissection. The pain of aortic dissection may mimic that of myocardial ischemia.
   - **Shock:** Cardiogenic or hypovolemic shock may be secondary to cardiac tamponade from aortic rupture into the pericardium, dissection or compression of the coronary arteries, acute aortic regurgitation, or acute blood loss.
   - **Pulse or blood pressure differential or deficit:** This occurs in approximately one-third to one-half of patients with proximal dissection and signifies the partial compression of the subclavian arteries. Only one-sixth of patients with a distal dissection have a pulse deficit.
   - **Hypertension:** More than 50% of patients with distal dissection are hypertensive, and severe hypertension with diastolic pressure as high as 160 mmHg may be encountered with distal dissection. Severe hypertension may be due to renal ischemia.
   - **Acute aortic regurgitation:** This may be present in 50% of patients with proximal dissection and may occur because of widening of the aortic annulus or actual disruption of the aortic valve leaflets.
   - **Pleural effusions:** Pleural effusions, which occur most frequently in the left chest, can be caused by rupture of the dissection into the pleural space or by weeping of fluid from the aorta as the result of an inflammatory reaction to the dissection.

- **Other:** Horner's syndrome, mesenteric ischemia, myocardial infarction, mottling of the flanks, vocal cord paralysis, compression of the pulmonary arteries, complete heart block, hemoptysis, and hematemesis have all been reported.

Hagan PG, Nienaber CA, Isselbacher EM: The International Registry of Acute Aortic Dissection (IRAD): New insights into an old disease. JAMA 283:897–903, 2000.

Khan IA, Nair CK: Clinical, diagnostic, and management perspectives of aortic dissection. Chest 122:311–328, 2002.

Klompas M: Does this patient have an acute thoracic aortic dissection? JAMA 287:2262–2272, 2002.

Nienaber CA, Eagle KA: Aortic dissection: New frontiers in diagnosis and management. Part I: From etiology to diagnostic strategies. Circulation 108:628–635, 2003. Available online at http://circ.ahajournals.org/cgi/content/full/108/5/628.

8. **What laboratory and other nonradiologic data are helpful in confirming the diagnosis of aortic dissection?**
Laboratory data are usually unrevealing. Anemia from loss of blood into the false lumen of the dissection can occur. A moderate leukocytosis (i.e., 10,000–14,000 white cells/mL) is sometimes seen. Lactic acid dehydrogenase and bilirubin levels may be elevated because of hemolysis within the false lumen. Disseminated intravascular coagulation has been reported. An electrocardiogram (ECG) without evidence of myocardial ischemia in a patient with severe chest pain may be suggestive of aortic dissection and should prompt further work-up. However, the presence of ischemia on an ECG does not rule out dissection, and two-thirds of patients with dissection have nonspecific ST-segment abnormalities on ECG.

9. **What procedures or imaging modalities are useful in confirming the diagnosis of aortic dissection?**
Although it lacks specificity, a chest radiograph should be obtained as part of the initial diagnostic evaluation. An abnormality revealed by chest x-ray is seen in 90% of patients with aortic dissection; most frequently, this is widening of the aorta and mediastinum. Other findings may include a localized hump on the aortic arch, displacement of calcification in the aortic knob, and the presence of pleural effusions.

Computed tomographic (CT) scanning, magnetic resonance imaging (MRI), and transesophageal echocardiography (TEE) are all highly accurate imaging modalities that can be used to make the diagnosis. Transthoracic echocardiography (TTE) has limited diagnostic accuracy. Aortography, which was once the test of choice, is invasive and time-consuming but is still used for patients undergoing elective operations on the thoracic aorta. Although there are advantages and disadvantages associated with each imaging modality, the choice among CT, MRI, and TEE should probably be based on which test is most readily available. Table 29-1 reviews the assets and limitations of the major diagnostic tests used in evaluating patients with suspected aortic dissection.

Khan, IA, Nair CK: Clinical, diagnostic, and management perspectives of aortic dissection. Chest 122:311–328, 2002.

Klompas M: Does this patient have an acute aortic dissection? JAMA 287:2262–2272, 2002.

10. **What should be considered in the differential diagnosis of aortic dissection?**
- Acute myocardial infarction
- Cerebrovascular accidents
- Thoracic nondissecting aneurysm
- Pericarditis
- Pleuritis
- Atherosclerotic emboli
- Pulmonary embolism
- Acute aortic regurgitation

- Mediastinal cysts or tumors
- Cholecystitis
- Musculoskeletal pain

Klompas M: Does this patient have an acute aortic dissection? JAMA 287:2262–2272, 2002.

TABLE 29-1. MAJOR CHARACTERISTICS OF COMMON TESTS USED IN THE DIAGNOSIS OF AORTIC DISSECTION

	Sensitivity	Specificity	Major Assets	Major Limitations
Angiography	80–90%	90–95%	Shows entry site	Time and personnel
			Shows aortic branches	Nephrotoxic agents
			Shows dependency of aortic branches	Misses intramural hematoma
Conventional CT	65–85%		Easiness and rapidity	Misses entry site
Ultrafast CT	80–100%	95–100%		Partial analysis of aortic branches
MRI	95–100%	95–100%	Precise flow analysis	Transfer of patient
			Shows aortic branches	Acquisition time and surveillance
			No contrast material	High cost
Echocardiography (transthoracic and transesophageal)	95–100%	85–90%	Rapidity	Misses the distal ascending aorta
			Assesses aortic regurgitation	Bedside examination
			Assesses pericardial effusion	Misses branch involvement
			Assesses myocardial function	Misses entry site
				Requires expertise Uncomfortable on the awake patient

CT = computed tomography, MRI = magnetic resonance imaging.

11. **What life-threatening problems can aortic dissection cause?**

The outer wall of the false channel may only be one-fourth as thick as the original media, which explains why aortic dissection frequently leads to rupture—often a catastrophic event. Rupture of the aortic arch occurs most frequently into the mediastinum, the descending thoracic aorta into the left pleural space, and the abdominal aorta into the retroperitoneum. Rupture of any portion of the ascending aorta can lead to cardiac tamponade from hemopericardium.

The dissection can also progress along the course of the aorta and occlude any of its arterial branches. Retrograde extension can lead to dissection of the coronaries with more frequent involvement of the right coronary artery than the left. Retrograde dissection can also result in loss of commissural support for one or more of the aortic valve cusps, causing acute aortic insufficiency.

12. **How should a Stanford type A dissection be managed?**
An acute type A dissection is a surgical emergency. However, medical management is critical to halt the progression of the dissection while the diagnostic work-up takes place and before the patient can be brought to the operating room for definitive treatment. While the diagnosis is being confirmed and a cardiothoracic surgeon is being consulted, patients should be carefully monitored and stabilized in an intensive care unit. Pain management and blood pressure control to a target systolic pressure of 110 mmHg are critical. Sufficient blood should be available in the event of aortic rupture.

13. **How should a Stanford type B dissection be managed?**
Patients with type B dissection are usually managed medically with beta blockers and other antihypertensive agents. These patients do better with medical therapy alone because they tend to be older, have extensive atherosclerotic vascular disease, and have other comorbidities including cardiac and pulmonary disease. Surgery may be indicated, however, if medical therapy fails, and in fact one-third of patients with distal dissection eventually require surgery. This is often due to continued dissection, rupture, end-organ or extremity ischemia resulting from the dissection, or intractable pain.

14. **What are the goals of medical therapy in acute aortic dissection? Which medications are commonly used?**
The goals of medical therapy are to treat pain and to control hypertension. The blood pressure should generally be lowered to a systolic of 100–120 mmHg and a mean of 60–65 mmHg, or to the lowest level that is compatible with perfusion of the vital organs.

The antihypertensive regimen must decrease blood pressure without increasing cardiac output. This is because an increase in cardiac output can increase flow rates, producing higher shear forces, thus propagating the dissection.

A standard regimen involves using a rapidly acting IV vasodilator such as nitroprusside to lower blood pressure in conjunction with an IV beta blocker such as esmolol. The beta blocker is used to prevent any reflex increase in cardiac output associated with the vasodilator therapy, and therefore adequate beta blockade must be established first, *before* the treatment with the vasodilator is initiated.

Alternatively, monotherapy is possible either with IV labetalol (a combination alpha and beta receptor antagonist) or less commonly with trimethaphan (a ganglionic blocker that produces vasodilation without causing any reflex increase in cardiac output).

Marino PL: The ICU Book, 2nd ed. Baltimore, Williams & Wilkins, 1998, pp 301–316.

15. **How does sodium nitroprusside work, how quickly does it work, and what is its dosing range?**
In contrast to pure arterial or venodilators, sodium nitroprusside is a balanced vasodilator that acts directly on both the arterial and venous circulations to concurrently decrease both afterload and preload (Table 29-2).

Nitroprusside is a carrier and donor of nitric oxide, and it is the spontaneous release of nitric oxide that mediates its vasodilatory action. Nitroprusside works rapidly to lower blood pressure within 1–2 minutes of initiating as infusion, and its effect is terminated equally as quickly after the drug is stopped. The initial dose is 0.25–0.5 µg/kg/min, which should be titrated slowly to a maximum of 10 µg/kg/min.

TABLE 29-2. CLASSIFICATION OF VASODILATOR DRUGS		
Arterial Dilators	**Balanced Dilators**	**Venodilators**
Hydralazine ACE inhibitors Nicardipine	Nitroprusside	Nitroglycerine

ACE = angiotensin-converting enzyme.

KEY POINTS: THE DIAGNOSIS AND TREATMENT OF ACUTE AORTIC DISSECTION

1. Aortic dissection is classically associated with sudden chest or back pain, a pulse deficit, and mediastinal widening exhibited on chest radiograph.

2. The imaging modality (i.e., CT, MRI, or TEE) that is most readily available should be the one selected to confirm the diagnosis of acute aortic dissection.

3. An acute type A aortic dissection is a surgical emergency. Although type B dissections are usually managed medically, one-third of the patients requiring this procedure eventually require surgery due to worsening of the dissection, rupture, end-organ or extremity ischemia, or intractable pain.

4. When managing acute aortic dissection, adequate beta blockade must be established *before* the initiation of nitroprusside to prevent propagation of the dissection from a reflex increase in cardiac output.

5. Cyanide toxicity from nitroprusside administration can be recognized by increasing tolerance to the drug (tachyphylaxis), an elevated mixed venous oxygen content, and the development of a metabolic (lactic) acidosis.

16. **What are the common side effects of nitroprusside?**
    These include nausea, restlessness, somnolence, and hypotension.

17. **What are the toxic complications of sodium nitroprusside therapy? How are they recognized and treated?**
    There is potential for cyanide and thiocyanate toxicity. It is recommended that doses no larger than 10 µg/kg/min be administered to patients and that the total dose given not exceed 3–3.5 mg/kg. Cyanide toxicity can be recognized by increasing tolerance to the drug (tachyphylaxis), elevated mixed venous oxygen content, and the development of lactic acidosis. Thiocyanate toxicity is characterized by muscle weakness, hyperreflexia, confusion, delirium, and coma. When the drug is being infused at rates higher than 3 µg/kg for periods exceeding 72 hours, thiocyanate levels should be measured. Cyanide poisoning can be treated with amyl nitrite, sodium nitrite, and sodium thiosulfate. For patients with severe thiocyanate toxicity, hemodialysis may be performed.

18. **What are the goals of surgery for type A dissection?**
    The goals are to resect the aortic segment containing the proximal intimal tear, to obliterate the false channel, and to restore aortic continuity with a graft or by reapproximating the transected ends of the aorta. For patients with aortic insufficiency, it may be possible to re-suspend the aortic valve, but in some cases, replacement of the aortic valve is necessary. In some cases of proximal dissection, reimplantation of the coronary arteries may be required. Surgery to repair an aortic dissection generally requires cardiopulmonary bypass and sometimes requires deep hypothermic circulatory arrest.

19. **What is a more recent alternative to surgical repair of aortic dissection?**
    An endovascular technique of stenting and/or balloon fenestration is now sometimes used to treat certain type A dissections and complicated type B dissections. For type B dissection, many reports have now demonstrated better results with endovascular repair versus surgery.

    Nienaber CA, Eagle KA: Aortic dissection: New frontiers in diagnosis and management. Part II: Therapeutic management and follow-up. Circulation 108:772–778, 2003.

ACKNOWLEDGMENTS

The authors gratefully acknowledge the contributions of Timothy R. White, MD, PhD, and David E. Schwartz, MD, FCCP, authors of this chapter in the third edition of *Critical Care Secrets*.

CHAPTER 30

VALVULAR HEART DISEASE

Rondall Lane, MD, and Peter M. Schulman, MD

MITRAL REGURGITATION

1. **What is the importance of the mitral valve apparatus?**

   Two papillary muscles, multiple chordae tendineae, an annulus, an anterior and posterior leaflet, and portions of the left ventricular wall make up the mitral valve. In addition to preventing regurgitation, the integration of the mitral valve apparatus into the left ventricle helps to maintain ventricular shape and to coordinate contraction. Abnormalities of the mitral valve lead to rapid and permanent left ventricular dysfunction.

   Soble JS, Neumann A: Valvular heart disease producing critical illness. In Parrillo JE, Dellinger RP (eds): Critical Care Medicine: Principles of Diagnosis and Management in the Adult, 2nd ed. St. Louis, Mosby, 2002, pp 638–657.

   Sorrentino M: Valvular heart disease. In Hall JB, Schmidt GA, Wood L (eds): Principles of Critical Care, 2nd ed. New York, McGraw-Hill, 1998, pp 467–482.

   Turgeman Y, Atar S, Rosenfeld T: The subvalvular apparatus in rheumatic mitral stenosis: Methods of assessment and therapeutic implications. Chest 124:1929–1936, 2003.

2. **Name some common causes of mitral regurgitation.**

   Chronic causes include elongation of the papillary muscles from chronic ischemia or scarring, left ventricular enlargement with dilatation of the annulus, and myomatous degeneration of the mitral valve, which is now more common than rheumatic heart disease as a cause of mitral regurgitation. Traumatic conditions usually cause acute mitral regurgitation and include fenestrations of a valve leaflet as a result of blunt trauma or endocarditis and rupture of the chordae or papillary muscle as a result of myocardial ischemia.

   Soble JS, Neumann A: Valvular heart disease producing critical illness. In Parrillo JE, Dellinger RP (eds): Critical Care Medicine: Principles of Diagnosis and Management in the Adult, 2nd ed. St. Louis, Mosby, 2002, pp 638–657.

3. **Describe the pathophysiology of mitral regurgitation.**

   Similar to aortic regurgitation, mitral regurgitation can develop from events that adversely affect leaflet integrity. Mitral regurgitation can develop from distortion of the mitral annulus or from functional or structural abnormalities of the submitral apparatus, including the chordae tendineae and the papillary muscles. Patients who present with severe acute mitral regurgitation commonly have myocardial infarctions, perivalvular abscesses, or endocarditis as the underlying etiologies. Endocarditis causes mitral regurgitation through leaflet destruction or through infection and rupture of the chordae muscles. Myocardial ischemia leads to impaired shortening of the papillary muscles, allowing regurgitant flow. Ischemia, particularly of the posteromedial papillary muscle, which receives its blood supply from the dominant coronary artery, can lead to infarction of papillary muscles and complete transection of the papillary muscle head with subsequent regurgitation through the mitral valve. Chronic mitral regurgitation is often due to mitral valve prolapse, rheumatic heart disease, left ventricular dysfunction, and ischemic or nonischemic dilated cardiomyopathy.

   Soble JS, Neumann A: Valvular heart disease producing critical illness. In Parrillo JE, Dellinger RP (eds): Critical Care Medicine: Principles of Diagnosis and Management in the Adult, 2nd ed. St. Louis, Mosby, 2002, pp 638–657.

4. **How does acute mitral regurgitation present?**
Acute mitral regurgitation usually presents with symptoms of congestive heart failure because the left ventricle, left atrium, and pulmonary vasculature have not had time to dilate and maintain forward flow. Subsequently, left atrium and pulmonary capillary wedge pressures increase strikingly. Cardiogenic shock may or may not be present. In patients with a diagnosis of myocardial infarction or endocarditis, mitral regurgitation should be suspected if the patient's condition deteriorates rapidly or if he or she develops acute pulmonary edema. In patients with an inferior wall myocardial infarction, papillary muscle rupture may occur several days into the course of disease and often occurs in the setting of multivessel disease. On examination, patients typically have a holosystolic murmur best heard at the apex. The murmur may muffle the first heart sound and continue through the second.

Soble JS, Neumann A: Valvular heart disease producing critical illness. In Parrillo JE, Dellinger RP (eds): Critical Care Medicine: Principles of Diagnosis and Management in the Adult, 2nd ed. St. Louis, Mosby, 2002, pp 638–657.

5. **Describe the reasons for decompensation in chronic mitral regurgitation.**
The hemodynamic consequences of mitral regurgitation include both volume overload of the left ventricle and pressure-volume overload of the left atrium. These changes lead to eccentric hypertrophy and eventually left ventricular dysfunction. Unlike aortic regurgitation, afterload is reduced in mitral regurgitation as a result of part of the cardiac output being ejected in the left atrium. This afterload reduction permits left ventricular ejection performance to be maintained even in the face of impaired contractility. In some cases, the actual amount of impaired contractility is not apparent until after valve replacement when the ejection fraction falls and the patient's condition declines hemodynamically.

Soble JS, Neumann A: Valvular heart disease producing critical illness. In Parrillo JE, Dellinger RP (eds): Critical Care Medicine: Principles of Diagnosis and Management in the Adult, 2nd ed. St. Louis, Mosby, 2002, pp 638–657.

6. **What diagnostic studies are available for mitral regurgitation?**
The chest radiograph will show pulmonary edema with a relatively normal heart size in severe acute mitral regurgitation. In chronic mitral regurgitation, cardiomegaly with left ventricular and left atrial enlargement and evidence of pulmonary venous hypertension or enlarged pulmonary arteries are suggestive of pulmonary arterial hypertension. Echocardiography allows for diagnosis and quantification of mitral regurgitation and the ruling out of other possible problems, including ventricular septal defect. Mean wedge pressure and V-wave height assessed by pulmonary artery catheterization can help determine the hemodynamic significance of the mitral regurgitation. Echocardiographic criteria for severe mitral regurgitation include color flow area > 40% of left atrial area, E velocity > 1.5 m/sec, effective regurgitant orifice (ERO) $\geq$ 0.40 cm^2, regurgitant volume $\geq$ 60 mL, and regurgitant fraction $\geq$ 55%.

Soble JS, Neumann A: Valvular heart disease producing critical illness. In Parrillo JE, Dellinger RP (eds): Critical Care Medicine: Principles of Diagnosis and Management in the Adult, 2nd ed. St. Louis, Mosby, 2002, pp 638–657.

Turgeman Y, Atar S, Rosenfeld T: The subvalvular apparatus in rheumatic mitral stenosis: Methods of assessment and therapeutic implications. Chest 124:1929–1936, 2003.

7. **What is the appropriate initial management of mitral regurgitation?**
Therapy for patients with acute mitral regurgitation is highly dependent on the presence or absence of shock. Patients with acute mitral regurgitation may be temporarily managed with inotropes (e.g., dopamine or dobutamine, if hypotension is absent) and reduction of afterload with vasodilators (e.g., angiotensin-converting enzyme inhibitors, nitrates), intra-aortic balloon counterpulsation, or a combination thereof. Examination of the valvular apparatus with echocardiography to determine left ventricular function assesses the possibility of valve repair and helps define the pathology leading to valvular dysfunction. IV nitroglycerin is helpful in patients who have mitral regurgitation resulting from ischemia.

American College of Cardiology and American Heart Association: Pocket Guidelines for Management of Patients with Valvular Heart Disease. AHA Journals, Lippincott Williams & Wilkins, 2000.

Lung B: Management of ischemic mitral regurgitation. Heart 89:459–464, 2003.

Soble JS, Neumann A: Valvular heart disease producing critical illness. In Parrillo JE, Dellinger RP (eds): Critical Care Medicine: Principles of Diagnosis and Management in the Adult, 2nd ed. St. Louis, Mosby, 2002, pp 638–657.

8. **What criteria would prompt you to refer a patient with mitral regurgitation to surgery?**

Surgery should be performed before the decline of left ventricular function. The onset of myocardial dysfunction is thought to have occurred when the ejection fraction falls to <0.60 or when end-systolic dimension approaches 45 mm. In severe acute mitral regurgitation, patients who present with pulmonary edema and shock are candidates for surgery. If ischemia is the underlying cause for mitral regurgitation, then percutaneous transluminal coronary angioplasty may be of benefit. The type of surgery depends on the overall clinical picture, with valve morphology and clinical circumstances being the most important determinants. Patients with endocarditis will need valve replacement. Women of childbearing years may benefit from valve repair or percutaneous balloon mitral valvuloplasty if circumstances allow because this allows them to avoid long-term anticoagulation and maintain chordal preservation. Asymptomatic patients who have an effective regurgitant orifice of at least 40 mm^2 have an increased risk of death from cardiac causes and should be considered as candidates for mitral valve surgery.

Carabello BA: Is it ever too late to operate on the patient with valvular heart disease? J Am Coll Cardiol 44:376–383, 2004.

Enriquez-Sarano M, Avierinos J, Messika-Zeitoun D, et al: Quantitative determinants of the outcome of asymptomatic mitral regurgitation. N Engl J Med 352:875–883, 2005.

Reimold S, Rutherford J: Valvular heart disease in pregnancy. N Engl J Med 349:52–59, 2003.

Soble JS, Neumann A: Valvular heart disease producing critical illness. In Parrillo JE, Dellinger RP (eds): Critical Care Medicine: Principles of Diagnosis and Management in the Adult, 2nd ed. St. Louis, Mosby, 2002, pp 638–657.

Talwalker N, Earle N, Earle E, Lawrie G: Mitral valve repair in patients with low left ventricular ejection fractions. Chest 126:709–715, 2004.

9. **Is the ejection fraction helpful in determining whether a patient is a candidate for mitral valve surgery?**

Initially, it was thought that surgical therapy for mitral regurgitation was synonymous with a postoperative reduction in ejection fraction resulting from removal of the favorable loading conditions that were a consequence of mitral regurgitation. It is now known that destruction of mitral apparatus during mitral valve replacement, and not the change in loading conditions, leads to loss of ventricular shape and loss of ventricular contractility. Hence, when the mitral apparatus is preserved, the ejection fraction is unchanged. Therefore, no matter how low the ejection fraction, almost no one should be excluded from surgery based on ejection fraction alone. If the mitral apparatus cannot be preserved, valve replacement for patients with ejection fractions < 0.35 is not recommended.

Carabello BA: Is it ever too late to operate on the patient with valvular heart disease? J Am Coll Cardiol 44:376–383, 2004.

Talwalker N, Earle N, Earle E, Lawrie G: Mitral valve repair in patients with low left ventricular ejection fractions. Chest 126:709–715, 2004.

MITRAL STENOSIS

10. **What is the etiology of mitral valve stenosis?**

Mitral valve stenosis can be caused by a variety of illnesses. Rheumatic heart disease was once a common cause of mitral valve stenosis. As the incidence of rheumatic fever has declined in developed nations, mitral valve stenosis has become mostly a disease of persons who have emigrated from areas where rheumatic fever is still endemic. Although mitral valve stenosis is due to rheumatic fever, it is two to three times more common in women. It is thought that the M protein antigen, shared by both the myocardium and group A hemolytic streptococci, leads to an autoimmune attack of heart muscle as the immune system reacts to the streptococcal infection. The disease predominantly affects the endocardium, leading to inflammation and scarring of the cardiac valves. Continued low-grade rheumatic process and/or hemodynamic stress on a damaged valve leads to chronic inflammation and scarring continuing after the initial attack, with subsequent valve damage eventually becoming severe. Stenosis results from leaflet thickening, commissural fusion, and chordal shortening and fusion. Other causes include mitral annular calcification, which is associated atherosclerosis rather than rheumatic fever.

Carabello B: Modern management of mitral stenosis. Circulation 112:432–437, 2005.

11. **What is the pathophysiology behind mitral valve stenosis?**
The normal orifice of the mitral valve is 4–5 cm^2, and it serves as the inlet valve to the left ventricle by essentially creating a common chamber between the left atrium and left ventricle during diastole. Normally, the mitral valve is a complex apparatus made up of an annulus and two leaflets that are attached by chordae tendineae to two papillary muscles. The papillary muscles originate from the walls of the left ventricle and secure the chordae and mitral leaflets, preventing prolapse of the valve during ventricular systole. Mitral valve stenosis results from any congenital or acquired pathologic process that narrows the effective mitral valve orifice at the supravalvular, valvular, or subvalvular levels. During ventricular filling, pressures are equal between the two chambers. As the mitral valve orifice narrows in mitral valve stenosis, a pressure gradient develops between the two chambers as a result of the inhibition of flow from the left atrium to the left ventricle. This pressure gradient is transmitted to the left ventricle diastolic pressure. This leads to an elevation of left atrial and pulmonary venous pressures. Enlarged bronchial veins may encroach on small bronchioles, with subsequent increase in airway resistance. Pulmonary edema occurs when pulmonary venous pressure is greater than plasma oncotic pressure. Pulmonary artery hypertension ensues with the compensatory vasoconstriction and medial hypertrophy and intimal thickening of the pulmonary arterioles. As the disease progresses, the right ventricle fails and pulmonary blood flow declines, decreasing systemic blood flow. If the fall in cardiac output is significant, end-organ failure, shock, and metabolic acidosis can occur. Right ventricular failure results in systemic venous congestion with development of hepatomegaly, ascites, and edema.

Carabello B: Modern management of mitral stenosis. Circulation 112:432–437, 2005.

12. **How is the diagnosis of mitral valve stenosis made?**
When the disease is mild, patients may be asymptomatic at rest and with exertion. As the stenosis worsens, dyspnea on exertion, orthopnea, and paroxysmal nocturnal dyspnea occur. Increased left atrial pressure may lead to hemoptysis as a result of rupture between bronchial veins. New-onset atrial fibrillation may be the presenting finding in some patients. Additionally, hoarseness resulting from an enlarged left atrium impinging on the left recurrent laryngeal nerve may develop in some patients (Ortner's syndrome). On physical examination, patients often have a reduced pulse pressure from reduced stroke volume, neck elevation from right heart failure, rales from left heart failure, or plethoric cheeks punctuated by bluish patches related to impaired cardiac output. A right ventricular lift may be present if pulmonary hypertension has developed.

Carabello B: Modern management of mitral stenosis. Circulation 112:432–437, 2005.
Chikwe J, Walther A, Pepper J: The surgical management of mitral valve disease. Br J Cardiol 11:42–48, 2004.

13. **Describe the classification for the severity of mitral valve stenosis.**
    - **Trivial mitral valve stenosis:** >2.0 cm^2 with a normal pressure gradient
    - **Mild mitral valve stenosis:** 1.0–2.5 cm^2 with a pressure gradient of 2.0–6.0 mmHg
    - **Moderate mitral valve stenosis:** 1.0–1.5 cm^2 with a pressure gradient of 6.0–12 mmHg
    - **Severe mitral valve stenosis:** <1.0 cm^2 with a pressure gradient of >12 mmHg

    Hartman GS, Thomas SJ: Valvular heart disease. In Yao FS, Artusio JF (eds): Yao and Artusio's Anesthesiology: Problem-Oriented Patient Management, 5th ed. Philadelphia, Lippincott Williams and Wilkins, pp 201–233.

14. **What is the differential diagnosis of mitral valve stenosis?**
    Left atrial myoma may demonstrate a similar clinical picture to mitral valve stenosis. Other lesions include the following:
    - **Cor-triatriatum sinister:** This is a rare congenital heart defect resulting from the division of the left atrium by a fibromuscular membrane. It is usual for patients to present with this defect in infancy and early childhood, although some cases remain undetected until adult life.
    - **Atrial myxoma**
    - **Pulmonary vein stenosis**
    - **Shone complex:** This congenital cardiac abnormality consists of supravalvular mitral ring, parachute mitral valve, subaortic stenosis, and aortic coarctation.

15. **When should surgery be considered in patients with mitral valve stenosis?**
    It may be as long as 20–40 years between the occurrence of rheumatic fever and the onset of symptomatic mitral valve stenosis. Once symptoms develop, it may be up to 10 years before they become disabling. In minimally symptomatic patients, the 10-year survival rate is 80%. However, this drops to 10–15% once symptoms become limiting. Hence, it is reasonable to offer surgery when more than mild symptoms have developed. The one exception to this would be an asymptomatic patient with pulmonary artery hypertension. Once there is severe pulmonary hypertension, mean survival drops to less than 3 years. Additionally, pulmonary hypertension increases the surgical mortality risk from approximately 3–8% to 12%. It appears best to offer surgery before the onset of pulmonary hypertension or just as soon as it is detected. Evidence suggests that patients with New York Heart Association functional class I–II symptoms, a mitral valve area <1.0 cm^2, and severe pulmonary artery hypertension (systolic pulmonary artery pressure $> 60–80$ mmHg) will still benefit from surgery. Pulmonary pressures usually return to normal or near normal after correction of mitral valve stenosis.

    Carabello B: Modern management of mitral stenosis. Circulation 112:432–437, 2005.
    Carabello BA: Is it ever too late to operate on the patient with valvular heart disease? J Am Coll Cardiol 44:376–383, 2004.
    Chikwe J, Walther A, Pepper J: The surgical management of mitral valve disease. Br J Cardiol 11:42–48, 2004.

AORTIC STENOSIS

16. **Describe the pathophysiology of aortic stenosis.**
    Aortic stenosis is the most frequent of all valvular abnormalities, estimated to occur in 2% of the population. Causes of aortic stenosis include both congenital and acquired etiologies. The most common form of acquired aortic stenosis is degeneration of previously normal tissue leading to calcification of the cuspal tissue or calcification of congenitally bicuspid valves, which occurs in approximately 1% of the population. The nidus for calcium and inorganic phosphate ions to crystallize and form hydroxyapatite crystals in the plasma membrane of dying cells is suggestive of a senile pathologic mechanism. Traditionally, it was believed that passive accumulation of hydroxyapatite mineral in the setting of sclerosis leads to calcification. However, it is now known that active processes similar to those involved

atherosclerotic arteries, including inflammation and lipid infiltration, play a significant role in aortic stenosis.

Mohler E: Mechanisms of aortic valve calcification. Am J Cardiol 94:1396–1402, 2004.

Schoen F: Cardiac valves and valvular pathology: Update on function, disease, repair and replacement. Cardiovasc Pathol 14:189–194, 2005.

17. **What are the two determinants of transvalvular flow?**
Transvalvular flow is determined by the pressure gradient and orifice area. Hence, the severity of aortic stenosis cannot be defined by a high pressure gradient alone as a number of patients with poor left ventricular systolic function, and thus low gradients, may be missed.

Carabello BA: Is it ever too late to operate on the patient with valvular heart disease? J Am Coll Cardiol 44:376–383, 2004.

18. **What do the terms *aortic pseudostenosis* and *inotropic reserve* mean?**
Patients with severe aortic stenosis (valve area < 1.0 cm^2) should undergo aortic valve replacement. A potential problem arises when a patient presents with a calculated valve area < 1.0 cm^2 and simultaneously has low cardiac output. Calculated valve area can be dramatically smaller in patients with low cardiac output. To establish whether truly severe aortic stenosis is present at low cardiac output, it is necessary to increase output pharmacologically with an agent such as dobutamine. If the gradient increases in concert with output, valve area will increase only slightly, and it is presumed that severe fixed obstruction is present.

Pseudostenosis occurs when increased output results in a simultaneous increase in valve area of > 0.3 cm^2 or when calculated valve area exceeds 1.0 cm^2. For such a result to occur, there has to be a large increase in output without a large increase in gradient, meaning that severe obstruction is not present. Hence, these patients are presumably less likely to benefit from aortic valve replacement. Additionally, if an inotropic challenge (dobutamine stress echo) is administered and cardiac output fails to increase, the prognosis is poor.

Compared with a 5–8% perioperative mortality rate observed in patients with an inotropic reserve, patients without an inotropic reserve experience a perioperative mortality rate as high as 33%. It has been suggested that patients with aortic stenosis whose cardiac output fails to increase by at least 25% during dobutamine challenge should be considered nonsurgical candidates because the absence of inotropic reserve signals severe and irreversible left ventricular dysfunction. However, a study has suggested that although the perioperative mortality for patients with severe aortic stenosis and a low transvalvular pressure gradient was significantly higher, those few who survived surgery had improvement in left ventricular ejection fraction and symptoms similar to those of patients with left ventricular contractile reserve.

Carabello BA: Is it ever too late to operate on the patient with valvular heart disease? J Am Coll Cardiol 44:376–383, 2004.

Quere J, Monin J, Levy F, et al: Influence of preoperative left ventricular contractile reserve on postoperative ejection fraction in low gradient aortic stenosis. Circulation 113:1738–1744, 2006.

19. **Describe the outcome predictors in severe asymptomatic aortic stenosis.**
Management of an asymptomatic patient with severe aortic is controversial. Currently, guidelines do not recommend surgery in asymptomatic patients. Additionally, clinical variables such as age, sex, hypertension, diabetes, left ventricular function, hypercholesterolemia, and coronary artery disease have all shown mixed results as predictors of outcome in asymptomatic severe aortic stenosis. In certain subgroups at increased risk of adverse cardiac events, early elective valve replacement may be a sensible consideration. Namely, those patients with moderate or severe valve calcification have worse event-free survival rates than those patients with mild or no calcification. Additional predictors include rate of progression of aortic jet

velocity. In one study, 79% of patients who had moderately or severely calcified valves and who had an increase of 0.3 m/sec or more within 1 year either developed symptoms and underwent surgery or died within 2 years.

Baumgartner H: Should early elective surgery be performed in patients with severe but asymptomatic aortic stenosis? Eur Heart J 23;1417–1421, 2002.

Rosenhek R, Binder T, Porenta G, et al: Predictors of outcome in severe, asymptomatic aortic stenosis. N Engl J Med 343:611–617, 2000.

20. **What are the symptoms of aortic stenosis?**
The principal manifestations of aortic stenosis include syncope, angina pectoris, and dyspnea. In general, symptoms can be attributed to aortic stenosis if the valve area is <1.0 cm^2 or if the mean transvalvular gradient exceeds 50 mmHg. The average time to death after the onset of angina, syncope, and dyspnea are 5, 3, and 2 years, respectively.

Carabello BA: Is it ever too late to operate on the patient with valvular heart disease? J Am Coll Cardiol 44:376–383, 2004.

Lester S, Heilbron B, Gin K: The natural history and rate of progression of aortic stenosis. Chest 113:1109–1114, 1998.

21. **What is the role of vasodilators in severe aortic stenosis associated with congestive heart failure?**
Vasodilators have traditionally been thought to be contraindicated in patients with severe aortic stenosis because they could lead to severe hypotension. The Use of Nitroprusside in Left Ventricular Dysfunction and Obstructive Aortic Valve Disease Study (UNLOAD) focused on patients who were admitted to the intensive care unit for invasive hemodynamic monitoring of heart failure; who had an ejection fraction of $\leq$0.35, an aortic valve area $\leq$1.0 cm^2 on echocardiography, and a cardiac index of $\leq$2.2 L/min per square meter by Fick; and who were not hypotensive (defined as a mean arterial pressure <60 mmHg or the need for pressor agents such as dobutamine, dopamine, epinephrine, milrinone, norepinephrine, or phenylephrine). Nitroprusside was started at a mean dose of 14 $\pm$ 10 μg/min titrated to keep mean arterial pressure between 60 and 70 mmHg. After 6 hours the mean dose was 103 μg/min and at 24 hours 128 μg/min. At 6 hours the cardiac index rose from 1.60 $\pm$ 0.35 to 2.22 $\pm$ 0.44 and at 24 hours to 2.52 $\pm$ 0.55. Systemic vascular resistance decreased from 1926 $\pm$ 543 to 1224 $\pm$ 242 at 6 hours and to 1042 $\pm$ 261 at 24 hours. In none of the patients did the cardiac index decrease. The authors concluded that in critically ill patients with severe aortic stenosis and severe left ventricular systolic function, nitroprusside consistently led to clinically significant and rapid improvement in cardiac output.

Khot U, Novaro G, Popvic Z, et al: Nitroprusside in critically ill patients with left ventricular dysfunction and aortic stenosis. N Engl J Med 348:1756–1763, 2003.

AORTIC REGURGITATION

22. **What are the most common causes of aortic regurgitation?**
In developing countries the most common cause of aortic regurgitation is rheumatic disease, and it presents in the second or third decade of life. Rheumatic disease in developed countries is less common. Etiologies for aortic regurgitation in developed countries include congenital (e.g., bicuspid valves) or degenerative (e.g., annuloaortic ectasia) diseases. The most common causes of acute aortic regurgitation are endocarditis, aortic dissection, and rupture or prolapse of an aortic valve leaflet. Other considerations include perforation or tear (the valve most commonly involved after blunt trauma to the chest), systemic hypertension, myxomatous degeneration, and Marfan's syndrome.

Carabello B, Crawford F: Valvular heart disease. N Engl J Med 337:32–41, 1997.

23. **What is the pathophysiology of aortic regurgitation?**

Lesions that result in aortic regurgitation create an orifice that allows regurgitant flow throughout diastole. In acute aortic regurgitation, a rapid increase in left ventricular filling pressures occurs due to the sudden increase in left ventricular volume without an increase in left ventricular compliance. Left ventricular stroke volume decreases as the regurgitant fraction increases. Tachycardia shortens the period of diastole and thereby reduces the regurgitant fraction. Diastolic filling of the ventricle may be compromised if left ventricular pressure exceeds left atrial pressure, leading to premature closure of the mitral valve. Increased systemic blood pressure increases systemic vascular resistance and can increase aortic regurgitation.

In chronic aortic regurgitation, ventricular remodeling occurs in response to the volume overload state. Remodeling is characterized by increased fiber length and subsequently increased end-diastolic volume. This leads to improved diastolic compliance, increased end-diastolic volume, and increased stroke volume without increasing filling pressures significantly. Over time, left ventricular contractility diminishes leading to increases in filling, end-diastolic, and systolic pressures, and to decreased ejection fractions.

24. **How is aortic regurgitation diagnosed?**

Aortic regurgitation is usually detected as an incidental finding on echocardiography. In acute aortic regurgitation, the electrocardiogram can appear normal. The chest radiograph usually shows pulmonary edema with normal heart size. The clinical examination findings include a decrescendo diastolic murmur, widened pulse pressure, and bounding pulses. Additional findings include a mid to late diastolic rumble (i.e., Austin flint murmur), Musset's sign (i.e., head bobbing), Quincke's pulse (i.e., alternating diastolic blanching and systolic reddening of a lightly compressed nail bed), signs of severe heart failure (e.g., tachycardia, tachypnea, and peripheral vasoconstriction), a right ventricular lift (resulting from pulmonary hypertension), and displaced apical impulse (chronic aortic regurgitation). Transesophageal echocardiography should be considered when aortic dissection or endocarditis is alleged to be the origin of aortic regurgitation and for classifying the severity of regurgitation. Echocardiographic findings suggestive of severe regurgitation include the following:

- Broad jet width on color flow imaging
- Steep jet velocity deceleration and prolonged diastolic flow reversal in the aorta
- Doppler echocardiography findings of a regurgitant orifice ≥ 30 cm^2
- Regurgitant volume ≥ 60 mL/beat

Carabello B, Crawford F: Valvular heart disease. N Engl J Med 337:32–41, 1997.

25. **Describe the natural history of aortic regurgitation.**

Fifty percent of patients will develop heart failure within 10 years after the diagnosis of severe aortic regurgitation. Persons with severe symptoms have an annual mortality rate of approximately 25%. Those with mild symptoms have an annual mortality rate of 6.3%. Asymptomatic patients with an end-systolic diameter of ≥ 25 mm/m^2 or whose ejection fraction is below 55% have an increased risk of death. Left ventricular dilatation of 80 mm or more is associated with sudden death.

26. **What are the medical treatment options for aortic regurgitation?**

For patients who are normotensive, diuresis and nitroprusside are first-line agents for reducing left ventricular filling pressures, decreasing the regurgitant fraction, and improving forward flow. Left ventricular function is often hyperdynamic, limiting the usefulness of inotropic agents. Bradycardia and the resultant increase in the diastolic filling period can be treated with dobutamine, isoproterenol, or transvenous pacing with the goal of increasing heart rate to shorten the diastolic filling period and subsequently reducing the regurgitant fraction. Intra-aortic balloon pumps are contraindicated. Once patients are stabilized, long-acting vasodilator therapy with hydralazine, angiotensin-converting enzymes inhibitors, calcium channel blockers, or alpha blockers can be used. Unfortunately, data are conflicting about the long-term use of vasodilator therapy in patients with severe aortic regurgitation, reducing or delaying the need for aortic valve replacement.

Evangelista A, Tornos P, Sambola A, et al: Long term vasodilator therapy in patients with severe aortic regurgitation. N Engl J Med 353:1342–1349, 2005.

Scognamiglio R, Negut C, Palisi M, et al: Long term survival and functional results after aortic valve replacement in asymptomatic patients with chronic severe aortic regurgitation and left ventricular dysfunction. J Am Coll Cardiol 45:1025–1030, 2005.

Scognamiglio R, Rahimtoola S, Fasoli G, et al: Nifedipine in asymptomatic patients with severe aortic regurgitation and normal left ventricular function. N Engl J Med 331:689–694, 1994.

27. **When is surgery indicated in aortic regurgitation?**
Early surgical intervention is indicated when patients present with heart failure resulting from valve dysfunction. This is particularly so when left ventricular pressures have increased to the point of mitral valve preclosure. In patients with chronic aortic regurgitation, acute illness can lead to decompensation. In these instances, the acute process should be treated and the need for valve replacement considered after recovery based on symptoms and left ventricular function. Persons who are without contraindications to surgery should proceed to early valve surgery because waiting until severe symptoms develop has been associated with excess mortality. In asymptomatic persons with aortic insufficiency, surgical intervention is warranted if frank left ventricular enlargement or moderate dysfunction is present. In general, aortic valve surgery should be considered before the ejection fraction falls below 55% or the end-systolic dimension becomes greater than 55 mm. Persons with a preoperative ejection fraction < 35% have a 10-year postoperative survival rate of 41%; with an ejection fraction of 35–49%, the 10-year postoperative survival rate is 56%; and if the ejection fraction is 50% or more, the 10-year postoperative survival rate is 70%. In patients who present with severe aortic insufficiency resulting from endocarditis, aortic valve replacement during active infection comes with <10% chance of infection. Therefore, in most patients, the possibility of sudden death from a cardiac source is greater than the risk of prosthetic valve infection, and valve replacement should proceed if warranted.

Carabello B, Crawford F: Valvular heart disease. N Engl J Med 337:32–41, 1997.

KEY POINTS: VALVULAR DISEASE

1. Acute severe mitral regurgitation presents with elevated pulmonary wedge pressures, pulmonary edema, and cardiogenic shock.

2. Consider surgery for mitral valve stenosis when patients are classified within New York Heart Association functional classes I–II and have a mitral valve area < 1.0 cm^2 and severe pulmonary artery hypertension (systolic pulmonary artery pressure > 60–80 mmHg). These patients will still benefit from surgery.

3. Aortic stenosis is the most common valvular abnormality and often occurs due to calcification of a bicuspid valve.

4. Calculated aortic valve area can be dramatically smaller in patients with low cardiac output. To establish whether truly severe aortic stenosis is present at low cardiac output, it is necessary to increase output pharmacologically with an agent such as dobutamine.

5. Surgery should be considered for aortic regurgitation when patients present with heart failure.

CHAPTER 31

PERICARDIAL DISEASE (PERICARDITIS AND PERICARDIAL TAMPONADE)

Stuart F. Sidlow, MD, and C. William Hanson, III, MD

1. **What is the structure of the pericardium?**

   The pericardium is a two-layered structure surrounding the heart and consisting of the fibrous and serous layers. The fibrous layer is a stiff, inelastic structure that has little ability to accommodate fluid accumulation over a short time. The serous layer consists of two layers, the parietal and visceral pericardium. The parietal layer is adherent to the fibrous pericardium, and the visceral layer is part of the epicardium or external layer of the heart wall. When pericardial effusion occurs, it normally is between the parietal and visceral layers of the serous pericardium. The pericardial space normally holds 15–50 mL of an ultrafiltrate of plasma.

   Moore K: Clinically Oriented Anatomy, 3rd ed. Baltimore, Williams & Wilkins, 1992.

2. **Why do hemodynamic changes occur with the buildup of fluid between the layers of the serous pericardium?**

   When fluid accumulates in the pericardial space, the fibrous pericardium has little ability to stretch. As the volume increases in this space, further inflow into the right side of the heart is impaired, which results in decrease in filling of the left heart, and thus preload is decreased.

   Moore K: Clinically Oriented Anatomy, 3rd ed. Baltimore, Williams & Wilkins, 1992.

3. **What general types of pericardial disease exist?**
   - Acute fibrinous pericarditis (acute pericarditis)
   - Pericardial effusion without hemodynamic compromise
   - Cardiac tamponade
   - Constrictive pericarditis

   Shabetai R, Soler-Soler J, Corey GR: Etiology of pericardial disease. Up To Date Online version 13.3: www.uptodate.com

4. **What are the major etiologies of acute pericarditis?**
   From most to least common:
   - Neoplastic/radiation
   - Viral-adenovirus, enterovirus, cytomegalovirus, influenza, hepatitis B virus, herpes simplex virus
   - Autoimmune/collagen vascular disease
   - Bacterial
   - Uremia
   - Tuberculosis (most common worldwide)
   - Idiopathic
   - Drugs or toxins

   Shabetai R, Soler-Soler J, Corey GR: Etiology of pericardial disease. Up To Date Online version 13.3: www.uptodate.com

5. **Describe the clinical manifestation of acute pericarditis (history and physical examination).**

   The patient may complain of pleuritic chest pain that gets worse on inspiration. Pain is exacerbated by the supine position and relieved by sitting up. Dyspnea may be present. A pericardial friction rub is highly specific to acute pericarditis. Many patients present with high fever ($>38°C$) and new cardiomegaly revealed by chest x-ray. Pleural effusions are frequently observed.

Shabetai R, Imazio M: Evaluation and management of acute pericarditis. Up To Date Online version 13.3: www.uptodate.com

6. **What is the differential diagnosis of acute pericarditis?**
   The differential diagnosis of acute pericarditis consists of acute myocardial infarction, pulmonary embolus, gastroesophageal reflux, and musculoskeletal pain.

   Benumof J (ed): Anesthesia and Uncommon Disease, 4th ed. Philadelphia, W.B. Saunders, 1998.

7. **How is acute pericarditis manifested on electrocardiography (ECG)?**
   There is a progression of four stages on ECG, but for diagnosis one should evaluate for concave-up ST segments throughout most leads (exceptions include aVr and V_1).

   Shabetai R, Imazio M: Evaluation and management of acute pericarditis. Up To Date Online version 13.3: www.uptodate.com

8. **What other diagnostic tests are useful in the diagnosis of acute pericarditis?**
   Serum cardiac troponin I and creatine kinase, myocardial bound (CKMB) levels should be evaluated. Usually mild troponin increases occur in the absence of increased CKMB levels. The increase is due to inflammation of myocardium. Based on suspicion and other findings, other tests may include analysis of antinuclear antibodies, tuberculin skin test, human immunodeficiency virus serology, and blood cultures.

   Shabetai R, Imazio M: Evaluation and management of acute pericarditis. Up To Date Online version 13.3: www.uptodate.com

9. **How is pericardiocentesis used in diagnosing or treating acute pericarditis?**
   Pericardiocentesis or surgical drainage should be performed for one of three reasons: (1) moderate to severe tamponade is present, resulting in hemodynamic compromise (class I recommendation), (2) purulent, tuberculous, or neoplastic effusion is suspected (class IIa recommendation), or (3) a persistently symptomatic effusion is present.

   Shabetai R, Imazio M: Evaluation and management of acute pericarditis. Up To Date Online version 13.3: www.uptodate.com

10. **Does echocardiography play a role in the diagnosis of acute pericarditis?**
    Echocardiography should be performed in all patients suspected of having acute pericarditis. The echocardiogram often has normal results, but when an effusion is seen, it supports the diagnosis of acute pericarditis. The absence of effusion does not rule it out. The use of echocardiography was given a class I recommendation by the American Heart Association, the American College of Cardiology, and the American Society of Echocardiography.

    Shabetai R, Imazio M: Evaluation and management of acute pericarditis. Up To Date Online version 13.3: www.uptodate.com

11. **How is therapy decided for the treatment of acute pericarditis?**
    Treatment is based on the cause of acute pericarditis, as follows:
    - **Neoplastic:** Drainage if hemodynamic compromise is present and appropriate chemotherapy
    - **Viral:** Symptomatic/supportive care
    - **Autoimmune:** Nonsteroidal anti-inflammatory drugs (NSAIDs) are the mainstay of treatment (class I); corticosteroids can be used in cases refractory to NSAID therapy
    - **Bacterial/tuberculous:** Antibiotics as appropriate by blood or pericardial fluid culture
    - **Uremic:** Reversal of uremic state

    Shabetai R, Imazio M: Evaluation and management of acute pericarditis. Up To Date Online version 13.3: www.uptodate.com

12. **What is constrictive pericarditis?**
    Constrictive pericarditis is a chronic condition in which the parietal and visceral layers of the pericardium fuse and are often calcified. Etiologies are similar to those with acute pericarditis. It is usually well tolerated until advanced stages, at which point diastolic filling becomes impaired. Patients are dyspneic and have Kussmaul's sign (described in question 15), peripheral edema is usually present, and a pericardial knock may be heard.

13. **What is pericardial tamponade?**
    Pericardial tamponade is a process in which fluid (blood or serous fluid) accumulates in the pericardial space, either acutely or over time.

    Moore K: Clinically Oriented Anatomy, 3rd ed. Baltimore, Williams & Wilkins, 1992.

14. **What is Beck's triad?**
    Beck's triad consists of falling arterial blood pressure, elevated systemic venous pressure (i.e., central venous pressure), and a small, quiet heart.

    Shebetai R, Hoit B: Cardiac tamponade. Up To Date Online version 13.3: www.uptodate.com

15. **What is Kussmaul's sign?**
    Kussmaul's sign is a paradoxical increase in central venous pressure with inspiration. It is observed in any condition that restricts venous return to the heart.

    Shebetai R, Hoit B: Cardiac tamponade. Up To Date Online version 13.3: www.uptodate.com

16. **List common settings for acute pericardial tamponade.**
    After cardiac operations, blunt or penetrating mediastinal trauma (especially stab wounds), acute myocardial infarction with free wall rupture, endovascular catheterization (including aortograms and carotid arteriograms) with perforation, and, uncommonly, central venous catheter placement (due to erosion of the catheter through a vessel wall).

    Murray M, Coursin R, Pearl R, Prough D (eds): Critical Care Medicine: Perioperative Management, 2nd ed. Philadelphia, Lippincott Williams & Wilkins, 2002.

17. **Describe the changes in hemodynamic monitoring seen in a patient with pericardial tamponade.**
    Generally referred to as *pulsus paradoxus* (Fig. 31-1), on arterial line tracing one may see first subtle then dramatic respiratory variation in the systolic pressure (>10 mmHg difference between expiration and inspiration). In a nonintubated patient, as venous return increases to the right heart with negative intrathoracic pressure during inspiration, the right ventricle's free wall cannot expand outward into the pericardial space due to the fluid accumulation. The intraventricular septum is displaced into the left ventricle as the right ventricle distends. As a

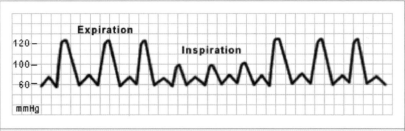

Figure 31-1. Pulsus paradoxus on arterial line tracing.

result, filling of the left ventricle is impaired, causing a decrease in left ventricular preload. During pulmonary artery catheter monitoring, one sees equalization of diastolic pressures. The pressure relationships are as follows: RA = RV = PAD = wedge pressure (difference < 5 mmHg).

Murray M, Coursin R, Pearl R, Prough D (eds): Critical Care Medicine: Perioperative Management, 2nd ed. Philadelphia, Lippincott Williams & Wilkins, 2002.

18. **What is the differential diagnosis in a patient with pulsus paradoxus by arterial line tracing?**
    - Obesity
    - Asthma
    - Pulmonary embolism
    - Constrictive pericarditis
    - Pericardial tamponade
    - Cardiogenic shock

    Sensitivity and specificity are 79% and 40%, respectively, for tamponade. Always use clinical suspicion when diagnosing this or other life-threatening conditions.

Murray M, Coursin R, Pearl R, Prough D (eds): Critical Care Medicine: Perioperative Management, 2nd ed. Philadelphia, Lippincott Williams & Wilkins, 2002.

19. **How is pericardial tamponade diagnosed?**
    Tamponade is a clinical diagnosis based on history and physical examination. It usually represents an emergency and can lead to pulseless electric activity cardiac arrest if left undiagnosed and untreated. Some common features include jugular venous distention with increased central venous pressure (Kussmaul's sign), faint heart sounds, sinus tachycardia, and pulsus paradoxus. If unsure of the diagnosis, some studies are helpful in diagnosis. The ECG may demonstrate electric alternans or sinus tachycardia with low-voltage QRS complexes. A chest x-ray may show an enlarged cardiac silhouette. Echocardiography is extremely useful in the diagnosis of this condition and has been given a class I recommendation. On echocardiography, right atrial collapse is more sensitive but less specific than right ventricular collapse. If tamponade is highly suspected, one should not wait for an echocardiogram before instituting therapy.

Schiller N, Foster E: Echocardiographic evaluation of the pericardium. Up To Date Online version 13.3: www.uptodate.com

KEY POINTS: CHARACTERISTICS OF PERICARDIAL TAMPONADE

1. Pericardial tamponade is usually a true medical emergency.

2. If left unnoticed or untreated, pericardial tamponade results in pulseless electric activity cardiac arrest.

3. Pericardial tamponade is a clinical diagnosis.

4. The most useful tool in diagnosing pericardial tamponade is echocardiography, if time permits.

5. For patients with pericardial tamponade in an emergent situation, a life-saving measure consists of needle pericardiocentesis.

20. **Briefly describe the hemodynamic strategy in a patient with suspected pericardial tamponade.**
    The hemodynamic strategy is denoted by the phrase "fast, full, and tight." *Fast* means the patient should be allowed to be tachycardic (no beta blockers, please), *full* means preload should be increased (fluids wide open), and *tight* means the patient's blood pressure should be allowed to rise either by volume resuscitation or vasopressor (e.g., norepinephrine, epinephrine, or phenylephrine, as indicated). This strategy should be used until definitive release of the tamponade can be performed. Intubation should be avoided until the last possible moment to avoid complete cardiovascular collapse during anesthetic induction.

    Benumof J (ed): Anesthesia and Uncommon Disease, 4th ed. Philadelphia, W.B. Saunders, 1998.

21. **Why should intubation be avoided during the initial treatment of tamponade?**
    Intubation should be deferred until the last possible moment because increasing intrathoracic pressure with positive pressure ventilation can decrease cardiac output by up to 25%, which may eliminate cardiac output in some patients.

22. **What therapeutic maneuvers should be performed on a patient with pericardial tamponade?**
    After determination of the cause and the rapidity with which the fluid accumulated, either pericardiocentesis or pericardial window (pericardotomy) should be performed.

    Benumof J (ed): Anesthesia and Uncommon Disease, 4th ed. Philadelphia, W.B. Saunders, 1998.

23. **List the contraindications for bedside pericardiocentesis.**
    - Severe coagulopathy or low platelet count
    - Stable effusion (i.e., blind, bedside pericardiocentesis should be performed only with impending cardiovascular collapse or during cardiopulmonary resuscitation)

    Murray M, Coursin R, Pearl R, Prough D (eds): Critical Care Medicine: Perioperative Management, 2nd ed. Philadelphia, Lippincott Williams & Wilkins, 2002.

24. **What other conditions are included in the differential diagnosis of pericardial tamponade?**
    Other conditions to be considered when tamponade is suspected include massive pulmonary embolus, tension pneumothorax, massive myocardial contusion or myocardial ischemia resulting in cardiogenic shock, exacerbation of severe chronic obstructive pulmonary disease with air trapping, and constrictive pericarditis (Fig. 31-2).

    Murray M, Coursin R, Pearl R, Prough D (eds): Critical Care Medicine: Perioperative Management, 2nd ed. Philadelphia, Lippincott Williams & Wilkins, 2002.

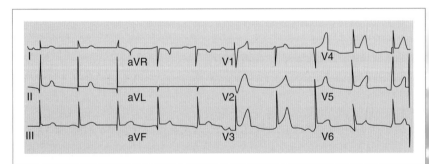

Figure 31-2. Electric alterans.

V. INFECTIOUS DISEASE

SEPSIS, SEVERE SEPSIS SYNDROME, AND SEPTIC SHOCK

Richard H. Savel, MD, and Michael A. Gropper, MD, PhD

CHAPTER 32

1. **What is sepsis?**
   Sepsis is an overwhelming inflammatory and coagulopathic response to a source of infection, usually from the lung or abdomen. If not recognized early, or not treated properly and aggressively, it is often a lethal syndrome. Please note that it is different from *bacteremia*, which only refers to the presence of bacteria in the bloodstream.

2. **Explain the nomenclature for disorders related to sepsis.**
   The nomenclature for disorders related to sepsis was defined in the 1990s by the American College of Chest Physicians and the Society of Critical Care Medicine. The following terms describe the progression of signs and symptoms regarding this somewhat confusing terminology:
   - **Systemic inflammatory response syndrome (SIRS):** SIRS is characterized by (1) temperature $> 38°C$ or $< 36°C$; (2) heart rate > 90 beats/min; (3) respiratory rate > 20 breaths/min or the need for mechanical ventilation; and (4) white blood cell count $> 12,000$ cells/mm^3 or < 4000 cells/mm^3.
   - **Sepsis:** Sepsis is defined as a suspected or documented source of infection plus two or more SIRS criteria.
   - **Severe sepsis syndrome (SSS):** Sepsis with acute sepsis-induced organ dysfunction of one or more organ systems is known as SSS.
   - **Septic shock:** Septic shock is a subset of SSS in which the organ dysfunction is cardiovascular; that is, sepsis-induced hypotension (mean arterial pressure [MAP] < 65 mmHg) that persists despite adequate and aggressive volume resuscitation. Patients will often require vasopressors to keep MAP ≥ 65 mmHg.
   - **Multiple organ dysfunction syndrome (MODS):** MODS is defined as failure in more than one organ system that requires acute intervention. Once the patient reaches this degree of illness, the chances of making a meaningful recovery can often be quite low.

   Bone RC, Balk RA, Cerra FB, et al: Definitions for sepsis and organ failure and guidelines for the use of innovative therapies in sepsis. The ACCP/SCCM Consensus Conference Committee. American College of Chest Physicians/Society of Critical Care Medicine. Chest 101:1644–1655, 1992.

3. **What is the incidence of sepsis?**
   SSS and septic shock are common and associated with substantial mortality and consumption of health care resources. There are an estimated 751,000 cases (3.0 cases per 1000 population) of sepsis or septic shock in the United States each year. Sepsis and septic shock are responsible for as many deaths each year as acute myocardial infarction (215,000, or 9.3% of all deaths). The incidence and mortality rate of sepsis are substantially higher in elderly than in younger persons. The projected growth of the elderly population in the United States will contribute to an increase in incidence of 1.5% per year, yielding an estimated 934,000 and 1,110,000 cases by the years 2010 and 2020, respectively. The present annual cost of sepsis and septic shock in the United States is estimated at $16.7 billion.

   Martin GS, Mannino DM, Eaton S, Moss M: The epidemiology of sepsis in the United States from 1979 through 2000. N Engl J Med 348:1546–1554, 2003.

4. **How does the nomenclature relate to outcome?**

Previous studies have shown that as the disorder progresses from SIRS to septic shock, the mortality rate increases. Interestingly, recent data support the concept that, although the degree of illness at presentation may have some correlation with outcomes, it is the change in clinical status from baseline to day 1 that may have the closest correlation with outcomes.

Sepsis progresses to MODS with tragic consequences. The mortality rate for patients with acute renal failure in the setting of sepsis ranges from 50% to 80%. For most patients with sepsis syndrome, the failure of three or more organ systems results in a mortality rate > 90%. The organ systems most often affected early in the process are pulmonary, hematologic, renal, and cardiovascular.

Levy MM, Macias WL, Vincent JL, et al: Early changes in organ function predict eventual survival in severe sepsis. Crit Care Med 33:2194–2201, 2005.

5. **Discuss the current understanding of the pathogenesis of sepsis and septic shock.**

Sepsis syndrome begins with the invasion and growth of microorganisms (i.e., gram-positive, gram-negative, fungal, or viral) in a normally sterile tissue space. The endothelium is damaged by infection, trauma, or other insult, and activation of the host immune response begins. Tumor necrosis factor alpha, interleukin (IL)-6, and IL-8 are associated with the activation of an inflammatory cascade and chemotaxis of leukocytes, monocytes, and macrophages. Anti-inflammatory substances such as IL-4, IL-10, prostaglandins, and other components of the immune system work to maintain homeostasis in the face of an infectious insult. Sepsis syndrome develops when the balance between the pro-inflammatory and anti-inflammatory substances is lost.

The coagulation pathway plays a critical role in sepsis. The complement system, vasoregulatory system (i.e., nitric oxide, bradykinin, prostaglandins), the coagulation cascade (i.e., tissue factor, protein C, thrombin, antithrombin III), and fibrinolysis (i.e., fibrin, plasmin, and plasminogen-activating factor) play a role as well. The result is the development of a vicious cycle that promotes, both locally and systemically, further inflammation, release of oxygen free radicals, and deposition of microvascular thrombi, resulting in ischemia, reperfusion injury, and tissue hypoxia. Global tissue hypoxia independently contributes to endothelial activation and further disruption of the homeostatic balance among coagulation, vascular permeability, and vascular tone. These are key mechanisms leading to microcirculatory failure, refractory tissue hypoxia, and organ dysfunction.

It is becoming clear that the processes of coagulation and inflammation are tightly linked. Recent studies have shown that patients with severe sepsis have depleted levels of protein C, protein S, and antithrombin III. Administration of protein C to patients with severe sepsis appears to decrease mortality by both regulating the coagulation pathway and decreasing inflammation.

Matthay MA: Severe sepsis—A new treatment with both anticoagulant and antiinflammatory properties. N Engl J Med 344:759–762, 2001.

6. **Which microorganisms are most commonly associated with sepsis?**

A recent study of nosocomial bloodstream infections found the following infecting organisms in the intensive care unit (ICU):

- **Gram-positive organisms (65%):** Coagulase-negative staphylococci (36% of isolates), *Staphylococcus aureus* (17%), enterococci (10%)
- **Gram-negative organisms (25%):** *Escherichia coli* (4%), *Klebsiella* species (4%), *Pseudomonas aeruginosa* (5%), *Enterobacter* species (5%), *Serratia* species (2%), *Acinetobacter* species (2%) (Clinically, however, the problem of resistant gram-negative organisms in the ICU is rapidly becoming a serious one nationwide.)
- **Fungi (9%):** Primarily *Candida* species (*Candida albicans* 54%, *Candida glabrata* 19%, *Candida parapsilosis* 11%, *Candida tropicalis* 11%)

Coagulase-negative staphylococci, *Pseudomonas* species, *Enterobacter* species, *Serratia* species, and *Acinetobacter* species were more likely to cause infections in patients in the ICU. The proportion of *S. aureus* isolates with methicillin resistance increased from 22% in 1995 to 57% in 2001.

Wisplinghoff H, Bischoff T, Tallent SM, et al: Nosocomial bloodstream infections in US hospitals: Analysis of 24,179 cases from a prospective nationwide surveillance study. Clin Infect Dis 39:309–317, 2004.

7. **What are the most common sources of infection?**
Lung (36%), blood (20%), abdomen (19%), urinary tract (13%), and skin (7%). Other sources comprised the last 5%.

Wheeler AP, Bernard GR: Treating patients with severe sepsis. N Engl J Med 340:207–214, 1999.

KEY POINTS: DIAGNOSIS AND MANAGEMENT OF SEVERE SEPSIS SYNDROME (SSS)

1. Sepsis = infection + two or more SIRS criteria.

2. *SSS* is defined as sepsis plus acute sepsis-induced organ dysfunction.

3. Early diagnosis and therapeutic interventions in patients with SSS are associated with better outcomes.

4. The Surviving Sepsis Campaign Guidelines provide a reasonable evidence-based approach to the current management of SSS.

5. Constant close communication between the critical care team and family members of the patient is key.

8. **What clinical signs and symptoms should raise suspicion of SIRS, sepsis, and underlying organ dysfunction?**
   - **Respiratory:** Cyanosis, tachypnea, orthopnea, increased sputum (yellow or green, frothy), hypoxemia ($PaO_2/FiO_2 < 300$), oxygen saturation < 90%.
   - **Cardiovascular:** Need for pressors, chest pain, pulmonary edema, arrhythmias, cardiac index < 2.5, heart rate > 100 beats/min, decreased systemic vascular resistance, increased cardiac output
   - **Renal:** Urine output < 0.5 mL/kg/h, increased blood urea nitrogen and creatinine concentrations, acute renal failure, acidosis, increasing base deficit, metabolic acidosis (usually lactate)
   - **Hepatic:** Elevated aspartate aminotransferase, alanine aminotransferase, or gamma-glutamyl transferase levels; prolonged bleeding time; asterixis; encephalopathy; elevated bilirubin. (This is often referred to as *ischemic hepatopathy* or "shock liver.")
   - **Immunologic:** Temperature > 38°C or hypothermia, chills, increased white blood cell count or left shift, neutropenia
   - **Hematologic:** Weakness, pallor, poor capillary refill, easy bruising, spontaneous bleeding, anemia, increased prothrombin or partial thromboplastin time, decreased fibrinogen, disseminated intravascular coagulation (elevated D-dimers)
   - **Gastrointestinal:** Anorexia, ileus, inability to tolerate tube feeds, nausea, vomiting, hypoalbuminemia
   - **Endocrine:** Hyperglycemia, hypoglycemia, adrenal insufficiency, weight loss

- **Neurologic:** Weakness, confusion, delirium, psychoses, seizures
- **Metabolic:** Serum lactate > 1.5 the upper limit of normal

Wheeler AP, Bernard GR: Treating patients with severe sepsis. N Engl J Med 340:207–214, 1999.

9. **What are the Surviving Sepsis Campaign Guidelines? What are some of the high points?**

This document was published in 2004 and was codified by 11 international critical care organizations. It provides a state-of-the-art, evidence-based approach to the management of SSS. Highlights of this important document are noted in Box 32-1.

Dellinger RP, Carlet JM, Masur H, et al: Surviving Sepsis Campaign Guidelines for management of severe sepsis and septic shock. Crit Care Med 32:858–873, 2004.

Gropper MA: Evidence-based management of critically ill patients: Analysis and implementation. Anesth Analg 99:566–572, 2004.

Savel RH, Matthay MA, Gropper MA: Management of the patient with shock, sepsis, and multiple organ failure. In George RB, Light RW, Matthay RA, Matthay MA (eds): Chest Medicine: Principles of Pulmonary and Critical Care Medicine, 5th ed. Philadelphia, Lippincott Williams & Wilkins, 2005, pp 589–607.

Society of Critical Care Medicine: www.sccm.org

Surviving Sepsis website: www.survivingsepsis.org

BOX 32-1.   HIGHLIGHTS OF THE SURVIVING SEPSIS CAMPAIGN GUIDELINES

Resuscitation

Current recommendations are to rapidly place a central venous catheter in most cases of septic shock. This should quickly be followed by aggressive volume resuscitation with fluid boluses of 500 mL to 1 L of crystalloid (usually normal saline) until the central venous pressure is between 8 and 12 mmHg. The goal blood pressure is a mean arterial pressure $\geq$ 65 mmHg. If after adequate volume resuscitation has occurred the patient remains hypovolemic, vasopressors should be started to keep the mean arterial pressure at the goal level. Recommended pressor agents are discussed below. At that point, a measurement of central venous saturation should be obtained. If this value is <70%, the patient is to be transfused with packed red blood cells until the hematocrit is $\geq$30%. If the central venous saturation remains below 70% after transfusion, consideration should be given to a trial of dobutamine as an inotrope to normalize oxygen delivery.*

Antibiotic therapy

While the patient is initially being treated for severe sepsis syndrome (SSS), appropriate culture specimens should be obtained—usually of blood, sputum, and urine. Then (preferably within 1 hour of initial evaluation), broad-spectrum antibiotics should be started. Whether the patient is considered at risk for nosocomial infections will determine how broad these antibiotics need to be. In general, gram-positive, gram-negative, and anaerobic coverage must be provided initially. If resistant gram-negative organisms are a possibility, many authors recommend providing two agents with gram-negative coverage (such as an antipseudomonal penicillin and an aminoglycoside). These antibiotics should be narrowed based on the results of the initial culture results within the next 48–72 hours.†

Source control

Although there are very few randomized trials in the area, it is considered standard practice in patients with SSS to quickly look for sources of infection (e.g., pneumonia, abdominal

BOX 32-1.   HIGHLIGHTS OF THE SURVIVING SEPSIS CAMPAIGN GUIDELINES—CONT'D

infection, infected hardware such as central venous catheters) and coordinate closely with the proper medical or surgical subspecialty to ensure that the sources of infection are properly drained and removed, if possible.[‡]

Fluid therapy

One of the most important controversies in the field of critical care is whether colloid volume resuscitation is superior to crystalloid. An important study was recently published documenting that although colloid (in this case albumin) did not appear to be better than crystalloid, it certainly did not appear to be associated with increased mortality, as had been suggested in previous studies.[§]

Vasopressors

Based on the literature, it is currently recommended that norepinephrine or dopamine be used as first-line agents when vasopressors are required for critically ill patients with SSS. These agents should be delivered through a central venous catheter as soon as is practical if resources are available. Low-dose dopamine should not be used for renal protection.[∥]

Inotropic therapy

As previously described, it is recommended that an inotrope (such as dobutamine) be administered to patients with SSS who have a decreased cardiac output and that the inotropic agent be titrated to a level that normalizes the cardiac output. The inotrope should not be used to generate a "supranormal" cardiac output. It has been shown in two randomized trials that doing so may be associated with increased mortality rates.[¶]

Steroids

It is currently recommended that patients with persistent vasopressor-dependent septic shock receive IV corticosteroids. Reasonable choices and dosages include hydrocortisone from 200 to 300 mg/day for 7 days given in three or four divided doses or as a continuous infusion. Doses higher than that should not be used. There are multiple controversies:

- Some experts consider tapering steroids at the end of therapy.
- Some experts add fludrocortisone (50 μg orally per day).
- Some experts would use a 250-μg adrenocorticotropic hormone (ACTH) stimulation test to identify responders (>9 μg/dL increase in cortisol 30–60 minutes after ACTH administration) and discontinue steroid therapy in these patients.[#]

Recombinant human activated protein C (Drotrecogin alfa activated)

An important randomized trial (Protein C Worldwide Evaluation in Severe Sepsis [PROWESS]) showed a significant improvement in 28-day mortality rates when recombinant human activated protein C (APC) was added to standard therapy in patients with SSS. This drug is currently recommended for patients with SSS and a high risk of death: examples include an Acute Physiology and Chronic Health Evaluation (APACHE) II score ≥ 25, sepsis-induced multiple organ failure, septic shock, or sepsis-induced acute respiratory distress syndrome (ARDS). APC has the potential to increase the risk of bleeding, and the risks and benefits should be carefully weighed before

Continued

BOX 32-1.   HIGHLIGHTS OF THE SURVIVING SEPSIS CAMPAIGN GUIDELINES—CONT'D

initiation of this agent. As previously described, the mechanisms behind the beneficial effects of APC are thought to be multifactorial and include the following: (1) its effects as a natural anticoagulant, (2) its ability to inhibit two important inhibitors of fibrinolysis (plasminogen activator inhibitor–1 and thrombin activatable fibrinolysis inhibitor), and (3) innate anti-inflammatory properties of APC itself. It does not appear to be efficacious in patients with SSS and low risk of death, nor in the pediatric population with this syndrome.[**]

Blood product administration

Once the initial phase of resuscitation is complete, red blood cell transfusion should only occur when the hemoglobin level has fallen to < 7.0 gm/dL, with a target hemoglobin level of 7.0–9.0 gm/dL. Examples of persons for whom these guidelines potentially should not be followed include patients with acute bleeding and those with acute myocardial infarction.[††]

Mechanical ventilation of sepsis-induced acute lung injury (ALI)/ARDS

The lungs are the most common organ system to fail in septic patients, and many such patients eventually require mechanical ventilation. The lungs are the most likely source of initial infection, and patients are at great risk for nosocomial and ventilator-associated pneumonias.

The recent definitions and guidelines for management of ALI and ARDS have made a significant impact on the identification of patients with these disorders. Diagnosis of ALI and ARDS are based on the following criteria: bilateral infiltrates, PaO_2/FiO_2 <300 (ALI) or < 200 (ARDS), and no evidence of a cardiac source (e.g., left atrial hypertension) for respiratory distress. Volutrauma caused by large tidal volumes not only leads to release of inflammatory mediators (e.g., IL-6) that can provoke a septic response but also allows translocation of bacteria across damaged alveolar membranes. The ARDS Network (a multicenter organization aimed at treating ARDS) has identified a protective ventilation strategy, based on lower tidal volumes and use of positive end-expiratory pressure, which significantly decreases the mortality rate of patients with ARDS. It is currently recommended that patients with ALI or ARDS be ventilated with a goal tidal volume of 6 mL/kg predicted body weight.

Another technique to decrease the number of days receiving respiratory assistance from the ventilator and the incidence of pneumonia and sepsis is the use of daily trials of spontaneous breathing (as opposed to pressure support or intermittent ventilation) to wean patients from ventilator dependence. Nearly all patients with respiratory failure should have such trials; if the trial results indicate success, patients should be extubated.[‡‡]

Sedation, analgesia, and neuromuscular blockade in sepsis

In general, patients who have sepsis and are intubated require some kind of analgesia and sedation. There are data to support the use of protocols for both the level of sedation and to ensure that the depth of or requirement for sedation is evaluated every day. Analgesia should be provided first; then, if need be, a sedative agent should be added. This often can be done—although it is not necessary—with a continuous IV infusion of an analgesic or analgesic/sedative combination. It is important to remember that most narcotic

BOX 32-1.   HIGHLIGHTS OF THE SURVIVING SEPSIS CAMPAIGN GUIDELINES—CONT'D

analgesics have sedative properties, but most sedatives (benzodiazepines) do not have analgesic properties.

Regarding neuromuscular blockade (i.e., paralysis): this should only be done as a therapeutic intervention of last resort for patients who are having extreme degrees of hypoxemia or ventilator dyssynchrony. The following cannot be overemphasized: if the patient is paralyzed, proper analgesia and sedation must be provided *before* the initiation of the muscle relaxant; some form of a nerve-twitch monitor is used to observe the level of paralysis. Once the patient is paralyzed, the airway must be frequently evaluated for safety reasons (because the patient has lost any ability to breathe on his or her own); in addition, the patient must be frequently turned to prevent skin breakdown.[§§]

Glucose control

Recent data in critically ill patients—primarily patients who have undergone cardiac surgery—revealed multiple improved outcomes with the use of "tight glucose control." Current recommendations for critically ill patients, including those with SSS, include some form of a glucose control protocol involving low-dose insulin infusion. Although the precise glucose target for critically ill patients remains controversial, $\leq$ 150 mg/dL is a current reasonable consensus.[||||]

Renal replacement

Patients with SSS who experience acute renal failure have a significantly worse outcome than similar patients without renal failure. There are no data to support the idea that administering diuretics in an attempt to convert oliguric into nonoliguric renal failure provides any benefit to the patient. This practice, however, remains common in many intensive care units (ICUs). In general, patients who require renal replacement therapy (RRT) should have early consultation with a nephrologist and, in general, should receive their RRT earlier rather than later in their ICU course. There are limited data to suggest that daily RRT is better than RRT administered every other day. There are no data supporting the idea that continuous RRT is associated with improved outcomes compared with intermittent RRT.[¶¶]

Bicarbonate therapy

It has been common practice to give bicarbonate therapy to vasopressor-dependent patients with SSS to improve hemodynamics. However, it is important to state that—to the extent that it has been studied—there are no data to support this intervention. Current recommendations are not to give bicarbonate for hypoperfusion-induced lactic acidosis unless the serum pH is < 7.15.[##]

Deep vein thrombosis (DVT) prophylaxis

Patients with SSS are at high risk for the development of DVT and should be administered subcutaneous heparin, either of the unfractionated or low-molecular-weight variety. For patients with an absolute contraindication to heparin (e.g., active bleeding, recent intracerebral hemorrhage, coagulopathy), mechanical DVT prophylaxis should be used,

Continued

BOX 32-1. HIGHLIGHTS OF THE SURVIVING SEPSIS CAMPAIGN GUIDELINES—CONT'D

examples of which include intermittent compression device or graduated compression stockings. A combination of mechanical and pharmacologic DVT prophylaxis should be considered in the patient at very high risk for DVT (i.e., history of DVT).***

Stress ulcer prophylaxis

All patients with SSS are at high risk for stress-related mucosal bleeding and, as such, should be given H_2-receptor inhibitors as the preferred agent. The proper role of a proton-pump inhibitor for this purpose has not been fully elucidated.[†††]

Consideration for limitation of support

SSS is a serious disease with a significant mortality. It is important for the multidisciplinary critical care team (MCCT) to be in frequent communication with the family, providing them with appropriate updates regarding the status and prognosis of their loved one. It is also paramount that the MCCT be aware of any previous wishes the patient may have had regarding resuscitation, heroic measures, and artificial life support because many people have strong opinions regarding these issues. It is also the job of the MCCT to recognize when the prognosis of the patient is becoming so poor (often described as a "prolongation of the dying process") that the focus of care should transition from aggressive life-sustaining treatment to aggressive comfort measures; the MCCT must guide the family through this emotionally challenging time. Recent data have shown that ICU clinicians must be supportive of whatever decision the families make and should not allow the patients to feel abandoned during the process. In addition, during family meetings, increased family satisfaction was associated with physicians who spent an increased proportion of the time in these meetings actively listening, rather than speaking.[‡‡‡]

*Rivers E, Nguyen B, Havstad S, et al: Early goal-directed therapy in the treatment of severe sepsis and septic shock. N Engl J Med 345:1368–1377, 2001.

[†]Ibrahim EH, Sherman G, Ward S, et al: The influence of inadequate antimicrobial treatment of bloodstream infections on patient outcomes in the ICU setting. Chest 118:146–155, 2000.

[‡]Marshall JC, Maier RV, Jimenez M, Dellinger EP: Source control in the management of severe sepsis and septic shock: An evidence-based review. Crit Care Med 32:S513–S526, 2004.

[§]Finfer S, Bellomo R, Boyce N, et al: A comparison of albumin and saline for fluid resuscitation in the intensive care unit. N Engl J Med 350:2247–2256, 2004.

[∥]Beale RJ, Hollenberg SM, Vincent JL, Parrillo JE: Vasopressor and inotropic support in septic shock: An evidence-based review. Crit Care Med 32:S455–S465, 2004.

[¶]Gattinoni L, Brazzi L, Pelosi P, et al: A trial of goal-oriented hemodynamic therapy in critically ill patients. SvO_2 Collaborative Group. N Engl J Med 333:1025–1032, 1995; Hayes MA, Timmins AC, Yau EH, et al: Elevation of systemic oxygen delivery in the treatment of critically ill patients. N Engl J Med 330:1717–1722, 1994.

[#]Gonzalez H, Nardi O, Annane D: Relative adrenal failure in the ICU: An identifiable problem requiring treatment. Crit Care Clin 22:105–118, 2006.

**Bernard GR, Vincent JL, Laterre PF, et al: Efficacy and safety of recombinant human activated protein C for severe sepsis. N Engl J Med 344:699–709, 2001.

[††]Hebert PC, Wells G, Blajchman MA, et al: A multicenter, randomized, controlled clinical trial of transfusion requirements in critical care. Transfusion Requirements in Critical Care Investigators, Canadian Critical Care Trials Group. N Engl J Med 340: 409–417, 1999.

[‡‡]Acute Respiratory Distress Syndrome Network: Ventilation with lower tidal volumes as compared with traditional tidal volumes for acute lung injury and the acute respiratory distress syndrome. N Engl J Med 342:1301–1308, 2000.

BOX 32-1. HIGHLIGHTS OF THE SURVIVING SEPSIS CAMPAIGN GUIDELINES—CONT'D

§§Brook AD, Ahrens TS, Schaiff R, et al: Effect of a nursing-implemented sedation protocol on the duration of mechanical ventilation. Crit Care Med 27:2609–2615, 1999; Kress JP, Pohlman AS, O'Connor MF, Hall JB: Daily interruption of sedative infusions in critically ill patients undergoing mechanical ventilation. N Engl J Med 342:1471–1477, 2000.

‖‖van den Berghe G, Wouters P, Weekers F, et al: Intensive insulin therapy in the critically ill patients. N Engl J Med 345:1359–1367, 2001.

¶¶Schiffl H, Lang SM, Fischer R: Daily hemodialysis and the outcome of acute renal failure. N Engl J Med 346:305–310, 2002.

##Mathieu D, Neviere R, Billard V, et al: Effects of bicarbonate therapy on hemodynamics and tissue oxygenation in patients with lactic acidosis: A prospective, controlled clinical study. Crit Care Med 19:1352–1356, 1991.

***Geerts WH, Pineo GF, Heit JA, et al: Prevention of venous thromboembolism: The Seventh ACCP Conference on Antithrombotic and Thrombolytic Therapy. Chest 126:338S–400S, 2004.

†††Daley RJ, Rebuck JA, Welage LS, Rogers FB: Prevention of stress ulceration: Current trends in critical care. Crit Care Med 32:2008–2013, 2004.

‡‡‡White DB, Curtis JR: Care near the end-of-life in critically ill patients: A North American perspective. Curr Opin Crit Care 11:610–615, 2005.

10. **What is an evidence-based approach to the use of the pulmonary artery catheter (PAC)?**

Since its initial description in *The New England Journal of Medicine* in 1970, the PAC has been an important tool for critical care clinicians. Its major roles have been as follows: (1) to distinguish cardiogenic from noncardiogenic pulmonary edema; (2) to determine which particular shock state (i.e., cardiogenic, distributive, hypovolemic) a patient may be experiencing; and (3) to serve as a guide for therapeutic interventions for patients in shock. Recent data from large randomized trials have been unable to document a particular subgroup of patients in whom the use of the PAC has been associated with improved outcomes. There are multiple complex reasons behind these results, which are still being debated in the literature. Nevertheless, it can be stated with some certainty that the placement of a PAC is no longer a requirement for the successful diagnosis and management of a patient with SSS.

Richard C, Warszawski J, Anguel N, et al: Early use of the pulmonary artery catheter and outcomes in patients with shock and acute respiratory distress syndrome: A randomized controlled trial. JAMA 290:2713–2720, 2003.

Sandham JD, Hull RD, Brant RF, et al: A randomized, controlled trial of the use of pulmonary-artery catheters in high-risk surgical patients. N Engl J Med 348:5–14, 2003.

CHAPTER 33

ENDOCARDITIS

Louis B. Polish, MD

1. **What are the Duke criteria for the diagnosis of endocarditis? How have they been modified?**

   The original Duke criteria for the diagnosis of infective endocarditis stratified patients into three categories:

   - **Definite:** Identified using clinical or pathologic criteria (Box 33-1)
   - **Possible:** Findings consistent with infective endocarditis that fall short of definite, but the diagnosis cannot be "rejected"
   - **Rejected:** Firm alternate diagnosis for manifestations of endocarditis *or* resolution of manifestations of endocarditis, with antibiotic therapy for 4 days or less, *or* no pathologic evidence of infective endocarditis at surgery or autopsy, after antibiotic therapy for 4 days or less

---

BOX 33-1. ORIGINAL DUKE PATHOLOGIC AND CLINICAL CRITERIA FOR DIAGNOSIS OF ENDOCARDITIS

1. **Pathologic criteria**

   Pathologic criteria include microorganisms demonstrated by culture *or* histology in a vegetation *or* in a vegetation that has embolized *or* in an intracardiac abscess *or* pathologic lesions, including vegetation or intracardiac abscess, confirmed by histology showing active endocarditis.

2. **Clinical criteria**

   Clinical criteria include either two major criteria *or* one major and three minor criteria *or* five minor criteria from the following list:

   Major criteria include:

   - Positive blood culture results with a typical microorganism for infective endocarditis from two separate blood cultures (viridans streptococci, including nutritionally variant strains; *Streptococcus bovis,* HACEK group, or community-acquired *Staphylococcus aureus* or enterococci in absence of a primary focus)
   - Persistently positive blood culture result, defined as recovery of a microorganism consistent with infective endocarditis from blood cultures drawn more than 12 hours apart *or* all of three or a majority of four or more separated blood cultures with first and last drawn at least 1 hour apart
   - Echocardiogram result positive for infective endocarditis, including one of the following:
     a. Oscillating intracardiac mass on valve or supporting structures, in the path of regurgitant jets, or on implanted material in the absence of an alternative anatomic explanation
     b. Abscess

Continued

> ## BOX 33-1.   ORIGINAL DUKE PATHOLOGIC AND CLINICAL CRITERIA FOR DIAGNOSIS OF ENDOCARDITIS—CONT'D
>
> c. New partial dehiscence of prosthetic valve
>
> d. New valvular regurgitation (increase or change in preexisting murmur not sufficient)
>
> Minor criteria include:
>
> - **Predisposition:** Predisposing heart condition or IV drug use
> - **Fever:** Body temperature > 38°C (100.4°F)
> - **Vascular phenomena:** Major arterial emboli, septic pulmonary infarcts, mycotic aneurysm, intracranial hemorrhage, conjunctival hemorrhages, Janeway lesions
> - **Immunologic phenomena:** Glomerulonephritis, Osler's nodes, Roth's spots, rheumatoid factor
> - **Microbiologic evidence:** Positive blood culture result but not meeting major criterion as noted previously *or* serologic evidence of active infection with organism consistent with infective endocarditis
> - **Echocardiogram:** Consistent with infective endocarditis but not meeting major criterion as noted previously

Since the original Duke criteria were published in 1994, several refinements have been made based on studies evaluating the sensitivity and specificity of the criteria:

- Bacteremia with *Staphylococcus aureus* was included as a major criterion only if it was community acquired. Subsequent research has shown that a significant proportion of patients with nosocomially acquired staphylococcal bacteremia will have documented infective endocarditis. Consequently, *S. aureus* bacteremia is now included as a major criterion regardless of whether the infection is nosocomial or community acquired.
- An additional major criterion was added as follows: Single blood culture result positive for *Coxiella burnetii* or anti-phase 1 immunoglobulin G antibody titer > 1:800.
- An additional statement was added to the major criteria regarding endocardial involvement and an echocardiogram positive for infective endocarditis. The statement now includes the following: Transesophageal echocardiography (TEE) is recommended for patients with prosthetic valves, diagnoses rated at least "possible infective endocarditis" by clinical criteria, or complicated infective endocarditis (paravalvular abscess); transthoracic echocardiography (TTE) should be the first test in other patients.
- The echocardiogram minor criterion was eliminated.
- The category of "possible endocarditis" was adjusted to include the following criteria: one major and one minor criterion or three minor criteria. This so-called "floor" was designated to reduce the proportion of patients assigned to the "possible" category.

Baddour LM, Wilson WR, Bayer AS, et al: Infective endocarditis: Diagnosis, antimicrobial therapy and management of complications. A statement from healthcare professionals from the Committee on Rheumatic Fever, Endocarditis and Kawasaki Disease, Council on Cardiovascular Disease in the Young, and the Councils on Clinical Cardiology, Stroke and Cardiovascular Surgery and Anesthesia, American Heart Association. Circulation 111:e394–e433, 2005.

2. **What are the HACEK organisms? How often do they cause endocarditis?**
   HACEK is an acronym for a group of fastidious, slow-growing, gram-negative bacteria:
   - **H:** *Haemophilus parainfluenzae, Haemophilus aphrophilus, Haemophilus paraphrophilus, Haemophilus influenzae*
   - **A:** *Actinobacillus actinomycetemcomitans*
   - **C:** *Cardiobacterium hominis*
   - **E:** *Eikenella corrodens*
   - **K:** *Kingella kingae, Kingella denitrificans*

These organisms account for approximately 5–10% of cases of community-acquired endocarditis. Because an increasing number of these organisms produce beta lactamase, they should be considered resistant to ampicillin. The treatment of choice is ceftriaxone or other third- or fourth-generation cephalosporins.

3. **What is the appropriate role of echocardiography in the diagnosis and management of endocarditis?**
   Echocardiography is an essential tool in the diagnostic work-up of a patient with suspected endocarditis. The primary objective is to identify, localize, and characterize valvular vegetations. However, echocardiography is also potentially important in the management of endocarditis. Identification of an abscess may indicate the need for surgical intervention. Patients may also benefit from repeating the echocardiography once a definitive diagnosis has been established to assess complications, including congestive heart failure and atrioventricular block, which suggest worsening valvular and myocardial function. It is important to emphasize that echocardiographic findings should always be interpreted in coordination with clinical information.
   The TEE is more sensitive than a TTE for the diagnosis of endocarditis. Sensitivities of the different modalities have ranged from 48% to 100% for TEE and from 18% to 63% for TTE. This is in part related to the fact that the transesophageal approach allows closer proximity to the heart and therefore can be performed at higher frequencies, providing greater spatial resolution. It can identify structures as small as 1 mm. TEE is the preferred modality in patients with prosthetic valves. The spatial resolution of the transthoracic echocardiography may be limited by overlying fat in obese patients or hyperinflated lungs from chronic obstructive pulmonary disease or mechanical ventilation. The TTE may only be able to identify structures as small as 5 mm.
   A cost-effectiveness analysis study conducted by Heidenreich and colleagues suggested that the prior probability of endocarditis was the most important factor in choosing the appropriate modality. Although echocardiography has become an essential diagnostic tool in patients with suspected endocarditis, there are no definitive echocardiographic features that can reliably distinguish infection from those lesions that are noninfective.

   Heidenreich PA, Massoudi FA, Maini B, et al: Echocardiography in patients with suspected endocarditis: A cost-effectiveness analysis. Am J Med 107:198–208, 1999.
   Sachdev M, Peterson GE, Jollis JG: Imaging techniques for diagnosis of infective endocarditis. Infect Dis Clin North Am 16:319–337, 2002.

4. **Is there a way to clinically predict the presence of a perivalvular abscess in patients with endocarditis?**
   The presence of a perivalvular abscess should be considered in patients with pericarditis, congestive heart failure (CHF), IV drug use, *S. aureus* infection, prosthetic valve endocarditis, aortic valve disease, or persistent fever or bacteremia while taking appropriate antibiotics. Formal evaluation has suggested that previously undetected atrioventricular or bundle-branch block may be a significant correlate of a perivalvular abscess. Aortic valve involvement and IV drug use have also been found to be significant factors in predicting the presence of a perivalvular abscess.

   Blumberg EA, Karalis DA, Chandrasekaran K, et al: Endocarditis-associated paravalvular abscesses: Do clinical parameters predict the presence of abscess? Chest 107:898–903, 1995.
   Omari B, Shapiro S, Ginzton L, et al: Predictive risk factors for periannular extension of native valve endocarditis: Clinical and echocardiographic analyses. Chest 96:1273–1279, 1989.

5. **What is the optimal timing, volume, and number of blood cultures for a patient suspected of having infective endocarditis?**
   Multiple blood cultures are necessary. Two blood cultures performed with adequate volumes of blood will identify approximately 99% of patients with culture-positive bacteremia.

However, this does not apply to patients who have received empiric antibiotics, patients with fungal endocarditis, or organisms that are difficult to culture. Multiple blood cultures increase the yield, help distinguish between contamination and true bacteremia, and prove continuous bacteremia characteristic of infective endocarditis. If the first set of blood culture results are negative, it is important to realize that repeating blood cultures may be important if the pretest probability of endocarditis remains high. If the clinical situation evolves and endocarditis appears less likely, repeating blood cultures may be counterproductive. Although it makes sense that the optimal time to obtain blood culture specimens is during the hour before the onset of chills or fever spikes, in reality this is not practical. Due to the continuous bacteremia associated with endocarditis, timing is less important, and waiting to initiate therapy in a patient with acute disease with a particularly virulent organism such as *S. aureus* is not warranted. Two to three blood cultures should be obtained within 5 minutes of each other before initiation of antimicrobial therapy. However, if the patient has a clinical course suggestive of subacute endocarditis, obtaining blood cultures over several hours to document continuous bacteremia would be prudent. In general, 20 mL of blood should be obtained for each two-bottle blood culture set. It should also be stressed that each blood culture set requires a separate venipuncture site.

Townes ML, Reller LB: Diagnostic methods: Current best practices and guidelines for isolation of bacteria and fungi in infective endocarditis. Infect Dis Clin North Am 16:363, 2002.

6. **How do you distinguish a case of *S. aureus* endocarditis from uncomplicated *S. aureus* bacteremia?**
   In a classic 1976 study, Nolan and Beaty suggested that among 105 patients with *S. aureus* bacteremia retrospectively identified, most of the 26 patients with endocarditis could be identified on the basis of three characteristics: community-acquired infection, absence of a primary focus of infection, and presence of metastatic foci of infection. However, in prospectively identified patients with *S. aureus* bacteremia who undergo early echocardiography, approximately 25% will have evidence of endocarditis by TEE. Clinical findings and predisposing heart disease did not distinguish those with or without endocarditis. In addition, a substantial portion of these patients had hospital-acquired *S. aureus* bacteremia. Similarly, TEE in one study appeared to be cost-effective in patients with catheter-associated *S. aureus* bacteremia in determining the appropriate length of therapy.

   Fowler VG Jr, Li J, Corey GR, et al: Role of echocardiography in evaluation of patients with *Staphylococcus aureus* bacteremia: Experience in 103 patients. J Am Coll Cardiol 30:1072–1078, 1997.
   Nolan CM, Beaty HN: *Staphylococcus* bacteremia—Current clinical patterns. Am J Med 60:495–500, 1976.
   Petti CA, Fowler VG Jr: *Staphylococcus aureus* bacteremia and endocarditis. Infect Dis Clin North Am 16:413–435, 2002.
   Rosen AB, Fowler AG, Corey GR, et al: Cost-effectiveness of transesophageal echocardiography to determine the duration of therapy for intravascular catheter-associated *Staphylococcus aureus* bacteremia. Ann Intern Med 130:810–820, 1999.

7. **What is nonbacterial thrombotic endocarditis (NBTE)?**
   NBTE refers to small, sterile vegetations on cardiac valves from platelet-fibrin deposits. The cardiac lesions most commonly resulting in NBTE include mitral regurgitation, aortic stenosis, aortic regurgitation, ventricular septal defect, and complex congenital heart disease. NBTE may also result from a hypercoagulable state, and sterile vegetations can be seen in systemic lupus erythematosus (i.e., Libman-Sacks endocarditis), antiphospholipid antibody syndrome, and collagen vascular diseases. Noninfectious vegetations can also be seen in patients with malignancy (e.g., renal cell carcinoma or melanoma), burns, or even acute septicemia. Other lesions that may be somewhat misleading include myxomatous valves, benign cardiac tumors, and degenerative thickening of the valves. Lambl's excrescences, which are multiple small tags on heart valves seen in a large number of adults at autopsy, can also be confused with infectious vegetations; however, these tend to be much more filamentous in appearance.

8. **What are the causes of culture-negative endocarditis?**

Approximately 2–30% of patients with infective endocarditis will have sterile blood culture specimens; however, it is more likely to be 5% using strict diagnosis criteria. Potential causes of culture-negative endocarditis include the following:

- Prior antibiotic usage
- NBTE or an incorrect diagnosis
- Slow growth of fastidious organisms, including anaerobes, HACEK organisms, nutritionally variant streptococci, or *Brucella* species
- Obligate intracellular organisms, including rickettsia, chlamydiae, *Tropheryma whippelii*, or viruses
- Other organisms, including *C. burnetii* (the etiologic agent of Q fever) and *Legionella, Bartonella,* or *Mycoplasma* species
- Subacute right-sided endocarditis
- Fungal endocarditis
- Mural endocarditis, as in patients with ventricular septal defects, post–myocardial infarction thrombi, or infection related to pacemaker wires
- Culture specimens taken at the end of a long course, usually >3 months

   Albrich WC, Kraft C, Fisk T, et al: A mechanic with a bad valve: Blood culture negative endocarditis. Lancet Infect Dis 4:777–784, 2004.

9. **What conduction abnormalities can be associated with endocarditis?**

Right and left bundle-branch blocks, second-degree atrioventricular block, and complete heart block. Heart block generally is the result of extension of infection to the atrioventricular node or the bundle of His. Most patients with heart block have involvement of the aortic valve. In one series, conduction abnormalities occurred in approximately 10% of patients with native valve endocarditis. Mitral valve endocarditis may cause first- or second-degree heart block, but third-degree heart block would be unusual. Aortic valve endocarditis can cause first- or second-degree heart block as well as bundle-branch blocks, hemiblocks, and complete heart blocks. It should be remembered that the electrocardiogram (ECG) is specific but not sensitive for involvement of the conduction system. Consequently, one could have a valve ring abscess but not have conduction abnormalities on the ECG. Complete heart block may be preceded by prolongation of the PR interval or a left bundle-branch block. Conduction abnormalities in the setting of endocarditis may occur for other reasons as well, including myocardial infarction (rarely), myocarditis, or pericarditis. ECG findings may also have prognostic implications because patients with persistent conduction abnormalities have an increased 1-year mortality compared with patients who have normal ECG findings.

   Mehta NJ, Nehra A: A 66 year old man with fever, hypotension and complete heart block. Chest 120:2053–2506, 2001.
   Sokil AB: Cardiac imaging in infective endocarditis. In Kaye K (ed): Infective Endocarditis, 2nd ed. New York, Raven, 1992, pp 125–150.

10. **What valves are most commonly affected in patients with endocarditis?**

This depends on the etiology of the endocarditis. In patients with native valve endocarditis, the mitral valve alone is involved in 28–45% of cases, 5%–36% for the aortic valve alone, and 0–35% for both valves combined. The tricuspid valve is involved alone 0–6% of the time, and the pulmonic valve is involved in <1% of the cases of endocarditis. Endocarditis occurs in approximately 5–15% of injection drug users admitted to the hospital for acute infection. In these patients, the frequency of valvular involvement is as follows: tricuspid valve alone or in combination, 50%; aortic valve alone, 19%; mitral valve alone, 11%; and aortic plus mitral, 12%. In patients with prosthetic valve endocarditis, there does not seem to be a difference in the incidence of endocarditis at the aortic compared with the mitral location. The overall risk of endocarditis is similar with a mechanical valve compared with a bioprosthetic valve; however, there are slight differences in the risk based on the length of time postoperatively. Within the first 6 months postoperatively, mechanical valves have a slightly increased risk of infection; however, there was no significant increased risk within the first 5 years postoperatively with mechanical valves compared with bioprosthetic valves. After 5 years, the risk of endocarditis for bioprosthetic valves is slightly greater than that for mechanical valves. In patients with fungal endocarditis, the aortic valve was involved 44% of the time either alone or in combination with other valves; the mitral valve, 26% alone or in combination; and the tricuspid valve, 7%; other locations were documented in 18% of patients.

Ellis ME, Al-Abdely H, Sandridge A, et al: Fungal endocarditis: Evidence in the world literature, 1965–1995. Clin Infect Dis 32:50–62, 2001.

Fowler V, Scheld WM, Bayer A: Endocarditis and intravascular infections. In Mandell GL, Bennett JE, Dolin R (eds): Principles and Practice of Infectious Diseases, 6th ed. New York, Churchill Livingstone, 2005, pp 975–1022.

11. **What are the clinical differences between right-sided and left-sided endocarditis?**
In patients with right-sided endocarditis (either the tricuspid or pulmonic valve), particularly injection drug users with tricuspid valve endocarditis, only 35% will have an audible murmur. In general, symptoms and complications arise from involvement of the pulmonary vasculature and are characterized by multiple pulmonary septic emboli that may cause pulmonary infarction, abscesses, pneumothoraces, pleural effusions, or empyema. In addition, multiple pulmonary emboli may result in right-sided heart failure with chamber dilatation and worsening tricuspid regurgitation. Clinical symptoms associated with these complications may include chest pain, dyspnea, cough, and hemoptysis. Peripheral embolic phenomena and neurologic involvement are generally absent in patients with right-sided endocarditis, and when they do occur in the setting of right-sided endocarditis, involvement of the left side or paradoxical embolization should be considered. Patients with left-sided endocarditis (aortic or mitral) generally have greater hemodynamic consequences and are more likely to have congestive heart failure. Systemic embolization (brain, kidney, spleen) is more common with left-sided lesions.

KEY POINTS: ENDOCARDITIS

1. The Duke criteria for the diagnosis of endocarditis include either two major criteria (i.e., positive blood culture results plus positive echocardiographic evidence of endocarditis), one major and three minor criteria (i.e., predisposition, fever, vascular or immunologic phenomena and microbiologic evidence), or five minor criteria.

2. The HACEK organisms are fastidious, slow-growing, gram-negative bacteria and include *Hemophilus, Actinobacillus, Cardiobacterium, Eikenella,* and *Kingella* species.

3. *S. aureus* endocarditis cannot be distinguished from bacteremia on the basis of community-acquired infection, lack of a primary focus, and presence of metastatic foci of infection.

4. Symptoms and complications of right-sided endocarditis generally result from involvement of the pulmonary vasculature, whereas complications of left-sided endocarditis are generally characterized by greater hemodynamic consequences, congestive heart failure, and systemic embolization.

5. Nervous system involvement occurs in 20–40% of patients and may be the presenting symptom in approximately 20% of the cases of infective endocarditis.

12. **What are the indications for surgical therapy? What is the optimal timing of surgery in the treatment of endocarditis?**

Clinical situations that warrant surgical intervention include moderate and severe (i.e., New York Heart Association class III or IV) or progressive and refractory CHF, valve dehiscence, rupture, or fistula. Although CHF has a worse prognosis with medical therapy alone, there is also an increased surgical risk. Delay in surgery may also lead to worsening cardiac decompensation or perivalvular extension, which will increase operative mortality as well as secondary complications. Several studies have shown benefits in mortality statistics with surgical intervention. Progressive heart failure in the presence of aortic or mitral valve regurgitation requires surgery. Right-sided endocarditis with tricuspid regurgitation is reasonably well tolerated if the pulmonary vascular resistance is not increased, and surgery is often not required. Other indications include perivalvular extension of infection, persistent bacteremia without evidence of an extracardiac source of bacteremia, mechanical valve obstruction, fungal endocarditis, prosthetic endocarditis, and difficult-to-treat organisms, including *Pseudomonas* species, *C. burnetii*, *Brucella* species, and *Staphylococcus lugdunensis*.

There are conflicting results regarding the correlation of vegetation size and the risk of embolization. Studies have indicated increased risk of embolization with mitral vegetations of >10 mm, whereas others have indicated increased risk with vegetations >20 mm. In several studies with small numbers of patients, vegetation size has not been identified as a risk for embolization. A study by DiSalvo found a higher incidence of embolism associated with vegetations >10 mm in size, mobile vegetations, and large (>15 mm) and mobile vegetations. *S. aureus* was also a risk factor; however, mitral location was not associated with embolism as it had been in previous studies. Conventional wisdom has been that indications for surgery to avoid embolization have been two or more major embolic events during therapy. However, determining the number and timing of embolic events may be difficult, given that the detection of damage may occur well after the actual embolism. The risk of embolization also decreases significantly during the first 1–2 weeks of antibiotic therapy.

Recent hemorrhage embolic stroke is a relative contraindication to surgery. Some experts delay surgery 10–14 days after the initial symptoms of stroke; however, in patients with ischemic stroke <1–2 cm, surgery may be safely performed according to some experts. Consequently, decisions regarding surgery should be individualized and based on the presence of heart failure, neurologic symptoms, and whether the infarct is hemorrhagic or ischemic. In general, a delay of approximately 2 weeks in patients with stroke may be preferable; however, the benefits may outweigh the risks, depending on the patient's clinical situation.

Does operative mortality depend on the duration of antibiotic therapy before surgery? In general, although it is important to have adequate antibiotic coverage during surgery, the duration of antibiotic therapy does not influence operative mortality. The incidence of reinfection of newly implanted valves is approximately 3% and may be as high as 10%.

DiSalvo G, Habib G, Pergola V, et al: Echocardiography predicts embolic events in infective endocarditis. J Am Coll Cardiol 37:1069–1076, 2001.

Olaison L, Pettersson G: Current best practices and guidelines: Indications for surgical intervention in infective endocarditis. Infect Dis Clin North Am 16:453–475, 2002.

13. **What are the neurologic manifestations of endocarditis? How often are they the presenting symptoms?**

Overall, the incidence of central nervous system involvement during the course of infective endocarditis ranges between 20% and 40%. Neurologic symptoms are the presenting manifestations in endocarditis approximately 16–23% of the time; however, there are generally other clues to the diagnosis. Neurologic complications usually occur within the first 2 weeks after starting antibiotics, but later complications—months to as long as 2 years after successful therapy—have been documented. The most common neurologic manifestation is stroke, and this accounts for approximately 50–60% of all neurologic complications. Stroke generally occurs from cerebral emboli with infarction, but hemorrhage or abscess may occur as well. Other neurologic manifestations with their associated main clinical presentations include encephalopathy (decreased level of consciousness), seizures, severe or localized headache, psychiatric syndromes from minor personality changes to more severe psychiatric syndromes (generally in elderly patients), various dyskinesias, visual disturbances, spinal cord involvement (para or tetraplegia), peripheral nerve involvement (mononeuropathy), and meningitis, which is more common with *S. aureus* and *Streptococcus pneumoniae* (with or without focal signs). Ocular complications include acute embolic occlusion of the central retinal artery, which may result in sudden vision loss. Other complications that have been well documented include involvement of cranial nerves III, IV, and VI, which can lead to diplopia, deviation of the eyes, nystagmus or unequal pupils, retinal hemorrhages, and endophthalmitis.

14. **How often do intracranial mycotic aneurysms (ICMAs) occur?**
ICMAs are uncommon, and although they constitute only 2–6% of all intracranial aneurysm, 80% of these are identified in the setting of infective endocarditis. Among patients with endocarditis, only 1–5% will have a recognized ICMA. The mortality rate is approximately 60%, and many patients present with a sudden subarachnoid or intracerebral hemorrhage. Rupture of an ICMA may occur while the patient is being treated for endocarditis or after completion of therapy.

Chun JY, Smith W, Halbach VV, et al: Current multimodality management of infectious intracranial aneurysms. Neurosurgery 48:1203–1213, 2001.

15. **What are the warning signs of ICMA? How is it diagnosed?**
Serious warning signs that should prompt further investigation for the possibility of an ICMA include severe localized headache and other focal neurologic signs, such as seizures, ischemic deficits, and cranial nerve abnormalities. Although sudden rupture is not an uncommon presentation of an ICMA, some aneurysms may leak slowly before rupture and produce meningeal irritation manifested by cerebrospinal fluid that is sterile but shows a moderate number of red cells and a neutrophilic reaction.

When hemorrhage is suspected, a computed tomography (CT) scan with and without contrast is the procedure of choice. If patients with focal neurologic findings are referred for magnetic resonance imaging or CT, magnetic resonance angiography (MRA) and CT angiography (CTA) should be part of the evaluation. These studies should include distal branches. Recent studies have shown that CTA and MRA have similar results in the detection of noninfectious intracranial aneurysms, and it is likely that the same would be true for infectious intracranial aneurysms. If hemorrhage has been confirmed and surgery is considered, conventional angiography is still the most appropriate diagnostic procedure to pinpoint location and anatomic relationships.

Chun JY, Smith W, Halbach VV, et al: Current multimodality management of infectious intracranial aneurysms. Neurosurgery 48:1203–1213, 2001.

16. **Describe the management of ICMAs.**
Optimal treatment is controversial. Medical management should include appropriate antibiotics and control of arterial pressure. ICMAs may resolve with antibiotic therapy alone; consequently, follow-up for unruptured ICMAs may be considered, particularly if multiple aneurysms are present or if they are in locations that are difficult to access. Conventional wisdom appears to dictate follow-up scans at 7- to 14-day intervals. In addition to antibiotics, endovascular approaches and surgical therapies are challenging, and factors that should be considered in making these clinical decisions include patient condition, location of the aneurysm, rupture, and hematomas with increased intracranial pressures. A recent algorithm has been proposed by Chun.

Chun JY, Smith W, Halbach VV, et al: Current multimodality management of infectious intracranial aneurysms. Neurosurgery 48:1203–1213, 2001.

17. **What are the organisms that most often cause endocarditis?**
    The etiologic agents of infective endocarditis include the following:
    - **Streptococci:** 60–80%
    - **Viridans streptococci:** 30–40%
    - **Enterococci:** 5–18%
    - **Other streptococci:** 15–25%
    - **Staphylococci:** 20–35%
    - **Coagulase-positive organisms:** 10–27%
    - **Coagulase-negative organisms:** 1–3%
    - **Gram-negative aerobic bacilli:** 1–13%
    - **Fungi:** 2–4%

    S. aureus tends to be the most common etiologic agent of infective endocarditis in IV drug users. *Pseudomonas aeruginosa* is also more commonly seen in patients using IV drugs. In patients with prosthetic valves, the microbiology is somewhat dependent on whether they have early (<2 months after valve replacement) versus late (>12 months) endocarditis. Staphylococci account for 40–60% of the cases of early-onset prosthetic valve endocarditis. Coagulase-negative staphylococci account for approximately 30–35% of cases, and *S. aureus* accounts for approximately 20–25%. Patients who have late-onset prosthetic valve endocarditis are more likely to have the organisms most commonly seen in patients with native valve endocarditis, with one exception: coagulase-negative staphylococci is seen more frequently (~10–12%) in patients with prosthetic valves. Patients who have fungal endocarditis are often IV drug users, have recently undergone cardiovascular surgery, or have received prolonged IV antibiotic therapy.

18. **What is the appropriate empiric therapy (cultures pending) for patients with presumptive infective endocarditis?**
    Several regimens considered by authorities to be appropriate would include the following:
    - **Acute:** Nafcillin or oxacillin, 2 gm IV every 4 hours, plus gentamicin or tobramycin, 1 mg/kg IV every 8 hours, *or* vancomycin, 15 mg/kg every 12 hours IV (dosing interval based on creatinine clearance) plus gentamicin, 1 mg/kg every 8 hours. Some experts would add ampicillin, 2 gm IV every 4 hours, to the previously described nafcillin regimen to cover the possibility of enterococci.
    - **Subacute:** Ampicillin/sulbactam, 3 gm IV every 4–6 hours, plus gentamicin or tobramycin, 1 mg/kg every 8 hours IV, *or* vancomycin, 15 mg/kg every 12 hours IV (dosing interval based on creatinine clearance), plus ceftriaxone, 2 gm every 12 hours IV.
    - **Prosthetic valve:** Vancomycin, 15 mg/kg every 12 hours (dosing interval based on creatinine clearance), plus gentamicin, 1 mg/kg every 8 hours IV, plus rifampin, 600 mg/day orally.

    Baddour LM, Wilson WR, Bayer AS, et al: Infective endocarditis: Diagnosis, antimicrobial therapy and management of complications. A statement for healthcare professionals from the Committee on Rheumatic Fever, Endocarditis and Kawasaki Disease, Council on Cardiovascular Disease in the Young, and the Councils on Clinical Cardiology, Stroke and Cardiovascular Surgery and Anesthesia, American Heart Association. Circulation 111:e394–e433, 2005.

19. **What are the important clinical manifestations of endocarditis? How often do they occur?**
    Several processes contribute to the clinical signs and symptoms of infective endocarditis, including valvular involvement with intracardiac complications, high-grade and persistent bacteremia (which may lead to metastatic foci), bland or septic embolization to any organ, and immune complex formation. Fever occurs in 80% of patients, and nonspecific symptoms, including anorexia, weight loss, malaise, fatigue, chills, weakness, nausea, vomiting, and night sweats, are very common. Although heart murmurs are common, the so-called "changing murmur" is relatively uncommon. The incidence of peripheral manifestations has decreased.

Osler's nodes, although not specific for endocarditis, may occur in 10–25% of all cases and are generally seen in subacute cases. Janeway lesions (i.e., macular, painless plaques on the palms and soles) are seen in fewer than 10% of cases. Clubbing may be seen if the disease is long-standing and may occur 10–20% of the time. Splenomegaly occurs in 25–60% of cases, generally those with subacute disease. Joint complaints may occur in approximately 40% of patients and may be relatively innocuous with low back pain or myalgias and arthralgias. Musculoskeletal symptoms may also be quite severe, including frank septic arthritis and severe low back pain. Other less common musculoskeletal manifestations include septic bursitis, sacroiliitis, septic diskitis, and polymyalgia rheumatica. Patients with long-standing subacute endocarditis may present as chronic wasting syndrome mimicking cancer or human immunodeficiency virus infection. Signs and symptoms of embolic episodes are determined by the location of the embolism. Patients with splenic emboli may develop left upper quadrant pain, left-sided pleural effusions, or a rub. Renal infarction from a septic embolus may present as flank pain and hematuria. Immune complex formation may lead to renal insufficiency. Cough and shortness of breath with chest pain often accompany pulmonary emboli. Coronary emboli occur rarely and may present with myocarditis, arrhythmias, myocardial infarction, or a combination thereof. Extension into the pericardial space may lead to purulent pericarditis with severe chest pain and hemodynamic compromise. Unexplained heart failure in a young patient without prior cardiac disease should prompt an investigation for infectious endocarditis.

Cavassini M, Meuli R, Francioli P: Complications of infective endocarditis. In Scheld, WM, Whitley RJ, Marra CM (eds): Infections of the Central Nervous System, 3rd ed. Philadelphia, Lippincott Williams & Wilkins, 2004, pp 537–568.

Crawford MH, Durack DT: Clinical presentation of infective endocarditis. Cardiol Clin 21:159–166, 2003.

Fowler VG Jr, Scheld WM, Bayer AS: Endocarditis and intravascular infections. In Mandell GL, Bennett JE, Dolin R (eds): Principles and Practice of Infectious Disease, 6th ed. New York, Churchill Livingstone, 2005, pp 975–1022.

Gonazales-Juanatey C, Gonzalez-Gay M, Llorca J, et al: Rheumatic manifestations of infective endocarditis in non-addicts: A 12 year study. Medicine 80:9–19, 2001.

20. **Are there differences in the manifestations of endocarditis in elderly patients?**
    There does appear to be an increased incidence of endocarditis in elderly patients that may be related to an increased life span in patients with rheumatic and other cardiovascular diseases, with a commensurate increase among patients with calcific and degenerative heart disease. In addition, the increase in prolonged catheter use, implantable devices, and dialysis catheters increases the incidence of nosocomial endocarditis. Endocarditis in elderly persons is more likely to occur in men, with a ratio of approximately 2–8:1 in patients older than 60 years of age. Staphylococci and streptococci account for approximately 80% of the cases in elderly persons, and *Streptococcus bovis* may be noted more frequently in elderly patients associated with underlying colonic malignancy. The clinical presentation of endocarditis may be nonspecific, including lethargy, fatigue, malaise, anorexia, failure to thrive, and weight loss (which may be attributed to aging or other medical illnesses common in the elderly). In addition, fever, which occurs in roughly 80% of patients with endocarditis, is more likely to be absent in elderly patients. Worsening heart failure and murmurs may be attributed to underlying disease and therefore erroneously neglected. Consequently, a high index of suspicion is necessary.

Dhawan VK: Infective endocarditis in the elderly. Clin Infect Dis 34:806–812, 2002.

CHAPTER 34

MENINGITIS

Shannon Kasperbauer, MD, and Randall Reves, MD

1. **Describe the clinical features of acute bacterial meningitis.**

   The classic triad of fever, neck stiffness, and altered mental status occurs in approximately two-thirds of cases, but 95% have two of the four symptoms of headache, fever, neck stiffness, or altered mental status. Up to 14% of patients may present in a coma, and some patients may have focal neurologic defects. Symptoms are more subtle in infants, the elderly, patients with neutropenia, and neurosurgical patients.

2. **What pathophysiologic features distinguish meningitis from other central nervous system infections?**

   Meningitis is an infection localized to the subarachnoid space, resulting in varying degrees of meningismus. With meningitis, neurologic dysfunction is usually limited to depressed sensorium and seizures. Focal cerebral signs or cranial nerve defects are seen in 14–33% of cases and result from the inflammation surrounding cranial nerves that traverse the subarachnoid space or increased intracranial pressure. Subdural empyema or epidural abscess within the cranium or spinal canal, brain abscess, encephalitis, myelitis, and neuritis tend to produce more localized signs or symptoms than those seen with meningitis. Viral pathogens can cause encephalitis, meningitis, or meningoencephalitis.

3. **Describe the differences in acute and chronic presentations of meningitis.**

   People presenting with a rapidly progressive illness of <24 hours' duration usually have bacterial meningitis. Although an acute or subacute presentation can be seen in most cases of bacterial or viral meningitis, the timing to seek medical attention may vary depending on the age of the patient and other medical comorbidities. Chronic meningitis is defined when signs, symptoms, and cerebrospinal fluid (CSF) abnormalities persist for at least 4 weeks and are usually due to mycobacteria, spirochetes, or fungi. Table 34-1 lists common pathogens by age group.

4. **What findings should prompt initiation of empiric antibiotics?**
   - **Patients with an acute, rapidly progressive course**
   - **Positive Gram stain results:** Gram stains of the CSF have positive results in 60–90% of culture-documented cases of meningitis and usually provide rapid information about likely etiologic agents.
   - **Pleocytosis with a polymorphonuclear predominance, low glucose, or elevated protein:** CSF cell count > 1000/mm^3, protein > 150 mg/dL, or glucose < 30 mg/dL indicates a high probability of bacterial meningitis and warrants appropriate antimicrobial therapy, pending the results of cultures and other studies.

TABLE 34-1.   COMMON PATHOGENS BY AGE GROUP

<1 Month	1–23 Months	2–50 Years	>50 Years
Streptococcus agalactiae	*S. agalactiae*	*Streptococcus pneumoniae*	*S. pneumoniae*
Escherichia coli	*E. coli*	*Neisseria meningitidis*	*N. meningitidis*
Listeria monocytogenes	*Haemophilus influenzae*		*L. monocytogenes*
Klebsiella pneumoniae	*S. pneumoniae*		Aerobic gram-negative bacilli
	N. meningitidis		

Data from Tunkel AR: Approach to the patient with central nervous system infection. In Mandell JL, Bennett JE, Dolin R (eds): Principles and Practice of Infectious Diseases, 6th ed. Philadelphia, Elsevier, 2005, pp 1083–1126.

KEY POINTS: ORDER OF THE DIAGNOSTIC WORK-UP IN SUSPECTED BACTERIAL MENINGITIS

1. Obtain two sets of blood culture specimens and a lumbar puncture sample immediately.

2. Administer dexamethasone and empiric antibiotics based on clinical and CSF findings.

or

1. Obtain two sets of blood culture specimens immediately.

2. Administer dexamethasone and empiric antibiotics before computed tomography (CT) scan.

3. Perform CT scan of the head (only if indicated).

4. Perform a lumbar puncture.

5. **Under what circumstances would you want to avoid a lumbar puncture?**
   Lumbar punctures generally should be avoided in the presence of brain abscess or other localized brain lesions in which the risk for herniation is deemed significant. Precautions should also be taken to avoid passing the spinal needle through an infected area such as infected skin or through an epidural abscess. In some situations, neurosurgical consultation may be required to sample CSF via cervical or cisternal approaches. Correction of coagulopathies or thrombocytopenia may be required before performing a spinal tap (generally recommended if there is active bleeding, if the platelet count is <50,000 or if the patient is receiving anticoagulation therapy).

6. **What are the indications for computed tomography (CT) of the head before lumbar puncture?**
   - Age older than 60 years
   - History of central nervous system disease
   - Immunocompromised state
   - Seizure within 1 week of presentation
   - Focal neurologic defects, papilledema, or decreased consciousness

In the study by Hasbun and colleagues, 59% of adult emergency department patients with suspected meningitis met the criteria for CT scanning before lumbar puncture, and only 27% of all patients were diagnosed with meningitis.

Hasbun R, Abrahams J, Jekel J, Quagliarello VJ: Computed tomography of the head before lumbar puncture in adults with suspected meningitis. N Engl J Med 345:1727–1733, 2001.

van Crevel H, Hijdra A, de Gans J: Lumbar puncture and the risk of herniation: When should we first perform CT? J Neurol 249:129–137, 2002.

7. **What is the mortality rate of bacterial meningitis?**
The overall mortality rate is approximately 20%. More specifically, the mortality rate is 30% in cases of *Streptococcus pneumoniae* meningitis, 7% with *Neisseria meningitidis* meningitis, and up to 40% for cases due to *Listeria monocytogenes*.

van de Beek D, de Gans J, Spanjaard L et al: Clinical features and prognostic factors in adults with bacterial meningitis. N Engl J Med 351:1849–1859, 2004.

8. **What features are consistent with a poor prognosis?**
Risk factors for an unfavorable outcome are advanced age, presence of otitis or sinusitis, absence of rash, a low score on the Glasgow Coma Scale on admission, tachycardia, a positive blood culture result, an elevated erythrocyte sedimentation rate, thrombocytopenia, and a low CSF white cell count. In summary, the risk factors listed here are consistent with systemic compromise, low level of consciousness, and infection with *S. pneumoniae*.

van de Beek D, de Gans J, Spanjaard L, et al: Clinical features and prognostic factors in adults with bacterial meningitis. N Engl J Med 351:1849–1859, 2004.

9. **What are the recommended antimicrobial agents for empiric therapy when the CSF Gram stain is nondiagnostic?**
The treatment of immunocompetent patients is a third-generation cephalosporin (cefotaxime or ceftriaxone) in addition to vancomycin. Vancomycin was added with the emergence of cephalosporin resistance in *S. pneumoniae*. Vancomycin should not be used as monotherapy. In patients at increased risk for *L. monocytogenes* infection, specifically infants younger than 2 months or adults older than 50 years of age, ampicillin should be added. Standard therapy for patients with *Streptococcus agalactiae* infection is ampicillin plus aminoglycoside. Patients who are immunocompromised have increased risk for *L. monocytogenes* infection and gram-negative bacilli and therefore should receive ampicillin, ceftazidime, and vancomycin. Staphylococci and gram-negative bacilli infections are more common after head trauma or neurosurgical procedures; empiric therapy should include vancomycin and ceftazidime, cefepime, or meropenem.

Tunkel AR, Hartman BJ, Kaplan SL, et al: Practice Guidelines for the Management of Bacterial Meningitis. Clin Infect Dis 39:1267–1284, 2004.

10. **Are steroids beneficial in the treatment of meningitis?**
Several controlled trials have demonstrated a benefit of using adjunctive dexamethasone to treat bacterial meningitis in children. With regard to adults, a recent randomized controlled trial showed early treatment with dexamethasone 10 mg every 6 hours for 4 days reduced mortality from 34% to 14% in patients with pneumococcal meningitis. Mortality rates were 4% and 3% for placebo and dexamethasone recipients, respectively, with meningococcal and all other etiologies. Dexamethasone also reduced mortality from 41.3% to 31.8% in patients with tuberculous meningitis (older than 14 years of age) but did not prevent severe disability.

de Gans J, van de Beek D: Dexamethasone in adults with bacterial meningitis. N Engl J Med 347:1549–1556, 2002.

Thwaites GE, Bang ND, Dung NH, et al: Dexamethasone for the treatment of tuberculous meningitis in adolescents and adults. N Engl J Med 351:1741–1751, 2004.

11. **What are the recommended antimicrobial agents for the treatment of meningitis when the Gram stain or culture identifies common bacterial pathogens?**
    - **Gram-positive cocci:** Vancomycin plus ceftriaxone (cefotaxime for neonates), pending susceptibility testing of the *S. pneumoniae*
    - **Gram-negative cocci *(N. meningitides)*:** Penicillin G
    - **Gram-positive bacilli *(L. monocytogenes)*:** Ampicillin plus gentamicin
    - **Gram-negative bacilli:** Broad-spectrum cephalosporin (cefotaxime or ceftriaxone) plus an aminoglycoside. For head trauma or neurosurgery patients, ceftazidime is the preferred cephalosporin. Cefotaxime or ceftriaxone is recommended for *Haemophilus influenzae* because of decreased rates of subsequent hearing loss.

    Tunkel AR, Hartman BJ, Kaplan SL, et al: Practice Guidelines for the Management of Bacterial Meningitis. Clin Infect Dis 39:1267–1284, 2004.

12. **How long should you treat bacterial meningitis?**
    Patients who present with a rapidly progressive illness have acute meningitis. Chronic meningitis appears with a more subacute presentation. Meningitis due to *N. meningitidis* and *H. influenzae* require 7 days of antibiotics in most cases. The recommended duration of therapy for *S. pneumoniae* is 10–14 days. The suggested duration of treatment for *S. agalactiae* is 14–21 days. Twenty-one days of therapy are recommended for *L. monocytogenes* and gram-negative bacilli other than *H. influenzae.* Treatment for neurosurgical patients, including those with ventricular shunt infections, must be individualized.

13. **Which empiric therapy should always be considered in chronic meningitis?**
    Acid-fast smears and cultures of CSF have negative results in up to 90% and 60% of patients, respectively, in cases of tuberculous meningitis. To avoid sequelae associated with delays in diagnosis and treatment of tuberculous meningitis, empiric therapy should be considered in any chronic, undiagnosed cases of meningitis, especially in patients at risk for tuberculosis (e.g., homeless, incarcerated, age older than 65 years, country of origin in Africa, Asia, or Latin America). The "typical" CSF parameters are notoriously nonspecific in tuberculous meningitis, and normal levels of CSF glucose do not exclude the diagnosis.

    Treatment for tuberculous meningitis is the same as for pulmonary tuberculosis, but systemic steroids may be considered. The recommended treatment for TB is Isoniazid 300 mg PO daily, Rifampin 600 mg PO daily, Pyrazinamide 25 mg/kg/day PO daily, Ethambutol 15 mg/kg/day PO daily, and Pyridoxine (vitamin B_6) 50 mg PO daily. However, an infectious disease consult is advised given the gravity of this infection.

14. **What are the causes of recurrent meningitis?**
    Recurrent bacterial meningitis can result from persistent unrecognized or undrained parameningeal foci. Recurrence can also result either from abnormal communications with the upper respiratory tract or skin. CSF leaks into the nasopharynx, middle ear, or paranasal sinuses can result from congenital defects or be acquired after trauma; pneumococci are the usual etiologic organism, except in patients receiving antibiotics, who are more likely to acquire gram-negative bacilli. Immunologic defects associated with recurrent meningitis include splenectomy, hypogammaglobulinemia, and inherited deficiencies of complement components.

15. **What is the aseptic meningitis syndrome?**
    Aseptic meningitis is a syndrome of meningitis with negative Gram stain and culture results and typically a normal CSF glucose level. It is not synonymous with viral meningitis, although viruses are the major cause of this syndrome.

KEY POINTS: VIRUSES MOST COMMONLY ASSOCIATED WITH ASEPTIC MENINGITIS

1. Enteroviruses are the most common viral etiology.

2. Arboviruses are more likely to cause an encephalitis than an aseptic meningitis.

3. Herpesviruses typically present as focal encephalitis, but may present as aseptic meningitis in immunocompromised patients.

4. Mumps virus is common in nonimmunized populations.

5. Human immunodeficiency virus infection should always be considered in patients at risk.

6. Lymphocytic choriomeningitis virus is a possibility in persons who have come in contact with rodents.

7. Aseptic meningitis due to West Nile virus presents in the summer months and may be associated with a flaccid paralysis or parkinsonian movement disorders. Severe neuropsychiatric sequelae are common in survivors.

16. **Which studies should be considered in the evaluation of aseptic meningitis?**

HIV, secondary syphilis, suppurative parameningeal foci, and bacterial meningitis may present as aseptic meningitis. The evaluation of aseptic meningitis should always include HIV testing as well as a serum rapid plasma reagin or Venereal Disease Research Laboratory test. Testing of CSF alone is inadequate because CSF usually tests negative in secondary syphilis. Sinus radiographs should be considered in all cases, and CT or magnetic resonance imaging scans of the head or spine may be indicated to rule out brain abscess, epidural abscess, and subdural empyema as parameningeal foci.

Tuberculosis, fungi, and some fastidious organisms such as *Leptospira, Borrelia,* and *Brucella* species may present with the aseptic meningitis syndrome and require repeat lumbar punctures or specific additional testing for diagnosis.

17. **What are the noninfectious causes of meningitis?**

There are several medications that can cause an acute meningitis syndrome, including antimicrobial agents such as trimethoprim/sulfamethoxazole, nonsteroidal anti-inflammatory agents, carbamazepine, muromonab-CD3 (OKT3), azathioprine, immune globulin, and ranitidine. Other noninfectious causes include carcinomatosis (usually with hypoglycorrhachia), inflammatory reactions to necrotic tumors, sarcoidosis, seizures, migraines, and connective tissue diseases.

A slowly leaking cerebral aneurysm may be responsible for aseptic meningitis with xanthochromic CSF.

18. **In the patient with human immunodeficiency virus (HIV) infection, what meningitides should be considered in the differential diagnosis?**

Cryptococcal meningitis and aseptic meningitis (possibly caused by HIV) are the most common HIV-related meningitides. Cryptococci are the most common cause of meningitis in patients with acquired immunodeficiency syndrome (AIDS), in whom it is common to find little or no indication of inflammation in the CSF. Other etiologies include tuberculosis, syphilis, herpes simplex, histoplasmosis, coccidioidomycosis (Fig. 34-1), metastatic lymphoma, and *L. monocytogenes*. The relative risk of purulent meningitis is 150 times greater in HIV-infected patients than in the general population.

19. **How sensitive are India ink examination and cryptococcal antigen testing for cryptococcal meningitis?**

The sensitivity of India ink examination of CSF for the diagnosis of cryptococcal meningitis is 50–70%, and the yield increases to 88% in patients with AIDS. Cryptococcal antigen testing of CSF has positive results in 85%, and the sensitivity is increased to 94% by testing both CSF and serum.

20. **Is meningitis contagious?**

Meningococcal meningitis is contagious. Among household members, the risk of secondary cases within a month of onset of the index case is <1% (about 6 per 1000). Two days of rifampin or a single dose of oral ciprofloxacin is recommended for household members, daycare contacts, and health care providers with contact to oral secretions to eradicate nasopharyngeal carriage. Cases should be reported promptly to the local/state public health department. The enteroviruses that cause the majority of cases of viral meningitis are contagious, but most infected contacts are either asymptomatic or manifest febrile illnesses other than meningitis.

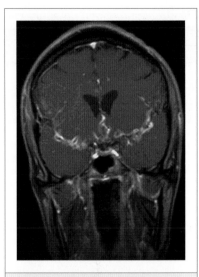

Figure 34-1. Magnetic resonance imaging of the brain revealing basilar meningitis in a patient with acquired immunodeficiency syndrome after highly active antiretroviral therapy was initiated. The cerebrospinal fluid findings included an elevated protein level and white blood cell count with a predominance of lymphocytes, but culture results were negative for routine bacteria, mycobacteria, and fungi. Coccidioidal meningitis was diagnosed based on a serum complement fixation titer of >1:256.

21. **In which populations should _N. meningitidis_ vaccine be used?**

- All children at their routine preadolescent visit
- College freshmen living in dormitories
- Persons with a terminal complement component or properdin deficiency or dysfunction
- Patients with anatomic or functional asplenia
- Persons traveling to areas with epidemic meningococcal disease
- Military recruits
- Close contacts of an index case as long as the serotype of the incident case is included in the quadrivalent vaccine (as an adjunct to chemoprophylaxis)

Centers for Disease Control and Prevention: Infectious Disease Information: www.cdc.gov/ncidod/diseases/submenus/sub_meningitis.htm

CHAPTER 35

DISSEMINATED FUNGAL INFECTIONS

Mark W. Bowyer, MD, DMCC, COL, USAF, MC

1. **How common are fungal infections in hospitalized patients?**
   In the last 25 years, the total number of fungal infections in hospitalized patients has increased from 6% in 1980 to 10.4 % in 1990 and may be as high as 25% in some hospitals in 2005. *Candida* species are currently the fourth most commonly recovered blood culture isolates.

2. **Why has the incidence of fungal infection increased so dramatically?**
   Fungi generally do not cause invasive infection in healthy persons. With the numbers of immunosuppressed patients increasing due to cancer and chemotherapy, transplantation, human immunodeficiency virus infection, vascular and urinary catheters, and the use of broad-spectrum antibacterial agents, there has been an explosion of deep-seated fungal infections in clinical practice.

3. **What fungi are responsible for invasive infection in humans?**
   More than 250 fungal species have been reported to produce human infections. Nearly 80% of these infections are caused by *Candida* species. *Candida albicans* had historically been the most common, resulting in the majority of all *Candida* infections. Other species such as *C. tropicalis, C. glabrata,* and *C. krusei* account for most of the remainder, and the incidence of these non-*albicans* species is on the increase. The other major fungal cause of human infection are the *Aspergillus* species, which account for 15–20% of infections. Other less common but increasing human mycoses include blastomycoses, coccidioidomycoses, cryptococcosis, histoplasmosis, and sporotrichosis.

   The Aspergillus Website: www.aspergillus.man.ac.uk
   Doctor Fungus Website: www.doctorfungus.org
   Segal E: Candida, still number one—What do we know and where are we going from there? Mycoses 48(Suppl 1):3–11, 2005.

4. **Describe the risk factors for disseminated fungal infection.**
   See Box 35-1.

5. **List the diagnostic criteria for disseminated fungal infection.**
   Definitive
   - Fungus cultured from tissue
   - Burn wound invasion
   - Endophthalmitis
   - Fungus cultured from peritoneal fluid

   Suggestive
   - Two positive blood culture results ≥24 hours apart (without a central line), *or* two positive blood culture results with the second obtained ≥24 hours after removal of a central line
   - Three confirmed colonized sites

BOX 35-1. RISK FACTORS FOR DISSEMINATED FUNGAL INFECTION

- Prolonged, multiple (≥3), or broad-spectrum antibiotics
- *Candida* organism isolated from multiple sites other than blood
- Hemodialysis
- Foreign bodies (e.g., central venous, arterial, or urinary catheters)
- Age older than 40 years
- Immunocompromise
  □ Diabetes mellitus
  □ Serum glucose >200 mg/dL
  □ Human immunodeficiency virus infection
  □ Hematologic malignancy
  □ Immunosuppressive therapy (for cancer or organ transplant)
  □ Acute renal failure
  □ Steroid therapy
  □ Parenteral nutrition (especially with high lipid content)
- Deep abdominal surgery
- Severe trauma
  □ Second- and third-degree burns
  □ Severe head injury
  □ Multiple organ system trauma
- Serious infection
  □ Gram-negative sepsis
  □ Acute peritonitis
  □ Intra-abdominal abscess
- Intensive care unit stay (especially if patient is mechanically ventilated)
- "Low risk" is defined as fewer than three risk factors.
- "High risk" is defined as three or more risk factors.

Doctor Fungus Website: www.doctorfungus.org

---

6. **How reliable are these diagnostic criteria?**
The previously mentioned criteria are positive in only 30–50% of patients with disseminated fungal infection. Therefore, a high index of suspicion must be maintained.

7. **If disseminated candidiasis is suspected, where should you look for it?**
In blood cultures, on the retina (endophthalmitis), heart valves (endocarditis), bone (osteomyelitis), wounds, liver, spleen, and kidneys (renal abscesses and candiduria).

8. **What is the overall mortality rate associated with candidemia?**
The overall mortality rate associated with candidemia is 40–60%, with an attributable mortality of 38%.

9. **Should antifungal therapy be delayed until blood culture results are positive for fungus?**
No. Blood cultures have been found to be only 40–68% sensitive. Systemic antifungal therapy should be strongly considered, especially in a patient that is at high risk for disseminated fungal infection, if:
- Fever persists despite antibiotics and negative blood culture results
- High-grade funguria occurs in the absence of a bladder catheter
- Funguria persists after removal of a bladder catheter

- Fungus is cultured from at least two body sites
- Visceral fungal lesions are confirmed

10. **What are the major classes of antifungal drugs in use today?**
    Antifungal drugs in clinical use today fall into three broad categories:
    - Polyene antifungals (amphotericin B)
    - Antifungal azoles (imidazoles and triazoles)
    - Echinocandins

11. **How does amphotericin B work?**
    Amphotericin B, a polyene, is fungicidal. It binds irreversibly to ergosterol (but not to cholesterol, the major sterol in mammalian cell membranes), creating a membrane channel that allows leakage of cytosol leading to cell death. Flucytosine is often used in conjunction with amphotericin B and is synergistic for *Candida* and *Cryptococcus* species. Flucytosine acts directly on fungal organisms by competitive inhibition of purine and pyrimidine uptake.

12. **What antifungal azoles are available? How do they work?**
    Fluconazole, voriconazole, and itraconazole, which are triazoles, are fungistatic. They inhibit C-14 α-demethylase, a cytochrome p450-dependent fungal enzyme required for the synthesis of ergosterol, the major sterol in the fungal cell membrane. This alters cell membrane fluidity, decreasing nutrient transport, increasing membrane permeability, and inhibiting cell growth and proliferation.

13. **How do echinocandins work? Are they being used?**
    The target for echinocandins is the complex of proteins responsible for synthesis of cell wall polysaccharides. Of these, caspofungin has been approved for therapy of aspergillosis and disseminated *Candida* infections. Two others, anidulafungin and micafungin, are in late-phase trials and show early promise.

    Morrison VA: Caspofungin: An overview. Expert Rev Anti Infect Ther 3:697–705, 2005.
    Vazquez JA: Anidulafungin: A new echinocandin with a novel profile. Clin Ther 27:657–673, 2005.
    Zaas AK, Alexander BD: Echinocandins: Role in antifungal therapy, 2005. Expert Opin Pharmacother 6:1657–1668, 2005.

14. **Compare the efficacy of fluconazole with that of amphotericin B in the treatment of candidemia.**
    Randomized multicenter trials have shown that there is no statistically significant difference in the efficacy of fluconazole versus amphotericin B against candidemia, in non-neutropenics, in terms of success in clearing fungemia and survival at the end of therapy. Meta-analysis has shown fluconazole to treat candidemia more successfully than amphotericin B in neutropenic patients.

    Rex JH, Bennett JE, Sugar AM, et al: A randomized trial comparing fluconazole with amphotericin B for the treatment of candidemia in patients without neutropenia. N Engl J Med 331:1325–1330, 1994.

15. **What advantages does fluconazole offer over amphotericin B in the treatment or prevention of disseminated fungal infections?**
    - Fluconazole is available in both IV and oral forms; patients have been successfully treated with 7 days of IV fluconazole followed by oral administration if the patient is able. Administration by mouth is both easier and less costly than IV administration.
    - Fluconazole is not nephrotoxic and has fewer overall adverse effects than amphotericin B, which can cause hypokalemia, fever, and chills.
    - Systemic fluconazole is equally effective against fungal urinary tract infections as amphotericin B bladder irrigation but has fewer of the previously mentioned adverse effects.

16. **Are there any limitations to the use of fluconazole?**
    Yes. Fluconazole is not active against *Aspergillus* species or *C. krusei*, whereas itraconazole and amphotericin B are. Also, remember that fluconazole may cause hepatotoxicity, increases phenytoin and cyclosporin levels, and potentiates Coumadin's anticoagulant effects. Fluconazole has fewer overall adverse effects than amphotericin B.

17. **What should be done when a candidal infection fails to respond to fluconazole?**
    If the diagnosis is confirmed, the underlying risk factors have been minimized, the regimen is being administered correctly, the dosage has been maximized (up to 800 mg/day), and drug-drug interactions are ruled out (rifampin decreases fluconazole levels), then try another azole such as voriconazole or itraconazole. Amphotericin B is a less desirable alternative, but one should not hesitate to use it in the case of life-threatening infections that do not respond to other means. Caspofungin may also be considered in this setting.

18. **Are less toxic forms of amphotericin B available?**
    Yes. To reduce the toxicity associated with amphotericin B, lipid formulations have been produced. The earliest and most widely studied of these is AmBisome, which in randomized trials was shown to be safer than amphotericin B with much fewer side effects. Other lipid-associated, nonliposomal products—amphotericin B lipid complex (Abelcet) and amphotericin B colloidal dispersion (Amphocil)—appear to be similar in efficacy and toxicity to AmBisome. The disadvantage of these alternative forms of amphotericin B is their currently high cost.

KEY POINTS: DISSEMINATED FUNGAL INFECTIONS

1. Fungal infections are an increasingly present source of morbidity and mortality in intensive care units.

2. Simple colonization does not require treatment.

3. *Candida* and *Aspergillus* species account for more than 90% of disseminated fungal infections.

4. Fluconazole is comparable to amphotericin B in the treatment of disseminated candidiasis, and it is less toxic.

5. Do not wait for confirmation by culture to initiate treatment because up to 50% of lethal infections may be culture-negative premortem.

6. Presumptive or preemptive therapy can be useful in selected high-risk groups.

19. **How can health care providers help to prevent the spread of fungal colonization in the intensive care unit (ICU)?**
    A simple solution is to wash your hands and wear gloves when working directly with patients. *Candida* species were found on the hands of 33–75% of ICU staff in one study.

CONTROVERSY

20. **Does the strategy of "presumptive" or "preemptive" treatment of high-risk patients prevent severe candidiasis in critically ill surgical patients?**
    The effectiveness of fluconazole in treating overt candidiasis has unfortunately provoked its widespread, unjustified use in non-neutropenic patients in the ICU setting. This practice has

likely led to an increase in non-*albicans* species that are resistant to fluconazole. Several studies have shown decreased incidence of colonization and the risk of candidiasis with such empiric therapy but have failed to show decreased mortality in any group other than high-risk transplant patients. Recent reviews have suggested that a targeted preemptive strategy may be of benefit in preventing candidiasis in the ICU. This concept requires further study before practice is instituted.

Piarroux R, Grenouillet F, Balvay P, et al: Assessment of preemptive treatment to prevent severe candidiasis in critically ill surgical patients. Crit Care Med 32:2443–2449, 2004.

CHAPTER 36

MULTIDRUG-RESISTANT BACTERIA

John W. Crommett, MD, and Mark W. Bowyer, MD, DMCC, COL, USAF, MC

1. What multidrug-resistant bacteria are of concern to critical care practitioners?

Of particular concern to critical care practitioners are gram-positive organisms such as vancomycin-resistant enterococci (VRE), methicillin-resistant *Staphylococcus aureus* (MRSA), and potentially, the emergence of vancomycin-resistant *S. aureus*. Multidrug-resistant gram-negative rods, particularly imipenem- and ceftazidime-resistant *Pseudomonas aeruginosa, Acinetobacter baumannii,* and *Stenotrophomonas* species are commonly encountered in intensive care units (ICUs). *Enterobacter cloacae, Serratia marcescens, Escherichia coli,* and *Klebsiella* species, among others, have also developed problematic multidrug resistance.

2. What are the major reasons for the development of antibiotic resistance?

- Overuse of antibiotics, in both inpatient and outpatient settings
- Immunosuppression
- Use of antibiotics in the agricultural industry
- Longer survival of critically ill patients
- Poor use of preventive infection control measures such as hand washing and strict isolation precautions
- Increased use of invasive procedures, particularly involving indwelling and prosthetic devices
- Congenital diseases such as cystic fibrosis

Alanis AJ: Resistance to antibiotics: Are we in the post-antibiotic era? Arch Med Res 36:697–705, 2005.

3. One of your patients has been found to be colonized or infected with VRE or MRSA. What isolation precautions should be taken to prevent patient-to-patient transmission?

- Place patients infected with VRE/MRSA in single rooms or in the same room with other patients colonized or infected with the same organism.
- All persons entering the room should wear disposable gloves. In addition, persons who will have substantial contact with the patient or environmental surfaces in the room should wear a disposable gown. These items should be removed before leaving the room, taking care that clothing does not come into contact with any surfaces or the patient.
- Wash hands vigorously with antiseptic soap for 30 seconds upon leaving the room. VRE can persist on hands for 1 hour and MRSA for more than 3 hours.
- Dedicate items such as stethoscopes, penlights, and sphygmomanometers to be used with the infected patient in his or her room during this particular admission. Dispose of the items or adequately clean them after the patient leaves.
- Obtain stool culture specimens or rectal swabs of roommates of patients found to be newly colonized or infected with VRE.
- Ensure that unit or floor staff caring for VRE-infected or colonized patients have as little contact as possible with other patients.

Hierholzer WJ, Garner JS, Adam AB, for the Hospital Infection Control Practices Advisory Committee: Recommendations for preventing the spread of vancomycin resistance: Recommendations of the Hospital Infection Control Practices Advisory Committee (HICPAC). Am J Infect Control 23:87–94, 1995.

Monteclavo MA, Jarvis WR, Ulman J, et al: Infection control measures reduce transmission of vancomycin-resistant enterococci in an endemic setting. Arch Intern Med 131:269–272, 1999.

4. **What is the anticipated role and spectrum of activity of tigecycline, the new glycylcycline antibiotic?**

Tigecycline, a semisynthetic glycylcycline related to minocycline and tetracycline in structure, is currently approved by the U.S. Food and Drug Administration for the treatment of skin, soft tissue, and intra-abdominal infections. It has potent *in vitro* activity against *S. aureus,* including MRSA; *Enterococcus,* including VRE; *Streptococcus pneumoniae; Haemophilus influenzae; Moraxella; Neisseria;* most Enterobacteriaceae organisms; and *Bacteroides fragilis.* It has limited or no activity against *P. aeruginosa* and reduced activity against *Proteus.* The role of tigecycline as part of combination therapy is yet to be determined.

Noskin GA: Tigecycline: A new glycylcycline for treatment of serious infections. Clin Infect Dis 41: S303–S314, 2005.

5. **What treatments are currently available against the emerging *A. baumannii– calcoaceticus* complex?**

Acinetobacter infections are becoming increasingly problematic due to their persistence in the environment and broad antimicrobial resistance patterns. Based on uncontrolled trials, agents with the most activity include imipenem/cilastatin, amikacin, ampicillin/sulbactam, colistin, and tetracyclines, but hospital and ICU-specific antibiograms should be consulted to develop a standard approach.

Navon-Venezia S, Ben-Ami R, Carmeli Y: Update on *Pseudomonas aeruginosa* and *Acinetobacter baumannii* infections in the healthcare setting. Curr Opin Infect Dis 18:306–313, 2005.

6. **Which cephalosporin demonstrates effectiveness against *Enterococcus* infections?**

This is a trick question—no cephalosporin has demonstrated activity against enterococci, and they should not be used to treat such infections.

7. **What new antibiotics are in the pipeline to help combat gram-positive, multidrug-resistant organisms?**

A few years ago quinupristin-dalfopristin and linezolid were introduced as effective new agents against gram-positive organisms, including VRE and MRSA. Since then, the aforementioned tigecycline has become available, and still newer agents are in development, including the cephalosporin, ceftobiprole, and the carbapenems doripenem and faropenem, as well as oritavancin, telavancin, and dalbavancin.

Bosso JA: The antimicrobial armamentarium: Evaluating current and future treatment options. Pharmacotherapy 25:55S–62S, 2005.

8. **What measures can be taken to help reduce selective pressures to antibiotic resistance?**

- Use antibacterial agents only to treat bacterial disease.
- Use appropriate dosage and duration of antibiotics.
- Stop antibiotic usage in animal husbandry for growth promotion.
- Establish antibiotic prescribing practices and regulations in countries where antibiotics are sold over the counter.
- Educate the public regarding the dangers of overuse and misuse of antibiotics.

Tenover FC, Hughes JM: The challenges of emerging infectious diseases: Development and spread of multiply-resistant bacterial pathogens. JAMA 275:300–304, 1996.

9. **Who is at risk for community-associated MRSA infections?**

About 1% of the population is colonized with MRSA. Clusters of these infections have occurred, in particular, in athletes, military recruits, children, nursing home residents, Pacific Islanders,

Alaskan natives, Native Americans, homosexual men, and prisoners. Risk factors in these clusters include close skin-to-skin contact, cuts or abrasions in the skin, contaminated items and surfaces, crowded living conditions, and poor hygiene.

Centers for Disease Control and Prevention: Community-associated MRSA information for the public: www.cdc.gov/ncidod/dhqp/ar_mrsa_ca_public.html

10. When is it permissible to take MRSA-infected patients out of isolation?

Individual hospitals have developed, in consultation with infection control teams and infectious disease specialists, requirements that must be met before patients are moved out of isolation. For example, three consecutive MRSA-negative cultures taken 72 hours apart from all sites previously found to be MRSA positive may be required before a patient may be moved out of isolation.

11. What is the significance of clearance in long-term care patients colonized with VRE?

Overall, little is known about the persistence of colonization with VRE in a patient who is not in the ICU and does not have cancer. A recent study revealed the following:

- Patients who receive long-term medical care, even without oncologic disease, may shed VRE for at least 5 years.
- Despite multiple negative VRE culture results, approximately 25% of patients remain colonized with VRE.
- Current culture techniques often fail to detect VRE.
- Recent antibiotic use leads to increased detection of VRE excretion.
- Criteria for determining genetic relationships in the long-term care setting must be developed because the criteria for outbreaks may be misleading.

Based on these findings, it is unclear what impact attempted clearance of VRE will have. If our detection techniques fail a significant portion of the time, we cannot reliably determine whether clearance has been achieved.

Baden LR, Thiemke W, Skolnik A, et al: Prolonged colonization with vancomycin-resistant *Enterococcus faecium* in long-term care patients and the significance of clearance. Clin Infect Dis 33:1654–1660, 2001.

12. What other problems with multidrug resistance are lurking on the horizon?

Of considerable concern are vancomycin-intermediate and vancomycin-resistant *S. aureus* and emerging imipenem resistance in some of the gram-negative rods such as *Pseudomonas* and *Acinetobacter* species. Most worrisome, however, is the development of resistance to the newer antibiotics (quinupristin-dalfopristin) and the oxazolidinones (linezolid). As always, development of new antibiotics is essential, but unless we continue to address inappropriate uses and infection control practices, the utility of new agents will be short-lived as the mechanisms for developing resistance persist.

Peterson LR: Squeezing the antibiotic balloon: The impact of antimicrobial classes on emerging resistance. Clin Microbiol Infect 11S5:4–16, 2005.

Pfeltz RF, Wilkinson BJ: The escalating challenge of vancomycin resistance in *Staphylococcus aureus*. Curr Drug Targets Infect Disord 4:273–294, 2004.

13. Should we be concerned about multidrug-resistant *S. pneumoniae*?

Once thought to be universally susceptible to penicillin, some strains of *S. pneumoniae* are now resistant to numerous antibiotics. In the United States, up to 35% of isolates are no longer susceptible to penicillin, and some strains are now susceptible only to vancomycin. Although not currently a major problem in ICUs, there are concerns that if vancomycin resistance should jump from enterococci to pneumococci, *S. pneumoniae* infection may become difficult to treat.

Metlay JP, Hofmann J, Cetron MS, et al: Impact of penicillin susceptibility on medical outcomes for adult patients with bacteremic pneumococcal pneumonia. Clin Infect Dis 30:520–528, 2000.

KEY POINTS: MULTIDRUG-RESISTANT BACTERIA

1. No cephalosporin is considered effective against *Enterococcus*.

2. Taking VRE-infected patients out of isolation is controversial because patients may remain colonized despite multiple negative VRE culture results.

3. Some organisms, such as *Stenotrophomonas,* have unique resistance patterns that need to be understood before empiric therapy is initiated.

4. *S. pneumoniae* is another organism that is beginning to develop resistance to commonly prescribed antibiotics, which may have a major impact on the treatment of community-acquired bacterial infections.

14. **How should MRSA and VRE infections be treated?**
    - **MRSA:** IV vancomycin is the drug of choice. Alternatives include the oxazolidinone compound, linezolid, as well as tigecycline, teicoplanin, which has the advantage of less frequent dosing and less nephrotoxicity and ototoxicity, and the streptogramin antibiotic combination quinupristin-dalfopristin.
    - **VRE:** Teicoplanin may be effective, but cross-resistance may occur in Van A or Van B types of enterococcal resistance. Linezolid, quinupristin-dalfopristin, or tigecycline should be strongly considered for patients with VRE infections. If an anatomic focus of infection can be found, surgical removal or drainage should be performed. Consultation with infectious disease specialists is prudent when a patient is first diagnosed with VRE colonization or infection.

    Mulligan ME, Murray-Leisure KA, Ribner BS, et al: Methicillin-resistant *Staphylococcus aureus:* A consensus review of the microbiology, pathogenesis, and epidemiology with implications for prevention and management. Am J Med 94:313–328, 1993.
    Murray BE: Vancomycin-resistant enterococci. Am J Med 102:284–293, 1997.

15. **What would be a good initial empiric treatment regimen in a patient with nosocomial pneumonia with *Stenotrophomonas maltophilia* if the sensitivities are not yet known?**
    Trimethoprim-sulfamethoxazole, gatifloxacin, and ticarcillin-clavulanate or piperacillin-tazobactam are all likely to be effective, as are cefepime and minocycline, depending on antibiogram results. Resistance to imipenem approaches 100%, and aminoglycosides and aztreonam are almost always ineffective. Ceftazidime may or may not be effective.

    Kaye KS, Engemann JJ, Fraimow HS et al: Pathogens resistant to antimicrobial agents: Epidemiology, molecular mechanisms, and clinical management. Infect Dis Clin North Am 18:467–511, 2004.

CHAPTER 37

CATHETER–RELATED INFECTIONS AND ASSOCIATED BACTEREMIA

Carlos E. Girod, MD

1. **Define the different types of catheter-related infections.**
   - **Catheter colonization:** Significant growth of a microorganism in a quantitative or semiquantitive culture of a catheter segment or section
   - **Catheter-related infection:** Presence of ≥15 colony-forming units (CFUs) in a semiquantitive culture or >10³ CFUs in a quantitative culture from a catheter segment *with* signs and symptoms of local and/or systemic infection
   - **Exit-site infection:** Erythema, tenderness, induration, or purulence within 2 cm of the exit site of the catheter or a positive culture of a microorganism from the exit site
   - **Tunnel infection:** Erythema, tenderness, and induration in the tissues overlying the catheter and >2 cm from the exit site
   - **Catheter-related bloodstream infection (CRBSI):** Isolation of the same organism from a semiquantitative culture of catheter segment and from blood (preferably a peripheral blood culture)

   Mermel LA, Farr BM, Sherertz RJ, et al: Guidelines for the management of intravascular catheter-related infections. Clin Infect Dis 32:1249–1272, 2001.

   Norwood S, Ruby A, Civetta J, Cortes V: Catheter-related infections and associated septicemia. Chest 99:968–975, 1991.

2. **Is catheter-related infection a rare syndrome associated only with inexperience?**
   No. Catheter-related infections remain among the top three causes of hospital-acquired infections, with an estimated incidence of 4–17%. In the United States, approximately 250,000 CRBSIs are reported each year. The case-fatality rate for catheter-related infections is approximately 14%, and 19% of these deaths are directly attributed to the catheter infection.

   Infectious Diseases Society of America: Practice Guidelines—Catheter-Related Infections: www.idsociety. org/Content/NavigationMenu/Practice_Guidelines/Guidelines_by_Topic/Practice_Guidelines_by_Topic. htm#Catheter_related.

   O'Grady NP, Alexander M, Dellinger EP, et al: Guidelines for the prevention of intravascular catheter-related infections. Centers for Disease Control and Prevention. MMWR Recomm Rep 2002;51 (RR-10):1–29, 2002.

3. **What are the portals of entry in catheter-related infections?**
   - The skin around the insertion site is the most common portal of entry of infection for nontunneled central venous catheters. Analysis of catheter segments by Gram stain and semiquantitative cultures shows predominance of bacteria along the outer surface of the catheter from tip to skin entry. The major mechanism for entry is bacterial adherence followed by migration along the catheter.
   - The second most common portal of entry of bacteria is via contamination of the catheter hub during its manipulation. It is typically seen in tunneled central venous catheters.

- Hematogenous dissemination from a distal infectious focus with catheter colonization is less common.
- Contaminated transducer kits, disinfectants, and infusion lines are rare sources of catheter-related infections.

Crnich CJ, Maki DG: Infections of vascular devices. In Cohen J, Powderly WG (eds): Infectious Diseases, 2nd ed. St. Louis, Mosby, 2004, pp 629–635.

Mermel LA, Farr BM, Sherertz RJ, et al: Guidelines for the management of intravascular catheter-related infections. Clin Infect Dis 32:1249–1272, 2001.

4. **What are important risk factors for catheter-related infections?**
   See Box 37-1. A review of the literature suggests that the presence of sepsis is the most important patient-related risk factor.

   Crnich CJ, Maki DG: Infections of vascular devices. In Cohen J, Powderly WG (eds): Infectious Diseases, 2nd ed. St. Louis, Mosby, 2004, pp 629–635.

   Safdar N, Maki DG: Risk of catheter-related bloodstream infection with peripherally inserted central venous catheters used in hospitalized patients. Chest 128:489–495, 2005.

BOX 37-1. IMPORTANT RISK FACTORS FOR CATHETER-RELATED INFECTIONS

- AIDS
- Diabetes mellitus
- Altered host defense
- Multiple medical problems
- Age <1 year, >60 years
- Immunosuppressive therapy
- Mechanical ventilation
- Granulocytopenia
- Loss of skin integrity
- Malnutrition
- Distal infection
- Total parenteral nutrition
- Sepsis

AIDS = acquired immunodeficiency syndrome.

---

5. **What are non–patient-related risk factors for catheter infections?**
   See Box 37-2. Duration of catheterization is the most important non–patient-related risk factor for catheter-related infection.

   Crnich CJ, Maki DG: Infections of vascular devices. In Cohen J, Powderly WG (eds): Infectious Diseases, 2nd ed. St. Louis, Mosby, 2004, pp 629–635.

6. **Is any specific type of catheter linked to increased infection?**
   - **Peripheral IV catheters:** These catheters have a significant risk for contamination 72 hours after insertion. Nevertheless, when changed every 72 hours, these catheters are less often associated with infection than central, pulmonary, and arterial catheters.

BOX 37-2.   NON–PATIENT-RELATED RISK FACTORS FOR CATHETER-RELATED INFECTIONS

- Alteration of skin flora
- Lack of sterile procedure
- Catheter adherence properties
- Catheter size
- Lumen number
- Inadequate maintenance
- Hypertonicity of infusate
- Skill of inserting physician
- Location and duration
- Type of catheter

KEY POINTS: HOST OR DEVICE FACTORS THAT POSE THE HIGHEST RELATIVE RISK (RR) FOR CATHETER-RELATED BLOODSTREAM INFECTION (CRBSI)

1. The RR for CRBSI in a patient with neutropenia is 1.0–15.1.

2. Other systemic or local infections carry an RR of 8.7–9.2.

3. The RR when a catheter is in place for >7 days is 1.0–8.7.

4. A prolonged hospital stay carries an RR of 1.0–6.7.

5. With multilumen catheter use, the RR for CRBSI is 6.5.

6. The RR for CRSBI is 5.4 in the case of a difficult catheter insertion.

7. Femoral vein catheterization carries an RR of 3.3–4.8.

- **Central venous catheters:** Central venous catheters definitely carry an increased risk of related infection and bacteremia compared with peripheral IV catheters. A meta-analysis demonstrated that multilumen central venous catheters have a higher risk of bloodstream infection than single-lumen catheters (odds ratio, 2.15; 95% confidence interval, 1.00–4.66). Nevertheless, the convenience of having multiple lumens for infusion may outweigh the risk of infection.
- **Pulmonary artery (PA) catheters:** PA catheters have an estimated incidence of bloodstream infection of 2% when left in place for <72 hours and 16% when left longer. This is due to the large number of manipulations performed with PA catheters.
- **Arterial catheters:** Arterial catheters are associated with rates of CRBSI similar to those seen with PA and central venous catheters.

Infectious Diseases Society of America: Practice Guidelines—Catheter-Related Infections: www.idsociety. org/Content/NavigationMenu/Practice_Guidelines/Guidelines_by_Topic/Practice_Guidelines_by_Topic. htm#Catheter_related

O'Grady NP, Alexander M, Dellinger EP, et al: Guidelines for the prevention of intravascular catheter-related infections. Centers for Disease Control and Prevention. MMWR Recomm Rep 51(RR-10):1–29, 2002.

7. **Are peripherally inserted central venous catheters (PICCs) less likely to cause bloodstream infection than catheters placed in the internal jugular or subclavian veins?**

   No. Because of their low risk of mechanical complications, PICCs are increasingly being used for intermediate- or long-range use at many medical centers. A recent prospective study by Maki with 251 PICC placements (mean duration of catheterization, 11.3 days) demonstrated a rate of CRBSI of 2.1–3.5 per 1000 catheter-days. This rate is comparable to that seen with internal jugular and subclavian central venous catheters (2–5 per 1000 catheter-days) and higher than that of tunneled and cuffed catheters (1 per 1000 catheter-days).

   Safdar N, Maki DG: Risk of catheter-related bloodstream infection with peripherally inserted central venous catheters used in hospitalized patients. Chest 128:489–495, 2005.

8. **Are physician experience and timing at insertion important?**

   Yes. Limited experience with fewer than 25 prior insertions carries an 18–20% incidence of catheter-related infection versus 8–12% for experienced operators with more than 25 prior insertions. A report by Sherertz and colleagues demonstrated that residents who attended a 1-day infection control course reduced their rate of subsequent catheter-related infections by 35%. The timing of insertion is also important, and an increased incidence of catheter-related infections is seen with catheters placed in patients that have been in the intensive care unit for more than 6 days.

   Sherertz RJ, Ely EW, Westbrook DM, et al: Education of physicians-in-training can decrease the risk for vascular catheter infection. Ann Intern Med 132:641–648, 2000.

9. **For how long should an intravascular catheter be used without increasing the risk for catheter-related infection?**

   Recommended duration of catheter use before removal should be determined on a patient-to-patient basis, taking into account the host and non–patient-related factors listed in questions 4 and 5. There are no available guidelines stating the "safe" duration of a venous or arterial catheter placement. It is well known that prolonged catheterization is the most important risk factor for catheter-related infections. As a rule, no catheter should be left in place any longer than absolutely necessary. The catheter should be removed or changed when clinically indicated.

   Crnich CJ, Maki DG: Infections of vascular devices. In Cohen J, Powderly WG (eds): Infectious Diseases, 2nd ed. St. Louis, Mosby, 2004, pp 629–635.

   Infectious Diseases Society of America: Practice Guidelines—Catheter-Related Infections: www.idsociety. org/Content/NavigationMenu/Practice_Guidelines/Guidelines_by_Topic/Practice_Guidelines_by_Topic. htm#Catheter_related.

   Mermel LA, Farr BM, Sherertz RJ, et al: Guidelines for the management of intravascular catheter-related infections. Clin Infect Dis 32:1249–1272, 2001.

   O'Grady NP, Alexander M, Dellinger EP, et al: Guidelines for the prevention of intravascular catheter-related infections. Centers for Disease Control and Prevention. MMWR Recomm Rep 51(RR-10):1–29, 2002.

10. **Do routine guidewire or new site changes every 3–7 days decrease the incidence of catheter-related infection?**

    A randomized controlled study of 160 patients demonstrated that routine replacement of central venous catheters every 3 days did not prevent the development of infection. This finding applied to both techniques of replacement: new site and guidewire exchanges. This study clearly demonstrated an increased risk for bleeding or pneumothorax in patients randomly assigned to receive routine new site catheter insertions. Further studies have compared scheduled routine catheter changes every 7 days to catheter changes when clinically indicated. No reduction in catheter-related bloodstream bacteremia was observed. Currently, routine replacement of catheters is not recommended. The catheter should be replaced when clinically indicated.

Cobb DK, High KP, Sawyer RG, et al: A controlled trial of scheduled replacement of central venous and pulmonary-artery catheters. N Engl J Med 327(15):1062–1068, 1992.

Infectious Diseases Society of America: Practice Guidelines—Catheter-Related Infections: www.idsociety. org/Content/NavigationMenu/Practice_Guidelines/Guidelines_by_Topic/Practice_Guidelines_by_Topic. htm#Catheter_related.

O'Grady NP, Alexander M, Dellinger EP, et al: Guidelines for the prevention of intravascular catheter-related infections. Centers for Disease Control and Prevention. MMWR Recomm Rep 51(RR-10):1–29, 2002.

11. **Is changing an intravascular catheter over a guidewire associated with less risk of related infection than a new site replacement?**
Recent studies have concluded that guidewire exchanges are associated with increased catheter colonization, exit site infection, and bacteremia. Nevertheless, guidewire changes are usually preferred over new site insertion because of a decreased risk of pneumothorax or bleeding complications. It is an effective method for ruling out catheter-related infection in febrile, nonseptic patients. Every attempt should be made to sterilize the entire external portion of the catheter, guidewire, and surrounding skin. The removed catheter should be cultured and, if infected, the guidewire-placed catheter must be removed. Guidewire exchanges should not be performed in patients with confirmed or suspected sepsis.

Infectious Diseases Society of America: Practice Guidelines—Catheter-Related Infections: www.idsociety. org/Content/NavigationMenu/Practice_Guidelines/Guidelines_by_Topic/Practice_Guidelines_by_Topic. htm#Catheter_related.

O'Grady NP, Alexander M, Dellinger EP, et al: Guidelines for the prevention of intravascular catheter-related infections. Centers for Disease Control and Prevention. MMWR Recomm Rep 51(RR-10):1–29, 2002.

Safdar N, Maki DG: Risk of catheter-related bloodstream infection with peripherally inserted central venous catheters used in hospitalized patients. Chest 128:489–495, 2005.

12. **Which site is more at risk for catheter-associated infection: internal jugular, femoral, or subclavian sites?**
The internal jugular site has a higher incidence of catheter-related infection than the subclavian site (relative risk, 1–3.3). The increased risk is likely due to the following factors:
- Increased oral and nasal secretions that pool in the neck site of a supine patient
- Inability to apply an occlusive dressing to the neck site
- Higher skin temperature

Femoral vein catheterization is the least preferred of the central venous catheter sites because of its increased risk of catheter-associated infection (relative risk, 3.3–4.8) and thrombotic complications. Femoral lines are in close anatomic proximity to the urogenital and rectal areas, with associated gram-negative bacterial colonization and infection. Moreover, a randomized clinical study demonstrated the presence of a deep vein thrombosis in 21.5% of patients with a femoral central line and 1.9% in patients with subclavian catheters ($P < 0.001$). Femoral vein catheterization may be used in emergency situations, such as hemodynamic instability, shock, or cardiac arrest.

Crnich CJ, Maki DG: Infections of vascular devices. In Cohen J, Powderly WG (eds): Infectious Diseases, 2nd ed. St. Louis, Mosby, 2004, pp 629–635.

McGee DC, Gould MK: Preventing complications of central venous catheterization. N Engl J Med 348:1123–1133, 2003.

Merrer J, De Jonghe B, Golliot F, et al: Complications of femoral and subclavian venous catheterization in critically ill patients: A randomized controlled trial. JAMA 286:700–707, 2001.

13. **What is the most sensitive and specific means of diagnosing catheter-related infections?**

    Physical examination is unreliable. Local inflammation or purulence at the entry site is seen in fewer than half of cases. Fever, leukocytosis, and positive peripheral blood culture results are also not reliable indicators of catheter-related infection. Nevertheless, two sets of blood culture specimens (at least one set from a percutaneous source) should be obtained in patients with suspected catheter-associated infection.

    The most widely used method for diagnosing a catheter-related infection is the "roll plate" method, which requires removal of the catheter and culture of its tip by rolling it over a blood-agar plate. Growth of ≥ 15 colonies per plate is associated with a sensitivity of 60% for CRBSI. A more sensitive technique is quantitative culture of the intravascular and subcutaneous catheter segments after sonication in broth. A greater than 10^3 CFU in culture has an 80% sensitivity for CRBSI.

    Crnich CJ, Maki DG: Infections of vascular devices. In Cohen J, Powderly WG (eds): Infectious Diseases, 2nd ed. St. Louis, Mosby, 2004, pp 629–635.

    Mermel LA, Farr BM, Sherertz RJ, et al: Guidelines for the management of intravascular catheter-related infections. Clin Infect Dis 32:1249–1272, 2001.

14. **What organisms cause catheter-related infections?**

    See Table 37-1. The most common organism leading to catheter-related infections is the coagulase-negative *Staphylococcus epidermidis*, accounting for 37% of these infections.

    Cobb DK, High KP, Sawyer RG, et al: A controlled trial of scheduled replacement of central venous and pulmonary-artery catheters. N Engl J Med 327:1062–1068, 1992.

    Mermel LA, Farr BM, Sherertz RJ, et al: Guidelines for the management of intravascular catheter-related infections. Clin Infect Dis 32:1249–1472, 2001.

    O'Grady NP, Alexander M, Dellinger EP, et al: Guidelines for the prevention of intravascular catheter-related infections. Centers for Disease Control and Prevention. MMWR Recomm Rep 51(RR-10):1–29, 2002.

    Raad II, Hanna HA: Intravascular catheter-related infections: new horizons and recent advances. Arch Intern Med 162:871–878, 2002.

15. **How should you treat nontunneled central venous catheter infections?**

    Treatment depends on the stage of infection and the pathogen. As a general rule, if CRBSI or bacteremia is strongly suspected, the catheter must be removed and replaced. For empiric antibiotic therapy, vancomycin is the drug of choice for covering methicillin-resistant staphylococci while culture results are awaited.

    Coagulase-negative staphylococci infections are treated with removal of the catheter and administration of IV antibiotics for 5–7 days.

    Staphylococcus aureus–associated bacteremia should be treated with removal of the catheter and administration of IV antibiotics for at least 2 weeks because of a higher association with endocarditis. Most experts recommend a transesophageal echocardiogram in these patients to exclude endocarditis.

    Catheter infections with *Candida* species should be treated with removal of the catheter and administration of IV antifungal agents for at least 14 days from the last positive blood culture result.

    Crnich CJ, Maki DG: Infections of vascular devices. In Cohen J, Powderly WG (eds): Infectious Diseases, 2nd ed. St. Louis, Mosby, 2004, pp 629–635.

    Mermel LA, Farr BM, Sherertz RJ, et al: Guidelines for the management of intravascular catheter-related infections. Clin Infect Dis 32:1249–1272, 2001.

    Raad, II, Hanna HA: Intravascular catheter-related infections: New horizons and recent advances. Arch Intern Med 162:871–878, 2002.

TABLE 37-1. MICROBIOLOGY OF VASCULAR CATHETER-RELATED COLONIZATION AND BLOODSTREAM INFECTIONS

Organism	No. (%) of Catheters Associated with:	
	Colonization	Bloodstream Infection
Coagulase-negative staphylococci	86 (54%)	7 (16%)
Staphylococcus aureus	20 (13%)	12 (27%)
Enterococci	3 (2%)	5 (11%)
Gram-negative bacilli	37 (23%)	15 (34%)
Gram-positive bacilli	3 (2%)	0
Mycobacterium chelonae	0	1 (2%)
Candida species	9 (6%)	4 (9%)
Total	**156 (100%)**	**44 (100%)**

Data from Raad II, Hanna HA: Intravascular catheter-related infections: New horizons and recent advances. Arch Intern Med 162:871–878, 2002.

16. **What is the standard of care for managing tunneled central venous catheter infections?**
Complicated infections at exit site or tunnel infection should be treated with removal of the tunneled catheter and 7–10 days of IV antibiotics targeting the offending microorganism. Occasionally, a tunneled central venous catheter associated with an uncomplicated infection may be salvaged with the use of antibiotics instilled through the catheter and the use of antibiotic "lock therapy" for at least 2 weeks. Antibiotic lock therapy is a technique that uses a small volume of high-concentration IV antibiotics instilled into the catheter lumen, and then the catheter is kept "locked" for at least 12 hours. This technique targets the bacteria colonizing the biofilm within the catheter. Studies have demonstrated successful clearance of infection in approximately 83% of uncomplicated tunneled catheter infections.

Mermel LA, Farr BM, Sherertz RJ, et al: Guidelines for the management of intravascular catheter-related infections. Clin Infect Dis 32:1249–1272, 2001.

Raad II, Hanna HA: Intravascular catheter-related infections: New horizons and recent advances. Arch Intern Med 162:871–878, 2002.

17. **What are other ways to prevent catheter infection?**
   - **Chlorhexidine gluconate:** Skin decontamination before insertion of the catheter leads to greater reduction of infection than with the use of iodine solutions.
   - **Povidone-iodine topical ointment:** Applied to the exit site, povidone-iodine topical ointment may not yield significant benefit in reducing catheter infection. There is a trend toward reduced staphylococcal bacteremia when the ointment is applied to hemodialysis catheters after completion of each hemodialysis session.
   - **Site dressings:** Site dressings are important, but a recent meta-analysis failed to demonstrate a significant reduction in central venous catheter–related bloodstream infection when transparent site dressings were compared with gauze dressings.

- **Vitacuff:** Use of this subcutaneous collagen cuff, which is impregnated with silver and placed at the catheter entry site, has been associated with a three- and fourfold reduction in colonization and bacteremia, respectively.
- **Antibiotic-impregnated catheters:** These minocycline-rifampin or chlorhexidine-silver sulfadiazine catheters have demonstrated a reduction in catheter colonization and associated bloodstream infections. Studies have demonstrated the cost-effectiveness of these catheters due to an observed reduction in nosocomial infection, leading to a $196 saving in direct medical costs per catheter placement despite the fact that these catheters are more expensive. Current guidelines recommend these antimicrobial-impregnated catheters for use in hospital units with greater than a 2% rate of catheter-related bacteremia or in immunocompromised hosts.
- **Specialized teams:** Eggimann and colleagues demonstrated a threefold reduction in catheter-related infection with a specialized team devoted to the placement and maintenance of central and peripheral venous catheters.
- **Mask and sterile gown and barrier:** There is a twofold reduction in catheter-associated infections when physicians use long-sleeved surgical gowns, masks, and full-length sterile drapes during insertion.

Darouiche RO, Raad, II, Heard SO, et al: A comparison of two antimicrobial-impregnated central venous catheters. Catheter Study Group. N Engl J Med 340:1–8, 1999.

Eggimann P, Harbarth S, Constantin MN, et al: Impact of a prevention strategy targeted at vascular-access care on incidence of infections acquired in intensive care. Lancet 355(9218):1864–1868, 2000.

McGee DC, Gould MK: Preventing complications of central venous catheterization. N Engl J Med 348:1123–1133, 2003.

O'Grady NP, Alexander M, Dellinger EP, et al: Guidelines for the prevention of intravascular catheter-related infections. Centers for Disease Control and Prevention. MMWR Recomm Rep 51(RR-10):1–29, 2002.

Rupp ME, Lisco SJ, Lipsett PA, et al: Effect of a second-generation venous catheter impregnated with chlorhexidine and silver sulfadiazine on central catheter-related infections: A randomized, controlled trial. Ann Intern Med 143:570–580, 2005.

Safdar N, Kluger DM, Maki DG: A review of risk factors for catheter-related bloodstream infection caused by percutaneously inserted, noncuffed central venous catheters: Implications for preventive strategies. Medicine (Baltimore) 81:466–479, 2002.

18. **What new methods allow for the diagnosis of CRBSIs without requiring catheter removal?**
Confirmation of catheter-related infection and associated bacteremia usually requires the removal of the catheter for culture. New methods for the diagnosis of CRBSIs are based on a difference in quantitative bacterial counts and the time to positivity between blood culture specimens drawn from a peripheral site versus those drawn from the central venous catheter. Quantitative blood culture specimens drawn from a central venous catheter that have 5–10 times greater colony counts than peripheral blood cultures are highly suggestive of a CRBSI. A study by Blot and colleagues suggested that CRBSI could be diagnosed by studying the differential time to positivity between a blood culture specimen obtained from the hub of the catheter and a peripheral blood culture site. A positive hub blood culture result at least 2 hours before a positive result from a peripheral blood culture had a sensitivity and specificity of 94% and 95%, respectively, for CRBSI.

Blot F, Nitenberg G, Chachaty E, et al: Diagnosis of catheter-related bacteraemia: A prospective comparison of the time to positivity of hub-blood versus peripheral-blood cultures. Lancet 354(9184):1071–1077, 1999.

Raad II, Hanna HA: Intravascular catheter-related infections: New horizons and recent advances. Arch Intern Med 162:871–878, 2002.

CHAPTER 38

BIOTERRORISM

Stanley L. Minken, MD, DMCC, and Mark W. Bowyer, MD, DMCC, COL, USAF, MC

1. **What is the definition of *bioterrorism*?**
   Bioterrorism is the deliberate use of biologic means to create and exploit a sense of fear and unrest within a defined population. It is aimed at undermining confidence in the current leadership with the goal of instituting political change.

2. **Who are the potential worldwide sources of a bioterrorist attack?**
   - Formal governments with biological warfare or nuclear development programs can use citizen scientists, immigrant scientists, spies, stolen documents, and/or stolen biomaterial.
   - Formal governments can use military delivery of bioweapons.
   - Nongovernmental terrorist organizations can use multiple national and international sympathizers, including sympathetic scientists, covert scientists, stolen documents, and purchased and donated biomaterials.
   - Terrorist organizations can use a worldwide network and employ unorthodox delivery methods of bioweapons.

3. **What constitutes a bioterrorism threat?**
   - Pathogenic bacteriologic, viral, and rickettsial agents introduced deliberately into the population
   - Chemical agents in gaseous, aerosolized, powdered, or liquid form exposed to an unsuspecting population
   - Nuclear debris exposed to the general population after a low-explosive-force detonation containing radioactive material

4. **What epidemiologic characteristics of a biologic outbreak should arouse suspicions of a bioattack?**
   - Emergence of an unusually large epidemic within a relatively defined population inconsistent with the health status of the general population
   - A high degree of disease severity out of proportion to usual patterns with unusual resistance to standard therapy
   - Emergence of synchronous epidemics of different pathogens
   - Emergence of synchronous epidemics of the same pathogen in discontinuous geographic areas
   - Diseases and pathogen strains unusual for the local geographic area
   - Development of concomitant disease syndromes in humans and animals
   - Intelligence data of a potential attack or specific claims of an attack
   - Proven data from investigational authorities of an agent's release or use

   Pavlin JA: Epidemiology of bioterrorism. Emerg Infect Dis 5:4, 1999: www.cdc.gov/ncidod/EID/vol5no4/pavlin.htm

5. **What are the common bacterial, viral, and rickettsial threats?**
   See Table 38-1.

TABLE 38-1.	COMMON BACTERIAL, VIRAL, AND RICKETTSIAL THREATS	
Bacterial	Viral	Rickettsial
Anthrax	Eastern equine encephalitis (EEE)	Q fever
Botulism	Rift Valley fever	Typhus
Plague	Venezuelan equine encephalitis (VEE)	
Typhoid	Viral hemorrhagic fevers (e.g., Marburg, Ebola, Lassa)	
	Western equine encephalitis (WEE)	
	Smallpox	

6. **What other experimental agents are being developed for biowarfare use?**
   - Smallpox plus Venezuelan equine encephalitis (VEEPOX)
   - Ebola plus smallpox (EBOLAPOX)

ANTHRAX

7. **What is anthrax?**
   Anthrax is a bacterial disease caused by a gram-positive, spore-forming bacillus. It presents 95% of the time as cutaneous anthrax contracted by direct contact. The inhalational variety, which is contracted by aerosol inhalation, represents 5% of cases and is the primary threat of bioterrorism among agents disseminated by powdered aerosol or contact with contaminated material.

   Dixon TC, Meselson M, Guillelin J, Hanna PC: Anthrax. N Engl J Med 341:815, 1999.

8. **Describe the clinical syndrome of cutaneous anthrax.**
   Lesions develop 2–5 days after exposure. They start as a papule and become a 1- to 2-cm vesicle with surrounding edema. The lesion is pruritic, not painful. The vesicle ruptures in 1 week, leaving an ulcer that becomes an eschar. The recovery rate is 85%, with a 2–15% death rate resulting from septicemia.

9. **What is the treatment of cutaneous anthrax?**
   - The disease responds well to penicillin, ciprofloxacin, or doxycycline.
   - Skin lesions should be treated with standard wound care.

10. **Describe the clinical syndrome of inhalational anthrax.**
    Spores deposit in the lower respiratory tract, causing fever, malaise, and nonproductive cough. Symptoms are mild for several days while spores are phagocytized by macrophages and transported to mediastinal lymph nodes. Spores germinate into multiplying bacilli and overwhelm the natural inflammatory response, with abrupt onset of respiratory distress. The infected person develops severe progressive pneumonia and necrotizing hemorrhagic mediastinitis. Death can occur in 24–48 hours with respiratory, meningeal, and septic symptoms. Laboratory diagnosis includes blood hematoxylin and eosin staining for bacillus and immunofluorescence.

    Inglesby TV, O'Toole T, Henderson DA, et al: Anthrax as a biological weapon. JAMA 160:287:2236–2252, 2001.

11. **What is the treatment of inhalational anthrax?**
    Treatment includes intubation with respiratory support. Naturally occurring strains respond to penicillin, streptomycin, erythromycin, and ciprofloxacin; fluoroquinolones are the drug of choice.

BOTULISM

12. What is botulism?

Botulism is a condition caused by a neurotoxin produced by *Clostridium botulinum* that inhibits the release of acetylcholine at the neuromuscular junction, resulting in a severe flaccid paralysis. The most common form is foodborne, but it may be aerosolized or spread by contaminated water. The bacterium is an anaerobic gram-positive spore that produces seven toxins (A–G). Type A toxin is the most potent and potentially lethal. The bioterrorism threat includes both foodborne and aerosolized toxin vaporization.

Shapiro RL, Hatheway C, Swerdlow DL: Botulism in the United States: A clinical and epidemiological review. Ann Intern Med 129:221–228, 1998.

13. What are the clinical syndromes of botulism?

See Table 38-2.

The primary triad includes the paresis and paralysis in an afebrile patient with no sensory changes. Death results from respiratory dysfunction. The foodborne variety is distinguished by the abdominal and gastrointestinal symptoms, absent in the respiratory variety.

TABLE 38-2. CLINICAL SYNDROMES OF BOTULISM

Foodborne	Inhalation
12- to 36-hour incubation period	24- to 72-hour incubation period
Symmetric descending weakness and paralysis	Symmetric descending weakness and paralysis
No sensory changes	No sensory changes
Alert patient without fever	Alert patient without fever
Abdominal pain	No abdominal pain
Nausea and vomiting	No nausea and vomiting
Ptosis, blurred vision, weak jaw, dysphagia	Ptosis, blurred vision, weak jaw, dysphagia
Respiratory dysfunction	Respiratory dysfunction
Ileus	Ileus

14. How can the diagnosis of botulism be confirmed?

Symptoms rapidly occurring in a widespread population rather than in an isolated group are highly suspicious of a bioattack. Confirmation of diagnosis rests on demonstrating the presence of toxin in feces, serum, or vomitus. Normal spinal fluid analysis will rule out more common neurologic processes such as stroke, Guillain-Barré syndrome, or polio.

15. How is botulism intoxication treated?

- Mechanical ventilation is required for respiratory function failure.
- Total neurodysfunction support for overall body functions is necessary.
- A trivalent antitoxin against types A, B, and E is commercially available and should be given in recommended dosage as soon as the diagnosis is confirmed. A multivalent antitoxin against all toxin types has recently been developed. Antitoxins are effective only against circulating toxins during the progressive stage of the disease process.
- Symptoms may last up to 3 months.

PLAGUE

16. **What is the causative agent of plague?**
    The etiologic agent is *Yersinia pestis* (Enterobacteriaceae). The disease vector is the Asiatic rat flea *(Xenopsylla cheopis)*.

    Centers for Disease Control and Prevention: Frequently asked questions about plague. 2005: www.bt.cdc. gov/agent/plague/faq.asp

17. **What are the common forms of the plague?**
    There are three forms of the disease:
    - **Bubonic:** Bubonic plague is the most common form, caused by trans-skin transmission. It appears with matted, painful, swollen lymph nodes.
    - **Pneumonic:** Pneumonic plague may occur as primary headache, weakness, and exhaustion; it results from lung infection or seeding from bubonic variety.
    - **Septicemic:** Septicemic plague may occur as a primary process or a complication of other varieties.

18. **What are the clinical presentations of bubonic and pneumonic plague?**
    See Table 38-3.

TABLE 38-3. CLINICAL PRESENTATIONS OF BUBONIC AND PNEUMONIC PLAGUE	
Bubonic	**Pneumonic**
Tender swollen lymph nodes	Rapid onset of dyspnea
Fever and chills	High fever
Headache, weakness, exhaustion	Headache, weakness, exhaustion
History of exposure	Chest pain with copious bloody sputum
Hemorrhagic pneumonia	Hemorrhagic pneumonia with respiratory failure
Septicemic shock	Septicemic shock
Death	Death

19. **What are the definitive diagnostic tests for plague?**
    - Bipolar rods (safety pin appearance) on light microscopy
    - Immunofluorescent antibody testing
    - Chemical assay: lactose-positive, urease-negative, and indole-negative results
    - Immunoglobulin M enzyme immunoassay

20. **What is the current treatment of choice for plague?**
    - Patients should be isolated when the disease is suspected.
    - All personnel should take respiratory precautions if pneumonic plague is suspected.
    - Effective antibiotic regimens include streptomycin, gentamicin, doxycycline, ciprofloxacin, and tetracycline.

21. **What is the prognosis after plague exposure?**
    - **Bubonic:** Mortality rate of 1–15% for treated cases, 40–60% for untreated cases
    - **Pneumonic:** Mortality rate of 100% if not vigorously treated within 24 hours
    - **Septic:** Mortality rate of 40% for treated cases, 100% for untreated cases
    Prophylactic antibiotic treatment for 1 week will protect against aerosolized exposure.
    A vaccine is available in limited supply, primarily for health care workers treating patients with the pneumonic form.

22. **Why is plague a potent biowarfare threat?**
    - Pneumonic plague is the primary biowarfare form.
    - The bacterium can be easily grown and made available to enemy forces.
    - Bacterial samples can be easily aerosolized and spread to large populations.
    - Easy patient-to-patient transmission creates a secondary epidemic mechanism. Resource use is overwhelming, with resultant high morbidity and mortality rates.

SALMONELLA

23. **What is the causative agent of *Salmonella* illness?**
    - *Salmonella* species are gram-negative, non–spore-forming, facultative anaerobes that produce endotoxins.
    - *Salmonella typhi* is the most virulent variant, causing typhoid fever.

24. **How are the *Salmonella* species biowarfare threats?**
    - Food and water sources can easily be contaminated by bacteria-infected material in localized or broad geographic areas.
    - Nontyphoid gastrointestinal infections are extremely labor and resource intensive, with large numbers of debilitated victims creating massive economic and service shutdowns.

25. **Can typhoid fever create a significant biothreat?**
    S. typhi is easily isolated and grown and can be used to cause bioepidemics. When recognized, the disease can be successfully treated with a low resulting mortality. Unrecognized and untreated cases can have a mortality rate up to 50%. Military personnel and at-risk populations can have prophylactic vaccinations.

    Olsen SJ, Bleasdale SC, Magnano AR, et al: Outbreaks of typhoid fever in the United States, 1960–1999. Epidemiol Infect 130:13–21, 2003.

26. **What is the clinical picture of typhoid fever?**
    The disease is contracted by the ingestion of infected material with an approximate 7- to 14-day incubation period. Rose spots develop on the chest area, associated with prolonged, high, and intermittent fevers and malaise. Within 2 weeks, green "pea soup" diarrhea develops with abdominal pain and distention; splenomegaly also develops. If untreated by the third week, toxemia, hemorrhage, perforation, and death occur.

27. **How is the diagnosis of typhoid fever made?**
    - Isolation and identification of the bacterium from the blood or marrow
    - Stool samples (may test positive in 50% of cases)

28. **What is the treatment of *Salmonella* infection and typhoid fever in particular?**
    - Early isolation and body fluid precautions are essential to control spread.
    - Antibiotics are effective, including fluoroquinolones, cephalosporins, and chloramphenicol.
    - Cardiorespiratory and metabolic support are necessary in advanced cases.

SMALLPOX

29. **What is the causative agent of smallpox?**
    The etiologic agent is the variola virus. Variola major produces the most severe form of the disease. Another variant, variola minor, causes a less severe syndrome. The disease is spread by saliva, body fluids, or pus from skin lesions. The most common form of transmission is via

droplets expelled through coughing. The virus remains viable in bedding and clothing. Humans are the only natural host.

World Health Organization: www.who.int/mediacertre/factsheets/smallpox/en/

30. **Describe the clinical presentation of smallpox.**
    See Table 38-4.

TABLE 38-4. CLINICAL PRESENTATION OF SMALLPOX

Prodromal Stage	Infectious (Eruptive) Stage
12- to 14-day incubation	Saliva contagious
High fever (101–104°F)	Intraoral and pharyngeal rash
Malaise with possible vomiting	Trunk and extremity rash (umbilicated bumps)
Headache and backache	Bumps break down into running pustules
	Pitted scars and scabs (contagious until scabs disappear in 3–4 weeks)

31. **What differentiates smallpox from chickenpox?**
    See Table 38-5.

TABLE 38-5. DIFFERENTIATION OF SMALLPOX AND CHICKENPOX

Smallpox	Chickenpox
Lesions feel deep	Lesions feel superficial
Painful lesions	Pruritic lesions
Centrifugal (face and extremities) lesions	Centripetal (primarily truncal) lesions
Involves palms and soles	Spares palms and soles
Vesicles develop uniformly	Vesicles develop in differing stages

32. **What are the major complications of smallpox?**
    - Sepsis is the primary cause of death, usually occurring during the second week of infection.
    - There is secondary bacterial infection of lesions, often involving *Staphylococcus aureus*.
    - Corneal ulcers requiring eventual transplant are present.
    - Rare cases of demyelinating encephalitis have been reported.

33. **How is the diagnosis of smallpox confirmed?**
    - Virus particle aggregates from lesions (Guarnieri bodies) are seen microscopically.
    - Cell culture growth is identified with positive polymerase chain reaction techniques.

34. **What is the treatment regimen for diagnosed or suspected smallpox?**
    Patients should be isolated immediately on suspicion of the disease. Treatment is supportive with ventilator assist, cardiac dynamics and blood pressure support, and volume and electrolyte replacement. There is no definitive chemotherapy or drug treatment. Antibiotics should be used against secondary infection with an organism such as *S. aureus*.

35. **What is the regimen for exposure or suspected exposure to smallpox?**
   - Vaccinate all exposed persons within 4 days of exposure. This will prevent development of the disease or lessen the severity two- to threefold and reduce mortality by 50%.
   - If available (only a limited supply may exist), give vaccinia immune globulin. This confers a passive immunity for 2 weeks, reducing incidence and mortality.

36. **Why does smallpox pose a major biowarfare threat?**
   - The disease is highly contagious with a high morbidity and mortality index with no specific treatment.
   - Large numbers of the current population have never been vaccinated. The vaccination fully protects for only 3–5 years and significantly immunodegrades over the next 10–20 years, rendering susceptible much of the population who were vaccinated more than 30 years ago.
   - Currently, there may not be enough vaccine available to provide mass vaccinations.

   Henderson DA, Inglesby TV, Bartlett JG, et al: Smallpox as a biological weapon: Medical and public health management. JAMA 281:2127–2137, 1999.

OTHER AGENTS

37. **What other viral and rickettsial diseases pose potential biothreats due to their degree of contagion and ability to disseminate?**

   Viral
   - Eastern equine encephalitis
   - Rift Valley fever
   - Venezuelan equine encephalitis
   - Viral hemorrhagic fevers
     (e.g., Marburg, Ebola, Lassa)
   - Western equine encephalitis

   Rickettsial
   - Q fever
   - Typhus

38. **Are there any new biothreats on the horizon?**
   Several potential biothreats are possible due to the ability to manipulate existing pathogens with biotechnology. Examples of this are VEEPOX and EBOLAPOX.

   Preston R: The bioweaponeers. Annals of Warfare, 1998: www.hackvan.com/pub/stig/articles/bioweapons.htm

39. **What is VEEPOX? What are its characteristics?**
   VEEPOX is a chimera of smallpox and Venezuelan equine encephalitis. This combination results in the following characteristics:
   - Highly disabling to populations
   - Headache, disorientation, severe malaise, near coma status
   - Disabling but not generally lethal

40. **What is EBOLAPOX? What are its characteristics?**
   EBOLAPOX is a chimera of the Ebola virus and the smallpox virus. This is a particularly nasty combination with the following characteristics:
   - It can be replicated in test tubes or animals.
   - It can produce a disease called *blackpox,* a form of hemorrhagic smallpox.
   - It combines the high mortality of Ebola virus with the high contagiousness of smallpox.

CHAPTER 39

SKIN AND SOFT TISSUE INFECTIONS

Richard Jacobs, MD, PhD, and Matthew J. Haight, DO

WOUND INFECTIONS

1. **What are the classic signs and symptoms of a wound infection?**
   Local signs include warmth, erythema, pain, swelling (calor, rubor, dolor, and tumor), and drainage that may be serosanguinous or purulent. Systemic signs are less common (15% of cases) but may include elevation in temperature and rigors.

2. **What are the risk factors for developing a postoperative wound infection?**
   At risk are elderly, debilitated, malnourished, and obese patients. Contributing factors include infection at a distant site, corticosteroid therapy, ascites, diabetes, and prior radiation therapy. Of ultimate importance, however, is the technical adequacy of the closure. Appropriate placement and tension of sutures are critical. It is unlikely, however, that interrupted versus running sutures or choice of incision (vertical versus transverse) contributes significantly to the incidence of dehiscence.

3. **What are the most common organisms implicated in postoperative wound infections?**
   The bacterial etiology depends, in part, on when the infection occurs. The majority of wound infections occur 1 to 2 weeks postoperatively and are most commonly due to *Staphylococcus aureus*, *Staphylococcus epidermidis* (especially in the presence of prosthetic material), enterococci, *Escherichia coli*, and *Pseudomonas aeruginosa*, although many other bacteria can potentially be pathogens. Infections that occur within a day or two of surgery are usually due to group A beta-hemolytic streptococcus or *Clostridium* species.

4. **When are prophylactic antibiotics indicated?**
   In cases where a clean incision is made and a contaminated area is exposed (i.e., clean contaminated cases), prophylactic antibiotics have been shown to decrease the incidence of postoperative wound infection. By definition, antibiotic administration in contaminated and dirty-infected wounds is therapeutic, not prophylactic. The routine administration of antibiotics for prophylaxis in clean cases continues to be controversial; however, a large, prospective randomized trial has demonstrated a 48% decrease in wound infection in breast biopsy and herniorrhaphy with antibiotic prophylaxis. Current consensus opinion recommends prophylaxis in high-risk clean operations in which foreign bodies are implanted (e.g., vascular graft, cardiac valve, and total joint replacement).

   Horan TC, Gaynes RP, Martone W, et al: CDC definitions of nosocomial surgical site infections, 1992: A modification of CDC definitions of surgical wound infections. Infect Control Hosp Epidemiol 13:606–608, 1992.

5. **Besides antibiotics, what other therapeutic interventions may limit the chance of a postoperative wound infection?**
   - Keep the patient's core temperature greater than 36°C during surgery. Maintenance of normothermia during colonic surgery has been shown to decrease wound infection rates threefold (6% versus 19%) in a recent randomized, prospective trial.

- Provide supplemental oxygen perioperatively. In a recent, prospective, randomized study of patients undergoing colorectal procedures, the perioperative administration of 80% oxygen decreased surgical wound infections by 50% (5.2% versus 11.2%).

Greif R, Akca O, Horn EP, et al: Supplemental perioperative oxygen to reduce the incidence of surgical-wound infection. The Outcomes Research Group. N Engl J Med 342:161–167, 2000.
Kurz A, Sessler DI, Lenhardt R: Perioperative normothermia to reduce the incidence of surgical-wound infection and shorten hospitalization. Study of Wound Infection and Temperature Group. N Engl J Med 334:1209–1216, 1996.

CELLULITIS

6. **Describe the bacteriology and treatment of cellulitis.**
Cellulitis presents with erythema (Fig. 39-1), warmth, and tenderness regardless of the bacterial etiology. The most important clinical determinant of bacteriology is the clinical setting in which the cellulitis occurs. See Table 39-1 for empiric and alternative therapies.

7. **What is the role of blood cultures in the diagnosis of cellulitis?**
The yield of blood cultures is very low, has a marginal impact on clinical management, and does not appear to be cost-effective for immunocompetent patients with community-acquired cellulitis and no signs of sepsis.

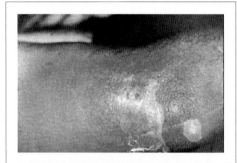

Figure 39-1. Hospital-associated cellulitis of the elbow demonstrating erythema and swelling.

Perl B, Gotteher NP, Raveh D, et al: Cost-effectiveness of blood cultures for adult patients with cellulitis. Clin Infect Dis 29:1483–1488, 1999.

8. **When should invasive procedures be considered in the diagnosis of cellulitis?**
If the patient does not respond to what appears to be appropriate antimicrobial therapy (clinical response is usually seen in 3 days), if the patient is immunocompromised (unusual organisms such as yeast, fungi, or *Mycobacterium* species can be pathogens in this setting), if there is crepitance or necrosis of the skin, or if a deep tissue infection is suspected, a biopsy or surgical exploration should be performed. Patients who are diabetic or immunocompromised can benefit from a leading-edge biopsy (70–100% isolation of an organism). Obtaining a needle aspirate or biopsy specimen from the leading edge of cellulitis is not recommended in immunocompetent patients because either technique isolates an organism <20% of the time and can potentially cause a superinfection.

Sachs M: The optimum use of needle aspiration in the bacteriologic diagnosis of cellulitis in adults. Arch Intern Med 150:1907–1912, 1990.

9. **What is appropriate therapy for diabetic and vascular insufficiency ulcers?**
Superficial ulcers with 3–4 cm of surrounding erythema without systemic toxicity is usually caused by group A streptococci or *S. aureus,* and therapy with an oral first-generation cephalosporin, clindamycin, or amoxicillin-clavulanic acid for 10–14 days is appropriate. For severe infections involving deeper tissues associated with systemic toxicity, IV broad-spectrum antibiotics and early surgical therapy are indicated (*see* Table 39-1).

TABLE 39-1. BACTERIOLOGY AND TREATMENT OF CELLULITIS

Clinical Setting	Microbiology	Empiric Therapy*	Alternative Therapy†
Outpatient cellulitis	Group A streptococci, *Staphylococcus aureus* (uncommon, but can occur secondarily and is difficult to exclude)	Vancomycin 10–15 mg/kg IV q12h	Daptomycin 4 mg/kg/day
Hospital-associated cellulitis (>72 hrs)	Group A streptococci, *S. aureus,* enterobacteriaceae	Vancomycin 10–15 mg/kg IV q12h with or without piperacillin/tazobactam 3.375 gm IV q6h *or* Vancomycin 10–15 mg/kg IV q12h with or without ceftriaxone 2 gm IV q24h	Vancomycin 10–15 mg/kg IV q12h with or without aztreonam 2 gm IV q8h
Decubitus/ venous stasis/arterial insufficiency/ diabetic ulcers	Polymicrobic, *Streptococcus pyogenes* (group A, C, G) enterococci, anaerobic streptococci, Enterobacteriaceae, *Pseudomonas* sp., *Bacteroides* sp., *S. aureus*	Vancomycin 10–15 mg/kg IV q12h *and* piperacillin/tazobactam 3.375 gm IV q6h *or* Vancomycin 10–15 mg/kg IV q12h *and* meropenem 1 gm IV q8h	Vancomycin 10–15 mg/kg IV q12h *and* metronidazole 500 mg IV q8h *and* aztreonam 2 gm IV q8h
Dog and cat bites	Viridans streptococci, *Streptococcus* sp., *Pasteurella multocida, S. aureus, Bacteroides* sp., *Fusobacterium* sp. (anaerobes)	Piperacillin/tazobactam 3.375 gm IV q6h	Clindamycin 600–900 mg IV q8h *and* ciprofloxacin 500 mg PO/IV q12h *or* clindamycin 600–900 mg IV q8h *and* levofloxacin 500 mg PO/IV q24h
Human bites	Viridans streptococci, *Eikenella* sp., streptococci, *S. aureus, S. epidermidis, Bacteroides* sp., peptostreptococci, *Corynebacterium* sp.	Piperacillin/tazobactam 3.375 gm IV q6h	Clindamycin 600–900 mg IV q8h *and* ciprofloxacin 500 mg IV q12h *or* clindamycin 600–900 mg IV q8h *and* levofloxacin 500 mg IV q24h
Deep tissue infection	Streptococci (group A, C, G), *Clostridium* sp., polymicrobic, aerobic, and anaerobic	Surgical débridement, vancomycin 10–15 mg/kg IV q12h *and* meropenem 1 gm IV q8h (if group A streptococci isolated, include clindamycin and consider IV immunoglobulin—see text)	Vancomycin 10–15 mg/kg IV q8h *and* clindamycin 600–900 mg IV q8h *and* aztreonam 2 gm IV q8h

IV = intravenous, PO = by mouth.
*Based on 70-kg person with normal renal function.
†Persons with immunoglobulin E-mediated reaction to penicillin.

10. **How does one diagnose osteomyelitis in the patient with a diabetic or vascular insufficiency ulcer?**
The simplest method is to probe the ulcer. If bone is felt, the presence of osteomyelitis is confirmed (89% positive predictive value). An alternative diagnostic modality is magnetic resonance imaging, which offers a 90% sensitivity and specificity. The gold standard is bone biopsy, which not only confirms the diagnosis but defines the bacteriology and allows rational therapy.

Lipsky BA, Berendt AR, Deery HG, et al: Diagnosis and treatment of diabetic foot infections. Clin Infect Dis 39:885–910, 2004.

11. **What other diseases must be considered when diagnosing cellulitis?**
See Table 39-2.

TABLE 39-2. IMPORTANT PROCESSES TO BE DISTINGUISHED FROM CELLULITIS	
Process	Clinical Clues
Infectious	
Necrotizing fasciitis	
Type I (mixture of anaerobes and facultative species such as streptococci or Enterobacteriaceae)	Acute, rapidly developing infection of deep fascia; marked pain, tenderness, swelling, and often crepitus; bullae and necrosis of underlying skin
Type II (infection with group A streptococci)	Acute infection, often accompanied by toxic shock syndrome; rapid progression of marked edema to violaceous bullae and necrosis of subcutaneous tissue; absence of crepitus
Anaerobic myonecrosis (gas gangrene due to *Clostridium perfringens*)	Rapidly progressive toxemic infection of previously injured muscle, producing marked edema, crepitus, and brown bullae (showing large gram-positive bacilli with scant polymorphonuclear cells); on radiographs, extensive gaseous dissection of muscle and fascial planes; bacteremic spread of *Clostridium septicum* from occult colon cancer can produce myonecrosis without penetrating trauma
Cutaneous anthrax	Gelatinous edema surrounding eschar of anthrax lesion may be mistaken for cellulites; anthrax lesion is painless or pruritic; epidemiologic factors are of paramount importance
Vaccinia vaccination	Erythema and induration around vaccination site reaches peak at 10–12 days (more slowly than cellulites); little toxicity
Inflammatory and neoplastic	
Insect bite (hypersensitivity response)	History of insect bite, local pruritus; absence of fever, toxicity, or leukocytosis

Continued

TABLE 39-2. IMPORTANT PROCESSES TO BE DISTINGUISHED FROM CELLULITIS—CONT'D	
Process	Clinical Clues
Inflammatory and neoplastic—cont'd	
Acute gout	Involvement of foot (podagra); joint pain, repeated attacks; increase in serum uric acid level
Deep venous thrombosis	Involvement of leg; sentinel venous cord and linear extent
Familial Mediterranean fever—associated cellulitis-like erythema	Occurs in persons of Sephardic Jewish descent and persons from the Middle East who have had previous episodes of recurrent fevers with or without episodes of acute abdominal pain
Fixed drug reaction	Skin erythema does not spread as rapidly as in cellulitis; if fever is present, temperature is not far above normal; history indicates medication use
Pyoderma gangrenosa (particularly lesions starting in subcutaneous fat as acute panniculitis)	Lesions become nodular or bullous and ulcerate; occurs particularly in patients with inflammatory bowel disease or collagen vascular disease
Sweet's syndrome (i.e., acute febrile neutropenic dermatosis)	Acute, tender erythematous pseudovesiculated plaques, fever, and neutrophilic leukocytosis; often associated with cancer (commonly hematologic); on face, may resemble erysipelas or periorbital cellulites; responds to corticosteroids
Kawasaki disease	Fever, conjunctivitis, acute cervical lymphadenopathy, oropharyngeal erythema; dermatitis of palms and soles; facial appearance may suggest periorbital cellulites; mainly in infancy and childhood
Wells' syndrome	Urticaria-like lesions with central clearing; lesions progress slowly and persist for weeks or months; histologically, infiltration with eosinophils; peripheral eosinophilia
Carcinoma erysipeloides	Form of metastatic carcinoma with lymphatic involvement; most often occurs on anterior chest wall with cancer of the breast but also may occur at sites of distant metastases; no fever; slower progression than cellulitis

Adapted from Swartz M: Clinical practice. Cellulitis. N Engl J Med 350:904–912, 2004.

DEEP TISSUE INFECTIONS

12. **What is necrotizing fasciitis?**
This worrisome diagnosis is characterized by widespread fascial necrosis and relative sparing of the skin and underlying muscle. It is fatal if left untreated and requires a high index of suspicion for diagnosis. Commonly, it presents as a slowly advancing cellulitis that progresses to a firm or "woody" induration of the subcutaneous tissues. A thin, brown exudate may be expressed from

the wound. A lack of response to nonoperative therapy, excruciating pain in the absence of clinical findings, or signs of systemic toxicity may be the only indication of underlying necrosis.

Necrotizing fasciitis may develop after relatively minor abrasions, insect bites, lacerations, or superficial wound infections in trauma or abdominal surgery. It is also seen in IV drug users. Ninety percent of cases are polymicrobial. Treatment relies primarily on early surgical débridement with time of onset to surgery correlating with a survival benefit. This is to be augmented by broad-spectrum antibiotics and supportive care. Antibiotics initially should be chosen to ensure coverage of aerobic gram-positive and gram-negative organisms and anaerobes, and then tailored to the specific organisms that are cultured. In a recent series, the mortality rate of necrotizing fasciitis approached 30% (*see* Table 39-1).

13. **When should necrotizing fasciitis be suspected?**
   In patients who present with cellulitis, deep tissue infection should be suspected if there is necrosis of the skin, drainage, or crepitance. Early in the pathophysiology of necrotizing fasciitis there may be necrosis of dermal nerves. Thus, the presence of anesthesia instead of hyperesthesia can be an early clue to diagnosis.

   Headley A: Necrotizing soft tissue infections: A primary care review. Am Fam Physician 68:323–328, 2003.

KEY POINTS: SKIN AND SOFT TISSUE INFECTIONS

1. Elderly, obese, and malnourished patients are at risk for postoperative wound infections.

2. Most postoperative wound infections occur 1–2 weeks after the operation.

3. Prophylactic antibiotics decrease wound infections when given for "clean" cases.

4. Necrotizing fasciitis can appear as slowly spreading cellulitis, with woody induration and severe pain.

5. Treatment for necrotizing fasciitis is rapid surgical débridement.

14. **What is the role of clindamycin and IV immunoglobulin (IVIG) in the therapy of these infections?**
   Clindamycin should be included in the empiric antibiotic regimen portion of the treatment of necrotizing fascistic due to group A streptococci and in the therapy of the streptococcal toxic shock syndrome. These infections are associated with a large number of bacteria that are in the stationary phase of growth and do not express penicillin-binding protein on their cell surface. Thus, penicillin and other beta lactams may be ineffective. The role of IVIG is unclear; small, uncontrolled studies indicate that it may be efficacious. If the patient's infection progresses despite antibiotics and surgery, IVIG is reasonable and should be given in large doses (*see* Table 39-1).

   Darenberg J, Ihendyane N, Sjolin J, et al: Intravenous immunoglobulin G therapy in streptococcal toxic shock syndrome: A European randomized, double-blind, placebo-controlled trial. Clin Infect Dis 37:333–340, 2003.

15. **What is Fournier's gangrene?**
   Necrotizing fasciitis of the perineum. Like other forms of necrotizing fasciitis, if left untreated it progresses to systemic sepsis, multiple organ failure, and death. Treatment consists of early diagnosis, early and repeated radical débridement, diversion of the fecal stream (i.e., colostomy), and broad-spectrum antibiotics.

16. **What are anaerobic cellulitis, synergistic necrotizing cellulitis, progressive bacterial synergistic gangrene, and clostridial myonecrosis?**

These are all deep tissue infections that have subtle differences in acuity, tissue involvement, type of discharge, and bacteriology. Clinically, if deep tissue infection is suspected, a course of broad-spectrum antibiotics should be started and débridement performed. Bacteriology is defined at the time of surgery and dictates future antibiotic therapy.

HYPERTENSION

Alan C. Pao, MD, and Stuart L. Linas, MD

CHAPTER 40

1. **What are the hemodynamic determinants of blood pressure (BP)?**
   Arterial BP is the product of cardiac output (CO) and systemic vascular resistance (SVR), or BP = CO × SVR (analogous to Ohm's law). Malignant hypertension is caused by increased SVR.

2. **What is the clinical spectrum of severe hypertension?**
   Severe hypertension can be classified in many ways, but there are three major categories:
   - **Hypertensive crisis (or hypertensive emergency):** This turning point in the course of hypertension occurs when the immediate management of elevated BP plays a decisive role in limiting or preventing target organ damage. The most common etiologies are accelerated and malignant hypertension. *Accelerated hypertension* is defined as severe hypertension (diastolic BP usually > 120 mmHg) in the setting of retinal hemorrhages and exudates (cotton wool spots). *Malignant hypertension* is accelerated hypertension with papilledema.
   - **Hypertension with end-organ dysfunction:** This form of severe hypertension involves evidence of end-organ damage, which can include cerebrovascular accident (CVA), myocardial infarction, congestive heart failure (CHF), and renal failure. BP reduction may be associated with relief of clinical signs and symptoms.
   - **Urgent hypertension (or hypertensive urgency):** Elevated BP in the absence of end-organ dysfunction define urgent hypertension. Because it is only an abnormal "number," urgent hypertension is not associated with the dire consequences of the other types of severe hypertension.

3. **What are the target organs affected by hypertensive crises?**
   Hypertensive crises can damage four main target organ systems:
   - **Eye/retina:** Retinal hemorrhages/exudates or papilledema
   - **Brain:** Hypertensive encephalopathy, atherothrombotic brain infarction, or intracerebral hemorrhage
   - **Heart:** Acute myocardial infarction, CHF, or aortic dissection
   - **Kidney:** Acute renal failure

   Kaplan NM: Hypertensive crises. In Kaplan NM (ed): Clinical Hypertension, 7th ed. Philadelphia, Lippincott Williams & Wilkins, 1998, pp 265–280.

4. **What are the potential complications of untreated malignant hypertension?**
   Studies from the 1950s and 1960s revealed that the mortality from untreated malignant hypertension was 80–90%. Most of the deaths were due to acute renal failure. With the initiation of prompt antihypertensive therapy and the availability of acute renal replacement therapy, the primary cause of morbidity and mortality has become cardiovascular disease (e.g., CVA, myocardial infarction, and CHF).

5. **What is the acute treatment of malignant hypertension?**
   The acute treatment of choice is IV sodium nitroprusside. The initial dose is 0.5 μg/kg/min, and this should be increased by 0.5 μg/kg/min every 2–3 minutes until a diastolic BP < 110 mmHg has been attained. Further acute decreases in BP may result in vital organ hypoperfusion

because blood flow autoregulation may have been altered to accommodate for chronically elevated BP. Acceptable alternative parenteral drugs for the acute treatment of malignant hypertension include labetalol, nicardipine, enalaprilat, or fenoldopam. BP should be monitored continuously during therapy with an indwelling arterial catheter.

Hirschl MM, Binder M, Bur A, et al: Clinical evaluation of different doses of intravenous enalaprilat in patients with hypertensive crises. Arch Intern Med 155:2217–2223, 1995.

Murphy MB, Murray C: Fenoldopam: A selective peripheral dopamine-receptor agonist for the treatment of severe hypertension. N Engl J Med 345:1548–1557, 2001.

Neutel JM, Smith DHG, Wallin D, et al: A comparison of intravenous nicardipine and sodium nitroprusside in the immediate treatment of severe hypertension. Am J Hypertens 7:623–628, 1994.

6. **Outline the typical chronic antihypertensive regimen following successful treatment of malignant hypertension.**
    Because malignant hypertension is mediated by increased SVR, it is recommended that chronic therapy include a vasodilator such as hydralazine or minoxidil. Vasodilators cause reflex tachycardia and sodium retention; therefore, it is usually also necessary to include a beta blocker and a diuretic agent. In some cases, chronic BP reduction may be achieved with less potent vasodilators, such as angiotensin-converting enzyme (ACE) inhibitors or calcium channel blockers.

7. **What is the appropriate acute treatment for hypertension in a patient with pheochromocytoma?**
    Hypertension from pheochromocytomas is caused by vascular smooth muscle alpha$_1$-receptor activation, which results in vasoconstriction. Thus, the best acute treatment is IV administration of the alpha$_1$ blocker phentolamine. Sodium nitroprusside is also a reasonable choice. Beta blockers should initially be avoided because they cause both unopposed peripheral alpha$_1$-receptor stimulation and decreased CO.

    Kaplan NM: Phecochromocytoma. In Kaplan NM (ed): Clinical Hypertension, 7th ed. Philadelphia, Lippincott Williams & Wilkins, 1998, pp 345–363.

8. **How is hypertension treated acutely in patients with aortic dissection?**
    The initial therapeutic aim is to decrease both BP and cardiac contractile force (dp/dt). This goal has traditionally been best achieved with sodium nitroprusside and esmolol. Labetalol alone is also effective in this setting.

    Vaughan CJ, Delanty N: Hypertensive emergencies. Lancet 356:411–417, 2000.

9. **Describe the acute treatment of cocaine-induced hypertensive crisis.**
    Cocaine causes hypertension by inhibiting catecholamine reuptake at nerve terminals. Therefore, drugs that can block alpha$_1$-receptors such as labetalol or phentolamine are effective. Selective beta blockers without alpha$_1$ blockade such as propranolol are not recommended because of the risk of unopposed alpha$_1$ action. If hypertension is severe, sodium nitroprusside is the drug of choice. In the setting of cocaine-related myocardial ischemia, nitroglycerin and benzodiazepines are effective against both cocaine-induced hypertension and vasoconstriction of the coronary arteries.

    Lange RA, Hillis LD: Cardiovascular complications of cocaine use. N Engl J Med 345:351–358, 2001.

10. **How should hypertension be treated acutely in patients with CVA?**
    Patients with acute CVA often have high BP for reasons not completely understood. BP <160/100 mmHg should not be treated because further BP reduction can result in hypoperfusion of vital organs, including the brain, that have adapted to a chronically elevated BP. BP >180/110 mmHg should be treated judiciously with parenteral agents such as sodium

nitroprusside. Rapid lowering should be avoided; the aim of therapy is to reduce mean arterial pressure by 25% or to lower diastolic BP to 100 mmHg—whichever is higher—during the first hour. If the patient's neurologic status deteriorates, the rate of BP reduction should be slowed. Oral therapy should be instituted before parenteral treatment is discontinued. Clonidine or alpha-methyldopa should be avoided because of the risk of impaired cerebral function.

Bath P, Chalmers J, Powers W, et al: International Society of Hypertension (ISH): Statement on the management of blood pressure in acute stroke. J Hypertens 21:665–672, 2003.

11. **Describe the acute treatment of hypertension in patients with ischemic heart disease and ongoing angina.**
Hypertension can precipitate ischemic chest pain in patients with severe coronary artery disease. Alternatively, hypertension can result from chest pain, which results in marked increases in catecholamines and secondary reactive hypertension. In either setting, hypertension is associated with an increase in SVR and increases in myocardial oxygen demand. Nitroglycerin and beta blockers are the initial agents of choice. Because nitroprusside increases heart rate and myocardial oxygen demand in this setting, it is considered a secondary agent.

Kitiyakara C, Guzman NJ: Malignant hypertension and hypertensive emergencies. J Am Soc Nephrol 9:133–142, 1998.
Vaughan CJ, Delanty N: Hypertensive emergencies. Lancet 356:411–417, 2000.

12. **How should hypertension associated with preeclampsia be treated?**
Preeclampsia is the combination of hypertension, proteinuria, and edema in pregnancy. It occurs after the 20th week of gestation. The traditional treatments of choice are hydralazine or alpha-methyldopa. If these drugs are ineffective or poorly tolerated, labetalol is a reasonably safe and effective alternative. Medications to be avoided because of potential teratogenesis include sodium nitroprusside, trimethaphan, diazoxide, ACE inhibitors, beta blockers, and calcium channel blockers. Unfortunately, the safety profile of many antihypertensive drugs during pregnancy is unknown. Because preeclampsia and eclampsia may be life threatening, it may be necessary to prescribe potent antihypertensive agents (sodium nitroprusside or minoxidil) with unclear fetal toxicity potential.

Duley L, Henderson-Smart DJ: Drugs for treatment of very high blood pressure during pregnancy. Cochrane Database Syst Rev 4:CD001449, 2002.

KEY POINTS: HYPERTENSION

1. Hypertensive crisis (or hypertensive emergency) is the turning point in the course of hypertension when the immediate management of elevated blood pressure plays a decisive role in limiting or preventing target organ damage.

2. Hypertensive crises can damage four main target organ systems: eye, brain, heart, and kidneys.

3. The acute treatment of choice for malignant hypertension is IV sodium nitroprusside.

4. Chronic therapy for malignant hypertension should include a vasodilator such as hydralazine or minoxidil, a beta blocker, and a diuretic agent.

5. Nitroglycerin and beta blockers are the initial agents of choice for patients with ischemic heart disease and angina.

13. **What is the role of sublingual nifedipine in the treatment of hypertensive crises?**
There is no role! The absorption of nifedipine from the buccal mucosa is poor and results in inconsistent systemic delivery. Serious and even fatal adverse effects have been reported when nifedipine has been administered acutely for the treatment of hypertensive crises. Nifedipine is contraindicated in these situations because of the unpredictability of the fall in arterial BP.

Grossman E, Messerli FH, Grodzicki T, et al: Should a moratorium be placed on sublingual nifedipine capsules given for hypertensive emergencies and pseudoemergencies? JAMA 276:1328–1331, 1996.

14. **In severe hypertension, why does lowering of BP potentially result in a decline in glomerular filtration rate (GFR)?**
Normally, GFR is maintained despite decreases in BP by compensatory increases in efferent arteriolar tone (Fig. 40-1). There are two major causes of loss of GFR after reduction of BP in the setting of severe hypertension:
- **Renal artery stenosis:** In a patient with a fixed atherosclerotic lesion of the main renal artery, a drop in BP can cause a fall in GFR because the fixed lesion limits afferent arteriolar flow to such an extent that even maximal elevation in efferent arteriolar tone cannot compensate and maintain GFR.

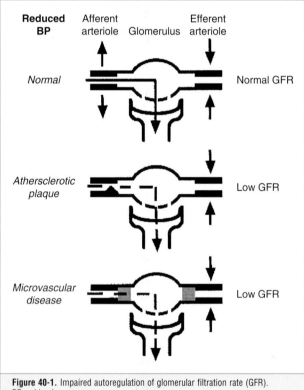

Figure 40-1. Impaired autoregulation of glomerular filtration rate (GFR). BP = blood pressure.

- **Long-standing essential hypertension:** In this setting, no macrovascular abnormalities are present; the problem is marked sclerosis of the microvasculature of the kidney, including the afferent artery. Because of afferent arteriolar sclerosis, the afferent artery is unable to vasodilate in response to a drop in BP. Hence, GFR falls when BP is lowered even with increases in efferent arteriolar tone that normally would offset, at least partially, decreases in BP.

15. **When should an evaluation for secondary hypertension be considered?**
    - At initial presentation of malignant hypertension (especially if the patient is Caucasian, younger than 30 years, or older than 50 years of age)
    - When rapid onset of severe hypertension occurs within less than 5 years
    - When an increase in serum creatinine level occurs after the initiation of ACE inhibitor treatment
    - In compliant patients whose BP is difficult to control after an adequate trial with a combination of diuretic, beta blocker, and potent vasodilator

    Pohl MA: Renal artery stenosis, renal vascular hypertension, and ischemic nephropathy. In: Schrier RW (ed): Diseases of the Kidney, 7th ed. Philadelphia, Lippincott Williams & Wilkins, 2001, pp 1399–1457.

16. **What are the important causes of secondary hypertension?**
    Secondary hypertension accounts for 5% of cases of hypertension.
    - **Renal:** Renovascular disease, renal parenchymal disease, polycystic kidney disease, Liddle syndrome, syndrome of apparent mineralocorticoid excess, hypercalcemia
    - **Endocrine:** Hyperthyroidism or hypothyroidism, primary hyperaldosteronism, Cushing's syndrome, pheochromocytoma, congenital adrenal hyperplasia
    - **Drugs:** Prescription (e.g., estrogen, cyclosporine, steroids), over-the-counter (e.g., pseudoephedrine, nonsteroidal anti-inflammatory drugs), illicit (e.g., tobacco smoking, ethanol, cocaine)
    - **Neurogenic:** Increased intracranial pressure, spinal cord section
    - **Miscellaneous:** Aortic coarctation, obstructive sleep apnea, polycythemia vera

CHAPTER 41

ACUTE RENAL FAILURE

Dinkar Kaw, MD, and Joseph I. Shapiro, MD

1. **How is acute renal failure (ARF) diagnosed?**
   ARF is a rapid loss of glomerular filtration rate (GFR) over a period of hours to a few days. This is usually determined by a sudden rise in plasma creatinine and blood urea nitrogen (BUN) levels. Until the patient achieves a steady state, the level of renal function cannot be assessed by the serum creatinine concentration. If a patient with previously normal renal function suddenly loses all renal function, serum creatinine will rise by only 1–2 mg/dL/day. However, patients with muscle wasting who make less creatinine may show smaller increases even with complete cessation of GFR. BUN is another indicator of decreasing glomerular filtration. Although a dramatic rise in BUN compared with creatinine may suggest a prerenal or obstructive (postrenal) etiology, one must also consider the possibility that creatinine production by the patient is limited. Measurement of timed creatinine and urea excretion rates allowing for calculation of creatinine and urea clearance are sometimes indicated to clarify this point. Serum cystatin C can detect minor reduction in GFR and therefore can be used to diagnose ARF in its early stages. It has been seen to detect ARF 1 or 2 days earlier than serum creatinine.

   Esson ML, Schrier RW: Diagnosis and treatment of acute tubular necrosis. Ann Intern Med 137:744–752, 2002.

   Herget-Rosenthal S, Marggraf G, Husing J, et al: Early detection of acute renal failure by serum cystatin C. Kidney Int 66:1115–1122, 2004.

2. **What features distinguish ARF from chronic renal failure?**
   When a patient presents some time after the onset of ARF, this distinction may not be easy. Chronic renal failure is more likely than ARF to be associated with anemia, hypocalcemia, normal urine output, and small shrunken kidneys on ultrasound examination. A kidney biopsy may be warranted if the kidneys are of normal size. It has been reported that chronic, but not acute, renal failure may be associated with an increase in the serum osmolal gap (i.e., the difference between measured and calculated serum osmolality).

   Toto RD: Approach to the patient with kidney disease. In Brenner BM (ed): Brenner & Rector's The Kidney, 7th ed. Philadelphia, Saunders, 2004, pp 1079–1106.

3. **How is ARF classified?**
   The main categories are prerenal, intrarenal or parenchymal, and postrenal or obstructive (Table 41-1).

TABLE 41-1. DIFFERENTIAL DIAGNOSIS OF ACUTE RENAL FAILURE		
Prerenal	Postrenal	Parenchymal
Dehydration	Ureter	Glomerular
Impaired cardiac function	Bladder	Interstitial
Vasodilation	Urethra	Allergic interstitial nephritis
Renal vascular obstruction		Vascular
Hepatorenal syndrome		Acute tubular necrosis

4. **How does examination of the urine help in the differential diagnosis of ARF?**
Laboratory evaluation begins with careful examination of the urine. A concentrated urine points more to prerenal causes, whereas isotonic urine suggests parenchymal or obstructive causes. Typically, the urine sediment of patients with prerenal azotemia demonstrates occasional hyaline casts or finely granular casts. In contrast, the presence of renal tubular epithelial cells and "muddy" granular casts strongly suggests acute tubular necrosis (ATN), microhematuria and red blood cell casts suggest glomerulonephritis, and white cell casts containing eosinophils suggest acute interstitial nephritis. As previously discussed, benign urine sediment is quite compatible with urinary obstruction.

5. **What are the implications of urinary electrolytes in the differential diagnosis of ARF?**
The determination of urine electrolyte and creatinine concentrations may be helpful in the differential diagnosis of ARF. When used with serum values, urinary diagnostic indices can be generated. Understanding the concepts behind the interpretation of these indices is easier and better than trying to remember specific numbers. Quite simply, if the tubule is working well in the setting of decreased GFR, tubular reabsorption of sodium and water is avid, and the relative clearance of sodium to creatinine is low. Conversely, if the tubule is injured and cannot reabsorb sodium well, the relative clearance of sodium to creatinine is not low. Therefore, with prerenal azotemia, the ratio of the clearance of sodium to the clearance of creatinine, which is also called the *fractional excretion of sodium* (FENa) (FENa = [urinary sodium]/[urinary creatinine] × [plasma creatinine]/[plasma sodium] × 100), is typically less than 1.0, whereas with parenchymal or obstructive causes of ARF, the FENa is generally greater than 2.0 (Fig. 41-1).

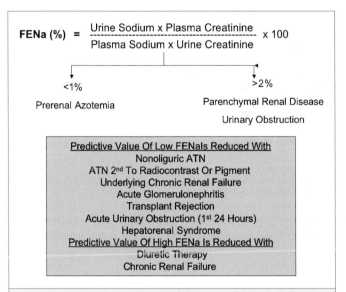

Figure 41-1. Fractional excretion of sodium (FENa), which measures the percent of filtered sodium that is excreted in the urine, helps to differentiate between prerenal causes of renal failure and both parenchymal renal diseases (e.g., acute tubular necrosis [ATN], allergic interstitial nephritis) and urinary obstruction. Under specific conditions, the predictive value of a low FENa (to diagnose prerenal azotemia) or a high FENa (to exclude prerenal azotemia) is limited.

The FENa test is much less useful when patients are nonoliguric. In this setting, the specificity of a low FENa for prerenal azotemia is markedly diminished. In addition to nonoliguria, several causes of ATN, specifically dye-induced ATN or ATN associated with hemolysis or rhabdomyolysis, may typically be associated with a low FENa. Patients who have prerenal azotemia but have either persistent diuretic effect, chronic tubulointerstitial injury, or bicarbonaturia may have a relatively high FENa. In the last case, the fractional excretion of chloride, which is calculated in an analogous way, will be appropriately low (<1%). Finally, the early stages of ARF from glomerulonephritis, transplant allograft rejection, or urinary obstruction may be associated with a low FENa.

Esson ML, Schrier RW: Diagnosis and treatment of acute tubular necrosis. Ann Intern Med 137:744–752, 2002.

Miller TR, Anderson RJ, Linas SL, et al: Urinary diagnostic indices in acute renal failure: A prospective study. Ann Intern Med 89:47–50, 1978.

6. **What is the pathophysiology of ATN?**
Renal ischemia, toxic injury to the kidney, or a combination of these insults can cause prolonged loss of renal function. Physiologically, decreased GFR must result from an alteration in glomerular hemodynamic factors, such as a decrease in the effective surface area or permeability of the glomerulus (Kf), a decrease in glomerular blood flow, or an abnormality in tubular integrity, including obstruction of tubular flow by cellular debris or back leak of ultrafiltrate through a porous tubule. In fact, each of these pathogenetic features can be shown to be operant in some experimental models of ARF.

Lameire N: The pathophysiology of acute renal failure. Crit Care Clin 21:197–210, 2005.

7. **How does ATN evolve?**
The major mechanism by which renal failure is induced may be different from the primary mechanism by which it is maintained. For example, in ischemic ARF, decreases in renal and glomerular blood flow may cause the initial loss of renal function. However, tubular necrosis, with its attendant obstructing debris and back leak of ultrafiltrate, maintains the low GFR. The tubular mechanisms are usually important in the maintenance of ARF from most causes seen clinically. Therefore, pharmacologic efforts to improve renal blood flow are not, by themselves, generally effective in shortening the duration of ARF. Interestingly, modern ATN appears to recover much less quickly than when the syndrome was first described. This slow recovery may be related to repeated bouts of renal ischemia, which can be attributed to altered renal vasodilation related to the initial ATN insult. Therefore, even mild degrees of hypotension should be avoided when treating patients with ATN.

Conger J: Hemodynamic factors in acute renal failure. Adv Ren Replace Ther 4:25–37, 1997.

Nowicki M, Zwiech R, Szklarek M: Acute renal failure: The new perspective. Annales Academiae Medicae Bialostocensis 49:145–150, 2004.

8. **How is ARF prevented?**
ATN usually occurs after surgery or preexisting dehydration. In these settings, nephrotoxic drugs, such as radiocontrast dye, aminoglycosides, amphotericin B, nonsteroidal anti-inflammatory agents, and some cancer chemotherapeutic agents (e.g., cisplatin, methotrexate), are far more potent in causing ARF. Optimizing volume status and establishing a relatively high rate of urine flow minimizes the risk of ARF. In specific situations, such as administration of radiocontrast dye or cisplatin and relatively high-risk surgery (e.g., open-heart or biliary tract surgery), mannitol (12.5–25 gm administered as an IV infusion) has been thought to be a useful adjunct in preventing ARF. However, subsequent studies showed that mannitol actually potentiates ARF after the administration of radiocontrast. Some recent studies suggest that administration of N-acetyl cysteine or sodium bicarbonate infusions may prevent contrast

nephropathy in high-risk patients, but the most accepted prophylaxis consists of iso-osmotic contrast media and cautious hydration before contrast administration.

Asif A, Epstein M: Prevention of radiocontrast induced nephropathy. Am J Kidney Dis 44:12–24, 2004.

9. **What are the treatment options in ATN?**
   ATN is best treated, as previously discussed, by prevention. Since nonoliguric ATN is associated with lower mortality and morbidity rates than oliguric ATN, there is some excitement about the administration of high-dose loop diuretics (1–3 gm/24 h given as an IV infusion or as repeated boluses) in concert with renal doses of dopamine (1–3 μg/kg/min). This therapy, which converts some patients with oliguric ATN to a nonoliguric state, certainly facilitates management of volume and nutritional status. Whether this approach actually improves the prognosis is not clear. Optimization of fluid status and avoidance of and/or therapy for electrolyte disorders are the mainstays of conservative management of ARF.

10. **Which critical electrolyte disorders accompany ARF?**
    The most common electrolyte disorders that accompany ARF include hyperkalemia, hypermagnesemia, hyperphosphatemia, hypocalcemia, and acidosis (Table 41-2). Of these disorders, hyperkalemia is the most common and probably the one that is usually most serious.
    Hyperkalemia most commonly occurs with oliguric ATN or urinary obstruction. It is truly a medical emergency. A serum potassium level above 6.0 mandates electrocardiography, searching for peaked T waves, diminished P-wave amplitude, or prolonged QRS complex. Any of these findings warrants the use of immediate measures to correct hyperkalemia.

TABLE 41-2. ELECTROLYTE DISTURBANCES IN ACUTE RENAL FAILURE (ARF)			
Disorder	Mechanism	Frequency	Clinical Importance
Hyperkalemia	Decreased K excretion Increased catabolism	Common, especially with oliguric ARF	Life threatening
Hypermagnesemia	Decreased Mg excretion	Common but not usually severe unless Mg is administered	Life threatening only if very severe
Hyperphosphatemia	Decreased phosphate excretion Increased catabolism	Universal	Serious only if very severe
Hypocalcemia	Calcium phosphate precipitation in tissues Loss of 1,25 vitamin D_3	Common but not usually severe	Life threatening if very severe
Acidosis	Decreased acid excretion Increased catabolism	Very common	Not usually life threatening

K = potassium, Mg = magnesium.

11. **What immediate measures are used to treat hyperkalemia?**
     The quickest-acting parenteral therapy is calcium, administered as chloride or gluconate salts.
     This therapy does not affect the serum potassium level but does antagonize the effects of
     hyperkalemia on the membrane potential of the heart and prevents, or reverses, the cardiac
     effects of hyperkalemia. Another rapidly effective approach is the administration of insulin,
     which drives potassium into cells and lowers the serum potassium level. In patients who have
     a normal serum glucose level, insulin (10 units IV) is generally administered with dextrose
     (one ampule of $D_{50}W$ or an infusion of $D_{10}W$). The effects of insulin last somewhat longer than
     those of calcium and can be prolonged by a constant infusion of insulin, usually administered
     with glucose to prevent hypoglycemia. Bicarbonate may also be used to raise arterial pH and to
     shift potassium into cells. Complications include potentially adverse hemodynamic effects of
     IV bicarbonate and volume expansion from sodium load.

     Wiseman AC, Linas S: Disorders of potassium and acid-base balance. Am J Kidney Dis 45:941–949, 2005.

12. **What is the uremic syndrome?**
     The uremic syndrome is a symptom complex associated with renal failure. It may occur with
     chronic and acute renal failure and involves virtually all organs of the body. Major manifestations
     are nausea and vomiting, pruritus, bleeding disorder, encephalopathy, and pericarditis. The
     syndrome generally mandates initiation of nonconservative therapy for ARF such as
     hemodialysis, peritoneal dialysis, or continuous arteriovenous hemofiltration. The pathogenesis
     of the uremic syndrome is still poorly understood; however, neither urea nor creatinine produces
     any of the known manifestations of uremia.

13. **What are the indications for nonconservative therapy of ARF?**
     Indications for nonconservative therapy, such as dialysis, include uremic signs or symptoms,
     fluid overload, and/or electrolyte abnormalities that are refractory to conservative management.
     It has become the standard of care to provide nonconservative therapy when the BUN level
     exceeds 100 mg/dL or the serum creatinine exceeds 10 mg/dL, especially in the setting of
     oliguric ATN. These latter guidelines are not absolute and must be interpreted in the light of
     other clinical features.

     Palevsky PM: Renal replacement therapy: Indications and timing. Crit Care Clin 21:347–356, 2005.

14. **What are the options for nonconservative therapy of ARF?**
     The three main options for nonconservative therapy of ARF are hemodialysis, peritoneal dialysis,
     and continuous renal replacement therapy (CRRT). Each option has advantages and
     disadvantages (Box 41-1), and there are, of course, variations of each of these modalities.
     Hemodialysis involves the pumping of blood through an artificial kidney that removes solutes
     primarily by dialysis along a concentration gradient; water is removed by ultrafiltration driven by
     a pressure gradient. Central venous access, anticoagulation, a skilled technician, and expensive
     equipment are mandatory for this process. Peritoneal dialysis involves the repetitive instillation
     and removal of fluid into and from the peritoneal cavity, respectively. Solute removal again
     results primarily by dialysis along a concentration gradient, and fluid removal occurs by
     ultrafiltration driven by an osmotic pressure gradient. Although this method is less efficient and
     less rapid than hemodialysis, no central venous access, anticoagulation, skilled technician, or
     expensive equipment is necessary.

     The amount of dialysis that needs to be prescribed is still somewhat controversial.
     Extrapolations from chronic renal failure prescription guidelines may not be sufficient to prevent
     the signs and symptoms of uremia in patients with ARF. A study suggests that a more intensive
     regimen of hemodialysis may actually improve survival in this setting.

     Briglia AE: Dialysis considerations in the patient with acute renal failure: ICU dialysis. In Henrich WL (ed):
     Principles and Practice of Dialysis, 3rd ed. Philadelphia, Lippincott Williams & Wilkins, 2004, pp 420–440.
     Schiffl H, Lang SM, Fischer R: Daily hemodialysis and the outcome of acute renal failure. N Engl J Med
     346:305–310, 2002.

BOX 41-1. DIALYSIS OPTIONS IN THE TREATMENT OF ACUTE RENAL FAILURE

Intermittent hemodialysis

Advantages

Efficient and intensive dialysis technique

Dialysis staff required for shorter period of time

Disadvantages

May cause hemodynamic instability

Relative need for anticoagulation

Potential for disequilibrium

Need for expensive machinery

Need for personnel to perform hemodialysis

Requirements

Venous access, anticoagulation, skilled staff, and expensive equipment

Peritoneal dialysis

Advantages

Slow, gentle form of dialysis

Provides better hemodynamic stability than intermittent hemodialysis

No need for anticoagulation

Disadvantages

Electrolyte disorders and volume corrected slowly

Many nursing units unfamiliar with methodology

Risk for leaks and peritoneal infection

Requirements

Peritoneal catheter, sterile peritoneal dialysis solutions, and trained staff

Continuous renal replacement therapy

Advantages

Slow continuous form of dialysis

Provides better hemodynamic stability than intermittent hemodialysis

Efficient solute removal and electrolyte balance

Round-the-clock maintenance of volume status

Nutrition and medications given while volume status is maintained

Disadvantages

Patient immobilization

Systemic anticoagulation

Nursing staff intensive

Expensive machinery

Requirements

Round-the-clock skilled nursing staff, vascular access, anticoagulation, and complex equipment

15. **What is CRRT?**

CRRT includes a number of treatments characterized by slow, gradual, continuous removal of fluid and electrolytes. Continuous venovenous hemodialysis (CVVHD) is the most widely used method. It involves solute removal by convection and fluid removal by hydrostatic pressure across high-flux membrane. Like conventional dialysis, CVVHD requires central venous access, anticoagulation, skilled staff, and complex equipment. Continuous arteriovenous hemofiltration/ dialysis is a technically simple but less efficient form of CRRT. Although each of these techniques has advantages and disadvantages, in general, the expertise of the professionals working at the center is probably the most important factor. Because of the difficulty in orienting nursing staff to continuous dialysis methods, slow low-efficiency daily dialysis has been developed that provides dialysis over approximately one-half of the hours of the day. Of interest, the biocompatibility of the hemodialysis membrane appears to be an important factor in determining outcome, whereas the intensity of the dialysis prescription (i.e., blood flow, dialysate flow) does not appear to be an important factor in determining patient outcomes.

Chanchairujira T, Mehta RL: Continuous dialysis therapeutic techniques. In Henrich WL (ed): Principles and Practice of Dialysis, 3rd ed. Philadelphia, Lippincott Williams & Wilkins, 2004, pp 162–180.

KEY POINTS: ACUTE RENAL FAILURE (ARF)

1. Serum creatinine concentration may be insensitive to the loss of renal function.

2. ARF due to acute tubular necrosis may be initiated by one mechanism and maintained by another different mechanism.

3. Results elicited by measures to prevent acute tubular necrosis are far superior to those yielded by efforts to provide treatment.

4. Urinalysis and urine electrolyte and creatinine estimation can provide important information about the cause of ARF.

5. Hyperkalemia is an important life-threatening complication of ARF requiring urgent management.

6. Renal replacement therapy, in the form of dialysis, may be required for correction of volume status, electrolyte imbalance, and acidosis, if conservative therapy fails.

CHAPTER 42

RENAL REPLACEMENT THERAPY AND RHABDOMYOLYSIS

Kathleen D. Liu, MD, PhD, and Glenn M. Chertow, MD, MPH

1. **What are the indications for renal replacement therapy?**
   Indications can be grouped using the AEIOU mnemonic:
   - **A:** Acidosis
   - **E:** Electrolyte imbalances—of these, hyperkalemia is the most life-threatening
   - **I:** Ingestions—dialysis will clear some drugs and toxins, including aspirin, lithium and methanol, or ethylene glycol as well as their toxic metabolites
   - **O:** Overload—dialysis can relieve volume overload leading to hypoxemia, which may be particularly problematic in the setting of oliguria/anuria
   - **U:** Uremia—complications of uremia can range from mild (e.g., decreased appetite, itching) to severe (e.g., altered mental status, pericardial effusion, pericarditis). Patients may also have clinical platelet dysfunction (bleeding) due to uremia.

   Palevsky PM: Renal replacement therapy: Indications and timing. Crit Care Clin 21:347–356, 2005.

2. **List the different modes of renal replacement therapy.**
   Intermittent renal replacement therapies
   - Peritoneal dialysis
   - Intermittent hemodialysis (IHD)
   - Ultrafiltration
   - Hybrid therapies: sustained low-efficiency dialysis (SLED), sustained low-efficiency diafiltration (SLEDF), extended daily dialysis (EDD), slow continuous dialysis (SCD)

   Continuous renal replacement therapies (CRRT)
   - Slow continuous ultrafiltration
   - Continuous arteriovenous hemofiltration (CAVH)
   - Continuous arteriovenous hemodialysis (CAVHD)
   - Continuous arteriovenous hemodiafiltration (CAVHDF)
   - Continuous venovenous hemofiltration (CVVH)
   - Continuous venovenous hemodialysis (CVVHD)
   - Continuous venovenous hemodiafiltration (CVVHDF)

3. **What are "hybrid therapies"?**
   SLED, SLEDF, EDD, and SCD are collectively referred to as *recently developed, hybrid modes of dialysis*. Dialysis can be delivered through a variety of conventional IHD machines (an advantage over CRRT), usually with some minor modifications to allow for slower dialysate flow rates compared with IHD. Therapy is delivered intermittently, but over a longer time period (8–12 hours/session) than conventional IHD (3–4 hours/session) and often on a daily basis. Thus, hybrid therapies have many of the benefits of CRRT, without some of the disadvantages (*see* question 5). These modalities are being actively developed and have a number of different names, so we will refer to them as *hybrid therapy*.

   Marshall MR, Golper TA: Sustained low efficiency or extended daily dialysis. UptoDate: www.utdol.com

4. **For whom should CRRT or hybrid therapy be considered?**
   CRRT or hybrid therapy may be considered in any critically ill patient with an indication for dialysis. CRRT/hybrid modalities tend to be better tolerated than intermittent dialysis from a hemodynamic standpoint because of slower fluid removal rates and lower rates of solute flux. Thus, CRRT or a hybrid modality should be considered in critically ill patients with hemodynamic instability. Furthermore, CRRT/hybrid modalities may allow for increased ultrafiltration compared with IHD because volume removal occurs slowly over many hours. In highly catabolic, critically ill patients, the increased clearance these modalities yield (compared with every other day IHD) may allow for better control of azotemia and acidosis. Last, patients with elevated intracranial pressure may not tolerate IHD due to rapid solute shifts; continuous/hybrid modalities are an alternative.

   Lamiere N, Van Biesen W, Vanholder R: Acute renal failure. Lancet 365:417–430, 2005.

5. **What are some disadvantages of CRRT?**
   Because of its continuous nature, CRRT requires long-term relative immobilization of the patient. Continuous anticoagulation is often used to prevent filter clotting and blood loss, but this may increase the bleeding risk. Last, CRRT frequently results in hypothermia and is highly labor intensive and therefore costly.

6. **Define *hemofiltration*, *hemodialysis*, and *hemodiafiltration*.**
   - **Hemofiltration:** Plasma is forced from the blood space into the effluent through a highly permeable membrane. This results in "convective" clearance of small and middle-sized molecules.
   - **Hemodialysis:** Blood flows on one side of a semipermeable membrane. The dialysate solution, which contains various electrolytes and glucose, is pumped along the other side of the membrane, usually in the opposite (i.e., countercurrent) direction. A concentration gradient drives electrolytes and water-soluble waste products from the plasma compartment into the dialysate. The dialysis machine generates transmembrane pressure to drive plasma water from the blood side to the dialysate side. Dialysis results in "diffusive" clearance, preferentially of small molecules.
   - **Hemodiafiltration:** Hemodiafiltration makes simultaneous use of hemofiltration and hemodialysis.

KEY POINTS: POTENTIAL ADVANTAGES OF CONTINUOUS RENAL REPLACEMENT THERAPIES (CRRT) AND HYBRID THERAPIES OVER INTERMITTENT HEMODIALYSIS (IHD)

1. CRRT and hybrid therapies are better tolerated hemodynamically than IHD.

2. An increased volume removal can occur with CRRT and hybrid therapies.

3. CRRT and hybrid therapies can yield an increased clearance of nitrogenous wastes.

4. Hybrid therapies and CRRT allow for more constant control of acidosis.

5. Fewer fluctuations in intracranial pressure may occur with CRRT and hybrid therapies.

7. **How are hemofiltration, hemodialysis, and hemodiafiltration used in IHD, hybrid therapy, and CRRT?**

IHD is exclusively hemodialysis. As the names imply, CVVH and CAVH use hemofiltration alone, CAVHD and CVVHD are hemodialysis modalities, and CAVHDF and CVVHDF use both hemofiltration and hemodialysis. Hybrid modalities consist of hemodialysis alone, or they may incorporate hemofiltration as well.

8. **What laboratory tests should be ordered regularly for patients receiving CRRT?**

Lab tests for sodium, potassium bicarbonate, calcium, and phosphates should be ordered regularly as concentrations of these electrolytes can change rapidly during CRRT. Hyper-phosphatemia frequently occurs during IHD because of inefficient clearance of phosphate, but hypophosphatemia is more common during CRRT. Hypocalcemia and hypomagnesemia are also seen, especially when these cations are complexed with citrate (e.g., when citrate is used as an anticoagulant). Patients with impaired lactate metabolism (e.g., due to severe sepsis or hepatic failure) may have high systemic lactate levels if the dialysate or replacement fluid contains lactate as a base equivalent. In these cases, high lactate levels or worsening acidosis should prompt the use of a bicarbonate-based dialysate or replacement fluid.

9. **What are the nutrition considerations for patients who experience acute renal failure (ARF) while receiving CRRT?**

- **Amino acids:** Amino acids are lost in both IHD and CRRT. Critically ill patients with ARF are frequently highly catabolic; patients treated with CRRT should receive protein in a dosage of at least 1.2 gm/kg/day, and many patients will require at least 1.5–1.8 gm/kg/day of protein or amino acids. These nutritional goals need to be serially reevaluated based on net nitrogen balance.
- **Vitamins:** *Water-soluble* vitamins are lost in both IHD and CRRT. These vitamins should be replaced, although excessive doses of vitamin C (>1 gm/day) should be avoided, given the impaired excretion of oxalate (a vitamin C by-product) in ARF. *Fat-soluble* vitamins are protein- or lipoprotein-bound and are therefore not significantly cleared by CRRT or IHD.
- **Minerals:** Trace minerals such as zinc may be dialyzed with IHD or CRRT; the benefit of supplementation in this situation remains unproven. Aluminum-containing products should be avoided due to central nervous system toxicity.

Bellomo R: Nutritional management of patients treated with continuous renal replacement therapy. In Kopple JD, and Masry SG (eds): Nutritional Management of Renal Disease, 2nd ed. Philadelphia, Lippincott Williams & Wilkins, 2004, pp 573–580.

10. **Discuss the role of CRRT in the management of septic shock.**

This is one of the most controversial issues related to CRRT. Theoretically, many inflammatory cytokines (including interleukins-1 and -6 and tumor necrosis factor alpha) are cleared by CRRT. Preliminary studies in animal models and humans were promising, but small randomized clinical trials have not shown consistent results. Further research has suggested that the decreased levels of inflammatory mediators seen in early trials were due to adsorption onto the filter membranes; this process is rapidly saturated and therefore an ineffective method of clearance. However, because of the theoretical possibilities of using CRRT to treat the systemic inflammatory response, and because of the ongoing development of new dialysis membranes with different filtration characteristics, this controversy is likely to continue.

Ratanarat R, Brendolan A, Piccini P, et al: Pulse high-volume hemofiltration for treatment of severe sepsis: Effects on hemodynamics and survival. Crit Care Forum 9:R294–R302, 2004.

11. **What kind of anticoagulation is required for the circuit in CRRT?**
    The anticoagulant is not typically administered systemically; rather, it is infused into the circuit just proximal to the filter, and the majority is removed via convective flow across the filter membrane. For patients in whom heparin is contraindicated, an alternative anticoagulant is trisodium citrate. Citrate infusion requires a post-filter calcium infusion to avoid systemic hypocalcemia and careful monitoring of serum ionized calcium levels. Prostacyclin has also been used as an anticoagulant, but it is associated with appreciable levels of systemic hypotension. CRRT may be done without anticoagulation; however, this results in a higher frequency of clotting episodes. The most common site of clotting is within the dialysis filter itself. Clotting should be avoided because a patient may lose 80–100 mL of blood if the entire CRRT circuit clots.

    Davenport A: Anticoagulation for continuous renal replacement therapy. Contrib Nephrol 144:228–238, 2004.

12. **What are the complications of CRRT?**
    Among the most important risks of CRRT are risks inherent in obtaining central venous access. In general, subclavian venous access should be avoided, given the risk of subclavian stenosis with an indwelling catheter, particularly among patients who might require long-term hemodialysis. If an arteriovenous mode of therapy is used, special attention must be paid to distal limb ischemia, given the large-bore size of the arterial catheters. However, with the advent of peristaltic blood flow pumps, arteriovenous modes are rarely used (rather, venovenous hemofiltration and hemodiafiltration are the modality of choice). Electrolyte abnormalities or hypovolemia may also develop with CRRT. Patients may become hypothermic due to heat loss and may not mount a normal febrile response to infection.

13. **What is the role of peritoneal dialysis in the critical care setting?**
    Peritoneal dialysis is contraindicated in patients with recent abdominal surgery and intra-abdominal infection or disease (e.g., peritonitis, ileus). These scenarios are common in critically ill patients. Patients lose a substantial amount of albumin to the dialysate solution, worsening protein-calorie malnutrition. Peritoneal dialysate solutions contain dextrose as the osmotic agent and can exacerbate hyperglycemia. The volume of the intraperitoneal solution (usually 2–3 L) can create problems with respiratory mechanics. A major advantage of peritoneal dialysis is that it is well tolerated from a hemodynamic standpoint. However, in an era when CRRT and hybrid modalities are often available, peritoneal dialysis is rarely indicated in the critical care setting.

RHABDOMYOLYSIS

14. **What causes rhabdomyolysis?**
    Muscle ischemia, damage, and eventual necrosis lead to rhabdomyolysis. The various etiologies are grouped into physical and nonphysical causes in Box 42-1. Both groups of causes probably share a common pathway in that increased demands on the muscle cells and their mitochondria, whether because of intrinsic deficiencies or extrinsic forces (i.e., decreased oxygen delivery or increased metabolic demands), lead to ischemia and eventual damage.

    Huerta-Alardin AL, Varon J, Marik PE: Bench-to-bedside review: Rhabdomyolysis—an overview for clinicians. Crit Care 9:158–169, 2005.

15. **Discuss the symptoms and signs of rhabdomyolysis.**
    The classic presentation of rhabdomyolysis, which consists of myalgia, weakness, and dark urine, is actually rare. Often, only one or two of these symptoms are present. However, a history suggestive of muscle compression, a physical examination demonstrating muscle tenderness, and laboratory test results confirming muscle damage lead to a strong presumptive diagnosis.

BOX 42-1. MAJOR CAUSES OF RHABDOMYOLYSIS

Physical causes

Trauma and compression

Occlusion or hypoperfusion of the muscular vessels

Excessive muscle strain: Exercise, seizure, tetanus, delirium tremens

Electrical current

Hyperthermia: Exercise, sepsis, neuroleptic malignant syndrome, malignant hyperthermia

Nonphysical causes

Metabolic myopathies, including McArdle disease, mitochondrial respiratory chain enzyme deficiencies, carnitine palmitoyl transferase deficiency, phosphofructokinase deficiency

Endocrinopathies, including hypothyroidism and diabetic ketoacidosis (due to electrolyte abnormalities)

Drugs and toxins, including medications (e.g., antimalarials, colchicines, corticosteroids, fibrates, HMG CoA reductase inhibitors, isoniazid, zidovudine), drugs of abuse (e.g., alcohol, heroin), and toxins (e.g., insect and snake venoms)

Infections (either local or systemic)

Electrolyte abnormalities: Hyperosmotic conditions, hypokalemia, hypophosphatemia, hyponatremia or hypernatremia,

Autoimmune diseases: Polymyositis or dermatomyositis

HMG CoA = 3-hydroxy-3-methylglutaryl coenzyme A.

16. **What laboratory tests should be ordered to diagnose rhabdomyolysis?**
    Lab tests for creatine phosphokinase should be ordered because creatine phosphokinase is the most sensitive indicator of muscle damage; it may continue to increase for several days after the original insult. Hyperkalemia, hyperuricemia, and hyperphosphatemia also occur. Hypocalcemia develops as calcium is chelated and deposited in the damaged muscle tissue. Lactic acidosis and an anion gap metabolic acidosis result from release of other organic acids.

17. **What are the complications of rhabdomyolysis?**
    The most immediate concern is hyperkalemia due to cell necrosis, particularly in the setting of ARF, which can be precipitated by rhabdomyolysis by several mechanisms. Damaged or dying myocytes release myoglobin and its metabolites, which can precipitate along with other cellular debris to form casts in the renal tubules. Tubular obstruction may be exacerbated by concomitant third-spacing of fluids leading to intravascular hypovolemia. Myoglobin also precipitates a cytokine cascade that leads to worsening renal vasoconstriction, which exacerbates acute renal failure. These processes result in the development of ARF and oliguria/anuria.
    Although patients usually are hypocalcemic, they are rarely symptomatic. Caution needs to be used when treating hypocalcemia because patients may have rebound hypercalcemia and soft tissue deposition, but symptoms of hypocalcemia such as tetany, Chvostek's sign, or cardiac

arrhythmias should be treated promptly. Other immediate concerns include hypovolemia, particularly in the setting of crush injuries or other causes of compression injury.

Vanholder R, Sever MS, Erek E, Lameire N: Rhabdomyolysis. J Am Soc Nephrol 11:1553–1561, 2000.

18. **What treatment options are available for a patient with rhabdomyolysis?**
Supportive care, with assurance of intravascular repletion and prevention of continued renal insult, is the main strategy. Although there is limited clinical evidence in support of these strategies, hydration with sodium bicarbonate–based crystalloids is often used to alkalinize the urine, which is thought to improve the solubility of myoglobin and decrease its direct tubular toxicity. Mannitol can be used to promote an osmotic diuresis. Allopurinol reduces the production of uric acid, which can crystallize in the tubules along with myoglobin. Control of hyperkalemia, which may require the provision of dialysis and treatment of symptomatic hypocalcemia, are important parts of the supportive care regimen.

Brown CVR, Rhee P, Chan L, et al: Preventing renal failure in patients with rhabdomyolysis: Do bicarbonate and mannitol make a difference?. J Trauma 56:1191–1196, 2004.
Malinoski DJ, Slater MS, Mullins RJ: Crush injury and rhabdomyolysis. Crit Care Clin 20:171–192, 2004.

KEY POINTS: MANAGEMENT OF RHABDOMYOLYSIS

1. Adequate resuscitation is critical.

2. Monitor for hyperkalemia and treat with dialysis or other supportive measures, if necessary.

3. Treat *symptomatic* hypocalcemia.

4. Alkalinization of urine with sodium bicarbonate is often used (although data are limited regarding this point).

19. **What kind of prophylactic management options are possible?**
Guidelines for the treatment of catastrophic crush injuries (developed in response to earthquake disasters) recommend the initiation of volume resuscitation with crystalloid even before extrication. In the first 24 hours, up to 10 L of intravascular volume may be lost as sequestrated fluid in the affected limb. Administration of up to 10–12 L of fluid may be required during this period, with careful monitoring of urine output.

Malinoski DJ, Slater MS, Mullins RJ: Crush injury and rhabdomyolysis. Crit Care Clin 20:171–192, 2004.

20. **What drugs need to be avoided in patients with rhabdomyolysis?**
Succinylcholine, a drug used for rapid muscle paralysis to achieve airway control, causes generalized depolarization of neuromuscular junctions and can cause hyperkalemia if the patient has abnormal proliferations of the motor end plates. Patients with rhabdomyolysis are often hyperkalemic, and therefore succinylcholine should generally be avoided, given the often lethal nature of these hyperkalemic events. In addition, medications that are known to be associated with rhabdomyolysis (e.g., 3-hydroxy-3-methylglutaryl coenzyme A [HMG CoA] reductase inhibitors) should be avoided, if possible.

CHAPTER 43

HYPOKALEMIA AND HYPERKALEMIA

Alan C. Pao, MD, and Stuart L. Linas, MD

1. **Is serum potassium an accurate estimate of total body potassium?**
   No. The majority of potassium is distributed in the intracellular fluid (ICF) compartment, with only about 2% of the total body potassium in the extracellular fluid (ECF) compartment. Alterations in serum potassium can result from transcellular potassium shift between ECF and ICF compartments or from actual changes in total body potassium.

   Rosa RM, Epstein FH: Extrarenal potassium metabolism. In Seldin DW, Giebisch G (eds): The Kidney. New York, Lippincott Williams & Wilkins, 2000, pp 1551–1552.

2. **When does serum potassium falsely estimate total body potassium?**
   Transcellular potassium shifts between ECF and ICF compartments can have profound effects on serum potassium. Buffering of the ECF compartment, with reciprocal movement of potassium and hydrogen across the cell membrane, can result in a rise in serum potassium in the case of acidemia and a fall in serum potassium in the case of alkalemia. Two important hormones that are known to drive potassium into the ICF compartment are insulin and catecholamines.

   The classic example of how serum potassium falsely estimates total body potassium is a patient who presents with diabetic ketoacidosis. Insulin deficiency and acidemia cause potassium to shift to the ECF compartment so that serum potassium may be normal despite profound total body potassium depletion (due to osmotic diuresis and hyperaldosteronemic state). Only after proper treatment of insulin deficiency and acidosis does the total body potassium depletion become apparent.

   Sterns RH, Cox M, Feig PU, et al: Internal potassium balance and the control of the plasma potassium concentration. Medicine 60:342–348, 1981.

3. **Why is tight regulation of serum potassium concentrations so critical?**
   Although a small fraction of total body potassium is in the ECF compartment, changes in ECF potassium, either by compartmental shifts or by net gain or loss, significantly alter the ratio of ECF to ICF potassium, which determines the cellular resting membrane potential. As a consequence, small fluctuations in ECF potassium can have profound effects on cardiac and neuromuscular excitability.

   Rosa RM, Epstein FH: Extrarenal potassium metabolism. In Seldin DW, Giebisch G (eds): The Kidney, 3rd ed. New York, Lippincott Williams & Wilkins, 2000, pp 1551–1552.

4. **How do you estimate the total body potassium deficit?**
   It is difficult to predict accurately the total body potassium deficit based on serum potassium, but in uncomplicated potassium depletion, a useful rule of thumb is as follows: For each 100-mEq potassium deficit, the fall in serum potassium is 0.27 mEq/L. Thus for a 70-kg patient, potassium = 3 mEq/L reflects a 300- to 400-mEq deficit, whereas potassium = 2 mEq/L reflects a 500- to 700-mEq deficit. In patients with acid–base disorders, this rule of thumb is not accurate due to shifts in compartmental potassium.

   Sterns RH, Cox M, Feig PU, et al: Internal potassium balance and the control of the plasma potassium concentration. Medicine 60:340–341, 1981.

5. **What is the relationship between potassium and magnesium?**
    Magnesium depletion typically occurs after diuretic use, sustained alcohol consumption, or diabetic ketoacidosis. Magnesium depletion can cause hypokalemia that is refractory to oral or IV potassium chloride therapy because severe magnesium depletion causes renal potassium wasting through undefined mechanisms. In the setting of severe magnesium and potassium depletion, magnesium and potassium must be replaced simultaneously.

    Whang R, Whang DD, Ryan MP: Refractory potassium repletion. Arch Intern Med 152:40–44, 1992.

6. **What are the factors that dictate urine potassium excretion?**
    Key factors influencing potassium secretion include adequate sodium delivery to the distal nephron and increased aldosterone action.

    Malnic G, Muto S, Giebisch G: Regulation of potassium excretion. In Seldin DW, Giebisch G (eds): The Kidney, 3rd ed. New York, Lippincott Williams & Wilkins, 2000, pp 1592–1601.

7. **What are the causes of hypokalemia?**
    Hypokalemia can be caused by low potassium intake, intracellular potassium redistribution, gastrointestinal potassium loss (i.e., diarrhea), and renal potassium loss. Intracellular potassium redistribution or shift can be caused by metabolic alkalosis, increased insulin availability, increased β-adrenergic activity, and periodic paralysis (classically associated with thyrotoxicosis). Renal potassium loss can be caused by diuretics, vomiting, states of mineralocorticoid excess (e.g., primary hyperaldosteronism, Cushing's disease, European licorice ingestion, and hyperreninemia), hypomagnesemia, and genetic diseases such as Bartter and Gitelman's syndromes.

8. **What are the clinical manifestations of hypokalemia?**
    By depressing neuromuscular excitability, hypokalemia leads to muscle weakness, which can include quadriplegia and hypoventilation. Severe hypokalemia disrupts cell integrity, leading to rhabdomyolysis. Among the most important manifestations of hypokalemia are cardiac arrhythmias, including paroxysmal atrial tachycardia with block, atrioventricular dissociation, first- and second-degree atrioventricular block with Wenckebach periods, and even ventricular tachycardia or fibrillation. Typical electrocardiographic (ECG) findings include ST-segment depression, flattened T waves, and prominent U waves.

    Chou TC: Electrolyte imbalance. In Chou TC, Knilans K (eds): Electrocardiography in Clinical Practice, 4th ed. Philadelphia, WB Saunders, 1996, pp 535–540.

9. **Which drugs can cause hypokalemia?**
    The most common drugs are diuretics—acetazolamide, loop diuretics, and thiazides. Increases in distal sodium delivery in the setting of high plasma aldosterone levels (due to lower blood volume) result in increases in urinary potassium and subsequent hypokalemia. Penicillin and penicillin analogs (e.g., carbenicillin, ticarcillin, piperacillin) also cause renal potassium wasting that is mediated by various mechanisms, including delivery of nonreabsorbable anions to the distal nephron, which results in potassium trapping in the urine. Drugs that damage renal tubular membranes such as amphotericin, cisplatinum, and aminoglycosides cause renal potassium wasting even in the absence of decreases in glomerular filtration rate (GFR).

    Weiner ID, Wingo CS: Hypokalemia: Consequences, causes, and correction. J Am Soc Nephrol 8:1183, 1997.

10. **What is the diagnostic approach to a patient with hypokalemia?**
    After eliminating spurious causes (such as leukocytosis), the diagnosis of true hypokalemia can be approached on the basis of urine potassium concentration, systemic acid–base status, urine chloride level, and blood pressure (Fig. 43-1). Urine potassium excretion is best measured by a

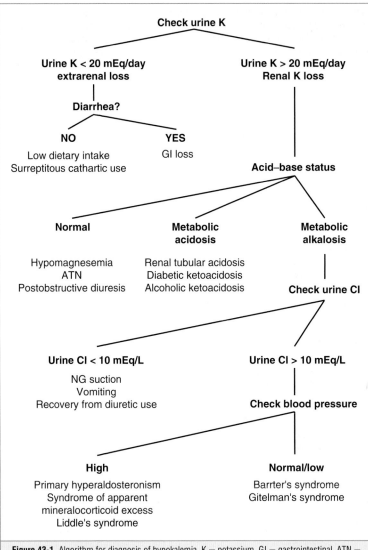

Figure 43-1. Algorithm for diagnosis of hypokalemia. K = potassium, GI = gastrointestinal, ATN = acute tubular necrosis, Cl = chloride, NG = nasogastric.

24-hour urine collection. A spot urine potassium concentration can also be measured (less accurate, but easier to obtain) with a value of <15 mEq/L indicating extrarenal loss and a value of >15 mEq/L indicating renal potassium wasting.

11. **How do you treat hypokalemia?**
Oral replacement is the safest route, and administration of doses of up to 40 mEq multiple times daily is allowed. In most cases, potassium chloride is used because metabolic alkalosis and chloride depletion often accompany hypokalemia, such as in patients who are taking diuretics or

who are vomiting. In these settings, coadministration of chloride is important for correction of both the metabolic alkalosis and hypokalemia. In other settings, potassium should be administered with other salt preparations. For example, in metabolic acidosis, replacement with potassium bicarbonate or bicarbonate equivalent (e.g., potassium citrate, acetate, or gluconate) is recommended to help alleviate the acidosis. Persons who abuse alcohol or who have diabetes with ketoacidosis often have concomitant phosphate deficiency and should receive some of the potassium in the form of potassium phosphate.

Rose B, Post TW: Hypokalemia. In Rose B, Post TW (eds): Clinical Physiology of Acid–Base and Electrolyte Disorders. New York, McGraw-Hill, 2001, pp 871–872.

12. **When is IV potassium replacement necessary? What are the risks?**
When oral administration is not possible, or in life-threatening situations such as severe weakness, respiratory distress, cardiac arrhythmias, or rhabdomyolysis, potassium must be replaced intravenously. Infusion rates in the intensive care unit should be limited to 20 mEq/h to prevent the potentially catastrophic effect of a potassium bolus to the heart.

Kruse JA, Carlson RW: Rapid correction of hypokalemia using concentrated intravenous potassium chloride infusions. Arch Intern Med 150:613–617, 1990.

KEY POINTS: CIRCUMSTANCES REQUIRING SPECIAL CARE IN MONITORING POTASSIUM REPLACEMENT

1. Patients with defects in potassium excretion (e.g., renal failure, use of potassium-sparing diuretics or angiotensin-converting enzyme inhibitors) must have their serum potassium concentrations monitored (i.e., daily laboratory checks) when potassium is being replaced to prevent overcorrection.

2. Patients who are receiving digitalis therapy and are experiencing hypokalemia are prone to having serious cardiac arrhythmias (especially in overdose situations) and must be treated urgently.

3. Patients with significant magnesium deficiency have renal potassium wasting and often must have their magnesium levels corrected before therapy for hypokalemia is initiated.

13. **What are the causes of hyperkalemia?**
Hyperkalemia can be caused by high potassium intake, extracellular potassium redistribution, and low renal potassium excretion. High potassium intake (e.g., oral potassium replacement, total parenteral nutrition, and high-dose potassium penicillin) can cause hyperkalemia, usually in the setting of low renal potassium excretion. Extracellular potassium redistribution or shift can be caused by metabolic acidosis, insulin deficiency, β-adrenergic blockade, rhabdomyolysis, massive hemolysis, tumor lysis syndrome, periodic paralysis (hyperkalemic form), and heavily catabolic states such as severe sepsis. Low renal potassium excretion can be caused by renal failure, decreased effective circulating volume (e.g., severe sepsis, congestive heart failure, cirrhosis), and states of hypoaldosteronism. States of hypoaldosteronism include decreased renin-angiotensin system activity (e.g., hyporeninemic hypoaldosteronism in diabetes, interstitial nephritis, angiotensin-converting enzyme [ACE] inhibitors, nonsteroidal anti-inflammatory drugs [NSAIDs], cyclosporine), decreased adrenal synthesis (e.g., Addison's disease, heparin), and aldosterone resistance (e.g., high-dose trimethoprim, potassium-sparing diuretic agents).

14. **Which drugs can cause hyperkalemia?**
Drugs that cause release of intracellular potassium include succinylcholine and, rarely, beta blockers. Drugs that block renin-angiotensin-aldosterone axis will result in decreased renal potassium excretion; these include spironolactone, ACE inhibitors, cyclosporine, heparin, and NSAIDs. Drugs that impair the process of sodium and potassium exchange include digitalis; drugs that block sodium and potassium exchange in the distal nephron include amiloride and trimethoprim.

15. **What are the clinical manifestations of hyperkalemia?**
The most serious manifestation of hyperkalemia involves the electrical conduction system of the heart. Profound hyperkalemia can lead to heart block and asystole. Initially, the ECG shows peaked T waves and decreased amplitude of P waves followed by prolongation of QRS waves. With severe hyperkalemia, QRS and T waves blend together into what appears to be a sine-wave pattern consistent with ventricular fibrillation. Because cardiac arrest can occur at any point in this progression, hyperkalemia with ECG changes constitutes a medical emergency. Other effects of hyperkalemia include weakness, neuromuscular paralysis (without central nervous system disturbances), and suppression of renal ammoniagenesis, which may result in metabolic acidosis.

> Chou TC: Electrolyte imbalance. In Chou TC, Knilans K (eds): Electrocardiography in Clinical Practice, 4th ed. Philadelphia, WB Saunders, 1996, pp 532–535.

16. **What degree of chronic kidney disease causes hyperkalemia?**
Chronic kidney disease *per se* is not associated with hyperkalemia until the GFR is reduced to about 75% of normal levels (serum creatinine > 4 mg/dL). Although more than 85% of filtered potassium is reabsorbed in the proximal tubule, urinary excretion of potassium is determined primarily by potassium secretion along the cortical collecting tubule. Hyperkalemia disproportionate to reductions in GFR usually results from decreases in potassium secretion (due to either decreases in aldosterone, as may occur in Addison's disease, or to diabetes with hyporeninemic hypoaldosteronism) or from marked decreases in sodium delivery to the distal nephron, as may occur in severe prerenal states.

17. **What is the transtubular potassium gradient (TTKG)? When should it be used?**
The TTKG is a semiquantitative index of the potassium secretory process and approximates the effect of aldosterone on distal tubular potassium (K) secretion. It is calculated as follows:

$$TTKG = U_K/(U_{Osm}/P_{Osm})/P_K$$

The TTKG provides a better clinical approach to uncover defects in urinary potassium (U_K) excretion as compared with U_K alone because the latter fails to account for plasma potassium concentration and for medullary water abstraction.

It is most commonly used in patients with hyperkalemia, where a TTKG < 5 suggests reduced renal mineralocorticoid activity. There are two limitations to using the TTKG: (1) urine sodium (U_{Na}) must be >25 mm (to ensure that sodium delivery is not the limiting factor) and (2) the urine must be hypertonic (to ensure that antidiuretic hormone is present for normal potassium conductance in the distal nephron).

> West ML, Marsden PA, Richardson RM, et al: New clinical approach to evaluate disorders of potassium excretion. Miner Electrolyte Metab 12:234–238, 1986.

18. **What is the diagnostic approach to treating a patient with hyperkalemia?**
The cause is often apparent after a careful history is taken, a review of medications is performed, and basic laboratory values are measured, including a chemistry panel with blood urea nitrogen and creatinine concentrations. Additional laboratory tests can be performed if there is clinical

suspicion for any of the following: pseudohyperkalemia (look for high white blood cell and platelet counts); rhabdomyolysis (look for high creatinine kinase concentration); tumor lysis syndrome (look for high lactate dehydrogenase, uric acid, and phosphorus, and low calcium levels); hypoaldosteronemic state (look for a TTKG < 5 in the setting of hyperkalemia).

19. What is pseudohyperkalemia?

Serum potassium measurements can be falsely elevated when potassium is released during the process of blood collection from the patient or during the process of clot formation in the specimen tube. In these situations, "pseudohyperkalemia" does not reflect true hyperkalemia. Potassium release from muscles distal to a tight tourniquet can artifactually elevate potassium by as much as 2.7 mEq/L. Potassium release during the process of clot formation in the specimen tube from leukocytes (white blood cell counts > 70,000/mm^3) or platelets (platelet count > 1,000,000/mm^3) can also become quite significant and distort serum potassium measurement results. In these circumstances, an unclotted blood sample (i.e., plasma potassium determination) should be obtained.

Bronson WR, DeVita VJ, Carbone PP, et al: Pseudohyperkalemia due to release of potassium from white blood cells during clotting. N Engl J Med 274:369–375, 1966.

Don BR, Sebastian A, Cheitlin M, et al: Pseudohyperkalemia caused by fist clenching during phlebotomy. N Engl J Med 322:1290–1292, 1990.

Hartman RC, Auditore JV, Jackson DP: Studies on thrombocytosis: 1. Hyperkalemia due to release of potassium from platelets during coagulation. J Clin Invest 37:699–707, 1958.

Hyman D, Kaplan NM: The difference between serum and plasma potassium. N Engl J Med 313:642, 1985.

Skinner SL: A cause of erroneous potassium levels. Lancet 1:478–480, 1961.

20. How do you treat hyperkalemia?

The presence of serum potassium > 6.5, ECG changes, or severe weakness mandates emergent therapy. The general approach is to use therapy involving each of the following:

- **Membrane stabilization:** Calcium raises the cell depolarization threshold and reduces myocardial irritability. One or two ampules of intravenous calcium chloride result in improvement in ECG changes within seconds, but the beneficial effect lasts only about 30 minutes.
- **Shift potassium into cells:** IV insulin (e.g., 10-unit bolus of regular insulin) with glucose administration begins to lower serum potassium levels in about 2–5 minutes and lasts a few hours. Correction of acidosis with IV sodium bicarbonate (e.g., two ampules) has a similar duration and time of onset. Nebulized β-adrenergic agonists such as albuterol can lower serum potassium by 0.5–1.5 mEq/L with an onset of 30 minutes and an effect lasting 2–4 hours.
- **Removal of potassium:** Loop diuretics can sometimes cause enough renal potassium loss in patients with intact renal function, but usually a potassium-binding resin must be used (e.g., Kayexalate, 30 gm taken orally or 50 gm administered by retention enema). Acute hemodialysis is quick and effective at removing potassium and must be used when the gastrointestinal tract is nonfunctional or when serious fluid overload is already present.

CHAPTER 44

HYPONATREMIA AND HYPERNATREMIA

Kathleen D. Liu, MD, PhD

1. **Why is sodium balance critical to volume control?**

   Sodium and its corresponding anions represent almost all of the osmotically active solutes in the extracellular fluid under normal conditions. Therefore, the serum concentration of sodium reflects the tonicity of body fluids. Small changes in tonicity are counteracted by thirst regulation, antidiuretic hormone (ADH) secretion, and renal concentrating or diluting mechanisms. Preservation of normal serum osmolality (i.e., 285–295 mOsm/L) guarantees cellular integrity by regulating net movement of water across cellular membranes.

   Adrogue HJ, Madias NE: Hyponatremia. N Engl J Med 342:1581–1589, 2000.

2. **What is another name for ADH? What is its mechanism of action?**

   ADH is also called *arginine vasopressin* or *vasopressin*. ADH is a small peptide hormone produced by the hypothalamus that binds to the vasopressin 1 and 2 receptors (V1 and V2). Vasopressin release is regulated by osmoreceptors in the hypothalamus, which are exquisitely sensitive to changes in plasma osmolality. Under hyperosmolar conditions, osmoreceptor stimulation leads to vasopressin release and stimulation of thirst. These two mechanisms result in increased water intake and retention. Vasopressin release is also regulated by baroreceptors in the carotid sinus and aortic arch; under conditions of hypovolemia, these receptors stimulate vasopressin release to increase water retention. At very high concentrations, vasopressin causes vascular smooth muscle constriction through the V1 receptor and increased vascular tone, resulting in increased blood pressure.

   Brenner BM (ed): Brenner and Rector's The Kidney, 7th ed. Philadelphia, Elsevier, 2004.

3. **Does hyponatremia simply represent a low sodium state?**

   No. *Hyponatremia* is defined as a serum sodium concentration < 135 mEq/L. However, serum sodium concentration does not correlate directly with volume status. Hyponatremia can occur in low total body sodium (hypovolemic), normal total body sodium (euvolemic), and excess total body sodium (hypervolemic) states. Determination of volume status is helpful in assessing a patient with hyponatremia because causes of hyponatremia can be classified based on volume status (Fig. 44-1). Helpful physical findings include tachycardia, dry mucous membranes, orthostatic hypotension, and increased skin turgor (associated with hypovolemia) or edema, S_3 heart sound, jugular venous distention, and ascites (present in hypervolemic states).

4. **How can hyponatremia develop in a patient with hypovolemia?**

   Hypovolemic hyponatremia represents a decrease in total body sodium in excess of a decrease in total body water. Simultaneous sodium and water loss can be due to renal or extrarenal causes. Hypovolemia results in a decrease in renal perfusion, a decrement in glomerular filtration rate, and an increase in proximal tubule reabsorption; all three mechanisms contribute to decreased water excretion. Furthermore, hypovolemia supersedes the expected inhibition of vasopressin release by hypotonicity and maintains the secretion of the hormone. In other words, the body protects volume at the expense of tonicity.

   Berl T, Verbalis J: Pathophysiology of water metabolism. In Brenner BM (ed): Brenner and Rector's The Kidney, 7th ed. Philadelphia, Elsevier, 2004, pp 858–907.

Serum Na⁺ <135 mmol/L

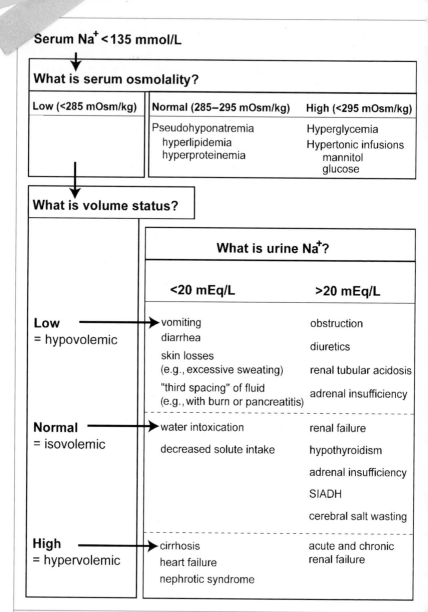

Figure 44-1. Diagnostic algorithm for hyponatremia. Na^+ = sodium concentration, SIADH = syndrome of inappropriate secretion of antidiuretic hormone.

5. **How does hypervolemic hyponatremia differ from hypovolemic hyponatremia?**
   In hypervolemic hyponatremia, the kidneys are at the center of the problem, either because of intrinsic renal disease or renal compensation for an extrarenal abnormality. Physical examination reveals edema and no evidence of volume depletion. Intrinsic renal disease with

markedly decreased glomerular filtration rate (acute or chronic) prevents the adequate excretion of sodium and water. Intake of sodium in excess of what can be excreted leads to hypervolemia (edema); excessive intake of water leads to hyponatremia. Homeostasis is lost, and volume overload, hyponatremia, and edema develop. In contrast, in congestive heart failure, hepatic cirrhosis, and nephrotic syndrome, the intrinsically normal kidney is stimulated to retain sodium and water, and hypervolemia and hyponatremia develop. In general, hypervolemic hypernatremia due to an extrarenal cause is characterized by a low urine sodium concentration ($\leq$10–20 mEq/L); this distinguishes it from hypervolemic hypernatremia due to intrinsic renal causes.

6. **What is the syndrome of inappropriate secretion of antidiuretic hormone (SIADH)?**
   SIADH is a common cause of euvolemic hyponatremia and is associated with malignancies, pulmonary disease, central nervous system disorders, and many drugs. The latter category includes hypoglycemic, psychotropic, narcotic, and chemotherapeutic agents. Other causes of euvolemic hyponatremia include psychogenic polydipsia, hypothyroidism, and adrenal insufficiency.

7. **What diagnostic tests are useful in the evaluation of hyponatremia?**
   The physical examination is critical to the determination of volume status, as previously described. Serum electrolyte and serum and urine osmolality measurements are useful. High urine osmolality despite low serum osmolality suggests SIADH in the euvolemic state or hypovolemic hyponatremia. Very low urine osmolality suggests excessive water intake, as in psychogenic polydipsia. Measurements of thyroid-stimulating hormone and cortisol can be used to assess endocrine causes of hyponatremia.

   Milionis HJ, Liamis GL, Elisaf MS: The hyponatremic patient: A systematic approach to laboratory diagnosis. Can Med Assoc J 166:1056–1062, 2002.

KEY POINTS: USEFUL DIAGNOSTIC TESTS IN HYPONATREMIA

1. Serum osmolality measurement is useful in the diagnosis of hyponatremia.

2. Determination of volume status is necessary.

3. If urine osmolality is inappropriately high, it is easier to differentiate causes of euvolemic hyponatremia. High urine osmolality implies inappropriate levels of antidiuretic hormone or antidiuretic hormone–like hormones.

4. Urine sodium needs to be interpreted with caution in cases of renal failure.

8. **Are *hyponatremia* and *hypo-osmolality* synonymous?**
   No. Hyponatremia can occur without a change in total body sodium or total body water in two settings. The first is pseudohyponatremia, which is only a laboratory abnormality in patients with severe hyperlipidemia or hyperproteinemia; lipids and proteins occupy an increasingly large volume in which the sodium determination is made. Serum sodium concentrations are low in these pathologic states when a flame photometry method is used but normal when an ion-specific electrode is used. Most clinical laboratories now use an ion-specific electrode. The second setting occurs when large quantities of osmotically active substances (such as glucose or mannitol) cause hyponatremia but not hypotonicity. This condition is known as

translocational hyponatremia. In such states, water is drawn out of cells into extracellular space, diluting the plasma solute and equilibrating osmolar differences. In addition, use of large quantities of irrigant solutions that do not contain sodium (but instead contain glycine, sorbitol, or mannitol) during gynecologic or urologic surgeries can also cause severe hyponatremia.

Adrogue HJ, Madias NE: Hyponatremia. N Engl J Med 342:1581–1589, 2000.

9. **Why do patients with diabetic ketoacidosis frequently present with hyponatremia?**
    Diabetic ketoacidosis is an example of hyperosmotic hyponatremia. In general, serum sodium concentrations decrease by approximately 1.6 mEq/L for every increase of 100 mg/dL over normal glucose levels. In this setting, the serum sodium level should not be interpreted without an accompanying serum glucose measurement, and the appropriate correction should be made if the glucose exceeds 200 mg/dL. Note that a recent study has suggested that this correction factor may be closer to 2.4 mEq/L; however, the key point here is to recognize that serum sodium should be corrected for hyperglycemia in patients with diabetic ketoacidosis, and to do this before any consideration of therapy for the "hyponatremia."

    Hillier TA, Abbott RD, Barrett EJ: Hyponatremia: Evaluating the correction factor for hyperglycemia. Am J Med 106:399–403, 1999.

10. **What is the difference between acute and chronic hyponatremia?**
    - **Acute hyponatremia:** A distinct entity in terms of morbidity and mortality as well as treatment strategies, acute hyponatremia most commonly occurs in the hospital (frequently in the postoperative setting), in psychogenic polydipsia, and in elderly women taking thiazide diuretic agents.
    - **Chronic hyponatremia:** Chronic hyponatremia is defined as having a duration > 48 hours. The majority of patients who present to physicians or to emergency departments with hyponatremia should be assumed to have chronic hyponatremia.

11. **What are the signs and symptoms of hyponatremia?**
    Hyponatremia is the most common electrolyte disorder in hospitalized patients, with a prevalence of about 2.5%. Although the majority of patients are asymptomatic, symptoms do develop in patients with a serum sodium concentration < 125 mEq/L or in whom the sodium has decreased rapidly. Gastrointestinal symptoms of nausea, vomiting, and anorexia occur early, but neuropsychiatric symptoms such as lethargy, confusion, agitation, psychosis, seizure, and coma are more common. Clinical symptoms roughly correlate with the amount and rate of decrease in serum sodium levels.

    Anderson RJ, Chung HM, Kluge R, Schrier RW: Hyponatremia: A prospective analysis of its epidemiology and the pathogenetic role of vasopressin. Ann Intern Med 102:164–168, 1985.

12. **What drugs, if any, are associated with hyponatremia?**
    Many drugs are associated with hyponatremia, but several warrant special note. Thiazide diuretics frequently cause hyponatremia by promoting sodium excretion in excess of water. Selective serotonin reuptake inhibitors cause hyponatremia, and this is thought to occur through the inappropriate release of ADH. Nonsteroidal anti-inflammatory drugs block the production of renal prostaglandins and allow the unopposed action of vasopressin in the kidney, which can lead to water retention. Tricyclic antidepressants and a number of anticonvulsants are associated with hyponatremia. Lastly, use of 3,4-methylenedioxymethamphetamine, or Ecstasy, in particular in combination with consumption of large volumes of water, is associated with severe, life-threatening hyponatremia.

    Adrogue HJ, Madias NE: Hyponatremia. N Engl J Med 342:1581–1589, 2000.
    Budisavljevic MN, Stewart L, Sahn SA, Ploth DW: Hyponatremia associated with 3–4-methylenedioxy-methylamphetamine ("Ectasy") abuse. Am J Med Sci 326:89–93, 2003.

13. Is there a standard therapy for hyponatremia?

Although controversy exists regarding treatment strategies, there is a consensus that not all hyponatremic patients should be treated alike! Duration (acute versus chronic) and the presence or absence of neurologic symptoms should direct therapy. The prescribed therapy must take into consideration the patient's current symptoms and the risk of a demyelinating syndrome with aggressive correction. In patients with acute symptomatic hyponatremia, the risk of delaying treatment and allowing the consequences of cerebral edema to culminate in a seizure and respiratory arrest clearly outweigh any risk of treatment. Hypertonic saline and furosemide (which promotes free water excretion), if needed, should be given until symptoms subside. It is possible to calculate the change in serum sodium concentration based on the amount and volume of sodium infused, and this should be done before the administration of hypertonic saline. In contrast, the asymptomatic chronic hyponatremia patient in high-risk categories (e.g., alcoholism, malnutrition, and liver disease) is at greatest risk for complications of the correction of hyponatremia, namely central pontine myelinolysis. Such patients are best treated with water restriction.

Berl T: Treating hyponatremia: Damned if we do and damned if we don't. Kidney Int 37:1006–1018, 1990.

14. What are some helpful guidelines for treatment of hyponatremia?

In chronic asymptomatic patients, simple free water restriction (i.e., 1000 mL/day) allows a slow and relatively safe correction of serum sodium levels. However, this strategy requires patient compliance, which may be particularly difficult in the outpatient setting. In selected patients who are resistant to free water restriction, an ADH antagonist (e.g., demeclocycline, 600–1200 mg/day) or a maneuver to increase urinary solute excretion may be necessary.

The most difficult therapeutic dilemma is posed by patients with cerebral symptoms and hyponatremia of unknown duration. Such patients are also at risk of a demyelinating disorder if treated too aggressively, yet the presence of symptoms is reflective of central nervous system dysfunction. These patients should be treated with careful (hourly) monitoring of serum sodium levels as hypertonic saline and furosemide are given. The rate of increase should not exceed 1.5 mEq/L/h, and the total increment should not exceed 8–10 mEq/24 h. Acute therapy can be slowed when one of the following endpoints is achieved: (1) symptoms are improved, (2) a "safe" serum sodium level (120–125 mEq/L) is attained (note that if the serum sodium level is extremely low, this may be too aggressive a correction for the first 24 hours).

Adrogue HJ, Madias NE: Hyponatremia. N Engl J Med 342:1581–1589, 2000.
Lin M, Liu SJ, Lim IT: Disorders of water imbalance. Emerg Med Clin North Am 23:749–770, 2005.

15. What is central pontine myelinolysis?

Central pontine myelinolysis is a rare neurologic disorder of unclear etiology characterized by symmetric midline demyelination of the central pons. Extrapontine lesions can occur in the basal ganglia, internal capsule, lateral geniculate body, and cortex. Symptoms include motor abnormalities that can progress to flaccid quadriplegia, respiratory paralysis, pseudobulbar palsy, mental status changes, and coma. Central pontine myelinolysis is often fatal in 3–5 weeks; of the patients who survive, many have significant residual deficits. Alterations in the white matter are best visualized by magnetic resonance imaging. Central pontine myelinolysis is one of the most feared complications of therapy for hyponatremia. Risk factors include a change in serum sodium level of >20–25 mEq/L in 24 hours, correction of serum sodium level to a normal or hypernatremic range, symptomatic and coexistent alcoholism, malnutrition, and liver disease.

Moritz ML, Ayus JC: The pathophysiology and treatment of hyponatremic encephalopathy: An update. Nephrol Dial Transplant 18:2486–2491, 2003.

16. **Can hypernatremia also occur in hypovolemic, euvolemic, and hypervolemic states?**

    Yes, and these categories, based on physical examination, provide a useful framework for understanding and treating patients. However, in contrast to hyponatremia, hypernatremia always reflects an excess of sodium relative to total body water content. Hypovolemic hypernatremia tends to occur in very young and very old persons. It is typically due to extracellular fluid losses and the inability to take in adequate amounts of free water. Febrile illnesses, vomiting, diarrhea, and renal losses are common causes.

    Euvolemic hypernatremia can also be due to extracellular loss of fluid without adequate access to water or from loss of control of water hemostasis. Diabetes insipidus, either central (i.e., inadequate ADH secretion) or nephrogenic (i.e., renal insensitivity to ADH), results in the inability to reabsorb filtered water, which causes systemic hypertonicity but hypo-osmolar urine. Hypervolemic hypernatremia, although uncommon, is iatrogenic. For example, sodium bicarbonate injection during cardiac arrest, administration of hypertonic saline, saline abortions, and inappropriately prepared infant formulas are several examples of induced hypernatremia.

    Adrogue HJ, Madias, NE: Hypernatremia. N Engl J Med 342:1493–1499, 2000.

17. **What are the causes of diabetes insipidus?**

    Central diabetes insipidus can result from trauma, tumors, strokes, granulomatous disease, and central nervous system infections, but it commonly occurs after neurosurgical procedures. Nephrogenic diabetes insipidus can occur in acute or chronic renal failure, hypercalcemia, hypokalemia, and sickle cell disease, or it may be related to drug use (e.g., lithium, demeclocycline).

    Verbalis J: Disorders of body water homeostasis. Best Pract Res Clin Endocrinol Metab 17:471–503, 2003.

18. **What are the signs and symptoms of hypernatremia?**

    In awake and alert patients, thirst is a prominent symptom. Anorexia, nausea, vomiting, altered mental status, agitation, irritability, lethargy, stupor, coma, and neuromuscular hyperactivity are also common symptoms.

19. **What is the best therapy for hypernatremia?**

    The first priority is circulatory stabilization with normal saline in patients with significant volume depletion. Once hypotension has been corrected, patients can be rehydrated with oral water, IV D_5W, or even one-half normal saline. Overly rapid correction of long-standing hypernatremia can result in cerebral edema. Water deficit can be calculated with the formula in question 20. Some investigators have suggested that in patients with long-standing hypernatremia, the water deficit should be corrected by no more than 10 mEq/day or 0.5 mmol/h. If the hypernatremia has occurred over a short period (hours), it can be corrected more rapidly, with the goal of correcting half of the water deficit in the first 24 hours. In patients with central diabetes insipidus, a synthetic analog of ADH (i.e., 1-deamino-8-D-arginine vasopressin [DDAVP]) can be administered, preferably by intranasal route.

20. **What are some helpful formulas for assessing sodium abnormalities?**

    - **Serum osmolality:** $2 [Na^+]$ + glucose/18 + (blood urea nitrogen)/2.8 + ethyl alcohol/4.6
    - **Total body water (TBW):** Body weight × 0.6
    - **TBW excess in hyponatremia:** TBW $(1 - [serum\ Na^+]/140)$
    - **TBW deficit in hypernatremia:** TBW $(serum\ [Na^+]/140 - 1)$

ACKNOWLEDGMENTS

The author would like to acknowledge the contributions of Drs. Stuart Senkfor and Tomas Berl.

UPPER AND LOWER GASTROINTESTINAL BLEEDING IN THE CRITICALLY ILL PATIENT

Jon Yang, MD, MPH, and Fernando Velayos, MD, MPH

CHAPTER 45

1. **What is the anatomic definition of** *upper gastrointestinal (GI) tract bleeding?* **of** *lower GI tract bleeding?*
   Upper GI tract bleeding is defined as hemorrhage originating proximal to the ligament of Treitz. *Lower GI tract bleeding* is defined as hemorrhage originating distal to this point.

2. **Define** *hematemesis, coffee-ground emesis, hematochezia,* **and** *melena.* **How does the presence of any of these features help determine the site and rate of bleeding?**
   Vomiting of blood is called *hematemesis* and indicates bleeding from the upper GI tract. The blood can be fresh and red in color or can be old and appear like coffee grounds. Melena is the passage of black, tarry, and foul-smelling bowel movements due to degradation of blood originating from the upper GI tract; it can rarely signify bleeding from the small bowel or right colon. Hematochezia is the passage of red blood through the rectum and indicates a lower GI tract source; it can indicate rapid transit of blood from the upper GI tract in 10% of cases.

   Rockey DC: Gastrointestinal bleeding. Gastroenterol Clin North Am 34:581–588, 2005.

3. **Is care in the intensive care unit (ICU) required for all patients with GI tract hemorrhage?**
   No. However, patients with evidence of active bleeding, significant abnormalities of vital signs, or other features associated with high mortality should be considered for admission to an ICU for close medical monitoring and urgent endoscopy.

4. **What is the relationship between vital sign abnormalities, volume of blood loss, and severity of bleeding?**
   See Table 45-1.

TABLE 45-1. VITAL SIGNS, VOLUME OF BLOOD LOSS, AND SEVERITY OF BLEEDING		
Vital Signs	Blood Loss (%)	Severity of Bleed
Resting hypotension (shock)	20–25	Massive
Orthostatic hypotension or tachycardia	10–20	Moderate
Normal	<10	Minor

5. **What factors are associated with high mortality rates in patients with upper GI tract hemorrhage?**
   - Age older than 60 years
   - Comorbid conditions (e.g., diabetes, renal failure, coronary artery disease, cancer, liver disease)

- Persistent hypotension
- More than 5 units of transfusion
- Bleeding or rebleeding during hospitalization
- Bloody nasogastric (NG) aspirate
- Need for emergency surgery
- Esophageal varices, bleeding ulcers or those with a visible clot, ulcers > 2 cm in size
- Ulcers located in the lesser curve of the stomach or in the posterior bulb of the duodenum
  Patients with these factors may benefit from early therapeutic endoscopy and ICU-level care.

KEY POINTS: FACTORS ASSOCIATED WITH HIGH MORTALITY RATES IN UPPER GASTROINTESTINAL (GI) TRACT BLEEDING

1. Patients who are older than 60 years tend to have higher mortality rates associated with upper GI tract bleeding.

2. Conditions associated with higher mortality rates include cardiopulmonary disease, liver disease, diabetes, and cancer.

3. Bleeding or rebleeding during hospitalization is associated with higher mortality rates.

4. Persistent hypotension in a patient experiencing upper GI tract bleeding is another factor associated with higher mortality rates.

5. Patients are also at risk for higher mortality rates if more than 5 units of blood are transfused.

6. **What are the top five causes of upper and lower GI tract bleeding?**
   Upper GI source
   - Duodenal ulcers (50%)
   - Gastric erosions (23%)
   - Varices (10%)
   - Mallory-Weiss tear (7%)
   - Esophagitis (6%)

   Lower GI source
   - Diverticulosis (43%)
   - Angiodysplasia (20%)
   - Undetermined (12%)
   - Neoplasia (9%)
   - Colitis (9%)

7. **What are important causes of GI tract bleeding in critically ill patients?**
   Although critically ill patients can have any of the typical causes of bleeding, they are at particular risk for developing stress-induced ulcers in the upper GI tract and hypotension-induced ischemia of the colon.

8. **What is unique about a hospitalized patient who develops GI tract bleeding?**
   Mortality increases to 25% compared with 3.5–7% if bleeding begins before admission. The cause of death typically is not due to the bleeding itself, but rather due to exacerbation of the primary disease process.

9. **What are nine key steps in the management of GI tract hemorrhage?**
   1. Place two large-bore (at least 18-gauge) IV catheters.
   2. Estimate the severity and acuity of bleeding based on vital signs, NG aspirate, and the results of rectal examination.
   3. Begin resuscitation with isotonic saline (and if appropriate, blood products) at a rate commensurate with estimation of blood loss, evidence of ongoing bleeding, and comorbidities.
   4. Consider fresh frozen plasma and platelet transfusions in patients with significant coagulopathy (international normalized ratio > 1.5) or thrombocytopenia (<50,000), respectively.
   5. Consider intubating uncooperative, agitated, or encephalopathic patients at high risk for aspiration from upper GI tract bleeding.
   6. Obtain an NG tube aspirate sample and perform a rectal examination to further localize the source (upper versus lower) and briskness of bleeding.
   7. Start medical therapy with a proton pump inhibitor.
   8. Consider giving a 50-μg IV bolus of octreotide followed by a continuous infusion of 50 μg/h if there is suspicion of bleeding varices.
   9. Perform appropriate diagnostic and therapeutic tests including endoscopy, radionuclide scanning, and angiography and consult with a gastroenterologist and surgeon.

10. **Does a nonbloody NG aspirate sample rule out upper GI tract bleeding?**
    No. Up to 15% of patients with upper GI bleeding may have a nonbloody NG aspirate specimen. This can occur when the tip of the NG tube is located in the esophagus or when a competent pyloric sphincter does not allow blood from a duodenal ulcer to reflux back into the stomach. Thus, patients with hematochezia, hemodynamic instability, and a negative NG aspirate test result should still be considered for immediate upper endoscopy.

11. **Does passage of an NG tube in a patient with varices precipitate bleeding?**
    No. There is no evidence to support the idea that passage of an NG tube precipitates bleeding by traumatizing a varix.

12. **What is the role of endoscopy in the management of upper GI tract bleeding?**
    Endoscopy is important in diagnosing and treating common causes of GI tract hemorrhage. Ulcers in the stomach or duodenum are treated either with thermal contact methods (e.g., heater probe, electrocoagulation) or injection with a variety of substances (e.g., epinephrine, saline, sclerosing agents such as alcohol). Varices are treated with endoscopic band ligation or with injection of sclerosing agents such as ethanolamine oleate. Urgent endoscopic therapy of varices and ulcers reduces length of hospital stay, incidence of further rebleeding, and need for surgery and improves survival rates.

13. **How does ulcer appearance help predict rebleeding/mortality and guide management?**
    See Table 45-2.

14. **What is the role of endoscopy in the management of lower GI tract bleeding?**
    Urgent colonoscopy for acute lower GI tract bleeding is less established than urgent esophagogastroduodenoscopy (EGD) is for acute upper GI tract bleeding. Diverticula and vascular ectasias may be scattered throughout the colon, and finding the culprit lesion can be difficult if there is active bleeding or if the colon is inadequately prepared. Forty-two percent of patients with acute lower GI tract bleeding have more than one potential bleeding source identified at colonoscopy. Some centers have investigated rapid purge followed by urgent colonoscopy within 12 hours of presentation and have reported success in identifying and treating the culprit lesion. Colonoscopy within 24 hours may be a more reasonable target

TABLE 45-2. ULCER APPEARANCE, REBLEEDING/MORTALITY, AND MANAGEMENT

	Appearance	Prevalence (%)	Rebleed (%)	Mortality (%)	Endoscopic Therapy	Medical Therapy
Lowest risk	Clean base	42	5	2	None needed	Oral PPI
	Flat spot	20	10	3	None needed	Oral PPI
	Adherent clot	17	22	7	Controversial	Oral/IV PPI
	Visible vessel	17	43	11	Yes	PPI infusion
Highest risk	Active bleeding	18	55	11	Yes	PPI infusion

PPI = proton pump inhibitor, IV = intravenous.
Adapted from Laine L, Peterson WL: Bleeding peptic ulcer. N Engl J Med 331:717–727, 1994.

whereby the patient can be adequately resuscitated and bowel preparation can be performed. Stratification into low- and high-risk groups for rebleeding has been established for EGD but not yet for colonoscopy.

Green BT, Rockey DC: Lower gastrointestinal bleeding-management. Gastroenterol Clin North Am 34:665–678, 2005.

15. **What is the role of tagged red blood cell (RBC) scan and angiography in the management of lower GI tract bleeding?**
    If blood loss is brisk enough to adversely affect the quality of the colonoscopy, a tagged RBC scan followed by angiography can assist in localizing and treating a bleeding lesion in the lower GI tract. Tagged RBC scan is more sensitive than angiography in detecting bleeding but is less accurate in localizing the bleeding. It does not provide therapeutic capabilities. It can detect 0.1 mL/min of blood loss. Angiography is superior to tagged RBC scan in localizing the source of bleeding and providing therapy but is less sensitive in detecting blood loss. It can detect 0.5 mL/min of blood loss.

16. **What is a "stress ulcer"?**
    A stress ulcer is part of a spectrum of mucosal lesions in the stomach and duodenum more currently named *stress-related mucosal disease* (SRMD). These lesions range from diffuse superficial erosions to deep ulcers.

17. **Who first described stress ulcers? Are these ulcers the same as those seen in SRMD?**
    Stress ulcers were initially described by Curling in patients with extensive burns and by Cushing in patients after severe central nervous system trauma. Cushing's ulcers are an interesting subset of SRMD because they are always associated with elevated gastrin and gastric acid secretion. In comparison, SRMD can occur with high, normal, or low acid output.

18. **How common is clinically important GI tract bleeding from SRMD?**
    In a prospective study of 2252 patients, the incidence of SRMD in an ICU population was 1.5%.

19. When should SRMD be suspected?
SRMD should be suspected in an ICU patient with overt bleeding complicated by hemodynamic instability or with occult bleeding resulting in a decrease in hematocrit or a need for blood transfusion.

20. What are the pathophysiologic factors contributing to SRMD?
Three important factors in SRMD are gastric acid secretion, mucosal ischemia, and reflux of bile into the stomach. Mucosal ischemia leads to impaired protection of the gastric epithelium against acid due to reduction in prostaglandins and the synthesis of alkaline-rich mucus.

21. What are risk factors for SRMD?
In a meta-analysis of 2252 patients, Cook and colleagues identified mechanical ventilation and coagulopathy as the two main risk factors for SRMD. The presence of additional risk factors such as hypotension, sepsis, liver failure, renal failure, extensive burns, or trauma proportionally increased the risk of significant stress-related hemorrhage. As may be expected, increasing severity of underlying illness correlates with increasing risk of clinically significant stress-related bleeding.

22. How can SRMD be prevented?
Maintaining a gastric pH above 4 has been shown to prevent SRMD. Antacids, H_2-receptor antagonists (H_2RA), and proton pump inhibitors (PPI) have all been investigated with this strategy in mind. Sucralfate is thought to work primarily as a cytoprotective agent, although stimulation of several growth factors implicated in ulcer healing may be its true mechanism of action. H_2RAs have been found to be significantly better than placebo, antacids, and sucralfate in reducing the incidence of clinically significant bleeding due to SRMD. Several small studies have suggested PPIs are superior to H_2RA for prophylaxis against SRMD. Unlike H_2RA, PPIs do not appear to develop tolerance with sustained therapy. Although the efficacy of PPIs is well recognized, they have not been approved as prophylaxis associated with stress ulceration.

Stollman N, Metz DC: Pathophysiology and prophylaxis of stress ulcer in intensive care unit patients. J Crit Care 20:35–45, 2005.

23. What is ischemic colitis?
Ischemic colitis constitutes a wide spectrum of injury to the colon due to compromised arterial inflow. The spectrum of injury extends from reversible colonopathy (e.g., submucosal or intramural hemorrhage, transient colitis) to irreversible disease (e.g., chronic ulcerating colitis, fulminant universal colitis, stricture, gangrene).

Brandt LJ, Boley SJ: AGA technical review on intestinal ischemia. American Gastrointestinal Association. Gastroenterology 118:954–968, 2000.

24. How is the diagnosis of ischemic colitis made?
Many features are variable and nonspecific. Clinically, patients often have crampy, left lower quadrant abdominal pain with passage of bright red or maroon blood usually not sufficient to require transfusion. Depending on whether the insult remains present, superficial ischemia can extend and produce transmural ischemia, abdominal distention, gangrene, and peritonitis. Plain abdominal film may demonstrate "thumb printing," indicating submucosal edema. A computed tomography scan of the abdomen may reveal a thickened colonic wall in the affected area or may demonstrate pneumatosis (i.e., air in the wall of the colon). There are no serum tests to help diagnose early ischemic colitis. Serum lactate, acidosis, lactate dehydrogenase, creatine phosphokinase, and amylase levels are typically elevated in the presence of advanced and severe ischemic damage. A colonoscopy or sigmoidoscopy can make the definitive diagnosis; however, these modalities are contraindicated if a patient has peritonitis or has significant colonic transmural involvement.

25. **What are the risk factors for ischemic colitis?**

In the ICU, ischemic colitis tends to occur in middle-aged or elderly patients with atherosclerotic disease (e.g., coronary artery disease, peripheral artery disease) in the setting of hypotension, shock in combination with vasoconstrictive drugs, or recent surgical repair of the aorta (particularly aneurysm repair). Ischemic colitis complicates 7% of elective aortic surgical repairs and 60% of surgeries for ruptured abdominal aortic aneurysms. Ischemic colitis is responsible for approximately 10% of deaths after aortic reconstruction.

26. **What areas of the colon are at greatest risk for ischemia?**

Colonic ischemia resulting from a low-flow state most commonly affects the right colon and is involved in 68% of hypotension-associated ischemic colitis. The arterial anatomy of the right colon contributes to this increased risk because a marginal artery formed from branches of the superior mesenteric artery is incompletely developed or absent in 25–75% of people. This results in fewer end vessels supplying oxygen to the right colon. Low-flow states can also affect the "watershed" areas in the splenic flexure or rectosigmoid junction because of poor collateral flow present in 10% of the population. Occlusion of the inferior mesenteric artery produces ischemia in the sigmoid colon, the area most remote from collateral flow.

27. **What area of the colon is at lowest risk for ischemia?**

The rectum rarely becomes ischemic because of its rich collateral flow between the inferior mesenteric artery and the internal iliac circulation.

28. **What is the treatment of ischemic colitis?**

Most ischemic colitis is reversible and associated with a low mortality. If there is no evidence of gangrene or perforation, treatment of suspected nonocclusive ischemic colitis is primarily supportive. Patients with iatrogenic occlusion, such as occurs after aortic surgery, may require repeat surgery and revascularization. Patients with evidence of transmural injury or perforation require emergent laparotomy. Mortality is greatly increased by the need for surgery.

CHAPTER 46

ACUTE PANCREATITIS

E. Matt Ritter, MD, MAJ, USAF, MC, and Mark W. Bowyer, MD, DMCC, COL, USAF, MC

1. **What is acute pancreatitis?**
   Acute pancreatitis is an acute noninfectious inflammatory condition of the pancreas caused by interstitial release of activated enzymes of the exocrine pancreas leading to autodigestion of the pancreas and surrounding tissues. The clinical course can range from a mild disease to multiorgan failure and sepsis.

2. **How is *severe acute pancreatitis* (SAP) defined?**
   SAP is an episode of acute pancreatitis associated with either local or systemic complications. Local complications include necrosis, hemorrhage, peripancreatic fluid collection, or pseudocyst. Systemic complications include the development of the systemic inflammatory response syndrome or the onset of organ system dysfunction associated with the episode of pancreatitis (i.e., renal failure or pulmonary failure). SAP should be treated in an intensive care setting.

   Nathens AB, Curtis JR, Beale RJ, et al: Management of the critically ill patient with acute pancreatitis. Crit Care Med 32:2524–2536, 2004.

3. **What are the causes of acute pancreatitis?**
   Variation in the frequency is quite marked from series to series and depends on the referral population. Gallstones (40–60%) and alcohol (35–70%) are the two most common etiologies in nearly all reported series. Miscellaneous causes of acute pancreatitis can include toxins, trauma, metabolic factors, or other less common causes. Toxins include methyl alcohol, organophosphorus insecticides, and scorpion venom. More than 80 different medications have been reported to cause pancreatitis including acetaminophen, angiotensin-converting enzyme inhibitors, furosemide, tetracycline, aminosalicylic acid, corticosteroids, procainamide, thiazides, metronidazole, and ranitidine, among others. The metabolic disorder most often associated with acute pancreatitis is hypertriglyceridemia (especially type V hyperlipoproteinemia) especially with levels in excess of 1000 mg/dL. Hypercalcemia has also been associated with pancreatitis in rare cases—typically in the setting of hyperparathyroidism.

KEY POINTS: "BAD TIME" MNEMONIC FOR COMMON CAUSES OF ACUTE PANCREATITIS

B: Biliary—gallstones, parasites, or malignancy

A: Alcohol

D: Drugs

T: Trauma, toxins

I: Idiopathic, ischemic, infectious, inherited

M: Metabolic—hyperlipidemia, hypercalcemia

E: Endoscopic retrograde cholangiopancreatography

4. **How does a patient with acute pancreatitis present?**
   A typical presentation for acute pancreatitis includes acute onset of severe epigastric pain boring through to the back. Associated symptoms frequently include nausea and vomiting. Classic physical findings of early acute pancreatitis include epigastric tenderness and elevated temperature or fever. Severe cases may present with signs and symptoms of septic shock including hemodynamic instability and organ system failure. Delayed physical finding in SAP can include Grey-Turner and Cullen's signs (*see* question 5).

5. **What is the Grey-Turner sign or Cullen's sign?**
   The Grey-Turner sign is the flank ecchymosis that is classically associated with retroperitoneal hemorrhage. This finding in the setting of acute pancreatitis is indicative of severe pancreatitis and will usually not be present for 3–7 days after onset of pain. Cullen's sign is the periumbilical ecchymosis that may be present in severe necrotizing pancreatitis or other causes of retroperitoneal hemorrhage. It is similar in significance to the Grey-Turner sign.

6. **What laboratory tests aid in the diagnosis of acute pancreatitis?**
   Serum amylase and lipase are the most commonly used *diagnostic* markers for acute pancreatitis. During the first 24 hours, an elevated amylase level has a sensitivity of 81–84%. By the second day, the sensitivity of amylase drops to 33%. The specificity of hyperamylasemia is low because it also may be caused by perforated peptic ulcers, bowel infarctions, salivary gland trauma, renal failure, and macroamylasemia. Serum lipase measurement is more specific than amylase and has a sensitivity of 85–100%; after 4 days it remains elevated in 90% of patients. Recent reports suggest that lipase is the more accurate test in acute pancreatitis, and some authors argue that obtaining both is not warranted. The degree of elevation of neither amylase nor lipase correlates with disease severity.

7. **How should imaging be used in the diagnosis of acute pancreatitis?**
   Imaging modalities can be used to confirm the diagnosis of acute pancreatitis, to search for etiologies, and to document and manage certain complications. Ultrasound interrogation of the abdomen can document the presence or absence of gallstones and biliary ductal dilation. Abdominal contrast-enhanced computed tomography (CT) can help differentiate acute pancreatitis from other causes of epigastric pain such as severe cholecystitis or complicated ulcer disease. CT scanning can also demonstrate complications of pancreatitis such as necrosis, abscess, or pseudocyst. Image-guided percutaneous interventions may be an option for the management of some of these conditions (*see* question 18).

   Romero-Urquhart G, Phillips J: Acute pancreatitis. eMedicine, June 23, 2004: www.emedicine.com/radio/topic521.htm

8. **When should imaging studies be performed?**
   If the diagnosis of acute pancreatitis is in doubt, imaging may be required immediately to exclude other causes of acute epigastric pain. In the setting of a known diagnosis, a delay in obtaining imaging, particularly CT scanning, is potentially beneficial. Delay of 48–72 hours after the onset of symptoms allows time for the demarcation of pancreatic necrosis, and the sensitivity of CT scanning for diagnosis of pancreatic necrosis approaches 100% after 4 days. Additionally, delay in CT imaging allows for fluid resuscitation and thus potentially reduces the likelihood of contrast-induced renal failure. There are also anecdotal reports of exacerbation of early pancreatic necrosis when scanning was obtained within the first 24 hours of illness.

   Clancy TE, Benoit EP, Ashley SW: Current management of acute pancreatitis. J Gastrointest Surg 9:440–452, 2005.

9. **What imaging options exist for patients with a contrast sensitivity or marginal renal function?**

   Magnetic resonance imaging (MRI) can detect the presence and extent of necrosis and peripancreatic fluid collections as well as CT. MRI requires the administration of gadolinium to detect necrosis. The fact that gadolinium is nontoxic in comparison with the ionized contrast agents required for CT increases the attractiveness of MRI in some patients. CT retains the advantages of lower cost, greater availability, and the ability to perform interventional procedures. MRI can also be cumbersome for critically ill patients due to the requirement for nonmetallic ventilators, beds, and infusion apparatus.

10. **What methods are available to estimate the severity and prognosis of acute pancreatitis?**

   The natural history of acute pancreatitis ranges from a mild self-limiting process to a fulminant, rapidly lethal disease. Early identification of the severity of disease, therefore, is important to permit the appropriate application of monitoring and invasive therapeutic measures. Several clinical criteria systems have been developed, including Ranson's criteria, Glasgow criteria, and the Acute Physiology and Chronic Health Evaluation (APACHE) II system. CT findings have also been used to estimate severity and have been correlated with mortality and complication rates. Ranson's criteria (Table 46-1) and the Balthazar CT severity index (Table 46-2) are the most

TABLE 46-1. RANSON'S PROGNOSTIC SIGNS

	Etiology of Pancreatitis	
	Nongallstone	Gallstone
At initial presentation		
Age (yr)	>55	>70
White blood cell count	>16 k	>18 k
Glucose (mg/dL)	>200	>220
Lactate dehydrogenase	>350	>400
Aspartate	>250	>250
During first 48 hours		
Decrease in hematocrit	>10	>10
Elevation in blood urea nitrogen (mg/dL)	>5	>2
Serum total calcium	<8.0	<8.0
Partial pressure of oxygen (mmHg)	<60	NA
Base deficit (mmol/L)	>4	>5
Fluid sequestration (L)	>6	>4

Prognosis	No. of Criteria Met	Predicted Mortality
	2 or less	0.9%
	3–4	16%
	5–6	40%
	7–8	100%

Adapted from Ranson JHC, Rifkind KM, Roses DF, et al: Prognostic signs and the role of operative management in acute pancreatitis. Surg Gynecol Obstet 139:69–81, 1974; and Ranson JHC: Etiological and prognostic factors in human acute pancreatitis: A review. Am J Gastroenterol 77:633–638, 1982.

TABLE 46-2. BALTHAZAR COMPUTED TOMOGRAPHY (CT) GRADING OF ACUTE PANCREATITIS AND CT SEVERITY INDEX

Grade	Description of CT Findings
A	Normal pancreas
B	Enlarged pancreas
C	Inflammation of pancreas or peripancreatic fat
D	One peripancreatic fluid collection
E	More than one peripancreatic fluid collection and/or air in retroperitoneum

		Necrosis Factor	
CT Grade	Points	% Necrosis	Points Added
A	0	0	0
B	1	0	0
C	2	<30	2
D	3	30–50	4
E	4	>50	6

Severity index = CT grade points + necrosis points

Severity index	% Morbidity	% Mortality
0–3	8	3
4–6	35	6
7–10	92	17

Adapted from Balthazar EJ: Acute pancreatitis: Assessment of severity with clinical and CT evaluation. Radiology 223:603–613, 2002.

commonly used systems. In addition to these scoring systems, several isolated indicators of prognosis have been reported. These include serum levels of C-reactive protein, interleukins 6 and 8, and trypsinogen activation peptide. Although many of these have shown promise, validation has been scant and assays for many of these markers are unreliable or not universally available.

11. **How is acute pancreatitis treated?**
Currently, the most important measures in the treatment of pancreatitis are supportive and symptomatic. The pain associated with acute pancreatitis may be severe, and IV narcotics are often required. Because pancreatitis is often associated with massive fluid shifts, monitoring and adequate replacement of intravascular fluid is essential. A urethral catheter should be placed; if the patient has underlying cardiovascular disease, invasive monitoring of intravascular volume status may be needed to ensure adequate resuscitation and to prevent renal failure. Because respiratory failure is a frequent feature of acute pancreatitis, serial arterial blood gas analyses

should be performed with early intubation and positive pressure ventilation, if needed, to maintain oxygenation. Nutritional depletion is very common in conjunction with severe acute pancreatitis, and nutritional support should be implemented early in the disease process.

2. How should nutritional support be delivered to patients with acute pancreatitis?
In patients with mild pancreatitis, enteral nutrition is routinely withheld for up to 7 days to allow pancreatic stimulation to be minimized. In patients with SAP, oral intake may not be possible for weeks and alternate nutritional support should be instituted. Traditionally, the parenteral route has been used in an attempt to minimize pancreatic stimulation, but benefits of enteral delivery include maintenance of intestinal immune function and potential reduction in bacterial translocation. Recently, several reports on the use of enteral jejunal feeding have shown that infection rates, requirement for surgical intervention, and length of hospital stay were lower in patients fed enterally without a clear benefit for mortality. Based on these data, many now feel that jejunal enteral feeding is the mode of choice in these patients.

Marik PE, Zaloga GP: Meta analysis of parenteral nutrition versus enteral nutrition in patients with acute pancreatitis. BMJ 328:1407, 2004.

3. Do antisecretory medications aid in the treatment of acute pancreatitis?
It has been postulated that the inhibition of pancreatic secretions ameliorates the course of pancreatitis. Inhibition of pancreatic secretions by anticholinergics or somatostatin has failed to show significant benefit in controlled clinical trials. Several agents, including apoprotein, soybean trypsin inhibitor, camostat, and fresh frozen plasma, have been studied as inhibitors of pancreatic enzymes without clear benefit.

4. What role do antibiotics play in the treatment of acute pancreatitis?
This is one of the most controversial topics to arise during discussion of the management of acute pancreatitis. When sterile pancreatic necrosis becomes infected pancreatic necrosis, the mortality rate rises from 10% to 25% to as high as 70%. Thus, prevention of the secondary infection of pancreatic necrosis is the main focus of the use of antibiotics for acute pancreatitis. Six randomized controlled trials have reported on the effect of various prophylactic regimens, with mixed results. The only double-blind study reported to date showed no decrease in infection rates or mortality with a prophylactic antibiotic regimen. Questions have been raised with regard to increased rates of fungal infection with routine prophylactic antibiotic use as well as development of antibiotic resistance. Currently there is no consensus among experts with respect to the routine use of prophylactic antibiotics, and this practice is not well supported by the currently available literature.

Golub R, Siddiqi F, Pohl D: Role of antibiotics in acute pancreatitis: A meta-analysis. J Gastrointest Surg 2:496–503, 1998.
Isenmann R, Runzi M, Kron M, et al: Prophylactic antibiotic treatment in patients with predicted severe acute pancreatitis: A placebo-controlled double-blind trial. Gastroenterology 126:997–1004, 2004.
Sharma VK, Howden CW: Prophylactic antibiotic administration reduces sepsis and mortality in acute necrotizing pancreatitis: A meta-analysis. Pancreas 22:28–31, 2001.

5. List the most common bacteria responsible for infected pancreatic necrosis.
Infection of pancreatic necrosis typically involves mono- or polymicrobial infections from gastrointestinal flora. The most common organisms include the following:
Escherichia coli (35%)
Klebsiella pneumoniae (24%)
Enterococcus species (24%)
Staphylococcus species (14%)
Pseudomonas species (11%)

Lumsden A, Bradley EL III: Secondary pancreatic infections. Surg Gynecol Obstet 170:459–467, 1990.

16. **When is surgery indicated in the treatment of acute pancreatitis?**

    In the majority of patients with mild pancreatitis, surgical intervention is typically reserved for the management of delayed complications such as a pseudocyst or prevention of recurrent disease through elective cholecystectomy. In patients with SAP, surgical intervention is typically reserved for the management of necrosis. When infected pancreatic necrosis is confirmed or strongly suspected on the basis of poor clinical response to treatment, surgical débridement (i.e., necrosectomy) should be performed. Although the simple presence of necrosis was a traditional indication for surgery, sterile necrosis is currently routinely managed nonoperatively. In all patients with SAP, operative placement of a feeding jejunostomy can greatly simplify nutritional support if enteral nutrition is to be used.

17. **How is pancreatic necrosectomy performed?**

    Tenants of surgical management of infected pancreatic necrosis include débridement of all infected necrotic material and drainage of the remaining pancreatic bed. Adequate débridement frequently requires multiple trips to the operating room. Drainage options include leaving the abdomen open with direct packing to the pancreatic bed and closure of the abdomen over multiple large closed sump drains with or without irrigation. Often some combination of the two techniques is used. These patients are usually critically ill and require vigorous supportive care.

18. **Is there a role for minimally invasive or image-guided therapy in the treatment of acute pancreatitis?**

    Image-guided techniques are being used increasingly often in patients with acute pancreatitis. CT-guided fine-needle aspiration of pancreatic necrosis is the method of choice to distinguish sterile from infected necrosis. Similarly, percutaneous image-guided drainage is used routinely to treat peripancreatic fluid collections that have developed into abscess. Flexible endoscopic and laparoscopic approaches are routinely used to manage delayed complications such as persistent pseudocyst. These less invasive approaches have been reported for the treatment of pancreatic necrosis but have not gained widespread acceptance. Open surgical necrosectomy and drainage is still considered the gold standard for the treatment of infected pancreatic necrosis.

19. **What is the role of early endoscopic retrograde cholangiopancreatography (ERCP) and sphincterotomy in the treatment of acute biliary pancreatitis?**

    A review of the available current literature yields the following recommendations with regard to the use of ERCP in the treatment of acute pancreatitis:

    - Early ERCP (within 24–72 hours of onset of symptoms) is safe in patients with a predicted severe episode of suspected acute biliary pancreatitis.
    - Early ERCP (and sphincterotomy, when bile duct stones are found) results in diminished biliary sepsis among patients with suspected biliary pancreatitis, especially those with a predicted severe attack. Diminished biliary sepsis, in turn, results in improved outcomes in this subgroup of patients.
    - Early ERCP (and sphincterotomy, when common bile duct stones are found) results in decreased complication rates in patients with acute biliary pancreatitis and a predicted severe attack.
    - At present, early ERCP should not be performed in patients with a predicted mild attack of acute pancreatitis of suspected biliary etiology.

    Barkun AN: Early endoscopic management of acute gallstone pancreatitis: An evidence-based review. J Gastrointest Surg 5:243–250, 2001.

20. **What are pancreatic pseudocysts?**

    Pancreatic pseudocysts are encapsulated collections of fluid with high enzyme concentrations that arise from the pancreas typically after either a bout of acute pancreatitis or pancreatic trauma. The walls of the pseudocyst are formed by inflammatory fibrosis of peritoneal, mesenteric, and serosal membranes. The term *pseudocyst* denotes the absence of an epithelial lining. Pseudocysts develop in about 2% of cases of acute pancreatitis. The cysts are single in 85% of cases and multiple in the remainder.

21. **How should pancreatic pseudocysts be managed?**
    Asymptomatic pseudocysts require no specific treatment. After acute pancreatitis, 25–50% of pseudocysts resolve spontaneously. Those that persist for more than 6 weeks may require treatment. Recent data based on two retrospective studies suggest that persistent pseudocysts of any size that remain asymptomatic require no treatment. Symptomatic pseudocysts typically are characterized by pain, fever, weight loss, tenderness, and a palpable mass. Symptomatic pseudocysts can be treated with internal drainage into the stomach or small bowel. Laparoscopic, flexible endoscopic, and open surgical approaches are all successfully used to perform either cyst gastrostomy, cyst duodenoscopy, or cyst jejunostomy. External drainage by image-guided percutaneous access is also reported but is generally less successful than the methods of internal drainage described previously.

CHAPTER 47

HEPATITIS AND CIRRHOSIS

Kullada O. Pichakron, MD, and Jon Perlstein, MD

1. **What is hepatitis?**
   Hepatitis is any inflammatory process that involves the liver parenchyma and may result in anything from mere laboratory abnormalities to a fulminant illness with mortality. The most common etiologic factor is viral.

2. **Which viruses are responsible for hepatitis?**
   Viral hepatitis may be caused by the A, B, C, D, and E hepatitis viruses; the Epstein-Barr virus; and the cytomegalovirus. A non-A–E hepatitis virus, hepatitis G, has been recently described. In general, it tends to yield clinical pictures similar to that of viruses A–E, ranging from asymptomatic to a rarely severe fulminant illness.

   Center for Disease Control: Viral hepatitis: www.cdc.gov/ncidod/diseases/hepatitis/
   Fox RK, Wright TL: Viral hepatitis. In Friedman SL, McQuaid KR, Grendell JH (eds): Current Diagnosis and Treatment in Gastroenterology, 2nd ed. New York, Lange, 2003, pp 546–549.

3. **What are the characteristics of hepatitis A?**
   The hepatitis A virus is an enterovirus of the family Picornaviridae, which causes an enterically transmitted disease acquired by ingestion of material that has had fecal contamination. The virus passes through the stomach, replicates in the lower intestine, is transported to the liver, and begins to replicate in the cytoplasm. Cellular damage in the parenchyma occurs as the body's immunologic defenses attempt to kill the virus.
   The average incubation period to onset of symptoms is about 32 days but ranges between 3 and 6 weeks. Classically, there is a prodromal phase during which malaise, anorexia, epigastric or right upper quadrant pain, fever, rashes, diarrhea, and constipation are frequent complaints. The disease is usually recognized during the icteric phase when dark urine and jaundice prompt patients to seek medical attention. Liver tests at this time reveal elevated transaminase and bilirubin levels, and the clinical diagnosis can be confirmed by the detection of the immunoglobulin M antibody to the virus.
   The severity of the illness is age related. Older adults tend to have worse symptoms than young adults. Most cases of acute hepatitis A resolve rapidly over several weeks with complete clinical and biochemical recovery.

   Fox RK, Wright TL: Viral hepatitis. In Friedman SL, McQuaid KR, Grendell JH (eds): Current Diagnosis and Treatment in Gastroenterology, 2nd ed. New York, Lange, 2003 pp 546–549.

4. **What are the characteristics of hepatitis B?**
   The hepatitis B virus (HBV) is the prototype of a new class of viruses, the Hepadnaviridae. Clinical expression of infection with HBV may range from a carrier state to fulminant hepatic failure (FHF). In classic acute hepatitis B, the incubation period varies from 60 to 180 days. As with hepatitis A, there is a prodromal phase. However, in HBV infection, this phase is more insidious and prolonged, with the addition of arthritis and urticarial rash as symptoms. As in hepatitis A, symptoms tend to improve with the onset of jaundice. During the icteric phase, the bilirubin tends to rise less steeply than in hepatitis A but reaches higher peak levels. The jaundice also lasts longer. There is a slower rise in the aminotransferase levels, which peak much later than in hepatitis A.

Unlike hepatitis A, acute hepatitis B may develop into chronic hepatitis and cirrhosis. Patients may also have an asymptomatic infection without liver disease (i.e., healthy carriers).

HBV infection can be spread via parenteral transmission. Blood is the most effective vehicle for transmission, but the virus is present in other bodily fluids as well (e.g., saliva and semen). HBV infection is a common problem among IV drug abusers, homosexual men, and the sexual partners of infected patients. Vertical transmission may occur to infants from mothers who experience hepatitis B infection during the last trimester of pregnancy.

Ganem D, Prince AM. Hepatitis B virus infection: Natural history and clinical consequences. N Engl J Med 350:1118–1129, 2004.

5. **What laboratory tests are available for hepatitis B? How are they interpreted?**
Sensitive immunoassays are available to measure the antigens associated with HBV and the antibodies it induces. The antigenic activity of the virus DNA core is designated HBc (core) antigen (Ag). The surface coat of the virus has distinctive antigenicity and is designated HBs (surface) Ag. These antigens evoke specific antibodies, and both constitute the important immunologic markers of the HBV infection and its course.

During a typical case of acute hepatitis B, HBsAg is first detected in the blood during the incubation period as early as 1 week after infection. The HBsAg level begins to decline after the onset of the illness and usually becomes undetectable within 3 months of exposure. The presence of HBsAg in serum indicates infectious potential. Anti-HBc appears in the serum toward the end of the incubation period and persists during the acute illness and for several months to years thereafter. Anti-HBs is detected during convalescence, several weeks to months after the disappearance of HBsAg. This persists for a prolonged time. A high titer of anti-HBs confirms immunity to HBV. The persistence of HBsAg is a sign of chronic hepatitis B.

Ganem D, Prince AM: Hepatitis B virus infection: Natural history and clinical consequences. N Engl J Med 350:1118–1129, 2004.

6. **What are the characteristics of hepatitis C?**
Hepatitis C is the name given to a single-stranded RNA virus distantly related to the flavivirus. The hepatitis C virus is the major cause of post-transfusion, community-acquired, cryptogenic hepatitis. Until the availability of serologic tests, it was responsible for 90–95% of all cases of post-transfusion hepatitis.

The incubation period to the rise in aminotransferases is 6–8 weeks. Symptoms are usually of moderate severity, but many cases (40–75%) are asymptomatic. Jaundice is uncommon (10%) and usually mild. There is a high rate of progression to chronic hepatitis and subsequent cirrhosis. Early identification of infection is difficult. Alanine aminotransferase levels are more likely to be elevated than aspartate aminotransferase.

7. **What laboratory test can be performed to detect the hepatitis C virus at the earliest point in the disease course?**
Hepatitis C RNA can be detected by polymerase chain reaction by 1 week after exposure.

Lauer GM, Walker BD: Hepatitis C virus infection. N Engl J Med 345:41–52, 2001.
Pearlman BL: Hepatitis C infection: A clinical review. South Med J 97:365–373, 2004.

8. **What are the characteristics of hepatitis D?**
Hepatitis D (delta agent) is an incomplete RNA viral particle similar to plant viruses that requires the presence of HBV for infection and replication to occur. Infection can occur only in HBsAg carriers exposed to the delta agent or in patients who are simultaneously infected with both HBV and hepatitis D virus. Acute simultaneous infection may be associated with fulminant hepatitis. Chronic infection with hepatitis D is frequently associated with chronic active hepatitis or cirrhosis.

9. **What is hepatitis E?**

   The hepatitis E virus produces a water-borne, fecal–oral-spread disease similar to, but generally milder than, hepatitis A. It has an average incubation period of 40 days and is epidemic in a number of developing countries. Fulminant hepatitis may occur, especially among pregnant women, with a mortality rate approaching 20%.

   World Health Organization: Hepatitis E: www.who.int/mediacentre/factsheets/fs280/en/

10. **What is hepatitis G?**

    Hepatitis G virus (HGV) is a unique virus that can be transmitted hematogenously. The association of hepatitis G with disease remains unclear, but it is estimated that approximately 0.3% of patients with acute viral hepatitis may be attributed solely to HGV. Persistent HGV infection appears to be quite prevalent in the general population; 1.2–13% of blood donors and 14–52% of patients with other forms of viral hepatitis test positive for HGV RNA.

    Alter HJ, Nakatsuji Y, Melpolder J, et al: The incidence of transfusion-associated hepatitis G virus infection and its relation to liver disease. N Engl J Med 336:747–754, 1997.
    Narayanan MKV: Non–A to E hepatitis. Curr Opin Infect Dis 15:529–534, 2002.

11. **What is cholestatic hepatitis?**

    Chronic viral hepatitis—or systemic inflammatory response syndrome—may result in a cholestatic process diagnosed by jaundice, pruritus, and elevated direct bilirubin and alkaline phosphatase levels. The etiology of this condition is canalicular dysfunction resulting from the viral infection and/or inflammatory response. Most episodes of cholestatic hepatitis are self-limited; however, extrahepatic biliary obstruction should be considered as a potential etiology as well.

12. **What is fulminant viral hepatitis?**

    Fulminant hepatitis occurs in about 1% of cases of acute viral hepatitis requiring hospitalization. In fulminant hepatitis, massive hepatocellular necrosis occurs and is thought to be related to an abnormally rapid clearance of the viral antigens. Hepatitis B accounts for approximately 50% of cases, hepatitis C for 45%, and hepatitis A for 5%. Fulminant hepatitis can also occur with a variety of hepatotoxic drugs and uncommon diseases. The end product is FHF. FHF is manifested by signs and symptoms of encephalopathy within 3–8 weeks of the onset of illness. A profound coagulopathy occurs as a result of poor hepatic synthetic function; this is best assessed with the prothrombin time. If the prothrombin time exceeds control by 10 seconds despite vitamin K supplementation, FHF has evolved. Renal failure due to volume depletion and cerebral edema are frequent sequelae of FHF.

13. **What are the cardiovascular changes associated with FHF? What is the treatment?**

    The typical cardiovascular changes associated with hepatic failure are decreased peripheral resistance and increased cardiac output (hyperdynamic state). The increased cardiac output is believed to be a result of the opening of myocutaneous vascular shunts. Pulmonary artery catheters are very useful in managing patients with this condition. Physiologically, the best method for treating the hyperdynamic state is by increasing peripheral vascular resistance. Dopamine and the α-adrenergic agents can be used, but one must monitor for tachyphylaxis and gastrointestinal bleeding. Clinical investigations are ongoing to study the use of levadopa to indirectly replete norepinephrine to the sympathetic nerve terminals.

    American College of Surgeons: Critical Care: Hepatic Failure: www.acssurgery.com/acs/pdf/ACS0809.pdf
    Keefe EB: Acute liver failure. In Friedman SL, McQuaid KR, Grendell JH (eds): Current Diagnosis and Treatment in Gastroenterology, 2nd ed. New York, Lange, 2003, pp 536–545.

14. **What are the electrolyte disturbances associated with FHF? What are the treatments?**

Electrolyte disorders associated with cirrhosis and hepatic failure are hyponatremia and hypokalemia. The hyponatremia is usually dilutional as a result of decreased renal water excretion. The hypokalemia results from increased urinary excretion of potassium secondary to the influence of aldosterone and gastrointestinal losses.

These abnormalities are best treated with fluid and sodium restriction. The aldosterone antagonist spironolactone increases water loss more than sodium loss. Additionally, it decreases renal potassium excretion. Combination therapy with loop diuretics (e.g., furosemide) and spironolactone can be used in refractory cases, but potassium levels must be monitored closely. The blood urea nitrogen and creatinine levels must be monitored closely; increasing levels should prompt discontinuation of diuretic therapy to prevent development of hepatorenal failure.

Cardenas A, Gines P: Pathogenesis and treatment of fluid and electrolyte imbalance in cirrhosis. Semin Nephrol 21:308–316, 2001.

15. **Describe the central nervous system changes seen with FHF. How are they treated?**

Hepatic encephalopathy and cerebral edema are commonly seen with fulminant hepatitis and hepatic failure. The clinical features of hepatic encephalopathy are mental status changes, asterixis, pre-coma, and coma. The cause of the encephalopathy is believed to be the increased serum levels of ammonia, which indirectly result in increased transport of amino acids across the blood–brain barrier.

The treatment of hepatic encephalopathy is based on reversing any precipitating factors and decreasing available amino acids for blood–brain barrier transport. If a specific medication is implicated, it should be discontinued. The primary treatment is catharsis with lactulose (15 mL t.i.d.) or magnesium citrate (240 mL daily) resulting in a lower stool pH and increased bacterial clearance. A reduction in the urease-producing bacteria via oral aminoglycosides (neomycin 1 gm q.i.d.) will also aid treatment. Patients with hepatic encephalopathy need a reduction in dietary protein and do not tolerate standard protein formulations of parenteral nutrition. Total parenteral nutrition designed for patients with liver failure should contain less aromatic, neutral amino acids. They should contain more branched-chain amino acids. Such solutions are better tolerated due to decreased neutral amino acids and increased protein production via branch-chained amino acids.

American College of Surgeons: Critical Care: Hepatic Failure: www.acssurgery.com/acs/pdf/ACS0809.pdf

16. **How is fulminant hepatitis treated?**

No specific form of treatment other than orthotopic liver transplantation (OLT) has been proved beneficial in fulminant hepatitis. The goal of current therapy is to sustain life and control hepatic failure over a period sufficient to allow hepatic regeneration before the patient succumbs to liver failure. Transplantation for fulminant hepatitis is still controversial. However, if OLT is considered, prompt surgical transplant consultation is critical because overall prognosis is related to the degree of encephalopathy.

17. **What is the prognosis for patients with fulminant hepatitis?**

The overall survival rate for patients with fulminant hepatitis is 20–25%. Survival correlates best with the age of the patient and the deepest level of encephalopathy reached. In patients who reach only stage II encephalopathy, more than 50% survive. In contrast, the survival rate of those patients who progress to stage IV encephalopathy is only 20%.

Shakil AO, Kramer D, Mazariegos GV, et al: Acute liver failure: Clinical features, outcome analysis, and applicability of prognostic criteria. Liver Transpl 6:163–169, 2000.

18. **What is chronic hepatitis?**

    Chronic hepatitis is defined as the presence of liver inflammation that persists for more than 6 months. There are two major variants: chronic persistent hepatitis and chronic active hepatitis. Chronic persistent hepatitis is a relapsing, remitting, benign, self-limited condition that is not associated with progressive liver damage. It does not lead to liver failure or cirrhosis. Chronic active hepatitis is a vicious disease characterized by progressive destruction of hepatocytes over a span of years with continued erosion of the hepatic functional reserve. Cirrhosis eventually develops. It is estimated that 5–10% of patients with acute hepatitis B and possibly as many as 33% of those with hepatitis C may experience chronic hepatitis.

19. **What are the nonviral causes of hepatitis?**

    Hepatic injury can be induced by a variety of chemical agents, drugs, and metabolic diseases. Drugs associated with chronic hepatitis or cirrhosis include acetaminophen, aspirin, chlorpromazine, dantrolene, ethanol, halothane, isoniazid, methyldopa, nitrofurantoin, propylthiouracil, and sulfonamides. Other hepatotoxins include carbon tetrachloride, phosphorus, tetracycline, chemotherapeutic agents, *Amanita phalloides* (mushroom toxin), and anabolic steroids. Metabolic diseases include Wilson's disease, alpha$_1$-antitrypsin deficiency, and autoimmune hepatitis.

20. **What is cirrhosis?**

    Cirrhosis is a diffuse process characterized by fibrosis and conversion of normal liver architecture into structurally abnormal nodules. The architectural disorganization of the liver is irreversible once established, and management is directed at both the prevention of further hepatocyte damage and the treatment of complications.

    Northrup PG, Wanamaker RC, Lee VD, et al: Model for end-stage liver disease (MELD) predicts nontransplant surgical mortality in patients with cirrhosis. Ann Surg 242:244–251, 2005.

21. **What are the major causes of cirrhosis?**

    Alcohol is by far the most common cause of cirrhosis, accounting for 60–70% of all cases of cirrhosis. Chronic viral hepatitis, autoimmune hepatitis, primary biliary cirrhosis, hemachromatosis, Wilson's disease, and idiopathic causes may also lead to the development of cirrhosis.

    Menon KV, Gores, GJ, Shah VH: Pathogenesis, diagnosis, and treatment of alcoholic liver disease. Mayo Clin Proc 76:1021–1029, 2001.

22. **What are the major complications of cirrhosis?**

    Progressive hepatocyte damage and portal hypertension are the sequelae of cirrhosis. These result in four major complications: ascites, spontaneous bacterial peritonitis, hepatic encephalopathy, and upper gastrointestinal tract hemorrhage. Each of these may lead to admission to an intensive care unit.

    Ginès P, Cárdenas A, Arroyo V, Rodés J: Current concepts: Management of cirrhosis and ascites. N Engl J Med 350:1646–1654, 2004.

    Talwalkar JA, Kamath PS: Influence of recent advances in medical management on clinical outcomes of cirrhosis. Mayo Clin Proc 80:1501–1508, 2005.

KEY POINTS: COMPLICATIONS OF CIRRHOSIS

1. Ascites is one possible complication of cirrhosis.

2. Spontaneous bacterial peritonitis has also been known to occur.

3. Hepatic encephalopathy is another possible complication.

4. Cirrhosis can also lead to upper gastrointestinal tract hemorrhage.

23. **How is cirrhotic ascites managed?**
The initial management of cirrhotic ascites is conservative, emphasizing sodium restriction and bed rest. Approximately 10–20% of patients will be adequately treated this way. Patients whose conditions fail to respond to conservative measures require diuretic therapy. Spironolactone is the agent of choice because of its physiologic actions, potassium-sparing effects, and relative safety. Combination therapy with furosemide is used in patients whose conditions fail to respond to spironolactone monotherapy. In cases of diuretic-resistant ascites, therapeutic paracentesis should be considered with possible albumin replacement. In truly unresponsive patients, the use of a peritoneovenous shunt should be considered. However, there is a high rate of complication associated with these shunts (e.g., disseminated intravascular coagulation and sepsis), and no proven benefit has been demonstrated with these devices.

Pamuk ON, Sonsuz A: The effect of mannitol infusion on the response to diuretic therapy in cirrhotic patients with ascites. J Clin Gastroenterol 35:403–405, 2002.
Talwalkar JA, Kamath PS: Influence of recent advances in medical management on clinical outcomes of cirrhosis. Mayo Clin Proc 80:1501–1508, 2005.

24. **How is primary spontaneous bacterial peritonitis differentiated from secondary bacterial peritonitis?**
The diagnosis of spontaneous bacterial peritonitis is confirmed by ascitic fluid analysis. The key tests are cell count, Gram stain, and measurements of total protein, lactate dehydrogenase, and glucose (Table 47-1).

American College of Surgeons: Critical Care: Hepatic Failure: www.acssurgery.com/acs/pdf/ACS0809.pdf

25. **What is portal hypertension?**
Portal hypertension is defined as portal venous pressure higher than 12 mmHg or a hepatic wedge venous pressure that exceeds the inferior vena cava pressure by more than 5 mmHg. It is classified as prehepatic, hepatic, or posthepatic according to the anatomic site of increased portal venous resistance. Hepatic portal hypertension resulting from cirrhosis is the most common type.

Garcia-Tsao G: Portal hypertension. Curr Opin Gastroenterol 21:313–322, 2005.
Nietsch HH: Management of portal hypertension. J Clin Gastroenterol 39:232–236, 2005.

26. **What is the appropriate management for upper gastrointestinal tract bleeding associated with cirrhosis?**
Approximately 70% of bleeding episodes in cirrhosis are due to variceal hemorrhage, but other etiologies such as gastritis, peptic ulcer, and Mallory-Weiss tears should be kept in mind. The

TABLE 47-1. ASCITIC FLUID ANALYSIS		
Fluid Test	Primary Spontaneous Bacterial Peritonitis	Secondary Bacterial Peritonitis
WBC (cells/mm³)	>500	>500
Total protein (gm/dL)	<1.0	>1.0
Glucose (mg/dL)	>50	<50
LDH (U/L)	<225	>225
Gram stain	Monomicrobial	Polymicrobial
LDH = lactate dehydrogenase.		

initial management is focused on volume resuscitation, correction of coagulopathy, and reduction in portal venous pressure. Vasopressin has been widely used to reduce portal pressure with high success rates. However, clinical trials have shown that somatostatin has similar results without the decreased coronary blood flow seen with vasopressin. Somatostatin has now become the drug of choice for acutely reducing portal pressure. Once the patient's condition has been stabilized, upper endoscopy is performed to define the etiology. If bleeding is due to esophageal varices, injection sclerotherapy or variceal banding is the preferred therapeutic method. Endoscopic methods have a success rate of 85% in arresting bleeding. If endoscopic measures fail, mechanical tamponade can be used via a Sengstaken-Blakemore tube. The Sengstaken-Blakemore tube is a temporizing device, not a definitive treatment. If variceal bleeding persists, portal hypertension must be relieved via a portosystemic shunt. Currently, transjugular intrahepatic portacaval shunt is considered a first choice. The portal venous system is decompressed to the systemic system via a stent placed across the hepatic parenchyma connecting a hepatic vein branch to a portal vein branch. If interventional radiology is not available, the portosystemic shunt may be achieved operatively in "good-risk" patients only. Alternatively, lower esophageal resection and/or esophagogastric devascularization (Sugiura procedure) can be performed. These have a high success in halting hemorrhage but are also associated with a high mortality.

Boyer TD, Haskal ZJ: American Association for the Study of Liver Diseases Practice Guidelines: The role of transjugular intrahepatic portosystemic shunt creation in the management of portal hypertension. J Vasc Interv Radiol 16:615–629, 2005.

Hassoun Z, Pomier-Layrargues G: The transjugular intrahepatic portosystemic shunt in the treatment of portal hypertension. Eur J Gastroenterol Hepatol 16:1–4, 2004.

Nietsch HH: Management of portal hypertension. J Clin Gastroenterol 39:232–236, 2005.

Ochs A, Rossle M, Haag K, et al: The transjugular intrahepatic portosystemic stent–shunt procedure for refractory ascites. N Engl J Med 332:1192, 1995. [Published erratum appears in N Engl J Med 332:1587, 1995.]

Samonakis DN, Triantos CK, Thalheimer U, et al: Management of portal hypertension. Postgrad Med J 80:634–641, 2004.

KEY POINTS: TREATMENT OF VARICEAL BLEEDING

1. Initiate volume resuscitation and correction of coagulopathy.

2. Reduce portal venous pressure with somatostatin.

3. Perform upper endoscopy for sclerotherapy and/or variceal banding.

4. If these methods are unsuccessful, do portosystemic shunt via transjugular intrahepatic portocaval shunt or operative portosystemic shunt.

5. Bleeding may be temporized with mechanical tamponade via Sengstaken-Blakemore tube.

27. **What is the role of orthotopic liver transplant (OLT) in cirrhosis?**
Liver transplantation has become the definitive treatment for end-stage cirrhosis. The 1- and 5-year survival rates are approximately 80% and 65%, respectively. The use of liver transplantation in patients with alcoholic cirrhosis is controversial. However, most transplant surgeons are willing to qualify the patients for transplantation if they prove they are abstinent from alcohol and are currently participating in rehabilitation. The use of OLT for patients with hepatitis B or C has now become standard for those patients with end-stage cirrhosis. With the use of hepatitis B immune globulin, reduction in the viral burden occurs, resulting in promising survival rates in patients with hepatitis B.

Brown RS: Hepatitis C and liver transplantation. Nature 436:973–978, 2005.

Keefe EB: Liver transplantation: Current status and novel approaches to liver replacement. Gastroenterology 120:749–762, 2001.

28. **Does xenograft transplantation play a role in the treatment of FHF?**

    Several case reports in the literature describe heterotopically transplanting porcine livers to provide metabolic support before transplantation with a human liver. The majority of these cases were unsuccessful in providing hepatic function for longer than 35–48 hours due to the onset of acute rejection. Despite the removal of anti-pig antibodies by plasmapheresis and *ex vivo* en bloc perfusion of the donor pig kidneys, antibody- and complement-mediated destruction of the xenografts occurred, rapidly resulting in graft loss and worsening hepatic failure.

    Chinnakotla S, Fox IJ: Prospects for xenotransplantation. Curr Opin Organ Transpl 7:35–40, 2002.

    Horslen SP, Hammel JM, Fristoe LW, et al: Extracorporeal liver perfusion using human and pig livers for acute liver failure. Transplantation 27:1472–1478, 2000.

29. **What advances have been made with regard to artificial liver support?**

    During the past few years, bioartificial liver support systems using hollow-fiber bioreactors, microcarrier cell culture techniques, and porcine hepatocytes have been transplanted in animals with acute liver failure. These have led to improved detoxification and synthetic function. Extracorporeal bioartificial liver systems using porcine hepatocytes have been tested *in vitro* and exhibit cytochrome p450 activity, protein synthesis, and bilirubin conjugation. *In vivo,* these systems provided substantial metabolic support to the animals, resulting in improved neurologic function. With further research, bioartificial livers may become an effective bridge to OLT for patients awaiting available donor organs.

    Mullin EJ, Metcalfe MS, Maddern GJ: Artificial liver support: Potential to retard regeneration? Arch Surg 139:670–677, 2004.

    van de Kerkhove MP, Hoekstra RP, Chamuleau RAFM, van Gulik TM: Clinical application of bioartificial liver support systems. Ann Surg 240:216–230, 2004.

CHAPTER 48

PERITONITIS

James P. Bonar, MD, and Mark W. Bowyer, MD, DMCC, COL, USAF, MC

1. **What is the peritoneum?**
   The abdominal cavity is lined by the peritoneum, which is composed of single sheet of flattened mesothelial cells that rest on a thin layer of fibroelastic tissue. The abdominal viscera are also covered by the peritoneum. The functions of the peritoneum are to maintain the surface integrity of the intra-abdominal structures and to provide a smooth lubricated surface so the intestines can move freely.

2. **What is the difference between the parietal and the visceral peritoneum?**
   The parietal peritoneum is the portion of the peritoneum that lines the entire abdominal cavity, covering the abdominal wall, diaphragm, and pelvic floor. The visceral peritoneum is the portion of the peritoneum that covers all of the intra-abdominal viscera and mesenteries.

3. **What features are unique to the parietal peritoneum overlying the diaphragm?**
   The peritoneum overlying the diaphragm is interrupted by intracellular pores called *stomata,* which serve as entrances into diaphragmatic lymphatic channels called *lacunae.* The lacunae drain into the substernal lymph nodes and then ultimately into the thoracic duct. The diaphragmatic stomata are also capable of absorbing particulate matter, including bacteria.

   Turnage RH, Li BDL, McDonald JC: Abdominal wall, umbilicus, peritoneum, mesenteries, omentum, and retroperitoneum. In Townsend MC, Beauchamp RD, Evers BM, Mattox KL (eds): Textbook of Surgery, 17th ed. Philadelphia, W.B. Saunders, 2004, pp 1171–1239.

4. **What is the general mechanism by which peritoneal fluid is moved throughout the abdominal cavity?**
   The peritoneal fluid contained in the peritoneal cavity moves systematically toward the diaphragm as a function of negative pressure that occurs with movement of the diaphragm.

5. **What is peritonitis?**
   The term *peritonitis* refers to an inflammation of the mesenchymal cells lining the peritoneal cavity and is due to either a localized or generalized intra-abdominal infection. Peritonitis has distinct phases that include contamination, dissemination, inflammation, and resolution or loculation.

   Sheer TA, Runyon BA: Spontaneous bacterial peritonitis. Dig Dis 23:39–46, 2005.

6. **What are the clinical manifestations of classic peritonitis?**
   Abdominal tenderness is the hallmark of peritonitis and can become steady, unrelenting, and burning. Patients with generalized peritonitis often have diffuse tenderness and will appear quite ill early in their clinical course. Characteristically, they lie quietly, supine, with knees flexed; they have shallow breathing because any motion intensifies their abdominal pain. Voluntary guarding produces rigidity of the abdominal muscles.

7. **How are peritoneal infections classified?**
   Primary (spontaneous), secondary (usually occurs in the setting of a gastrointestinal perforation), and tertiary (recurrent or persistent infection after adequate initial treatment).

8. **What are the typical features of primary peritonitis?**
   Primary peritonitis is characterized by a diffuse microbiologic infection of the peritoneal cavity that occurs in the absence of a perforation or disruption of the gastrointestinal tract. Often, it is a consequence of peritoneal contamination arising from a remote source. The peritonitis begins when microorganisms become embedded within the peritoneal cavity due to translocation of bacteria across the gut wall or via hematogenous seeding.

   Rimola A, Garcia-Tsao G, Navasa M, et al: Diagnosis, treatment and prophylaxis of spontaneous bacterial peritonitis: A consensus document. J Hepatol 32:142–153, 2000.

9. **What is the most common etiology of primary peritonitis?**
   The most common cause of primary peritonitis is spontaneous bacterial peritonitis (SBP), which is commonly caused by chronic liver disease with ascites. Ascites is the pathologic accumulation of fluid within the peritoneal space. Approximately 10–30% of patients with cirrhotic liver disease who have ascites will experience peritonitis.

   Sandhu BS, Sanyal AJ: Management of ascites in cirrhosis. Clin Liver Dis 9:715–732, 2005.

10. **Name two other causes of primary peritonitis.**
    Tuberculous peritonitis and chronic ambulatory peritoneal dialysis. In patients with chronic renal failure, primary peritonitis is a common complication when patients are undergoing chronic ambulatory peritoneal dialysis. Another etiology is tuberculous peritonitis, which occurs as a reactivation of latent peritoneal disease that had been previously established due to hematogenous or lymphatic spread. Although rare in the United States, it continues to be a significant problem in underdeveloped countries.

    Nannini EC, Paphitou NI, Ostrosky-Zeichner L: Peritonitis due to *Aspergillus* and zygomycetes in patients undergoing peritoneal dialysis: Report of 2 cases and review of the literature. Diagn Microbiol Infect Dis 46:49–54, 2003.
    Pereira JM, Madureira AJ, Vieira A, Ramos I: Abdominal tuberculosis: Imaging features. Eur J Radiol 55:173–180, 2005.

11. **Which organisms are commonly associated with primary peritonitis?**
    In patients with cirrhosis, more than 90% of infections are monomicrobial. The most common pathogens include gram-negative organisms with enteric organisms predominating— particularly *Escherichia coli* and *Klebsiella pneumoniae*. Anaerobic organisms are uncommon in primary peritonitis, and polymicrobial infections occur in fewer than 10% of cases. However, opportunistic organisms, including cytomegalovirus and *Mycobacterium tuberculosis,* can be cultured in immunocompromised patients.

    Peritonitis and abdominal sepsis: www.emedicine.com

12. **Describe the clinical features of SBP.**
    Jaundice, hepatic encephalopathy, and abdominal pain are common clinical findings, yet one-third to one-half of the patients may not exhibit any abdominal tenderness. The most common symptom is fever, but this may be absent in more than 30% of patients. The clinical presentation of SBP can be subtle. Ascites is essentially always present, but the volume can vary greatly.

    Johnson CC, Baldessarre J, Levinson ME: Peritonitis: Update on pathophysiology, clinical manifestations, and management. Clin Infect Dis 24:1035, 1997.

13. **How is SBP diagnosed?**
    The key to the diagnosis of SBP is examination of the ascitic fluid from a diagnostic paracentesis. The fluid should be examined for pH, lactate, and protein levels and cell count with differential. A Gram stain and culture are also essential.

KEY POINTS: PERITONEAL FLUID GRAM STAIN AND ETIOLOGY OF PERITONITIS

1. Gram-positive cocci found on Gram stain suggest likely spontaneous bacterial peritonitis.

2. Gram-negative rods indicate either primary or secondary peritonitis.

3. Mixed flora suggest likely bowel perforation (secondary peritonitis).

4. Antimicrobial therapy should be adjusted when the results of culture and sensitivity of peritoneal fluid become available.

14. **What is the best single laboratory predictor of SBP?**
    The absolute polymorphonuclear leukocyte (PMN) count of the sampled ascetic fluid is the best predictor of infection. An accurate method of culturing ascitic fluid is to place 10–20 mL into both aerobic and anaerobic blood culture bottles at the bedside to improve the sensitivity of the test.

    Blondeau JM, Pylypchuk GB, Kappel E, et al: Comparison of bedside- and laboratory-inoculated Bactec high- and low-volume resin bottles for the recovery of microorganisms causing peritonitis in CAPD patients. Diagn Microbiol Infect Dis 31:281–287, 1998.

15. **What are the laboratory values of ascetic fluid that suggest infection?**
    Generally, a PMN count > 250 cells/mm^3 *suggests* a diagnosis of SBP. PMN counts > 500 cells/mm^3 are *highly* suggestive of SBP, and patients with these counts should be treated as if SBP was present, pending culture results. If the PMN count is >1000 cells/mm^3, treatment for SBP should be continued *regardless* of culture results. A Gram stain is useful because the visualization of a single bacterial type would be consistent with SBP. In contrast, a Gram stain showing multiple bacterial forms would suggest a secondary peritonitis.

    Rimola A, Garcia-Tsao G, Navasa M, et al: Diagnosis, treatment of spontaneous bacterial peritonitis: A consensus document. J Hepatol 32:142–153, 2000.

16. **How is SBP treated?**
    Specific antimicrobial agents must be selected before culture results are available. The Gram stain of the centrifuged ascites is the most useful test to guide the initial selection of an antimicrobial regimen. If the Gram stain is unrevealing or there is no obvious organism or potential source, treatment should be broad spectrum and empiric. The suggested initial empiric treatment is cefotaxime 2.0 gm q8h given intravenously; alternatively, other useful agents include ticarcillin/clavulanate, piperacillin/tazobactam, or ampicillin/sulbactam.

    Ricart E, Soriano G, Novella MT, et al: Amoxicillin-clavulanic acid versus cefotaxime in the therapy of bacterial infections in cirrhotic patients. J Hepatol 32:596–602, 2000.

17. **How long should antibiotic therapy continue in patients being treated for SBP?**
    Traditionally, IV antibiotics have been administered for 10–14 days. Recently, shorter courses of therapy (5 days) have been shown to be as effective. However, the patient must be doing well

clinically, and the results of repeated culture of their ascetic fluid must be negative with a PMN count below 250 cells/mm^3.

Terg R, Cobas S, Fassio E, et al: Oral ciprofloxacin after a short course of intravenous ciprofloxacin in the treatment of spontaneous bacterial peritonitis: Results of a multicenter, randomized study. J Hepatol 33:564–569, 2000.

18. What is secondary peritonitis?

Secondary bacterial peritonitis or *classic peritonitis* is defined as a peritoneal infection that begins with the perforation of the gastrointestinal tract with subsequent contamination of the peritoneal cavity. It can occur with trauma, eroded gastrointestinal tract neoplasms, or other inflammatory processes such as perforated appendicitis, perforated duodenal ulcer, or perforated colon resulting from diverticulitis. Additionally, postoperative gastrointestinal tract anastomotic disruption will cause peritonitis.

Newton E, Mandavia S: Surgical complications of selected gastrointestinal emergencies: Pitfalls in management of the acute abdomen. Emerg Med Clin North Am 21:873–907, 2003.
Surgical Tutor: www.surgical-tutor.org.uk

19. How is secondary peritonitis diagnosed?

The diagnosis is usually a clinical one, although some patients may require abdominal computed tomography (CT) scan. The classic findings along with abdominal pain are peritoneal signs, such as tenderness, guarding, and increased abdominal wall tone. Leukocytosis with white blood cell count $> 11,000/mm^3$ and a left shift, free air under the diaphragm, or evidence of ileus supports the clinical diagnosis of peritonitis. If an abdominal CT scan is unavailable or impractical, peritoneal lavage may be useful. The presence of > 500 white blood cells/mm^3 in the lavage fluid strongly suggests the presence of intra-abdominal pathology.

Christau NV: Intraabdominal infections. In Cameron JL (ed): Current Surgical Therapy, 8th ed. Philadelphia, Elsevier, 2004, pp 1118–1121.
eMedicine: www.emedicine.com
Malangoni MA: Contributions to the management of intraabdominal infections. Am J Surg 190:255–259, 2005.

20. How should secondary peritonitis be managed?

The treatment of secondary peritonitis is primarily operative. The goals of the operative management of peritonitis are to eliminate the source of contamination, reduce the bacterial inoculum, and prevent recurrent or persistent sepsis. Infections within the peritoneal cavity are almost always polymicrobial in nature and contain a mixture of aerobic and anaerobic bacteria.

Lee S-C, Fung C-P, Chen H-Y, et al: Candida peritonitis due to peptic ulcer perforation: Incidence rate, risk factors, prognosis and susceptibility to fluconazole and amphotericin B. Diagn Microbiol Infect Dis 44:23–27, 2002.

21. What is tertiary peritonitis?

Secondary peritonitis that cannot be controlled, whether due to impaired host defense mechanisms or overwhelming infection, progresses to diffuse persistent (i.e., tertiary) peritonitis. The clinical picture is one of occult sepsis without a well-defined focus of infection. Despite aggressive management, progressive multiple-system organ failure frequently develops.

Nathens AB, Rotstein OD, Marshall JC: Tertiary peritonitis: Clinical features of a complex nosocomial infection. World J Surg 22:158–163, 1998.

22. What are the characteristics of intraperitoneal abscesses?

Intraperitoneal abscesses arise during the resolution of generalized peritonitis and most commonly occur in the pelvis or subphrenic regions. These locations are a reflection of the anatomy of the peritoneum, which permits gravity-dependent flow of infected material into these dependent areas. Clinical symptoms may be vague early on but may include paralytic ileus, anorexia, abdominal distention, recurrent or persistent fever, chills, abdominal pain, and tachycardia.

Christau NV: Intraabdominal infections. In Cameron JL (ed): Current Surgical Therapy, 8th ed. Philadelphia, Elsevier, 2004, pp 1118–1121.

DIABETIC KETOACIDOSIS

Jeanne M. Rozwadowski, MD, and Philip S. Mehler, MD

CHAPTER 49

1. What is diabetic ketoacidosis (DKA)?

DKA is a serious metabolic complication of diabetes mellitus (DM) resulting from a combination of insulin deficiency (either relative or absolute) and an increase in glucose counter-regulatory hormones (i.e., catecholamines, glucagon, cortisol, and growth hormones). A triad of metabolic acidosis, ketosis, and hyperglycemia characterizes DKA.

Cateels K, Mathieu C: Diabetic ketoacidosis. Rev Endocrinol Metab Disord 4:159–166, 2003.

2. Describe the pathophysiologic basis of DKA.

Insulin deficiency is the focal point of the disorder and causes both the hyperglycemia and ketonemia. In a normal state, insulin ensures the storage of glucose as glucagon in the liver. With a deficiency of insulin, there is both increased hepatic glucose production through increased glycogenolysis and gluconeogenesis as well as decreased glucose use. The result is hyperglycemia.

The ketonemia is similarly due to a state of insulin deficiency. Under normal conditions, insulin allows free fatty acids, as triglycerides, to be stored in adipose tissue. As a result of the reduced insulin levels and the concomitantly elevated levels of glucose counter-regulatory hormones, there is excessive production of free fatty acids from the breakdown of triglycerides. Free fatty acids are converted to ketone bodies in the liver. In addition, decreased ketone use contributes to the ketonemia.

Cateels K, Mathieu C: Diabetic ketoacidosis. Rev Endocrinol Metab Disord 4:159–166, 2003.

3. Is DKA a complication of type 1 DM only?

Although DKA is generally considered a consequence of absolute insulin deficiency that reflects the irreversible beta-cell damage seen in type 1 DM, studies have shown that DKA occurs in patients with type 2 DM as well, especially in nonwhite persons. A study evaluated 138 patients admitted for moderate to severe DKA to a diabetes unit at an inner-city hospital. Twenty-two percent of the patients had type 2 diabetes. On presentation, the patients with type 2 DM were less acidotic, were more likely to present with normal potassium levels, and required a longer treatment time to clear their acidemia. The theory is that these patients with type 2 DM do not have enough insulin production to prevent DKA; however, they do have sufficient insulin production to prevent a more severe level of acidosis.

Newton CA, Raskin P: Diabetic ketoacidosis in type 1 and type 2 diabetes mellitus. Arch Intern Med 64:1925–1931, 2004.

4. How is DKA diagnosed?

The combination of hyperglycemia, anion-gap metabolic acidosis, and elevated blood ketone levels are needed to diagnose DKA. DKA is usually suspected from the history, especially in a person with known diabetes who presents with an acute illness or a history of missed medications.

American Diabetes Association: Hyperglycemic crises in diabetes. Diabetes Care 27(Suppl 1):S94–S102, 2004.

5. **What are the common signs and symptoms of DKA?**
Patients with DKA often present with the symptoms of hyperglycemia, which are polyuria, polydipsia, polyphagia, lassitude, weight loss, and blurry vision. There can be mental status changes ranging from lethargy to deep coma; 20% of patients present in a stuporous state. Nausea, vomiting, and abdominal pain, which are not usually due to definite intra-abdominal pathology, frequently complicate the early course of DKA. Acidosis is also responsible for one of the classic signs of DKA: Kussmaul respirations, which are long, deep, sighing breaths, made in an attempt to compensate for the metabolic acidosis by lowering the arterial PCO_2. An odor of decaying apples or fruity gum on the patient's breath is another sign of DKA and is caused by acetone, as the other ketones are odorless.

Patients with DKA are generally volume depleted and have electrolyte disturbances, predominantly a result of hyperglycemia. Hyperglycemia causes glucosuria and, subsequently, an osmotic diuresis with loss of volume and electrolytes. In the average 70-kg man with DKA, there is a 3- to 5-L saline deficiency, a 300- to 500-mEq sodium deficiency, and a 150- to 250-mEq potassium deficiency. Furthermore, patients with DKA are often hypothermic because of the unavailability of substrate to generate heat as well as peripheral vasodilation.

American Diabetes Association: Hyperglycemic crises in diabetes. Diabetes Care 27(Suppl 1):S94–S10, 2004.

6. **What is the significance of abdominal pain in DKA?**
Abdominal pain is a common complaint in patients presenting with DKA, occurring in almost half of cases of DKA in one recent study. The definitive cause is not known; however, gastric distention and stretching of the liver capsule have been offered as explanations for the pain. Generally the pain resolves promptly with the treatment of DKA. In the aforementioned study, the abdominal pain was due to the DKA in 35% of patients. The severity of the acidosis and a history of alcohol or cocaine use were associated with the presence of pain; the severity of hyperglycemia and dehydration was not. However, if there are signs of intra-abdominal pathology at presentation, they should be immediately investigated. Certainly, if the abdominal pain does not resolve with the treatment of the volume depletion and the resolution of the acidosis, it is important to investigate further.

Umpierrez G, Freire AX: Abdominal pain in patients with hyperglycemic crisis. J Crit Care 17:63–67, 2002.

7. **Does a patient with abdominal pain and elevated amylase level in the presence of DKA have pancreatitis?**
In patients with DKA, it is common to find a mildly elevated amylase level. The pancreas produces about 40–50% of the body's amylase; the remainder is produced in the salivary glands. Also, in a volume-depleted state (as in DKA), there is reduced renal clearance of amylase. Elevations in lipase levels are thought to be more specific for the diagnosis of pancreatitis. In one prospective study of 100 consecutive patients presenting to a single hospital, the relationship between DKA and acute pancreatitis was studied. The authors found acute pancreatitis in 15% of the patients with DKA. They also found that amylase was a sensitive and specific marker of pancreatitis as long as the levels were at least three times normal, and a computed tomography scan is recommended in any patient with amylase or lipase levels three times normal.

Nair S, Yadav D, Pitchumoni CS: Association of diabetic ketoacidosis and acute pancreatitis: Observations in 100 consecutive episodes. Am J Gastroenterol 95:2795–2800, 2000.

8. **What is the differential diagnosis of DKA?**
Starvation ketosis and alcoholic ketoacidosis cause a ketosis and a metabolic acidosis; however, in both, the blood glucose is either only mildly elevated or is decreased. Other causes of an anion-gap acidosis include ingestion of drugs (e.g., salicylate, methanol, ethylene glycol, and

paraldehyde), lactic acidosis, and chronic renal insufficiency. It is also important to consider the hyperosmolar hyperglycemic state in any patient who is hyperglycemic because it too can cause a mild increase in the anion gap.

Charfen MA, Fernandez-Frackelton M: Diabetic ketoacidosis. Emerg Med Clin North Am 23:609–628, 2005.

9. **What are the usual laboratory findings in the presence of DKA?**
   DKA is characterized by hyperglycemia, anion-gap metabolic acidosis, bicarbonate level < 15 mEq/L, and positive serum ketones. Hyperglycemia need not be impressive. Fifteen percent of the patients with DKA have a glucose level < 300 mg/dL. The vast majority of the patients with DKA have an anion-gap metabolic acidosis, although some can have a nongap hyperchloremic acidosis. The type of acidosis the patient presents with is linked to his or her volume status at the time of presentation. Some patients can present with a mixed acid–base problem of a metabolic acidosis, a metabolic alkalosis, and a respiratory alkalosis. This "triple" acid–base disorder can occur when there is DKA along with intractable vomiting (producing a metabolic alkalosis) and severe abdominal pain (causing hyperventilation), and thus a respiratory alkalosis.

Charfen MA, Fernandez-Frackelton M: Diabetic ketoacidosis. Emerg Med Clin North Am 23:609–628, 2005.

10. **What happens to potassium levels in DKA?**
    In all patients with DKA, there is total body potassium depletion. However, on presentation, potassium levels can be elevated when measured. This is explained by the state of insulin deficiency and acidosis, causing a transcellular shift of potassium out of cells. During the course of therapy, serum potassium levels drop rapidly because of the combination of insulin therapy and the resolution of the acidosis driving the potassium into cells, as well as the osmotic diuresis from the volume restoration used to treat the volume depletion. Once the potassium level is 5.5 mEq/L or less, there should be potassium replacement added to the patient's IV fluids to prevent serious hypokalemia. Thus, a "normal" potassium level on presentation of DKA generally indicates profound potassium depletion.

Charfen MA, Fernandez-Frackelton M: Diabetic ketoacidosis. Emerg Med Clin North Am 23:609–628, 2005.

11. **Why is hyponatremia common in DKA?**
    The serum sodium level is low in more than half of the patients who present with DKA. Generally, it is not true hyponatremia; rather, it is pseudohyponatremia. The elevated serum glucose level shifts water into cells, which creates a dilutional effect and results in hyponatremia. One can correct for the hyperglycemia by adding 1.6 mEq/L to the sodium for every 100 mg/dL the glucose is above the normal range.

Charfen MA, Fernandez-Frackelton M: Diabetic ketoacidosis. Emerg Med Clin North Am 23:609–628, 2005.

12. **What happens to phosphate levels in DKA?**
    Most patients with DKA are hyperphosphatemic on presentation to the hospital, although generally there is a total body depletion of phosphate in these patients. However, randomized clinical trials of phosphate repletion have not shown benefit in outcome in DKA. In severe depletion careful replacement is warranted, especially in patients with cardiac dysfunction, anemia, respiratory depression, and very low serum phosphate concentrations (<1.0 mg/dL). Once the DKA is treated, phosphate levels will reach nadir 24–36 hours later and should be regularly checked.

Fisher J, Kitabchi A: A randomized study of phosphate therapy in treatment of diabetic ketoacidosis. J Clin Endocrinol Metab 57:177–180, 1983.
Trachtenbarg DE: Diabetic ketoacidosis. Am Fam Physician 71:1705–1714, 2005.

13. **Is the determination of serum ketone levels helpful in the treatment of patients with DKA?**

Serum ketones are helpful in the initial diagnosis of DKA and should be measured once at the time the patient presents. There are three blood ketones: β-hydroxybutyrate, acetoacetone, and acetone. In DKA, the great majority of the ketones may exist as β-hydroxybutyrate, which is not picked up by the qualitative ketone measurements on the urine dipstick. These dipsticks only detect acetoacetone. Thus, ketone measurements may be falsely low or negative. In fact, during successful therapy of DKA, levels of these serum ketones may paradoxically rise (or fail to fall), which is a result of the conversion of β-hydroxybutyrate (not measured) to acetoacetone (measured) before its use. Therefore, following serum ketone levels can be misleading and is not recommended. Rather, successful treatment of DKA is defined by normalization of the anion gap.

Cateels K, Mathieu C: Diabetic ketoacidosis. Rev Endocrinol Metabolic Disord 4:159–166, 2003.

14. **Why are fluids important in the initial treatment of DKA?**

The majority of patients with DKA have a fluid deficit of 100 mL per kilogram of body weight. Studies using tracers have found that up to 80% of the hyperglycemia is cleared by rehydration. Of course, in DKA, insulin is also required because the bottom-line problem is insulin deficiency. Initially, isotonic saline should be infused until the intravascular volume is replete. Once the patient is euvolemic, switching to half-normal saline is recommended unless the patient is hyponatremic.

American Diabetes Association: Hyperglycemic crises in diabetes. Diabetes Care 27(Suppl 1):S94–S102, 2004.

Trachtenbarg DE: Diabetic ketoacidosis. Am Fam Physician 71:1705–1714, 2005.

15. **How is DKA treated?**

Insulin, fluids, and potassium supplementation are the cornerstones of therapy. To avoid potential complications, meticulous attention to detail is essential. The goal of therapy is correction of the metabolic acidosis and the hyperglycemia. Unless insulin resistance is severe, the amount of insulin required is 0.1 U/kg/h.

After a rapid IV infusion of 0.15 U per kilogram of regular insulin, an insulin drip at 0.1 U/kg/h (i.e., 7 U/h in a 70-kg person) should be initiated, and the plasma glucose concentration should be measured 1 hour after the drip is started. If the glucose concentration does not fall by 50–70 mg/day, the patient is insulin resistant and the infusion should be doubled. Do not discontinue the drip even if the blood sugar falls to <250 mg/dL.

When this glucose level is reached, add 5% dextrose to the IV fluids and continue the infusion at the previous rate. Remember that it takes longer to clear the ketoacidosis (10–20 hours) than it does to correct the hyperglycemia (4–8 hours).

American Diabetes Association: Hyperglycemic crises in diabetes. Diabetes Care 27(Suppl 1):S94–S102, 2004.

16. **Can subcutaneous insulin be used to treat DKA?**

There are controlled studies that have shown subcutaneous regular insulin to be effective in the treatment of DKA. The concern with using subcutaneous insulin is the variable uptake and onset of action. Studies that have compared the use of regular insulin—given intravenously, subcutaneously, and intramuscularly—have shown a more rapid and predictable decrease in hyperglycemia and ketonemia with the IV administration. There are newer studies evaluating the use of lispro insulin subcutaneously with equivalent effect to IV regular insulin. Although it is not yet a standard of care, there may be a future trend of treating DKA in a non–intensive care unit setting with subcutaneous lispro insulin.

Trachtenbarg DE: Diabetic ketoacidosis. Am Fam Physician 71:1705–1714, 2005.

Umpierrez GE, Latif K, Stoever J, et al: Efficacy of subcutaneous lispro insulin versus continuous intravenous regular insulin for the treatment of patients with diabetic ketoacidosis. Am J Med 117:291–296, 2004.

17. **What is the best indicator of resolution of DKA, given that it may be misleading to follow serial ketone measurements?**
The most reliable indicator of DKA resolution is the anion gap. Glucose corrects simply and rapidly as a consequence of fluid repletion and thus cannot be relied on to determine whether DKA is resolved. Urinary ketones tend to remain detectable long after the resolution of DKA (*see* question 13). Therefore, these are not a good predictor of resolution of DKA either. However, when the anion gap returns to normal, ketoacid production has ceased.

Cateels K, Mathieu C: Diabetic ketoacidosis. Rev Endocrinol Metab Disord 4:159–166, 2003.

18. **How do you transition the patient away from IV insulin administration?**
Once the electrolyte measurements demonstrate a normal anion gap, continue the insulin infusion for a few more hours to ensure that control has been achieved. After that, if the patient can eat, the patient's previous insulin administration can be reinstituted (if known and satisfactory) and the insulin infusion can be discontinued. It is important to overlap the IV and subcutaneous insulin to prevent worsening of blood sugar control.

American Diabetes Association: Hyperglycemic crises in diabetes. Diabetes Care 27(Suppl 1):S94–S102, 2004.

19. **Why do most patients develop a hyperchloremic nongap acidosis after therapy for DKA?**
Chloride from the IV fluids used to treat DKA replaces the ketoacids, which are excreted during the osmotic diuresis. Because the renal threshold for ketones is quite low, with volume expansion, excretion of the ketones in the urine is increased. These excreted ketones are "bicarbonate equivalents" that limit the availability of substrate to regenerate bicarbonate. Therefore, the majority of patients develop a hyperchloremic nongap metabolic acidosis, which is transient and clinically insignificant.

American Diabetes Association: Hyperglycemic crises in diabetes. Diabetes Care 27(Suppl 1):S94–S102, 2004.

20. **What are the most common precipitating events for development of DKA?**
When a precipitating cause can be found, the most common one is infection, accounting for 30–50% of the cases with pneumonia. Urinary tract infections are most common. The next most common precipitating cause of DKA is noncompliance or undertreatment with insulin, especially in urban African-American populations. A significant portion of patients presenting with DKA have new-onset diabetes. Other, less common precipitating causes include myocardial infarction, cerebrovascular accident, alcohol abuse, pancreatitis, gastrointestinal bleeding, and trauma. In up to 10% of patients, no precipitating cause is identified. There are some drugs that can precipitate DKA, including corticosteroids, thiazides, and sympathomimetic agents.

Goldberg PA, Inzucchi SE: Critical issues in endocrinology. Clin Chest Med 24:583–606, 2003.

KEY POINTS: DIABETIC KETOACIDOSIS (DKA)

1. The diagnosis of DKA requires hyperglycemia, an anion-gap metabolic acidosis, and elevated blood ketone levels.

2. An elevated amylase level is nonspecific for pancreatitis in a patient with DKA unless it is three times the normal level.

3. A "normal" potassium level on presentation of DKA generally indicates profound potassium depletion.

4. During treatment of DKA, switch the patient's IV fluids to 5% dextrose when the blood sugar level falls to <250 mg/dL.

5. There is no benefit to bicarbonate therapy if the patient's pH is >6.9.

21. **Is leukocytosis a sensitive indicator of infection in DKA?**
No. Leukocytosis by itself is not a sensitive or specific indicator of infection in DKA because leukocyte counts in the 20,000-cells/mm^3 range are commonly seen in DKA due to stress and hemoconcentration. It has been shown that an elevated band count (10% or greater) is a sensitive and significant indicator of occult coexisting infection. Total leukocyte count, blood glucose level, serum bicarbonate level, and temperature have little value in predicting covert infection in DKA.

Slivos CM, Mork EG, Bain RP: Diabetic ketoacidosis and infection. Am J Emerg Med 5:1–5, 1987.

22. **What are the major complications in DKA?**
The mortality rate of DKA is <5%. Hypotension and coma, as well as the extremes of age, carry a negative prognosis. A few complications are potentially associated with the therapy for DKA. The easily treatable ones are hypoglycemia, hypokalemia, and hypophosphatemia. Cerebral edema is a very rare complication in adults; however, it is commonly fatal and should be considered in any DKA patient with rapid neurologic deterioration. It seems to be associated with a rapid decline in plasma osmolality; gradual replacement of sodium and water is therefore recommended. Hypoxia and/or noncardiogenic pulmonary edema can also complicate the treatment of DKA.

American Diabetes Association: Hyperglycemic crises in diabetes. Diabetes Care 27(Suppl 1):S94–S102, 2004.

23. **What is the role of bicarbonate therapy in DKA?**
There is much controversy regarding the use of bicarbonate therapy in the treatment of DKA. Many studies have been performed and have not shown a benefit in using bicarbonate for patients with a pH > 6.9. Although there are no randomized trails involving patients with pH < 6.9, some clinicians think the severity of the acidosis warrants the use of bicarbonate in that situation. If used, the dose is 100 mmol of sodium bicarbonate infused at 200 mL/h.

American Diabetes Association: Hyperglycemic crises in diabetes. Diabetes Care 27(Suppl 1):S94–S102, 2004.

HYPERGLYCEMIC HYPEROSMOLAR SYNDROME

CHAPTER 50

Joshua Blum, MD, and Philip S. Mehler, MD

1. **How is hyperglycemic hyperosmolar syndrome (HHS) defined?**
   HHS is characterized by marked hyperglycemia (plasma glucose $\geq$ 600 mg/dL) along with hyperosmolarity (effective serum osmolarity $\geq$ 320 mOsm/L) and severe dehydration in the absence of significant ketoacidosis.

2. **What are the major differences between HHS and diabetic ketoacidosis (DKA)?**
   See Table 50-1.

3. **Why do some persons with diabetes develop DKA and others HHS?**
   The mechanism may be multifactorial. First, patients with HHS have been shown to have higher portal vein concentrations of insulin than patients with DKA. These higher insulin levels may be sufficient to suppress release of free fatty acids, but not enough to facilitate glucose transport and metabolism. Second, in DKA, higher glucagon levels increase the availability of free fatty acids, and thus the development of ketone bodies and subsequent metabolic acidosis. Finally, hyperosmolarity itself suppresses lipolysis. In truth, considerable overlap occurs among these entities. In one series, 22% of patients presented with DKA, 45% with HHS, and 33% with features of both (Fig. 50-1).

   Wachtel TJ, Tet-Mouradian LM, Goldman DL, et al: Hyperosmolarity and acidosis in diabetes mellitus: A three-year experience in Rhode Island. J Gen Intern Med 6:495–502, 1991.

4. **How does one calculate effective osmolarity? How does it differ from serum osmolarity?**
   Serum osmolarity is approximated by the following calculation:

   $$2 \times [\text{Na (mEq/L)} + \text{K (mEq/L)}] + \text{plasma glucose (mg/dL)}/18 + \text{blood urea nitrogen (mg/dL)}/2.8$$

   The normal range for serum osmolarity is 280–295 mOsm/L. However, because urea is freely permeable across cell membranes, it does not contribute to the serum *tonicity,* also referred to as the *effective* osmolarity, relative to the intracellular space. Effective osmolarity (Eosm) is therefore calculated by:

TABLE 50-1. HYPERGLYCEMIC HYPEROSMOLAR SYNDROME VERSUS DIABETIC KETOACIDOSIS

	Hyperglycemic Hyperosmolar Syndrome	Diabetic Ketoacidosis
Age	Middle-aged or elderly	Young or middle-aged
Hyperglycemia	Severe ($\geq$600 mg/dL)	Moderate ($\geq$300 mg/dL)
Ketosis/acidosis	None to minimal (pH $\geq$ 7.3)	Severe (pH $\leq$ 7.3)
Onset	Prolonged, insidious (days to weeks)	Rapid (hours to days)
Dehydration	Very severe	Moderate to severe

$$2 \times [\text{Na (mEq/L)} + \text{K (mEq/L)}] + \text{plasma glucose (mg/dL)}/18$$

Significant hyperosmolarity is present when the Eosm exceeds 320, and severe hyperosmolarity is defined as an Eosm $\geq$ 350.

5. **What are the most common precipitating causes of HHS and DKA?**
Infections top the list, with pneumonias and urinary tract infections most common. Another very common cause is inadequately treated or untreated diabetes. Up to 40% of older adults with a hyperglycemia syndrome do not have a prior diabetes diagnosis. Other inciting events include vascular events, such as myocardial infarction and cerebral vascular accident. Rounding out the list of common causes are gastrointestinal tract conditions (such as pancreatitis or cholecystitis), trauma, burns, drugs, and medications.

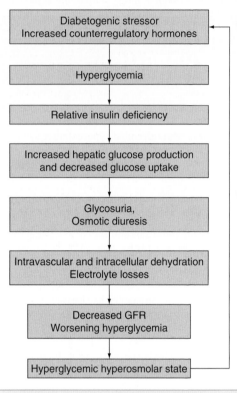

Figure 50-1. Pathogenesis of hyperglycemic hyperosmolar syndrome. GFR = glomerular filtration rate.

6. **Which medications are most frequently associated with the development of hyperglycemic crises?**
Diuretics (especially thiazides and loop diuretics), beta blockers, steroids, phenytoin, sympathomimetic agents, H_2 blockers, calcium channel blockers, interferon-α, ribavirin, pentamidine, and antipsychotics have all been linked to severe hyperglycemia. Recently, the newer, "atypical" antipsychotics have been associated with significantly increased risk for the development of type 2 diabetes.

7. **What are the symptoms of HHS?**
The history is usually notable for complaints of progressive weakness, malaise, and perhaps hints of possible precipitating events. Patients may complain of new-onset urinary incontinence resulting from marked polyuria due to the osmotic diuresis.

8. **What other questions are vital to the history in a patient with suspected HHS?**
A thorough history is essential to diagnosing and managing this potentially life-threatening complication. The history should include a careful review of possible precipitating events or illnesses; a description of the patient's diabetes history, including medications, symptoms, and diabetes-related complications; a review of medication adherence; a complete past medical history; a social history including alcohol and other drug use; and an assessment of gastrointestinal symptoms including vomiting and the ability to take fluids orally.

9. **What physical findings should one expect in a patient with suspected HHS?**
Patients with DKA and patients with HHS have profound volume depletion. As a result, it is imperative to assess hemodynamic status and degree of dehydration. Hypotension and tachycardia are common, as are diminished skin turgor and dry mucous membranes. Normothermia is common, even in the setting of infection. Patients need to be examined for any infectious or ischemic complications and for any evidence of overt or subtle cognitive deficits. A depressed cognitive state ranging from profound stupor to mild clouding of the sensorium may be present. Focal neurologic abnormalities may also be noted. Symptoms and findings tend to be more severe in elderly persons and in those with baseline cognitive dysfunction. The degree of alteration of mental status correlates with the severity of the hyperosmolarity, but not with acidosis.

Gaglia JL, Wyckoff J, Abrahamson MJ: Acute hyperglycemic crisis in the elderly. Med Clin North Am 88:1063–1084, 2004.

10. **What laboratory tests should be ordered in a patient with suspected HHS?**
Initial laboratory evaluation should include a Sequential Multiple Analysis for seven different serum tests (SMA-7), hepatic panel, complete blood count, urinalysis, urine culture, and measurement of phosphorus, magnesium, calcium, and serum ketone levels. Other tests to consider include blood cultures, arterial blood gas analysis, and cardiac enzyme measurement. Patients should also undergo electrocardiography and chest radiography.

11. **What abnormalities should one expect to see among the laboratory test results of a patient with suspected HHS?**
Because intracellular dehydration and acidosis typically lead to potassium loss, total body stores are often significantly depleted. However, hypokalemia may not be present on initial laboratory evaluation because of the extracellular potassium shift caused by acidemia. Other common electrolyte disturbances include hypophosphatemia, hypomagnesemia, and hypocalcemia. Hemoconcentration usually results in a hematocrit in the range of 55–60%, and the white blood cell count is typically elevated to between 12,000 and 20,000.

12. **How is HHS treated?**
The primary goals of treatment are to rapidly restore intravascular volume and to identify and rapidly correct any precipitating illnesses. Fluid resuscitation lowers blood glucose levels independent of insulin by diluting serum glucose and by improving renal perfusion, which leads to increased glycosuria. Fluid resuscitation also reduces levels of counter-regulatory hormones, thereby improving insulin sensitivity.

13. **What is the best way to replace fluids?**
The first step is to determine the patient's fluid deficit, which can be calculated using the patient's corrected serum sodium and weight (*see* question 15). Many authorities recommend correction of the fluid deficit relatively slowly, with half the deficit replaced in the first 12 hours and the second half over the next 12–24 hours.

14. **Should one use isotonic or hypotonic fluids?**
Some experts recommend starting with isotonic fluids such as normal saline because these fluids are still hypotonic relative to the patient's serum osmolality and they remain within the intravascular space more than hypotonic solutions. Because hemodynamic stability is of foremost importance, normal saline should always be used in patients with significant hypotension. Other authorities advocate using hypotonic fluids such as 0.45% NaCl or balanced solutions such as lactated Ringer's solution even at the outset because the patient is losing fluids that are relatively hypotonic with respect to electrolytes. The argument against isotonic solutions is that they provide excessive amounts of sodium and chloride,

which can lead to persistent hypernatremia, exacerbated by continued loss of isotonic fluids even after fluid resuscitation has begun. Hypotonic solutions are avoided by some since they could lead to a risk of cerebral edema, although this has not been the case in clinical practice. A reasonable approach is to administer normal saline for the first 1–4 hours to improve hemodynamic status. Once intravascular volume is restored, as reflected by an increase in supine blood pressure and a decrease in resting pulse, one should switch to half normal saline.

KEY POINTS: HYPEROSMOTIC HYPERGLYCEMIC SYNDROME (HHS)

1. HHS is defined by an effective serum osmolarity ≥ 320 mOsm/L and a plasma glucose ≥ 600 in the absence of significant acidosis.

2. HHS is differentiated from diabetic ketoacidosis by a more insidious onset, an older average patient age, extreme hyperglycemia, and severe dehydration.

3. Common precipitating causes of HHS include unknown diabetes or inadequate diabetic treatment, infections, myocardial infarction and other vascular events, drugs and medications, and pancreatitis.

4. Volume resuscitation is the cornerstone of treatment! Fluids alone will correct much of the hyperglycemia and hyperosmolality.

5. Using isotonic versus hypotonic fluids for initial treatment is controversial, although either option is reasonable.

15. **What is the conversion for corrected serum sodium in the setting of severe hyperglycemia?**
    The low measured serum sodium observed in the presence of severely elevated glucose levels is termed *pseudohyponatremia*. Corrected serum sodium can be calculated using the following formula:

    Corrected Na $= (Na) + 1.6$(gloucose in mg/dL $- 100)/100 + 0.002$(triglycerides in mg/dL)

    For simplicity, a reasonable rule is that for each 100-mg/dL increase in serum glucose above normal, the measured serum sodium concentration decreases by approximately 2 mEq/L.

16. **Why can insulin be harmful early in the treatment of HHS?**
    With chronic severe volume depletion, a large amount of fluid is held in the intravascular space by the osmotic effects of glucose. When insulin is administered to patients early in the treatment of HHS, glucose moves rapidly into cells, causing fluid to follow. This rapid decrease in intravascular volume can lead to hypotension and shock. Because glucose levels show a marked improvement with fluid replacement alone, insulin should be administered only after sufficient volume has been infused to replenish intravascular volume. Once the patient has been adequately resuscitated, an insulin infusion may be used similar to its use in patients with DKA, although the doses needed are typically lower.

Matz R: Hyperglycemic hyperosmolar syndrome. In Porte D, Sherwin RS, Baron A (eds): Ellenberg and Rifkin's Diabetes Mellitus, 6th ed. New York, McGraw-Hill, 2003, pp 587–599.

17. **How does one determine a patient's total body water (TBW) deficit?**
The water deficit can be calculated based on the "true" serum sodium concentration, working on the assumption that 60% of the body's weight is water (or about 50% in women). In the following example, a 70-kg male has a corrected serum sodium of 154 mEq/L, with a goal sodium level of 140 mEq/L. His TBW is therefore:

$$70 \text{ kg} \times 0.6 = 42 \text{ L water}$$

His expected TBW can be calculated by:

$$(154 \text{ mEq/L Na}) \times (42 \text{ L actual TBW}) = (140 \text{ mEq/L}) \times (\text{expected TBW})$$
$$\text{expected TBW} = (154) \times (42)/(140) = 46.2 \text{ L}$$
$$\text{Fluid deficit} = \text{expected TBW} - \text{actual TBW}$$
$$= 46.2 \text{ L} - 42 \text{ L} = 4.2\text{-L deficit}$$

The TBW deficit may also be calculated by the following formula:

$$\text{TBW deficit (in liters)} = 0.6 \times (\text{body weight in kilograms}) \times (1 - 140/[\text{Na}])$$

18. **How should one treat the electrolyte abnormalities associated with HHS?**
Because the total body potassium level is usually low despite normal serum levels, potassium should be administered to patients with levels < 5.5. Potassium may be added to the patient's IV fluids or may be taken by mouth. Phosphate should not be replaced unless losses are severe (≤1.5) because of the risk of causing hypocalcemia.

Wyckoff J, Abrahamson MJ: Diabetic ketoacidosis and hyperosmolar hyperglycemic state. In Kahn CR, Weir GC, King GL, et al (eds): Joslin's Diabetes Mellitus, 14th ed. Philadelphia, Lippincott Williams & Wilkins, 2005, pp 887–899.

19. **What are some of the complications associated with HHS?**
Thrombotic events may be seen in the setting of hyperviscosity and low flow related to the severe dehydration of HHS. Subclinical rhabdomyolysis with creatine kinase elevations ≥ 1000 IU/L may be relatively common. However, acute renal failure from acute tubular necrosis is very rare, probably because of the concomitant high-volume osmotic diuresis. Disseminated intravascular coagulation is another rare but potentially fatal complication. Pulmonary aspiration resulting from gastroparesis and altered mental status is another potential consequence of HHS, as is pancreatitis. Cerebral edema is an extremely rare complication, occurring more frequently in younger patients with DKA.

CHAPTER 51

ADRENAL INSUFFICIENCY IN THE INTENSIVE CARE UNIT

Michael Young, MD

1. **Is adrenal insufficiency common among patients in the intensive care unit (ICU)?**
   The incidence of adrenal insufficiency in the ICU population is 1–6% and may be as high as 74% for patients with severe sepsis and septic shock. However, there is no agreed-upon gold standard for confirming adrenal insufficiency among most ICU patients.

   Cooper MS, Stewart PM: Corticosteroid insufficiency in acutely ill patients. N Engl J Med 348:727–734, 2003.

2. **Describe the main types of adrenal insufficiency seen in patients in the ICU.**
   1. **Relative adrenal insufficiency:** This is the most common and perplexing type of adrenal insufficiency seen in patients in the ICU. Patients with relative adrenal insufficiency may present with vasopressor dependency, multiple organ dysfunction, hypothermia, or an inability to wean from mechanical ventilation. These patients can be identified by their limited response to adrenal stimulation tests or lower-than-expected basal cortisol levels despite critical illness (Fig. 51-1).
   2. **Acute adrenal crisis/insufficiency:** Acute clinical presentation includes profound hypotension, fever, and hypovolemia. These patients have very low cortisol levels (≤ 3 µg/dL).
   3. **Chronic adrenal insufficiency**
      - **Primary adrenal insufficiency (Addison's disease):** The most common causes are autoimmune diseases (70%) and tuberculosis (10%). Rare causes include adrenal hemorrhage, adrenal metastasis, cytomegalovirus, human immunodeficiency virus (HIV) disease, amyloidosis, and sarcoidosis.
      - **Secondary adrenal insufficiency:** This condition is caused by inadequate production of adrenocorticotropic hormone (ACTH) due to chronic use of exogenous steroids (most common cause), hypopituitary state, or isolated ACTH deficiency.

3. **What are the clinical markers of acute adrenal insufficiency?**
   Acute adrenal insufficiency presents with various combinations of hypotension, tachycardia, severe hypovolemia, respiratory failure, nausea, vomiting, diarrhea, lethargy, and weakness. Patients with acute adrenal insufficiency due to chronic exogenous replacement may not initially exhibit hypotension because mineralocorticoid secretion can be intact until late-stage illness.

4. **List the laboratory abnormalities associated with adrenal insufficiency.**
   - Hyponatremia is most common.
   - Low levels of chloride and bicarbonate and high levels of potassium occur frequently.
   - Also seen are moderate eosinophilia, lymphocytosis, hypercalcemia, and hypoglycemia.

5. **How is adrenal insufficiency diagnosed?**
   - **In ICU patients:** The use of provocative adrenal stimulation tests in critically ill patients remains controversial. Perhaps the most widely used protocol (from Annane et al.) identifies patients with severe sepsis and septic shock as having relative adrenal insufficiency if their

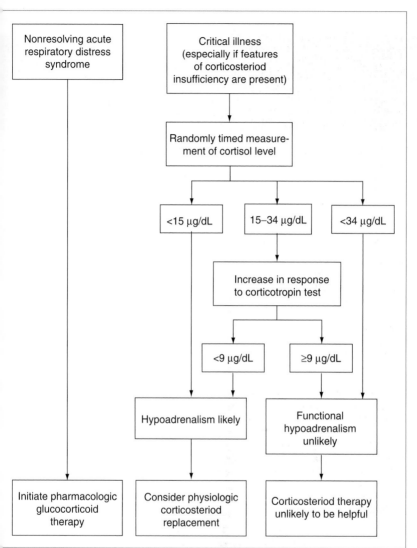

Figure 51-1. Steroid replacement in severe sepsis and septic shock. Steroid use for "late acute respiratory distress syndrome" is controversial (see www.ardsnet.org/). (From Cooper MS, Stewart PM: Corticosteroid insufficiency in acutely ill patients. N Engl J Med 348:727–734, 2003, with permission.)

baseline cortisol level is <35 μg/dL and they respond to an ACTH stimulation test (250 μg corticotropin) with a bump in cortisol of <10 μg/dL (see Fig. 51-1). Other authors caution that "free cortisol" levels, rather than the standard cortisol levels, should be used to avoid the overdiagnosis of relative adrenal insufficiency. Still others argue that 250 μg corticotropin far exceeds the test dose that should be used.

- **In non-ICU patients:** In a nonstressed patient, a random cortisol level >20 μg/dL may rule out the diagnosis of adrenal insufficiency. A random cortisol level <3 μg/dL confirms the diagnosis of adrenal insufficiency.

  Annane D, Sebille V, Charpentier C, et al: Effect of treatment with low doses of hydrocortisone and fludrocortisone on mortality in patients with septic shock. JAMA 288:862–871, 2005.

  Hamrahian AH, Oseni TS, Arafah BM: Measurements of serum free cortisol in critically ill patients. N Eng J Med 350:1629–1638, 2004

  Zaloga GP, Marik P: Hypothalamic-pituitary-adrenal insufficiency. Crit Car Clin 17:25–41, 2001.

6. **How should one use the ACTH stimulation test?**
   Cortisol levels are measured before and 30–60 minutes after a supraphysiologic dose of ACTH (250 μg corticotropin given intravenously). In patients who are not critically ill, a normal response generates a poststimulation cortisol level ≥20 μg/dL. For critically ill patients, see Fig. 51-1.

7. **What about corticotropin-releasing hormone (CHR) stimulation?**
   CHR is given to stimulate cortisol levels. Unlike the ACTH stimulation test, CHR stimulation can rule out central adrenal insufficiency. A normal response generates a poststimulation cortisol level ≥20 μg/dL or a 30- to 60-minute rise in cortisol ≥7.

8. **Should the low-dose ACTH (1-μG) stimulation test be used?**
   This test may detect adrenal atrophy associated with adrenal insufficiency. There is no consensus on how to determine the lower level that equates with a normal cortisol response.

9. **How does one distinguish between acute adrenal insufficiency and other illness states in the ICU?**
   The clinical findings and laboratory findings found among patients with acute adrenal insufficiency are also common in the ICU population. Distinguishing between adrenal insufficiency and other illnesses in critically ill patients requires clinical suspicion and at least one of the following:
   - Failure to respond adequately to an adrenal stimulation test
   - Inappropriately low basal cortisol levels
   - An unequivocal clinical response to empiric exogenous steroids

10. **Should steroids be administered to ICU patients with a history of chronic steroid use?**
    Patients may become adrenally insufficient after taking the equivalent of 20 mg/day of prednisone for just 5 days, but adrenal insufficiency is rare among patients taking steroids for <7 days. Patients can become adrenally insufficient after taking very-low-dose steroids for months to years (>5 mg/day prednisone equivalent). Fearing life-threatening adrenal impairment, many physicians give "stress doses" (hydrocortisone, 300–400 mg/day or equivalent) to critically ill patients who received chronic steroids before their admission to the ICU.

    Krasner AS: Glucocorticoid-induced adrenal insufficiency. JAMA 282:671–676, 1999.

11. **What ICU patient groups are at high risk for adrenal insufficiency?**
    - Patients with severe sepsis and septic shock
    - Patients taking chronic steroids: See question 10.
    - Patients with HIV disease: The adrenal gland may be involved in >50% of patients infected with HIV. However, because adrenal function requires <20% of the gland to function, adrenal insufficiency in this population is uncommon (3%).
    - Patients with cancer: Even when cancers metastasize to the adrenal gland, adrenal dysfunction is uncommon.

KEY POINTS: ADRENAL INSUFFICIENCY

1. Relative adrenal insufficiency exists in a majority of ICU patients with severe sepsis or septic shock.

2. Newly critically ill ICU patients who recently received a prednisone equivalent to ≥ 5 mg/day for ≥ 7 days should probably receive stress-dose steroid coverage.

3. To detect relative adrenal insufficiency among critically ill ICU patients requires at least one of the following:
   - Clinical suspicion
   - Patient's failure to respond to an adrenal stimulation test
   - Inappropriately low basal cortisol levels
   - An unequivocal clinical response to exogenous steroids

4. Stress-dose steroids should be given to most patients with severe sepsis or septic shock and relative adrenal insufficiency.

- High-risk postoperative patients: Patients >55 years old, patients undergoing major operations (e.g., coronary artery bypass grafting, abdominal aortic aneurysm repair, Whipple procedure), patients with multiple trauma, and postoperative patients requiring vasopressors or failing to wean from mechanical ventilation appear to be at higher risk for adrenal insufficiency.

    Brown CJ, Buie WD: Perioperative stress dose steroids: Do they make a difference?. J Am Coll Surg 193:678–686, 2001.
    Mayo J, Collazos J, Martinez E, Ibarra S: Adrenal function in the human immunodeficiency virus–infected patient. Arch Intern Med 162:1095–1098, 2002.
    Rivers EP, Gaspari M, Saad GA, et al: Adrenal insufficiency in high-risk surgical ICU patients. Chest 119:889–896, 2001.

2. **Do neurotrauma patients have special problems with adrenal insufficiency?**
   Fifty percent of patients suffering moderate to severe traumatic head injury have cortisol levels ≤ 15 µg/dL. This is especially true among patients receiving pentobarbital or propofol. These patients often require vasopressors. Thus, monitoring cortisol levels in patients with moderate to severe head injury may be warranted. Steroid supplementation can be considered in patients with head trauma who have relative adrenal insufficiency and sustained hypotension.

    Cohan C, Wang, C, McArthur D, et al: Acute secondary adrenal insufficiency after traumatic brain injury: A prospective study. Crit Care Med 22:2358–2366, 2005.

3. **Should every critically ill ICU patient with relative adrenal insufficiency receive stress-dose steroids?**
   The evidence for steroid use to treat relative adrenal insufficiency is strongest among ICU patients with severe sepsis and septic shock. There have been no randomized trials to guide clinicians when confronted with nonseptic critically ill ICU patients with evidence of relative adrenal insufficiency, such as postoperative surgical patients, patients with severe pancreatitis, and patients with moderate to severe traumatic head injury.

4. **What are the indicated therapies for ICU patients with severe sepsis or septic shock suspected to have adrenal insufficiency?**
   - **Fluid resuscitation:** When septic patients with known or strongly suspected adrenal insufficiency do not respond adequately to repeated large boluses of isotonic fluid, and/or when they require vasopressors, the administration of stress-dose steroids should be started immediately.

- **Steroid dosing:** Administration of hydrocortisone, 300–400 mg/day given intravenously in three or four divided doses with or without fludrocortisone (50 μg enterally every day), is accepted practice, but the dose and frequency are not evidence based.
- **Steroid duration:** For relative adrenal insufficiency associated with severe sepsis or septic shock, the author recommends administration of stress-dose hydrocortisone (300 mg/day) for 72 hours. If the patient shows rapid clinical improvement, the steroids may be tapered over 1–2 days. If significant hypotension recurs, steroid dosing should return to the initial stress doses, and a rapid taper can be undertaken after 7 days.

15. **Should stress-dose steroid supplementation be strongly considered in all patients with severe sepsis or septic shock?**
    Opinions on this point differ.
    - **Yes, of course:** A majority of patients with severe sepsis or septic shock have relative adrenal insufficiency. The mortality rate for such patients is 40–60%. A recent randomized control trial found an absolute mortality reduction of 10% among patients with severe sepsis or septic shock and relative adrenal insufficiency who received stress-dose steroids versus placebo. This finding is supported by multiple animal and human models. Steroid supplementation for most patients with severe sepsis or sepsis shock makes sense given the modest risk of a short course of low-dose steroids.

        Annane D, Sebille V, Charpentier C, et al: Effect of treatment with low doses of hydrocortisone and fludrocortisone on mortality in patients with septic shock. JAMA 288:862–871, 2005.
        Balk RB: Steroids for septic shock. Back from the dead? (pro) Chest 123:490S, 2003. [An earlier randomized controlled trial (Sprung et al.) used superphysiologic doses, p 499S.].
    - **No, data are still too mixed:** A randomized trial using superphysiologic doses of steroids among patients with septic shock found an increased rate of late infections and no mortality reduction. The "might help, can't hurt" argument for steroids in this setting is problematic. The Annane trial did not demonstrate across-the-board mortality reduction in the steroid group with severe sepsis and septic shock. In addition, there is insufficient understanding of the implication of relatively low cortisol levels or an inadequate response to cosyntropin stimulation among patients with severe sepsis or septic shock.

        Sessler CN: Steroids for septic shock: Back from the dead (con). Chest 123:482S–489S, 2003.
        Sprung CL, Caralis PV, Marcial EH, et al: The effects of high-dose corticosteroids in patients with septic shock: A prospective, controlled study. N Engl J Med 311:1137–1143, 1984.

THYROID DISEASE IN THE INTENSIVE CARE UNIT

Michael T. McDermott, MD

CHAPTER 52

1. **What is the euthyroid sick syndrome?**

   Euthyroid sick syndrome refers to changes in serum thyroid hormone and thyroid-stimulating hormone (TSH) levels that occur in patients with a variety of nonthyroidal illnesses, including infections, malignancies, inflammatory conditions, myocardial infarction, surgery, trauma, and starvation. This condition is also called the *nonthyroidal illness syndrome*. It is not a primary thyroid disorder but instead results from changes in peripheral thyroid hormone metabolism and transport induced by the nonthyroidal illness.

   Brennan MD, Bahn RS: Thyroid hormones and illness. Endocr Pract 4:396–403, 1998.

   Cerillo AG, Storti S, Mariani M, et al: The non-thyroidal illness syndrome after coronary artery bypass grafting: A 6-month follow-up study. Clin Chem Lab Med 43:289–293, 2005.

   Den Brinker M, Joosten KF, Visser TJ, et al: Euthyroid sick syndrome in meningococcal sepsis: The impact of peripheral thyroid hormone metabolism and binding proteins. J Clin Endocrinol Metab. 90:5613–5620, 2005.

2. **What hormone changes characterize the euthyroid sick syndrome?**

   - **Mild to moderate illnesses:** Serum triiodothyronine (T3) (total and free) levels decrease due to decreased conversion of thyroxine (T4) to T3 in peripheral tissues. Serum free T4 and TSH levels usually remain within the reference range.
   - **Moderate to severe illnesses:** Serum T3 (total and free) levels decrease further; total T4 decreases and T3 resin uptake (T3RU) increases because of reduced thyroid hormone binding to transport proteins due both to impaired protein synthesis and the presence of circulating inhibitors of binding. Free T4 may be normal, decreased, or increased. Serum TSH levels are normal or slightly decreased at this stage.
   - **Recovery from illnesses:** Free T4 decreases and TSH increases (and may be transiently elevated) as hepatic protein synthesis improves and circulating inhibitors of protein binding disappear.

   McIver B, Gorman CA: Euthyroid sick syndrome: An overview. Thyroid 7:125–132, 1997.

3. **How can the euthyroid sick syndrome be distinguished from hypothyroidism?**

   In the euthyroid sick syndrome, the serum T3 level is decreased proportionately more than T4, the T3RU level tends to be high, and the TSH level is normal or mildly decreased. In primary hypothyroidism, the serum T4 level is reduced proportionately more than T3, the T3RU level tends to be low, and the TSH level is increased. Other tests also may be helpful. In the euthyroid sick syndrome, free T4 is usually at a normal level and reverse T3 (RT3) is increased; in hypothyroidism, both free T4 and RT3 levels are decreased.

4. **What causes the euthyroid sick syndrome?**

   The euthyroid sick syndrome is believed to be caused by increased circulating levels of cytokines and other inflammation mediators resulting from the underlying nonthyroidal illness. These mediators can inhibit the thyroid axis at multiple levels, including the pituitary (decreased TSH secretion), the thyroid (decreased T4 and T3 responses to TSH), peripheral tissues (decreased conversion of T4 to T3; decreased responses to T3), and transport proteins (decreased thyroid hormone binding).

Kimura T, Kanda T, Kotajima N, et al: Involvement of circulating interleukin-6 and its receptor in the development of euthyroid sick syndrome in patients with acute myocardial infarction. Eur J Endocrinol 143:179–184, 2000.

Nagaya T, Fujieda M, Otsuka G, et al: A potential role of activated NF-kappa B in the pathogenesis of euthyroid sick syndrome. J Clin Invest 106:393–402, 2000.

Peeters RP, Wouters PJ, Kaptein E, et al: Reduced activation and increased inactivation of thyroid hormone in tissues of critically ill patients. J Clin Endocrinol Metab 88:3202–3211, 2003.

5. **Is the euthyroid sick syndrome an adaptive mechanism, or is it harmful?**
   Many experts consider the euthyroid sick syndrome to be an adaptive mechanism that may reduce peripheral tissue energy expenditure during nonthyroidal illness. Conversely, others argue that the alterations in circulating thyroid hormone levels may themselves be harmful and may accentuate the effects of the nonthyroidal illness. This issue is likely to remain controversial for years to come.

Iervasi G, Pingatore A, Landi P, et al: Low-T3 syndrome: A strong prognostic predictor of death in patients with heart disease. Circulation 107:708–711, 2003.

Peeters RP, Wouters PJ, van Toor H, et al: Serum 3,3′,5′-triiodothyronine (rT3) and 3,5,3′-triiodothyronine/rT3 are prognostic markers in critically ill patients and are associated with postmortem tissue deiodinase activities. J Clin Endocrinol Metab 90:4559–4565, 2005.

Pingitore A, Landi P, Taddei MC, et al: Triiodothyronine levels for risk stratification of patients with chronic heart failure. Am J Med 118:132–136, 2005.

6. **Should patients with the euthyroid sick syndrome be treated with thyroid hormones?**
   Management of the euthyroid sick syndrome is also highly controversial. Currently, there are no consistent or convincing data demonstrating a recovery or survival benefit from treating euthyroid sick syndrome patients with either levothyroxine (LT4) or liothyronine (LT3). Experts continue to debate this issue, however, and agree that large, prospective studies are needed to answer this question. In the absence of more definitive data, thyroid hormone therapy is not recommended at this time.

Bartalena L: The dilemma of non-thyroidal illness syndrome: To treat or not to treat? J Endocrinol Invest 26:1162, 2003.

Brent GA, Hershman JM: Thyroxine therapy in patients with severe nonthyroidal illness and low serum thyroxine concentration. J Clin Endocrinol Metab 63:1–8, 1986.

Camacho PM, Dwarkanathan A: Sick euthyroid syndrome. What to do when thyroid function tests are abnormal in critically ill patients. Postgrad Med 105:215–219, 1999.

DeGroot L: "Non-thyroidal illness syndrome" is functional central hypothyroidism, and if severe, hormone replacement is appropriate in light of present knowledge. J Endocrinol Invest 26:1162, 2003.

Stathatos N, Wartofsky L: The euthyroid sick syndrome: Is there a physiologic rationale for thyroid hormone treatment?. J Endocrinol Invest 26:1174–1179, 2003.

7. **Are levels of thyroid hormone ever elevated in patients with nonthyroidal diseases?**
   The serum T4 level may be transiently elevated in patients with acute psychiatric illnesses and various acute medical illnesses. The mechanisms underlying such elevations of T4 are not well understood, but they may be mediated by alterations in neurotransmitters or cytokines. This condition must be distinguished from true thyrotoxicosis.

8. **What is thyroid storm?**
   Thyroid storm or crisis is a life-threatening condition characterized by an exaggeration of the manifestations of thyrotoxicosis.

Burch HD, Wartofsky L: Life threatening thyrotoxicosis: Thyroid storm. Endocrinol Metab Clin North Am 22:263–278, 1993.

Tietgens ST, Leinung MC: Thyroid storm. Med Clin North Am 79:169–184, 1995.

9. **How do patients develop thyroid storm?**
   Thyroid storm usually occurs in patients who have unrecognized or inadequately treated thyrotoxicosis and a superimposed precipitating event, such as thyroid surgery, nonthyroidal surgery, infection, or trauma.

10. **What are the clinical manifestations of thyroid storm?**
    Fever (temperature $> 102°F$) is the cardinal manifestation. Tachycardia is usually present and tachypnea is common, but the blood pressure is variable. Cardiac arrhythmias, congestive heart failure, and ischemic heart symptoms may develop. Nausea, vomiting, diarrhea, and abdominal pain are frequent features. Central nervous system manifestations include hyperkinesis, psychosis, and coma. A goiter is a helpful finding but is not always present.

11. **What laboratory abnormalities are seen in thyroid storm?**
    Serum T4 (total and free) and T3 (total and free) levels are usually significantly elevated, and the serum TSH is undetectable. Other common laboratory abnormalities include anemia, leukocytosis, hyperglycemia, azotemia, hypercalcemia, and elevated levels of liver-associated enzymes.

12. **How is the diagnosis of thyroid storm made?**
    The diagnosis must be made on the basis of suspicious but nonspecific clinical findings. Serum thyroid hormone levels are elevated, but if the diagnosis is strongly suspected, waiting for the results of tests may cause a critical delay in the initiation of effective life-saving therapy. Furthermore, thyroid hormone levels do not reliably distinguish patients with thyroid storm from those who have uncomplicated thyrotoxicosis as a coincident disorder. Clinical features are therefore the key.

    Brooks MH, Waldstein SS: Free thyroxine concentrations in thyroid storm. Ann Intern Med 93:694–697, 1980.

13. **What other conditions may mimic thyroid storm?**
    Similar presentations may be seen with sepsis, pheochromocytoma, and malignant hyperthermia.

14. **How should patients with thyroid storm be treated?**
    The immediate goals are to decrease thyroid hormone synthesis, to inhibit thyroid hormone release, to reduce the heart rate, to support the circulation, and to treat the precipitating condition. Because β_1-adrenergic receptors are significantly increased in patients with this condition, β_1-selective blockers are the preferred agents for heart rate control. Recommended medications are listed in Table 52-1.

    Dillmann WH: Thyroid storm. Curr Ther Endocrinol Metab 6:81–85, 1997.
    Yeung S-CJ, Go R, Balasubramanyam A: Rectal administration of iodide and propylthiouracil in the treatment of thyroid storm. Thyroid 5:403–405, 1995.

15. **What is myxedema coma?**
    Myxedema coma is a life-threatening condition characterized by an exaggeration of the manifestations of hypothyroidism.

    Nicoloff JT: Myxedema coma: A form of decompensated hypothyroidism. Endocrinol Metab Clin North Am 22:279–290, 1993.
    Tsitouras PD: Myxedema coma. Clin Geriatr Med 11:251–258, 1995.

16. **How does myxedema coma develop?**
    Myxedema coma usually occurs in elderly patients who have inadequately treated or untreated hypothyroidism and a superimposed precipitating event. Important events include prolonged cold exposure, infection, trauma, surgery, myocardial infarction, congestive heart failure, pulmonary embolism, stroke, respiratory failure, gastrointestinal bleeding, and

TABLE 52-1. RECOMMENDED MEDICATIONS FOR TREATMENT OF THYROID STORM

Medication	Dosage
Decrease thyroid hormone synthesis	
Propylthiouracil	200 mg q4h (orally, rectally or NG tube)
Methimazole (Tapazole)	20 mg q4h (orally, rectally, or NG tube)
Inhibit thyroid hormone release	
Sodium iodide (NaI)	1 gm over 24 hours IV
Potassium iodide (SSKI)	5 drops q8h orally
Lugol's solution	10 drops q8h orally
Reduce the heart rate	
Esmolol	500 μg/kg over 1 min IV, then
	50–300 μg/kg/min by infusion
Metoprolol	5–10 mg IV q2–4h
Diltiazem	60–90 mg q6–8h orally *or*
	0.25 mg/kg over 2 min IV, then 10 mg/min by infusion
Support the circulation	
Dexamethasone	2 mg q6h IV *or*
Hydrocortisone	100 mg q8h IV
Intravenous fluids	
Treat the precipitating condition	

NG = nasogastric, SSKI = saturated solution of potassium iodide.

administration of various drugs, particularly those that have a depressive effect on the central nervous system.

17. **What are the clinical manifestations of myxedema coma?**
Hypothermia, bradycardia, and hypoventilation are common; blood pressure, while generally reduced, is more variable. Pericardial, pleural, and peritoneal effusions are often found. An ileus is present in about two-thirds of patients, and acute urinary retention also may be seen. Central nervous system manifestations include seizures, stupor, and coma; deep tendon reflexes are absent or exhibit a delayed relaxation phase. Typical hypothyroid skin and hair changes may be apparent. A goiter, although frequently absent, is a helpful finding; a thyroidectomy scar also may be an important clue.

18. **What laboratory abnormalities are seen in myxedema coma?**
Serum T4 (total and free) and T3 (total and free) levels are usually low, and the TSH level is significantly elevated. Other frequent abnormalities include anemia, hyponatremia,

hypoglycemia, and elevated serum levels of cholesterol and creatine kinase. Arterial blood gases often reveal carbon dioxide retention and hypoxemia. The electrocardiogram often shows sinus bradycardia, various types and degrees of heart block, low voltage, and T-wave flattening.

9. **How is the diagnosis of myxedema coma made?**
The diagnosis must be made on clinical grounds based on the findings described previously. Serum levels of thyroid hormone levels are reduced and the TSH level is elevated, but the delay involved in waiting for test results may unnecessarily postpone the initiation of effective therapy.

KEY POINTS: THYROID DISORDERS

1. The euthyroid sick syndrome is not a thyroid disorder but is instead a group of changes in serum thyroid hormone and thyroid-stimulating hormone levels that result from cytokines and inflammatory mediators produced in patients with nonthyroidal illnesses.

2. The most common feature of the euthyroid sick syndrome is a decrease in serum triiodothyronine (T3) levels due to reduced conversion of thyroxine (T4) to T3 in the liver and other tissues.

3. The euthyroid sick syndrome appears to be an adaptive response to reduce tissue metabolism and preserve energy during systemic illnesses, and therefore treatment with thyroid hormone is not currently recommended for this condition.

4. Thyroid storm is a life-threatening form of severe thyrotoxicosis that usually has an identifiable precipitating factor and has a high mortality rate if not treated promptly and appropriately.

5. When thyroid storm is diagnosed or suspected, treatment with antithyroid drugs, cold iodine, beta blockers, and stress doses of glucocorticoids, along with management of any precipitating factors, should be promptly initiated.

6. Myxedema coma is a life-threatening form of severe hypothyroidism that often has an identifiable precipitating cause and has a high mortality rate if not promptly and adequately treated.

7. When myxedema coma is diagnosed or suspected, management should include rapid repletion of the thyroid hormone deficit, stress doses of glucocorticoids, and treatment of any precipitating causes.

20. **How should patients with myxedema coma be treated?**
The goals are to rapidly replace the depleted thyroid hormone pool, to replace glucocorticoids, to support vital functions, and to treat any precipitating conditions. The normal total body pool of T4 is about 1000 μg (500 μg in the thyroid and 500 μg in the rest of the body). Whether to use levothyroxine (LT4), liothyronine (LT3), or both remains controversial, but this author favors the combination of LT4 plus LT3. Regimens for LT4 alone, LT3 then LT4, and LT4 plus LT3 are in Table 52-2.

Jordan RM: Myxedema coma. Pathophysiology, therapy, and factors affecting prognosis. Med Clin North Am 79:185–194, 1995.

Pittman CS, Zayed AA: Myxedema coma. Curr Ther Endocrinol Metab 6:98–101, 1997.

Yamamoto T, Fukuyama J, Fujiyoshi A: Factors associated with mortality of myxedema coma: Report of eight cases and literature survey. Thyroid 9:1167–1174, 1999.

TABLE 52-2. REGIMENS FOR TREATMENT OF MYXEDEMA COMA

Regimen	Dosage
Provide rapid repletion of circulating thyroid hormones	
LT4 alone	LT4 200–500 μg over 5 min IV, then
	LT4 50–100 μg q.d. orally or IV
LT3 then LT4	LT3 50–100 μg over 5 min IV, then
	LT4 50–100 μg q.d. orally or IV
LT4 plus LT3	LT4 200–500 μg over 5 min IV, plus
	LT3 20–50 μg over 5 min IV, then
	LT4 50–100 μg q.d. and LT3 20–30 μg q.d. orally or IV
Replace glucocorticoids	
Hydrocortisone	100 mg q8h IV
Support vital functions	
Oxygen	
IV fluids	
Rewarming (blankets or central rewarming)	
Mechanical ventilation (if needed)	
Treat the precipitating condition	

LT4 = levothyroxine, LT3 = liothyronine.

BLOOD PRODUCTS AND COAGULATION

David G. Burris, MD, DMCC, COL, USA, MC, and Mark W. Bowyer, MD, DMCC, COL, USAF, MC

CHAPTER 53

1. **What is the best fluid with which to treat shock due to acute blood loss?**
   Warm fresh whole blood, if it can be obtained, because it contains red cells for oxygen transport, coagulation factors, and platelets. It is usually not available because of its short storage life. It is a matter of paramount importance to stop hemorrhage as quickly as possible to keep the patient's own blood.

2. **How is blood preserved?**
   Banked blood contains CPDA-1 (or CAPD or CPD), which contains **C**itrate to prevent coagulation and **P**hosphate, **D**extrose, and **A**denine as energy sources for the cells. Blood is stored at 4–7°C to prevent bacterial growth.

3. **What components of blood are available?**
   Packed red blood cells (PRBCs), fresh frozen plasma (FFP), cryoprecipitate, platelets, and white cell preparations.

4. **What are PRBCs?**
   PRBCs remain after the centrifugation of whole blood and the removal of plasma. One unit of PRBCs raises the hemoglobin level by 1 mg/dL or the hematocrit by an average of three points.

5. **How long can RBCs be stored?**
   Forty-two days. Although up to 80% of the RBCs are still viable after 42 days, the white cells and platelets are not, and clotting factors have minimal activity.

6. **Discuss the indications for RBC transfusions in critically ill patients.**
   RBC transfusions are used to maximize oxygen delivery to the tissues (the primary purpose for transfusions). The only absolute indications for transfusion are clinical evidence of tissue hypoxia or a hemoglobin level less than 7 mg/dL (hematocrit < 21). Transfusion at higher hemoglobin levels may be required based on patient age, chronic anemia, and coexisting disease that leads to tissue ischemia, including coronary artery disease, pulmonary insufficiency, and occlusive vascular disease.

7. **What is the ideal hematocrit level in critically ill patients?**
   Recent work suggests that survival may be impaired by transfusing patients to achieve a hematocrit level greater than 25.

8. **Define *hemolytic transfusion reaction*.**
   Hemolytic transfusion reactions occur when ABO- or Rh-mismatched blood is given. (Avoid clerical error!) It may occur when as little as 10 mL of blood is infused; the reaction causes fulminant disseminated intravascular coagulation (DIC) and is associated with a mortality rate of about 35%. Significant morbidity also may occur; acute renal failure may result from acute tubular necrosis.

9. **List the classic findings in hemolytic transfusion reaction.**

   Fever, chills, back or flank pain, chest pain, dyspnea, hypotension, oliguria, and hemoglobinuria Intraoperatively, this reaction may be heralded by sudden hemorrhage in a previously dry field

10. **How is a hemolytic transfusion reaction treated?**

    First and foremost, stop the transfusion. Support the patient with IV fluids, diuretics (e.g., mannitol), inotropes, plasma products, and monitoring in the intensive care unit (ICU).

11. **What are the infectious risks of transfusion?**

    Although the risk depends on the prevalence of infection in the donating population, the overal risk of infection from a transfused unit in the United States is about 1:2,000,000 for hepatitis B hepatitis C, and human immunodeficiency virus.

    Sandler SG, Yu H, Rassai N: Risks of blood transfusions and their prevention. Clin Adv Hematol Oncol 1:307–313, 2003.

12. **What can be done to restore oxygen-carrying capacity while limiting the risk of transfusion?**

    - Autologous transfusion
    - Erythropoietin administration
    - Administration of oxygen-carrying solutions or "blood substitutes"
    - Hemorrhage control

13. **List common techniques of autologous transfusion.**

    - **Preoperative autologous blood donation:** Blood is donated beginning 4–6 weeks before surgery, as frequently as every 3 days, and is transfused postoperatively only as indicated.
    - **Acute normovolemic hemodilution (ANH):** Blood is withdrawn immediately before surgery, and intravascular volume is maintained intraoperatively by using crystalloid or colloid before surgical blood loss. The removed blood is transfused during or after surgery, as needed, to maintain the desired post-ANH hemoglobin concentration.
    - **Intraoperative blood salvage:** Blood is collected intraoperatively and centrifuged; RBCs are washed and then reinfused.

    Coursin DB, Monk TG: Extreme normovolemic hemodilution: How low can you go and other alternatives to transfusion. Crit Care Med 29:908–910, 2001.

14. **Which "blood substitutes" can be used in critically ill patients?**

    - **Perfluorochemical emulsions:** Fluoridation of hydrocarbons generates a biologically inert liquid with high oxygen solubility. Oxygen is dissolved in these solutions in a linear relationship to inspired oxygen. High levels of supplemental oxygen are required to provide clinically useful oxygen delivery. Newer formulations may overcome the adverse reactions and carry more oxygen. These products are not clinically available.
    - **Hemoglobin-based oxygen-carrying solutions:** Free hemoglobin leads to an unfavorable oxygen dissociation curve, nephrotoxicity, and hypertension, probably mediated by nitric oxide scavenging. Modifications of free hemoglobin, such as cross-linkage of the tetramer, conjugation with large molecules, polymerization, and liposome encapsulation, seem to resolve these problems. The hemoglobin for these solutions can be obtained from human, bovine, porcine, and bacterial sources (using recombinant techniques). A polymerized bovine solution has been approved for veterinary use in the United States and for human use in South Africa, and approval is being sought from the U.S. Food and Drug Administration. A polymerized human solution has shown much promise in U.S. phase I and II trauma trials and is undergoing a phase III prehospital trial.

    Creteur J, Vincent J-L: Hemoglobin solutions. Crit Care Med 31(12 Suppl):S698–S707, 2003.
    Moore FA, Moore, McKinley BA, Moore EE: The next generation in shock resuscitation. Lancet 363:1988–1996, 2004.

15. **What is the role of erythropoietin in critically ill patients?**
ICU patients lose blood through repeated sampling, bleeding, drug reactions, and breakdown due to chronic illness. Previously, these patients were given transfusions. The use of erythropoietin in critically ill patients has led to decreased blood transfusions and possibly increased survival. Erythropoietin does not work quickly enough to have a role in the treatment of acute hemorrhage.

16. **What is FFP?**
FFP is plasma separated from the blood cells and placed immediately at or below $-18°C$ to preserve the coagulation factors, which are labile. FFP contains fibrinogen; prothrombin; factors V, VII, VIII, IX, and XIII; antithrombin III; and proteins C and S.

17. **List the indications for FFP.**
   - Coagulopathy due to a congenital deficiency, especially of factor II, V, VII, VIII, X, XI, or XIII
   - Coagulopathy due to an acquired deficiency of multiple factors, such as severe liver disease, DIC, or vitamin K depletion
   - Dilutional coagulopathy in a massively transfused patient (more than one blood volume); monitor with coagulation studies and thromboelastography
   - Reversal of warfarin effect (1 unit of FFP decrease the prothrombin time by 2 seconds)
   - Treatment of antithrombin III deficiency

18. **What is cryoprecipitate?**
Cryoprecipitate (also called *cryo*) is prepared from FFP by slow thawing at $4–6°C$. Cryoprecipitate contains high concentrations of factor VIII, von Willebrand factor, fibrinogen, and factor XIII.

19. **List the indications for giving cryoprecipitate.**
   - Hypofibrinogenemia (fibrinogen level less than 100 mg/dL)
   - Von Willebrand's disease
   - Hemophilia A (factor VIII deficiency)
   - Bleeding due to thrombolytic therapy
   Cryoprecipitate can be used to promote hemostasis in a bleeding patient; in most circumstances, however, it is preferable to give FFP, which contains more of the essential clotting factors.

20. **List some other hemostatic agents and their actions and indications.**
   - **Aprotinin:** Serine protease inhibitor blocking inflammation and clot breakdown. Indications include cardiac, hip, and spine surgery.
   - **Epsilon-aminocaproic acid and tranexamic acid:** Synthetic lysine analogs that inhibit fibrinolysis. These agents are indicated in cardiac surgery.
   - **Desmopressin (DDAVP):** Useful in the treatment of von Willebrand's disease and sometimes in platelet dysfunction due to uremia, cirrhosis, or aspirin consumption.
   - **Recombinant human factor VIIa:** Genetically engineered human protein from cultured hamster kidney cells. The main indication for this treatment is hemophilia. Off-label use in severe hemorrhage, including trauma and battlefield trauma, is reportedly successful. More controlled studies have been requested. Recombinant human factor VIIa does not work in extremely cold and acidotic patients.

Enomoto TM, Thorborg P: Emerging off-label uses for recombinant activated factor VII: Grading the evidence. Crit Care Clin 21:611–631, 2005.

Kokoszka A, Kuflik P, Bitan F, et al: Evidence-based review of the role of aprotinin in blood conservation during orthopaedic surgery. J Bone Joint Surg Am 87A(5):1129–1136, 2005.

Levy JH: Hemostatic agents. Transfusion 44:58S–62S, 2004.

21. **Describe a method to diminish blood loss in uncontrolled hemorrhage.**
Controlled resuscitation (also known as *balanced resuscitation, hypotensive resuscitation,* and *permissive hypotension*) is the resuscitation strategy that attempts to balance the risk of increased bleeding with the needs of tissue perfusion. A less than normal blood pressure is accepted, attempting to diminish blood loss and allow the use of less resuscitation fluid. This is guided by signs of organ perfusion. This method is terminated when hemorrhage control is achieved and is used in patients who have undergone trauma and in patients with rupturing aortic aneurysms. This method may not allow adequate resuscitation in patients with brain injury.

KEY POINTS: BLOOD PRODUCTS AND COAGULATION

1. Blood products have a finite but definite risk to the patient.

2. Stop the hemorrhage! This is more important than replacing the losses. The patient's own blood is best. Help the patient keep it in.

3. Know the indications, contraindications, and actions of therapeutic options and tailor them to the patient's needs to diminish the risk.

4. Avoid overuse of fluids.

22. **What is measured by prothrombin time (PT)?**
PT assesses the activity of factor VII, which is involved in the extrinsic coagulation pathway only. It is prolonged in patients with liver disease and patients who are deficient in vitamin K.

23. **What is measured by partial thromboplastin time (PTT)?**
PTT assesses activities of the intrinsic coagulation pathway, which includes factors XII, XI, IX, and VIII. A prolonged PTT with a normal PT suggests an inherited defect in coagulation.

24. **What is the most common inherited factor deficiency?**
Hemophilia A, a deficiency of factor VIII (about 75%), followed by hemophilia B, a deficiency of factor IX (about 20%).

25. **How does warfarin work?**
Warfarin (Coumadin) inhibits the conversion of vitamin K to its active form. This inhibition interferes with the hepatic synthesis of vitamin K–dependent clotting factors II, VII, IX, and X. Warfarin primarily prolongs PT but may have an effect on PTT.

26. **How does heparin work?**
Heparin binds to and activates antithrombin III, which in turn inhibits several coagulation enzymes, including thrombin and activated factors X, XII, XI, and IX. The biological half-life of heparin is 30–60 minutes; its effects can be reversed within 2–4 hours after an infusion is stopped. Heparin prolongs PTT.

27. **What is low-molecular-weight heparin (LMWH)?**
LMWH is a fragment produced by the chemical breakdown of heparin. It exerts its anticoagulant effect by binding with antithrombin III and inhibiting several coagulation enzymes. LMWH principally inhibits activated factor X.

28. **What are the major differences between standard heparin and LMWH?**
    - LMWH has a longer half-life and thus can be administered once daily.
    - LMWH gives a more predictable anticoagulant response at high doses and thus can be administered without monitoring (i.e., serial activated PTTs).
    - LMWH produces fewer bleeding complications than standard heparin at equivalent antithrombotic doses.

CHAPTER 54

THROMBOCYTOPENIA AND PLATELETS

Hasan B. Alam, MD, and Mark W. Bowyer, MD, DMCC, COL, USAF, MC

1. **What are two principal functions of platelets in effecting hemostasis?**
   Platelets function to effect hemostasis (1) by formation of an initial platelet plug and (2) by degranulation and secretion of proteins and catalysts for the clotting cascade. The initial platelet plug is due to loose aggregation of platelets in an area of injury and requires the presence of von Willebrand factor. Heparin does not affect this primary hemostasis, which explains why hemostasis can still occur in heparinized patients.

2. **What is the most common congenital platelet deficiency?**
   Von Willebrand's disease. The absence of this factor disrupts the formation of platelet aggregates (*see* question 1).

3. **Define *thrombocytopenia*.**
   A platelet count of less than 100,000 per cubic millimeter is considered to constitute thrombocytopenia. Thrombocytopenia is the most common platelet disorder in surgical patients.

4. **What are the basic mechanisms of thrombocytopenia?**
   Thrombocytopenia can be caused by decreased platelet production (marrow failure or replacement by cancerous cells or fibrosis), disordered platelet distribution/sequestration (hypersplenism), or increased platelet destruction (e.g., antibody-mediated, prosthetic valves, extracorporeal bypass, disseminated intravascular coagulation [DIC]). These mechanisms can occur in isolation or in combination.

5. **What is hypersplenism?**
   Hypersplenism refers only to excessive splenic function leading to accelerated destruction of circulating cellular elements; varying degrees of anemia, leukopenia, and thrombocytopenia will be present. Hypersplenism can occur in the absence of splenomegaly, as in chronic immune thrombocytopenic purpura (ITP). If splenomegaly is present, the condition is referred to as *secondary hypersplenism*.

6. **What are different treatment options for patients with ITP?**
   ITP is caused by immunoglobulin G antibodies against the platelet glycoproteins (i.e., GPIIb/IIIa and GP Ib/IX). Corticosteroids have been the mainstay of therapy for a long time, but alternative therapies are now commonly prescribed. These include intravenous gamma globulins (IVIG) and intravenous anti-D immunoglobulin (IV anti-D). Both cause "Fc receptor blockade" as an important mechanism of acute platelet increase. IVIG works fast (24 hours) and can be used in Rh-negative and splenectomized patients, whereas IV anti-D causes a slower rate of platelet increase (72 hours) and is relatively ineffective in Rh-negative and splenectomized patients. It is, however, effective in patients infected with the human immunodeficiency virus. Patients who initially respond to medical management but have a relapse within 1–3 months may be considered candidates for splenectomy. For refractory ITP, combination chemotherapies are used (cyclophosphamide, hydroxydaunomycin, Oncovin, and prednisone [CHOP],

vincristine–IVIG–Solu-Medrol) followed by maintenance therapy (using combinations of steroids, danazol, Imuran, Cellcept, and cyclosporin, among others).

7. **How does one differentiate between thrombotic thrombocytopenic purpura (TTP) and hemolytic uremic syndrome (HUS)?**
   ITP and HUS share thrombocytopenia, hemolytic anemia, and thrombotic occlusions in terminal arterioles and capillaries. Differentiating clinical features are the presence of focal neurologic symptoms in TTP and renal impairment in HUS. Additionally, levels of plasma von Willebrand factor–cleaving protease are low in TTP and normal in HUS.

8. **What is heparin-induced thrombocytopenia (HIT)?**
   HIT is a life- and limb-threatening prothrombotic complication of heparin administration (absolute risk of 2.6% with unfractionated heparin and 0.2% with low–molecular-weight heparin in a large meta-analysis). It results from an immune response triggered by the interaction of heparin with a specific platelet protein, platelet factor 4. Up to 8% of patients on unfractionated heparin will develop antibodies, and approximately 3% will develop thrombocytopenia, with about 1% manifesting thrombotic complications of HIT. HIT with thrombotic complication has a mortality rate of 20%, with about 20–30% of patients suffering permanent disability (e.g., amputations, stroke).

9. **When should a patient be worked up for HIT?**
   The diagnosis must be considered in any patient who develops thrombocytopenia, has an unexplained fall in platelet count of 30–40%, or has a thrombotic complication 5–10 days (may be as late as 20 days) after heparin exposure. Two clinically distinct types of HIT have been described (Table 54-1).

TABLE 54-1. HEPARIN-INDUCED THROMBOCYTOPENIA		
	Type I	**Type II***
Platelet count	Rarely <100,000	Commonly <100,000
Onset (after heparin exposure)	1–4 days	Typically 5–14 days
Mechanism	Non–immune-mediated; direct effect of heparin on platelet activation	Immune mediated
Outcome	Usually resolves spontaneously, despite continuation of heparin	Does not resolve unless heparin exposure is eliminated
Complications	Usually benign	Thrombosis and organ damage

*Type II HIT is now synonymous with "heparin-induced thrombocytopenia."

10. **How is HIT diagnosed?**
    Almost all patients with HIT have circulating antibodies to complexes between platelet factor 4 (PF4) and heparin. However, most of the patients who have circulating antibodies do not

clinically develop HIT. Therefore, it is currently not indicated to screen asymptomatic patients for these antibodies. Two different types of assays are available:

- **Functional assays:** These assays measure heparin-dependent platelet activation by PF4-heparin antibody *in vitro*. One of the functional assays, [14]serotonin-release assay (SRA), is considered the gold standard in diagnosis with a positive predictive value of almost 100% (but a negative predictive value of about 20%).
- **Immunoassays:** Immunoassays (e.g., enzyme-linked immunosorbent assay [ELISA]) measure the levels of antibodies in circulation (sensitivity, 93–97%; positive predictive value, 93–100%; specificity, 86–100%; negative predictive value, 88–95%). ELISA is easy and rapid to perform, but only 25% of the ELISA-positive specimens are SRA positive.

11. **Is repeating HIT testing useful?**
If an ELISA yields negative but borderline results, it should be repeated. The chances of a negative test result turning positive 3 days later depend on the titer levels. About 45% of high titer results that are negative but almost positive may turn positive, whereas approximately 15% and 5% of the medium and low titer results, respectively, are likely to turn positive.

12. **How is HIT treated?**
Type I HIT requires no specific treatment. Type II HIT requires immediate withdrawal of all heparin and treatment with anticoagulation agents. Because distinguishing type I from type II HIT can be difficult, the decision to stop the administration of heparin should be carefully contemplated based on the clinical scenario. The Warkentin criteria may be used to determine the patient's pretest probability of HIT (Table 54-2). All patients (with or without thrombosis) with type II HIT must be anticoagulated because the risk of thrombosis is >50% without anticoagulation. Do not transfuse platelets unless clearly indicated because platelet transfusion

TABLE 54-2. WARKENTIN CRITERIA TO DETERMINE THE PROBABILITY OF HIT			
Criteria	2 Points	1 Point	0 Point
Thrombocytopenia	>50% fall or platelet nadir of 20–100 × 10⁹/L	30–50% fall or platelet nadir of 10–19 × 10⁹/L	<30% fall or platelet nadir of <10 ×10⁹/L
Timing of platelet drop	Clear onset day 5–10 or <1 day (if heparin exposure within past 100 days)	Consistent with immune activation but not clear (e.g., missing data) or onset after day 10	Platelet count fall too early (without recent heparin exposure)
Thrombosis or other sequelae	New thrombosis; skin necrosis; post-heparin bolus acute reaction	Progressive or recurrent thrombosis; erythematous skin lesions; suspected thrombosis (not yet proven)	None
Other causes for thrombocytopenia	No other cause for platelet count drop evident	Possible other causes	Definite other cause present

HIT = heparin-induced thrombocytopenia.
Pretest probability score: 6–8 = high; 4–5 = intermediate; 0–3 = low.

actually increases the amount of PF4 and may exaggerate the antigen response. If continued anticoagulation is required, a vitamin K antagonist (warfarin) should be initiated *after* the patient is fully treated with one of the following agents:

- **Danaparoid** (low-molecular-weight glycosaminoglycan composed of heparin sulfate, dermatan sulfate, and chondroitin sulfate): This drug has mostly anti–factor Xa activity with a limited antithrombin action. The dose is titrated to keep anti–factor Xa levels between 0.5 and 0.8 U/mL. There is no antidote for bleeding.
- **Recombinant hirudin** (lepirudin, Refludan): This 7-kDa peptide acts directly on circulating and clot-bound thrombin. Anticoagulant effects last about 40 minutes. It is given as a slow bolus (0.4 mg/kg) followed by continuous infusion at 0.15 mg/kg to maintain activated partial thromboplastin time (aPTT) between 1.5 and 2.5 times baseline. This is a good choice for patients who will need to be transitioned to warfarin. Lepirudin does not alter the interpretation of international normalized ratio (INR) as significantly as argatroban.
- **Argatroban:** This 509-Dalton, arginine-based direct thrombin inhibitor inhibits both soluble and clot-bound thrombin. Its half-life is 46.2 ± 10.2 minutes, and steady-state activity is achieved within 1–2 hours of continuous infusion. The recommended dose is 2.0 µg/kg/min and is adjusted to keep aPTT between 1.5 and 3 times baseline (maximum, 10 µg/kg/min).
- **Fondaparinux:** This newer drug is given via subcutaneous route. The recommended dosage is 7.5 mg once a day.

13. **How should one monitor warfarin effect when it is coadministered with argatroban?**
Use chromogenic factor X assay while the patient is taking argatroban, and switch to the measurement of INR 3 hours after discontinuation of argatroban.

14. **Is heparin therapy ever an option once a patient has tested positive for HIT?**
Yes. Antibodies are usually no longer detected 50–85 days after cessation of heparin. Heparin *may* be safe when used for a short time if given >100 days after heparin exposure and if a current HIT antibody test result is negative.

15. **What are some causes of platelet dysfunction in the intensive care unit (ICU)?**
The principal causes of platelet dysfunction and thrombocytopenia in the ICU are drug side effects, uremia, and sepsis. Antibiotics, nitrates, local anesthetics, α- and β-adrenergic blockers, xanthine derivatives, diuretics, H_2-receptor blockers, and dextran are some examples of drugs that can impair platelet activity. Uremia, also a common finding among patients in the ICU, is an important cause of platelet dysfunction.

16. **What are the indications for platelet transfusion?**
The platelet counts that should serve as a trigger for platelet transfusion have evolved over the last 2 decades. Although somewhat controversial, the following threshold levels have been proposed in the literature:
- **Bleeding prophylaxis in a stable oncologic patient:** $10,000/mm^3$ (previously, $<20,000/mm^3$)
- **Lumbar puncture in a patient with leukemia:** $10,000/mm^3$
- **Stable HIT:** $10,000/mm^3$
- **Bone marrow aspiration:** $20,000/mm^3$
- **Gastrointestinal endoscopy in cancer:** $20,000–40,000/mm^3$
- **DIC:** $20,000–50,000/mm^3$
- **Fiberoptic bronchoscopy:** $20,000–50,000/mm^3$
- **Major surgery:** $50,000/mm^3$
- **Thrombocytopenia resulting from massive transfusion:** $50,000/mm^3$
- **Invasive procedures in cirrhosis:** $50,000/mm^3$
- **Cardiopulmonary bypass:** $50,000–60,000/mm^3$

- **Neurosurgical procedures:** 100,000/mm^3
- **Thrombocytopenia and bleeding** (intracerebral, gastrointestinal, genitourinary, or retinal hemorrhage): 100,000/mm^3

  There is no specific count at which bleeding is completely prevented. In addition to the count, the quality and function of the platelets are also important. However, life-threatening bleeding can occur with platelet counts < 5000/mm^3, and spontaneous bleeding with counts < 10,000–20,000/mm^3.

KEY POINTS: THROMBOCYTOPENIA AND PLATELETS

1. Thrombocytopenia is a common finding in the patients in the ICU, and the basic rule for management is to treat the underlying cause.

2. Transfuse platelets only if needed or if the platelet count is <10,000/mm^3.

3. Heparin-induced thrombocytopenia (HIT) is a relatively uncommon but potentially serious complication of heparin administration.

4. Platelets counts should be monitored in all patients who are receiving heparin (unfractionated or low molecular weight). A drop in platelet count (>50% from baseline or below 100,000/mm^3) is reason to suspect HIT.

5. Most of the patients who have circulating antibodies to PF4 do not clinically develop HIT. Therefore, only screen patients for these antibodies when clinically indicated.

6. All patients (with or without thrombosis) with HIT (type II) must be anticoagulated because the risk of thrombosis is >50% without anticoagulation.

17. **How does aspirin affect platelet function?**

    Aspirin irreversibly inhibits platelet cyclo-oxygenase, resulting in a functional defect that lasts the duration of the platelets' life span (8–9 days).

18. **What laboratory test measures platelet function?**

    Bleeding time is a sensitive indicator of overall platelet function.

19. **How are platelet disorders managed?**

    The patient's drug regimen should be carefully scrutinized, and medications implicated in thrombocytopenia should be eliminated or substituted. Platelet transfusion may be required (*see* question 16). Uremia-associated thrombocytopenia can be treated with hemodialysis. Cryoprecipitate, 1-desamino-8-D arginine vasopressin (DDAVP), and conjugated estrogens have also been used with good results.

BIBLIOGRAPHY

1. AuBuchon JP: Platelet transfusion therapy. Clin Lab Med 16:797–816, 1996.

2. Chong BH, Eisbacher M: Pathophysiology and laboratory testing of heparin-induced thrombocytopenia. Semin Hematol 35:3–8, 1998.

3. Fuse I: Disorders of platelet function. Crit Rev Oncol/Hematol 22:1–25, 1996.

4. Greinacher A, Warkentin TE: Recognition, treatment, and prevention of heparin-induced thrombocytopenia: Review and update. Thromb Res 118:165–176, 2006.

5. Lipsett PA, Perler BA: The use of blood products for surgical bleeding. Semin Vasc Surg 9:347–353, 1996.
6. Martel N, Lee J, Wells PS: Risk for heparin-induced thrombocytopenia with unfractionated and low molecular weight heparin thromboprophylaxis: A meta-analysis. Blood 106:2710–2715, 2005.
7. McCrae KR, Bussel JB, Mannucci PM, et al: Platelets: An update on diagnosis and management of thrombocytopenic disorders. Hematology Am Soc Hematol Edu Progr 282–305, 2001.
8. NIH consensus statement: Platelet transfusion therapy 6:1–6, 1986.
9. Rebulla P: Platelet transfusion trigger in difficult patients. Transfus Clin Biol 8:249–254, 2001.

CHAPTER 55

DISSEMINATED INTRAVASCULAR COAGULATION

Andrea Harzstark, MD, and Patrick F. Fogarty, MD

1. **What is disseminated intravascular coagulation (DIC)?**

   DIC occurs when coagulation is activated inappropriately, leading to thrombin generation and fibrin deposition in small vessels. Usually, an underlying causative disorder is present (*see* question 4). Because coagulation proteins and platelets are consumed by the ongoing prothrombotic process, they can become depleted, leading to bleeding. Thus, in DIC, hemorrhage and thrombosis can occur simultaneously. Although DIC is usually recognized to occur acutely and systemically, local or chronic DIC is also possible. Hereafter, the discussion will focus primarily on acute DIC.

2. **Why is DIC important?**

   DIC is a common cause of concurrent thrombocytopenia and prolonged clotting times (i.e., activated partial thromboplastin time [aPTT] and prothrombin time [PT]) in hospitalized patients. In certain populations, it is also an independent predictor of mortality. DIC leads to fibrin deposition in small vessels, which can cause tissue ischemia and result in organ dysfunction. The consumptive coagulopathy can lead to clinically significant bleeding.

3. **What is the pathophysiology of DIC?**

   The inciting event in most cases of DIC is unknown, but entities such as tissue factor or exogenous procoagulant molecules (e.g., bacterial lipopolysaccharide) are thought to initiate the coagulation cascade, resulting in thrombin generation. This process may be mediated by interleukin 6. As thrombin generation proceeds, fibrin is deposited in small blood vessels. In acute DIC, clotting factors and platelets are consumed, which can result in systemic bleeding. However, if this process occurs chronically or slowly, clotting factors and platelets are replaced and bleeding does not occur; instead, thrombosis predominates. For instance, Trousseau syndrome, which typically occurs in the setting of an underlying visceral cancer, presents with peripheral venous thrombosis or migratory thrombophlebitis.

   Stouthard JM, Levi M, Hack CE, et al: Interleukin-6 stimulates coagulation, not fibrinolysis, in humans. Thromb Haemost 76:738–742, 1996.

4. **In critical care patients, what conditions are associated with DIC?**
   - **Sepsis:** Gram-negative or gram-positive bacterial infections, rickettsial or viral infections
   - **Trauma:** Fracture of long bones, head trauma
   - **Malignancy:** Adenocarcinoma, acute promyelocytic leukemia (incidence approaches 100%)
   - **Obstetric:** Hemolysis, elevated liver enzymes, and low platelets (HELLP syndrome); retained uterine placental or fetal tissue; placental abruption or previa
   - **Vascular:** Vasculitis, abdominal aortic aneurysm, cavernous hemangiomas
   - **Miscellaneous:** Burns, anaphylaxis, transfusion reaction, snake bite, acute pancreatitis, transplant rejection

5. **How does DIC present clinically?**

   In acutely ill hospitalized patients, DIC usually presents with prolongations in the PT and aPTT and concurrently decreased fibrinogen and platelets; systemic bleeding may or may not be present. Typically, bleeding manifests as ecchymoses, purpura, and petechiae; it also occurs at surgical incisions or insertion sites of vascular access catheters. Mucosal and urinary bleeding are common, whereas pulmonary, gastrointestinal, and central nervous system bleeding occur less frequently. Due to widespread intravascular coagulation, tissue ischemia can occur, resulting in cyanosis, delirium, oliguria, hypoxia, and frank tissue necrosis.

6. **What laboratory abnormalities are typical of DIC?**
   Thrombocytopenia, hypofibrinogenemia, and prolongation of the PT, aPTT, and thrombin time are characteristic, but in compensated (i.e., chronic) DIC, levels can be normal. Early in the course of DIC, the platelet count may be in the normal range but is often decreased from baseline. Platelet counts are rarely less than 20,000/μL. D-dimer and levels of fibrin degradation products are almost always elevated.

7. **Is a peripheral blood smear useful in the diagnosis of DIC?**
   The peripheral blood smear from a patient with DIC typically shows mild to moderate thrombocytopenia. The finding of schistocytes (red blood cell fragments created by intravascular hemolysis) are neither sensitive nor specific and are present in only 10–50% of cases of acute DIC. See www.ashimagebank.org/ for a blood smear demonstrating schistocytes.
   Schmaier AH: Correspondence. N Engl J Med 341:1937–1938, 1999.

8. **What conditions make interpretation of laboratory abnormalities in DIC more difficult?**
   Fibrinogen is an acute-phase reactant. As such, measurements of this factor can be within the normal range in a patient with acute DIC, especially if there is an underlying inflammatory disorder. In this case, assessment of the trend of fibrinogen levels over time can reveal a decrease from the baseline value.

9. **Why is it difficult to make the diagnosis of DIC in patients with advanced liver disease?**
   The liver produces most coagulation proteins, and most cases of advanced liver disease feature a prolonged PT and aPTT and a decreased fibrinogen level. Additionally, the platelet count may be reduced in cirrhotic patients because of hypersplenism. Laboratory abnormalities in liver disease tend to be relatively stable, however, whereas in acute DIC, abnormalities tend to worsen over time.

10. **When and how is DIC treated?**
    Because DIC tends to be a secondary process, treatment of the underlying disorder is mandatory and must underlie any other DIC-specific intervention. Blood products should be administered only in cases of DIC complicated by clinically significant bleeding or significantly elevated risk of bleeding (e.g., thrombocytopenia in a patient with recent vascular surgery) and are not typically required. Blood components should not be given solely in response to laboratory abnormalities. Transfusion of blood products is associated with a measurable risk of transfusion-related complications (including viral infections and transfusion reactions), and administration of blood components to a nonbleeding patient with DIC usually represents a poor use of vital resources.

11. **How should blood products be administered in cases of acute DIC?**
    If they are to be used, platelet transfusions may be given to a platelet count goal of >20,000/μL for bleeding associated with acute DIC or >50,000/μL in cases of life-threatening bleeding or intracranial hemorrhage. Cryoprecipitate may be administered to keep the fibrinogen level

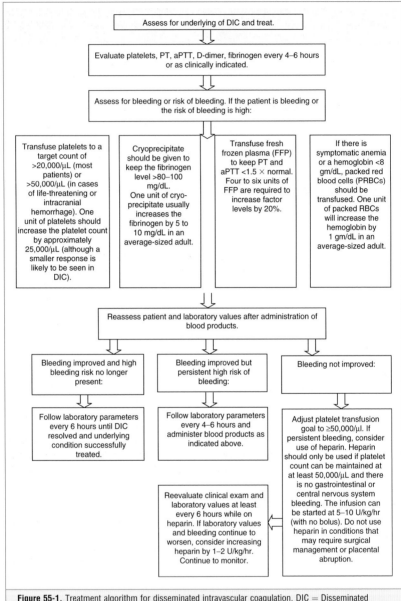

Figure 55-1. Treatment algorithm for disseminated intravascular coagulation. DIC = Disseminated intravascular coagulation, PT = prothrombin time, aPTT = activated partial thromboplastin time.

> 80–100 mg/dL. Fresh frozen plasma should be given only if clinically significant bleeding is present; it should not be used solely to "correct" a prolonged PT or aPTT. Major hemorrhage should be treated with transfusion of red blood cells if symptomatic anemia occurs or the hemoglobin declines to <8 gm/dL. See Fig. 55-1 for additional details.

KEY POINTS: DISSEMINATED INTRAVASCULAR COAGULATION (DIC)

1. DIC is a syndrome involving the activation of coagulation, resulting in the intravascular deposition of fibrin and the consumption of coagulation proteins and platelets, which commonly leads to bleeding.

2. DIC can lead to organ dysfunction and is associated with high mortality rates.

3. No single laboratory test can be used to diagnose DIC. Instead, a combination of a prolonged aPTT and PT, decreased fibrinogen, decreased platelets, increased D-dimer or fibrin degradation products, and schistocytes on a blood smear in an appropriate clinical context may suggest the diagnosis.

4. Management of DIC should focus primarily on treatment of the underlying disorder.

12. **What are other special causes of DIC that require specific treatment?**
    - HELLP syndrome is a peripartum form of DIC, resulting in clinically significant hepatic injury and hemolytic anemia. In addition to supportive care, treatment for HELLP includes either delivery of the fetus or dilatation and curettage to remove retained fetal or placental fragments.
    - Acute promyelocytic leukemia is almost always associated with DIC, likely because of procoagulants expressed by circulating promyelocytes. In addition to appropriate transfusions for the treatment of DIC, urgent initiation of chemotherapy—which should include all transretinoic acid—is indicated.

13. **In what scenarios should heparin be considered for the treatment of DIC?**
    In cases of acute DIC characterized by ongoing, clinically significant bleeding despite administration of platelets and cryoprecipitate, heparin may be considered, although its use should be weighed carefully because it can exacerbate bleeding. Use of heparin requires that the platelet count be maintained at >50,000/μL and that there be no concurrent gastrointestinal or central nervous system bleeding. Heparin is contraindicated in conditions that require surgical management, such as retained uterine placental tissue. In addition, its use should be avoided in patients with placental abruption.

14. **How should heparin be administered?**
    A continuous infusion of unfractionated heparin (5–10 U/kg/h) is reasonable, until the bleeding has lessened or stopped and/or the underlying clinical condition has been effectively treated. No bolus dose should be given. Low-molecular-weight heparin (LMWH) is not appropriate for the treatment of acute DIC complicated by bleeding. Heparin or LMWH, however, is the preferred treatment for chronic DIC leading to Trousseau syndrome (*see* question 17).

15. **What other agents have been considered for use in DIC?**
    Fibrinolytic inhibitors, such as ε-aminocaproic acid (Amicar), can be used to treat DIC-associated refractory bleeding by preventing systemic fibrinolysis. However, use of these inhibitors should be considered carefully in DIC because they can worsen systemic fibrin deposition. It should be noted that the manufacturer of recombinant coagulation factor VIIa (rhVIIa; NovoSeven) has indicated in its product insert that patients with DIC may be at an increased risk of thrombotic events after the administration of rhVIIa.

    www.us.novoseven.com/pdf/00609_novose_pi_fa.pdf

16. **How is the efficacy of DIC treatment evaluated?**
Laboratory parameters, including the PT, aPTT, fibrinogen, and platelet count, should be monitored at least every 6 hours and should return to baseline levels as the disorder is effectively treated. In addition, clinical bleeding should improve.

17. **How does chronic DIC differ from the acute form?**
In chronic DIC, coagulation proteins may be replaced as quickly as they are consumed, leading to reduced or absent bleeding and a preponderance of thrombotic events. The platelet count may be normal or only slightly decreased, and the fibrinogen level may be normal or elevated. The PT and aPTT may be normal. Trousseau syndrome (*see* question 14) is usually treated with an LMWH such as enoxaparin, 1 mg/kg every 12 hours, for at least 3–6 months after the initial thrombotic event or as long as malignancy is present, whichever is longer. Warfarin does not appear to be as effective as LMWH for secondary prevention of thrombosis in patients with Trousseau syndrome.

Prandoni P: How I treat venous thromboembolism in patients with cancer. Blood 106:4027–4033, 2005.

18. **What treatments are controversial in DIC?**
Randomized trials in patients with DIC are lacking. However, several novel agents that may have clinical applications in the management of DIC have recently become available. For instance, recombinant activated protein C (drotrecogin alfa) has been approved for use in severe sepsis with organ failure based on a 20% relative survival advantage at 28 days in one randomized prospective double-blinded trial consisting of 1690 patients. However, use of the agent is associated with an increased risk of bleeding (3.5% versus 2% in placebo group; $P = 0.06$).

Bernard GR, Vincent JL, Laterre PF, et al: Efficacy and safety of recombinant human activated protein C for severe sepsis. N Engl J Med 344:699–709, 2001.

19. **What new treatments may be available in the future for DIC?**
Antithrombin III concentrates have not yet been shown to confer a survival advantage in patients with severe sepsis resulting from infection, but they continue to be evaluated. Other molecules that have been suggested as potential treatments or targets in the management of acute DIC include recombinant nematode anticoagulant protein c2 (via inhibition of the factor Xa complex), tissue factor pathway inhibitor, and hirudin (via inhibition of thrombin and subsequent control of activation of coagulation).

Abraham E, Reinhardt K, Svoboda P, et al: Assessment of the safety of recombinant tissue factor pathway inhibitor in patients with severe sepsis: A multicenter, randomized, placebo-controlled, single-blind, dose escalation study. Crit Care Med 29:2081–2089, 2001.

Creasey AA, Chang AC, Feigen L, et al: Tissue factor pathway inhibitor reduces mortality from *Escherichia coli* septic shock. J Clin Invest 91:2850–2860, 1993.

Fourrier F, Chopin C, Huart J, et al: Double blind, placebo-controlled trial of antithrombin III concentrates in septic shock with disseminated intravascular coagulation. Chest 104:882–888, 1993.

Fuse S, Tomita H, Yoshida M, et al: High dose of intravenous antithrombin III without heparin in the treatment of disseminated intravascular coagulation and organ failure in four children. Am J Hematol 53:18–21, 1996.

Hermida J, Montes R, Paramo JA, et al: Endotoxin-induced disseminated intravascular coagulation in rabbits: Effect of recombinant hirudin on hemostatic parameters, fibrin deposits, and mortality. J Lab Clin Med 131:77–83, 1998.

Moons AH, Peters RJ, Cate H, et al: Recombinant nematode anticoagulant protein c2, a novel inhibitor of tissue factor–factor VIIa activity, abrogates endotoxin-induced coagulation in chimpanzees. Thromb Haemost 88:627–631, 2002.

Warren BL, KyberSept Trial Study Group: High-dose antithrombin III for severe sepsis, a randomized controlled trial. JAMA 286:1869–1878, 2001.

CHAPTER 56

SICKLE CELL DISEASE

Kathryn L. Hassell, MD

1. **What is sickle cell disease?**

   The term *sickle cell disease* refers to a group of inherited hemoglobinopathies in which abnormal hemoglobin β-chains are produced. They occur when one β-globin gene has the sickle cell mutation (i.e., valine substituted for glutamic acid in the sixth position of the β chain) and the other β-globin gene is abnormal. When sickle cells are exposed to extreme conditions, such as hypoxia or osmotic changes (e.g., dehydration), the sickle hemoglobin (Hb S) can polymerize, and the red blood cell reversibly assumes a sickled shape. These red blood cells, whether sickled or unsickled, can adhere to vascular endothelium, resulting in acute and chronic vaso-occlusion, vascular injury, and organ damage.

   Chiang EY, Frenette PS: Sickle cell vaso-occlusion. Hematol Oncol Clin North Am 19:771–784, 2005.

2. **What are the different types of sickle cell disease?**

   ■ Patients with two Hb S genes have sickle cell anemia (HbSS), which is characterized by hemolytic anemia with baseline elevation in reticulocyte count and indirect bilirubin as well as episodic painful vaso-occlusive events. Even in the absence of pain, chronic organ damage often occurs, especially in the spleen, lungs, kidneys, retina, and femoral and humeral heads.

   ■ Patients who have one Hb S gene and one Hb C gene have HbSC disease, which usually is associated with milder anemia, fewer painful episodes, and less chronic organ injury than HbSS.

   ■ Patients with one gene for Hb S and one gene with a mutation for β-thalassemia have HbSβ⁻ or HbSβ⁺ thalassemia. HbSβ⁻ thalassemia clinically resembles HbSS in severity, but HbSβ⁺ thalassemia is usually less severe. The mean corpuscular volume is low, reflecting the thalassemic component.

   Powars DR, Chan LS, Hiti A, et al: Outcome of sickle cell anemia: A 4-decade observational study of 1056 patients. Medicine (Baltimore) 84:363, 2005.

3. **Is sickle cell trait the same as sickle cell disease?**

   No. People who carry one Hb S gene and one normal gene have sickle cell trait (HbAS). They do not have classic signs or symptoms of sickle cell disease and have a completely normal hematologic picture. However, concentrating defects in the kidney, occasional hematuria, papillary necrosis, and, less commonly, splenic infarction at high altitude may occur.

   Lane PA, Githens JH: Splenic crises at mountain altitudes in sickle cell trait. Its occurrence in nonblack persons. JAMA 253:2251–2254, 1985.

4. **How is sickle cell disease diagnosed?**

   Sickle cell disease is diagnosed by hemoglobin electrophoresis. Because of the differences in charges, Hb S and other abnormal hemoglobins migrate differently from normal Hb A. Use of "sickle cell prep," which detects the presence of hemoglobin S, cannot distinguish between sickle cell trait (AS), sickle cell anemia (HbSS), HgbSC disease, HbSβ⁻ thalassemia, or HbSβ⁺ thalassemia, because it does not quantitate the amount of sickle hemoglobin or detect other abnormal hemoglobins.

   National Institutes of Health: The Management of Sickle Cell Disease, 4th ed. Bethesda, MD, National Institutes of Health, National Heart, Lung, and Blood Institute, 2002.

5. **What is a painful sickle cell crisis?**

A painful crisis, often characterized by pain in the back, abdomen, or extremities, represents acute vaso-occlusion likely triggered by many pathophysiologic factors, including red blood cell adhesion, inflammation, endothelial injury, and vasoconstriction. Extremes of temperature, heavy physical exertion, and infection may predispose to crises; dehydration can occur easily with poor oral intake or excessive fluid losses due to the renal concentrating defect induced by chronic ischemia to the renal medulla. Despite thorough evaluation, the precipitating event of some crises cannot be determined.

6. **What evaluation should be done for patients presenting with a painful sickle cell crisis?**

Evaluation should include careful history-taking and a thorough physical examination with attention to possible sites of infection. Laboratory studies should include complete blood count with a reticulocyte count to confirm that the patient is producing red blood cells in response to the increased red blood cell destruction. Baseline chemistry testing should be done to assess hepatic and renal function. Cultures of urine, sputum, and blood, followed by empiric antibiotic coverage, should be done for fever. A chest x-ray is useful in patients with hypoxia, a history of pulmonary disease, or pulmonary signs or symptoms.

7. **What infections are common in sickle cell disease?**

Because most patients with sickle cell anemia (HbSS) and HbSβ° thalassemia have an infarcted spleen by the age of 3 or 4 years, they are susceptible to encapsulated organisms, including *Haemophilus influenzae, Streptococcus pneumoniae,* and *Neisseria meningitidis.* Pyelonephritis is also common and may be associated with bacteremia. Osteomyelitis can also develop and is most commonly caused by staphylococci, although the incidence of osteomyelitis due to *Salmonella* species is increased in sickle cell patients compared with other patients.

8. **How are painful sickle cell crises treated?**

The usual approach to painful crisis includes IV and oral fluids to attain and maintain adequate, but not excessive, hydration. Supplemental oxygen is given if hypoxia is present that may precipitate red blood cell adhesion and sickling. Parenteral analgesics, usually morphine sulfate, are given intravenously on a fixed schedule (not "as needed") until the pain has subsided enough to warrant the use of oral analgesics. Evidence of infection (positive urinalysis or culture results) is treated appropriately, and in the setting of fever, empiric IV antibiotic coverage is recommended. Transfusion therapy is not indicated for uncomplicated pain events or mild decreases in hemoglobin in the absence of acute end-organ injury.

Ballas S: Pain management of sickle cell disease. Hematol Oncol Clin North Am 19:785–802, 2005.

9. **Define *acute chest syndrome* (ACS).**

ACS is characterized by chest pain, fever, increasing hypoxia, and, ultimately, development of pulmonary infiltrates, identified on chest radiograph, associated with leaky vascular endothelium and ischemia of the lung due to sickled and/or adherent red blood cells. ACS is more commonly associated with infection in children and with pulmonary fat emboli in adults. Pulmonary embolism (not associated with sickle cell disease) may be an appropriate consideration; if present, it should be treated with anticoagulation. Otherwise, anticoagulation has not been shown to be an effective therapy for ACS. Treatment may involve simple or exchange red blood cell transfusion (*see* questions 12 and 14). Because it is often difficult to differentiate between worsening pneumonia and ACS, IV antibiotics should be given.

Vichinsky EP, Neumayr L, Earles A, et al: Causes and outcomes of the acute chest syndrome in sickle cell disease. National Acute Chest Syndrome Study Group. N Engl J Med 342:1855–1865, 2000.

10. **What is aplastic crisis?**

Aplastic crisis is characterized by a rapid fall in hemoglobin levels associated with few or no reticulocytes, indicating a failure of the bone marrow to respond to increased cell turnover. Folate deficiency can occur in the setting of chronic hemolytic anemia in some patients unless supplemental folate is taken. Parvovirus (B19) has been associated with bone marrow suppression and subsequent aplastic crisis; other viral infections or severe bacterial infections may also suppress the bone marrow. Treatment of aplastic crisis may be necessary when the hematocrit level becomes dangerously low. Packed red blood cells are given to support an adequate hematocrit until bone marrow suppression is resolved, folate is repleted, and the reticulocyte count improves.

11. **What is splenic sequestration?**

Splenic sequestration is characterized by rapid, painful enlargement of the spleen, with rapid fall in hemoglobin and occasionally platelets due to sickling and sudden intravascular pooling of blood in the spleen. Splenic sequestration is a significant cause of morbidity in young children but usually does not occur in adults with HbSS or HbSβ° thalassemia because the spleen has infarcted by the age of 3–4 years. In HbSC disease or HbSβ+ thalassemia, however, the disease is less severe and splenic function can be preserved into adulthood. In adults, the sequestration is often relatively mild, with only a 1- to 2-gm/dL drop in hemoglobin; transfusion is rarely required for support. On rare occasions, the spleen may become so massive and/or necrotic that splenectomy is required.

12. **What cerebrovascular complications can occur with sickle cell disease?**

Thrombotic stroke affects 6–12% of children and adolescents with sickle cell anemia (HbSS) or HbSβ⁻ thalassemia. These strokes are usually due to large-vessel disease, which may be seen with magnetic resonance angiography and detected by transcranial Doppler scan. Acute management involves red blood cell exchange transfusion to remove sickle red blood cells and enhance oxygen-carrying capacity. Acute simple transfusions are not recommended because blood viscosity may be increased with increased hematocrit if sickled cells are not removed. Anticonvulsants are sometimes needed because seizures can occur during acute infarction. Adults tend to have hemorrhagic strokes, which may be associated with aneurysms and moyamoya malformations; thrombotic strokes may also occur.

Ohene-Frempong K, Weiner S, Sleeper LA, et al: Cerebrovascular accidents in sickle cell disease: Rates and risk factors. Blood 91:288–294, 1998.

13. **What other acute complications may develop with sickle cell disease?**

Acute multiorgan failure syndrome, characterized by acute pulmonary, hepatic, and renal failure thought to be due to diffuse vaso-occlusion, can occur but may be rapidly reversed with exchange or simple transfusion. Pulmonary hypertension, likely related to chronic lung injury by sickle red blood cells, is a leading cause of death in adults with sickle cell disease; patients may present with right heart failure, arrhythmias, and other associated acute complications. Chronic renal disease, which occurs in 10% of adult patients with sickle cell disease, is underestimated by serum creatinine values and may be exacerbated by acute illness or interventions (e.g., dye load). Intrahepatic sickling can occur, with rapid rises in liver enzymes, a fall in hemoglobin due to sequestration in the liver, and, in severe cases, an extreme rise in conjugated bilirubin level and prothrombin time. More commonly, liver disease due to underlying iron overload and/or hepatitis C from previous transfusion can be exacerbated during acute illness. Gallstones are common due to chronic hyperbilirubinemia and may cause acute cholecystitis or common bile duct obstruction. Sustained priapism requires acute urologic intervention. Acute myocardial infarction is not more common in patients with sickle cell disease than in the general population.

Ataga K, Orringer E: Renal abnormalities in sickle cell disease. Am J Hematol 63:205–211, 2000.

Hassell KL, Eckman JR, Lane PA: Acute multiorgan failure syndrome: A potentially catastrophic complication of severe sickle cell pain episodes. Am J Med 96:155–162, 1994.

Machado RF, Gladwin MT: Chronic sickle cell lung disease: New insights into the diagnosis, pathogenesis and treatment of pulmonary hypertension. Br J Haematol 129:449–464, 2005.

Scheinman JI: Sickle cell disease and the kidney. Semin Nephrol 23:66–76, 2003.

Tsironi M, Aessopos A: The heart in sickle cell disease. Acta Cardiol 60:589–598, 2005.

KEY POINTS: CAUSES OF SEVERE ACUTE ILLNESS IN SICKLE CELL DISEASE

1. Acute chest syndrome, which resembles noncardiogenic pulmonary edema, is a potential cause of illness in sickle cell disease.

2. Acute multiorgan failure syndrome due to diffuse vaso-occlusion is another possible cause.

3. Illness can result from exacerbation of chronic pulmonary hypertension with right heart failure.

4. Exacerbation of chronic renal failure, despite apparently normal serum creatinine, is another risk factor.

5. Patients with sickle cell disease may become ill as a result of decompensation of chronic liver disease caused by transfusional iron overload.

6. Sepsis associated with pneumonia or pyelonephritis can also cause illness in this population.

14. **What are the surgical risks for patients with sickle cell disease?**
Patients with sickle cell anemia (HbSS) or HbSβ° who undergo general anesthesia may be at increased risk for development of acute painful crisis and ACS. Simple transfusion therapy, with a goal of reducing the percentage of sickle hemoglobin to 60%, was as effective as exchange transfusion (with <30% HbS) in preventing perioperative complications in a randomized trial in sickle cell anemia. Patients should be carefully monitored for hypoxia to avoid precipitation of acute vaso-occlusion. Adequate hydration should be carefully maintained.

Vichinsky EP, Haberkern CM, Neumayr L, et al: A comparison of conservative and aggressive transfusion regimens in the perioperative management of sickle cell disease. The Preoperative Transfusion in Sickle Cell Disease Study Group. N Engl J Med 333:206, 1995.

15. **Discuss the role of acute transfusion in sickle cell disease.**
Packed red blood cell transfusions are indicated in the setting of severe anemia with hemodynamic instability, severe hypoxia, or acute end-organ injury. The final hematocrit measurement after transfusion should not exceed a value > 30% because blood viscosity will increase at higher values. In patients with a baseline hematocrit > 30%, transfusion therapy should result in a return to baseline hematocrit level. If life-threatening events such as acute stroke, ACS, or acute multiorgan failure syndrome develop, red blood cell exchange transfusion should be considered, especially if the hematocrit has not fallen significantly below baseline values. An apheresis instrument can be used for an automated exchange procedure using a double-lumen dialysis catheter. Alternatively, aliquots of blood are removed through an arterial or venous line and replaced with whole blood or "reconstituted" packed red blood cells. In all cases, an effort should be made to match transfused units to minor antigens on the patient's red blood cells (i.e., minor antigen match); otherwise, patients with sickle cell disease tend to develop multiple alloantibodies, making future crossmatching difficult.

16. **Discuss the role of hydroxyurea (Hydrea) in the treatment of sickle cell disease.**
    In some patients with sickle cell disease, there is persistent production of fetal hemoglobin
    (Hb F). These patients have been observed to have a milder form of sickle cell disease.
    Hydroxyurea therapy is associated with increased production of hemoglobin F in patients with
    sickle cell disease. A placebo-controlled trial of hydroxyurea in adults with severe sickle cell
    anemia (HbSS) or HbSβ⁻ thalassemia demonstrated a 50% reduction in pain events, ACS, and
    reduced mortality. However, it has not been shown to offer protection against stroke or chronic
    organ injury, nor to have benefits in the treatment of other forms of sickle cell disease.

    Charache S, Terrin ML, Moore RD, et al: Effect of hydroxyurea on the frequency of painful crises in sickle
    cell anemia. Investigators of the Multicenter Study of Hydroxyurea in Sickle Cell Anemia. N Engl J Med
    332:1317–1322, 1995.

    Steinberg MH, Barton F, Castro O, et al: Effect of hydroxyurea on mortality and morbidity in adult sickle cell
    anemia: Risks and benefits up to 9 years of treatment. JAMA 289:1645–1651, 2003.

CONTROVERSIES

17. **Is pulse oximetry reliable in patients with sickle cell disease?**
    Accurate assessment of oxygenation in patients with sickle cell disease may be difficult. Pulse
    oximetry may be off by as much as $\pm$ 4% compared with measured oxygen saturation by blood
    gas analysis, especially in those with hemoglobin levels < 11 gm/dL. If there is doubt about
    hypoxia, an arterial blood gas analysis with direct measurement of PO_2 is indicated.

    Comber JT, Lopez BL: Evaluation of pulse oximetry in sickle cell anemia patients presenting to the
    emergency department in acute vasooclussive crisis. Am J Emerg Med 14:16–18, 1996.

18. **What is the role of bone marrow transplant in the treatment of sickle cell
    disease?**
    Allogeneic bone marrow transplant has been successfully performed in children with severe
    sickle cell disease using matched sibling bone marrow or cord blood. Appropriate selection
    of candidates for transplant, application to adult patients, and the role of unrelated donors or
    mini-allogeneic transplantation have yet to be determined.

    Iannone R, Ohene-Frempong K, Fuchs EJ, et al: Bone marrow transplantation for sickle cell anemia:
    Progress and prospects. Pediatr Blood Cancer 44:436–440, 2005.

CHAPTER 57

ONCOLOGIC EMERGENCIES (INCLUDING HYPERCALCEMIA)

Deborah R. Cook, MD, and William Eng Lee, MD

1. **List important oncologic emergencies.**
   - Spinal cord compression
   - Hypercalcemia
   - Brain metastases
   - Tumor lysis
   - Neutropenic fever
   - Malignant pericardial effusion
   - Superior vena cava (SVC) syndrome

2. **Why is it important to identify and treat spinal cord compression quickly?**
   In most cases, neurologic deficits present at the time of diagnosis cannot be reversed with treatment. Rapid treatment is needed to prevent further loss of function.

3. **What are the common clinical features of spinal cord compression?**
   Back pain usually precedes motor weakness, which tends to precede sensory changes and sphincter dysfunction. Pain is often present for 4–6 weeks before diagnosis and is characteristically worse during recumbency.

4. **Which cancers commonly cause spinal cord compression?**
   Prostate, breast, and lung cancers account for more than 60%. Non-Hodgkin's lymphoma, multiple myeloma, and kidney cancer each account for an additional 5–10%.

5. **Which imaging study is used to diagnose spinal cord compression?**
   Magnetic resonance imaging (MRI). MRI and computed tomography (CT) myelography are superior to plain films, bone scans, and CT as diagnostic imaging methods. The advantages of MRI include the following:
   - The entire thecal sac can be imaged, regardless of spinal block.
   - MRI is not contraindicated in patients with large brain metastases, thrombocytopenia, or coagulopathy.
   - It is less invasive than myelography.

6. **Discuss the treatment options for spinal cord compression.**
   - **Corticosteroids:** Dosing should begin immediately for pain reduction and to improve neurologic symptoms. Dexamethasone (16–96 mg daily in divided doses) is acceptable. Higher doses have not been shown to have additional effect and have increased risk of complications.
   - **Radiation:** Radiation prevents further tumor growth and neurologic damage. This treatment generally produces minimal adverse effects.
   - **Surgery:** Direct decompressive surgery plus postoperative radiotherapy is thought to be superior to treatment with radiotherapy alone. However, studies have included very specific patient populations (i.e., able to undergo surgery, expected survival of 3 months, and only a single area of metastatic spinal cord compression).

   Patchell RA, Tibbs PA, Regine WF, et al: Direct decompressive surgical resection in the treatment of spinal cord compression caused by metastatic cancer: A randomised trial. Lancet 366:643–648, 2005.

7. **List the three major types of hypercalcemia and the cancers with which they are associated.**
    See Table 57-1.

TABLE 57-1.	THREE MAJOR TYPES OF HYPERCALCEMIA		
Type	Cause	Frequency	Cancers
Humoral	PTH-related protein	80%	NSCLC, cervical, esophageal, head and neck, renal cancer
Osteolytic	Cytokines, PTHrP	20%	Breast, myeloma, NHL
Calcitriol	1,25(OH)2D secretion	<1%	Lymphomas

PTHrP = parathyroid hormone–related protein, NSCLC = non–small cell lung cancer, NHL = non-Hodgkin's lymphoma, 1,25(OH)2D = 1,25-dihydroxyvitamin D.

8. **List the available therapies for hypercalcemia.**
    ▪ IV hydration with isotonic saline (200–500 mL/h unless cardiac or renal disease prevents) is one option.
    ▪ Loop diuretics such as furosemide enhance the calciuric effects of volume expansion. Thiazide diuretics are *absolutely contraindicated* because they increase the distal tubular reabsorption of calcium.
    ▪ Bisphosphonates such as pamidronate and zoledronate block osteoclastic bone resorption. Administration of these drugs should be started early because they require 2 to 4 days to elicit a significant response.
    ▪ Calcitonin inhibits bone resorption and increases renal excretion of calcium. Its onset of action is rapid but short lived.
    ▪ Oral phosphate repletion for low phosphorus levels will improve the efficacy of the previously discussed treatments.
    Stewart A: Hypercalcemia associated with cancer. N Engl J Med 352:373–379, 2005.

9. **What goes up and what goes down in tumor lysis syndrome?**

Up	Down
Potassium	Calcium
Uric acid	
Phosphorus	
Blood urea nitrogen	

10. **What are the risk factors for tumor lysis syndrome?**
    The risk factors include rapidly dividing tumor, large tumor burden, and tumors that are highly responsive to chemotherapy. Examples include acute lymphoblastic leukemia, Burkitt's lymphoma, acute myelogenous leukemia, and multiple myeloma. Other predisposing factors are dehydration, obstructive uropathy, renal insufficiency, and increased levels of lactate dehydrogenase or uric acid before initiation of chemotherapy.

11. **Describe the treatment for tumor lysis syndrome.**
    The best treatment is prevention. Patients at risk for tumor lysis syndrome should be pretreated with allopurinol and IV hydration to maintain a high urine output. If the uric acid levels are very high on presentation, urate oxidase (rasburicase) may be used to break down the uric

acid to allantoin, which is much more soluble in urine. Frequent monitoring of blood urea nitrogen, creatinine, uric acid, calcium, phosphate, and potassium levels is required to detect metabolic abnormalities early.

Cairo M, Bishop M: Tumour lysis syndrome: New therapeutic strategies and classification. Br J Haematol 127:3–11, 2004.

12. **What are the predisposing factors for infection in patients with cancer?**
Patients with cancer are "compromised hosts" at risk for infection due to the underlying malignancy and as a result of anticancer therapy. Risk factors for infection include defects in cellular and humoral immunity, disruption of mucosal and skin integrity, tumor-related obstruction, granulocytopenia, and iatrogenic procedures.

13. **What is the major source of infection?**
The patient's endogenous flora.

14. **Describe the evaluation of febrile, neutropenic patients.**
A careful history and physical examination should include an evaluation of all potential mucosal and epithelial portals of entry. The sinuses, oral cavity, and perirectal areas are important sources of infection in neutropenic patients. Any indwelling venous catheters should be inspected and palpated. The laboratory evaluation should include Gram stain and cultures of blood, urine, sputum, throat, stool, and other available fluids. Lumbar puncture should be performed if central nervous system infection is suspected. Chest radiographs should always be obtained along with radiologic evaluation of the paranasal sinuses, abdomen, and other sites, as clinically indicated.

15. **Describe the treatment for fever in a patient with neutropenia.**
After cultures have been obtained, empiric broad-spectrum antibiotic coverage should be initiated promptly. The institution's predominant pathogens and resistance pattern will guide the therapy. Vancomycin should only be added to the empiric regimens if gram-positive bacteria are common causes of serious infections, catheter-related infection is highly suspected, the patient is colonized with resistant strains of pneumococci or *Staphylococcus aureus*, blood culture results are positive for gram-positive organisms, or there is evidence of sepsis. Acceptable initial empiric regimens are listed in Table 57-2.

Crawford J, Dale DC, Lyman GH: Chemotherapy-induced neutropenia: Risks, consequences, and new directions for its management. Cancer 100:228–327, 2004.

Hughes WT, Armstrong D, Bodey GP, et al: 2002 guidelines for the use of antimicrobial agents in neutropenic patients with cancer. Clin Infect Dis 34:730–751, 2002.

TABLE 57-2. INITIAL THERAPY FOR FEVER IN A PATIENT WITH NEUTROPENIA	
Monotherapy	Two-Drug Combinations
Cefepime	Aminoglycoside *plus*
Ceftazidime	Antipseudomonal penicillin *or*
Imipenem-cilastatin or meropenem	Cefepime *or*
Piperacillin-tazobactam	Ceftazidime *or*
	Carbapenem
	Ciprofloxacin *plus*
	Piperacillin-tazobactam

16. **What are the common clinical features of a malignant pericardial effusion?**
Acute-onset dyspnea, orthopnea, cough, chest discomfort, jugular venous distention, hepatomegaly, and edema. If the effusion develops slowly, symptoms may be minimal.

17. **What are the most common cancers that involve the pericardium?**
Carcinomas of the lung and breast, melanoma, and the lymphomas.

18. **What is the treatment for malignant pericardial effusion?**
- **Pericardiocentesis:** Performed immediately, it can be lifesaving as well as diagnostic.
- **Chemotherapy and radiation:** This treatment is most effective in cancers that are sensitive.
- **Intrapericardial instillation:** Use of sclerosing agents such as tetracycline, bleomycin, OK-432, thiotepa, and cisplatin can prevent reaccumulation of the effusion.
- **Indwelling pericardial catheters:** These can be placed with local anesthesia and are associated with lower morbidity rates.
- **Balloon pericardiotomy**: This treatment can be performed in cardiac catheterization laboratories under fluoroscopy.
- **Surgery:** This modality involves the surgical creation of a pericardial window or pericardiectomy.

   Karam N, Patel P, deFilippi C: Diagnosis and management of chronic pericardial effusions. Am J Med Sci 322:79–87, 2001.

19. **Brain metastases commonly originate from which cancers?**
Lung, breast, melanoma, and kidney cancers.

20. **What acute neurologic symptoms are concerning for brain metastases?**
Headaches, cognitive impairment, focal neurologic deficits, and seizures.

KEY POINTS: BRAIN METASTASES AND SPINAL CORD COMPRESSION

1. Start the administration of steroids right away.

2. MRI is the imaging of choice.

3. Radiation therapy will always be part of the treatment plan.

21. **Which imaging studies are diagnostic? What are the characteristic findings?**
MRI with gadolinium is more sensitive than CT with contrast. The typical findings are multiple ring-enhancing round lesions with edema.

22. **What are the treatment options?**
- **Corticosteroids:** The administration of corticosteroids should be started immediately to decrease cerebral edema.
- **Anticonvulsants:** Use *only* in patients who develop seizures, not as prophylaxis.
- **Surgery:** Reserve for single, large, accessible metastasis causing significant obstructive hydrocephalus.
- **Whole brain radiation therapy (WBRT):** Widely available, principal therapy for multiple metastases
- **Stereotactic radiosurgery:** A single high dose of radiation using multiple cobalt sources or a linear accelerator is typically used in patients with four or fewer brain lesions that are <3 cm

in size. When combined with WBRT in these patients, stereotactic radiosurgery improves brain control, and in some cases overall survival, better than WBRT alone.

- **Chemotherapy:** Chemotherapy is limited by the blood–brain barrier but can be effective as sole therapy in chemosensitive cancers such as small-cell lung cancer or germ cell cancers

Andrews DW, Scott CB, Sperduto PW, et al: Whole brain radiation therapy with or without stereotactic radiosurgery boost for patients with one to three brain metastases: Phase III results of the RTOG 9508 randomized trial. Lancet 363(9422):1665–1672, 2004.

Soffietti R, Ruda R, Mitani R: Management of brain metastases. J Neurol 249:1357–1369, 2002.

23. **What are the clinical manifestations of SVC syndrome?**
    The most common symptom is dyspnea. Patients may also complain of facial swelling, fullness in the head, cough, and facial plethora. Physical findings most often include distended neck veins, distention of the superficial veins of the chest wall, and facial edema.

24. **What causes SVC syndrome?**
    Malignant tumors cause up to 85% of the cases of SVC syndrome. Infection and clot (often from a central venous catheter) account for most of the rest. Lung cancer and lymphoma are the most common malignant causes. Oddly enough, almost 60% of patients diagnosed with SVC syndrome are not yet diagnosed with cancer.

25. **How do we treat SVC syndrome?**
    A quick way to relieve symptoms is with intraluminal stenting. This is being used more often as upfront treatment while the underlying etiology is pursued. Accurate diagnosis of the cause of the SVC syndrome is important in determining treatment with radiation versus chemotherapy. Non-Hodgkin's lymphomas, germ cell cancers, and small cell lung cancer all respond very well to chemotherapy. On the other hand, non–small cell lung cancer may respond to chemotherapy or radiation.

Rowell NP, Gleeson FV: Steroids, radiotherapy, chemotherapy and stents for superior vena caval obstruction in carcinoma of the bronchus: A systematic review. Clin Oncol 14:338–351, 2002.

RHEUMATOLOGIC DISEASE IN THE INTENSIVE CARE UNIT

Danny C. Williams, MD

1. **What is the differential diagnosis for acute inflammatory arthritis in the critical care setting?**
   See Table 58-1.

   Harris ED, Budd RC, Genovese MC, et al (eds): Kelly's Textbook of Rheumatology, 7th ed. Philadelphia, W.B. Saunders, 2005.

TABLE 58-1. DIFFERENTIAL DIAGNOSIS FOR ACUTE INFLAMMATORY ARTHRITIS	
Monoarthritis (Single Joint)*	**Polyarthritis (Multiple Joints)***
Septic arthritis	Infective endocarditis
Crystalline arthritis	Viral arthritis
Traumatic arthritis	Gonococcal arthritis
Hemarthrosis	Reactive arthritis
Osteonecrosis	Rheumatoid arthritis
Septic prosthetic joint	Systemic lupus erythematosus
Neuropathic joint	Enteropathic arthritis
Steroid injection synovitis	Psoriatic arthritis
Iatrogenic infection	Systemic vasculitis
	Serum sickness
	Sickle cell disease
	Cancer
	Sarcoid

*Classification of these disorders by the number of involved joints reflects their most common pattern of clinical presentation.

2. **In evaluating articular pain, what physical features can differentiate inflammatory arthritis from bursitis, tendinitis, or cellulitis?**
   See Table 58-2.

   Polly HF, Hunder GG: Rheumatologic Interviewing and Physical Examination of the Joints, 2nd ed. Philadelphia, W.B. Saunders, 1978.

TABLE 58-2. PHYSICAL FEATURES DIFFERENTIATING ARTHRITIS, BURSITIS, TENDINITIS, AND CELLULITIS

Feature*	Arthritis	Bursitis	Tendinitis	Cellulitis
Erythema	Often	Often	Seldom	Always
Warmth	Often	Often	Seldom	Always
Swelling	Global	Focal	Linear	Focal
Subjective pain	Global	Focal	Focal	Focal
Joint-line tenderness	Always	None	None	None
Joint stress pain	Always	None	None	None
Joint flexion deformity	Often	Seldom	Seldom	None
Loss of range	Global	Partial	Partial	None
Active range of motion	Limited	Limited	Limited	Normal
Passive range of motion	Limited	Normal	Normal	Normal
Effusion	Often	Often	Seldom	None
Crepitance	Often	Seldom	Seldom	Seldom
Skinfold tenderness	Seldom	Seldom	Seldom	Always

*In the absence of nonsteroidal anti-inflammatory drugs or corticosteroids.
Caution: Arthritis, bursitis, tendinitis, and cellulitis may coexist in the same patient.

KEY POINTS: BEST PHYSICAL INDICATORS OF INFLAMMATORY ARTHRITIS

1. Warmth, with or without erythema

2. A distended joint capsule, with or without effusion

3. A tender joint line

4. Equal limitation of active and passive range of motion

5. Global articular pain elicited by stressing the joint

3. **What are the indications for arthrocentesis?**
See Table 58-3.

4. **How do you perform arthrocentesis of the knee (Fig. 58-1)?**
In the critical care setting, the knee is a frequent target of arthritis. Thus, proficiency in knee arthrocentesis is essential. The joint space can be accessed at one of six points circumscribing the patella. Visualizing the patella as a clock face is helpful. Large suprapatellar compartment effusions should be aspirated at the 11- or 1-o'clock position, with the knee in slight flexion. If the lateral or medial approach (8- or 4-o'clock) is used, simultaneous compression of the suprapatellar compartment may enhance synovial fluid collection. The inferior approach

TABLE 58-3. INDICATIONS FOR ARTHROCENTESIS

Diagnostic	Therapeutic
Septic arthritis*	Pus drainage
Crystalline arthritis	Crystal depletion
Hemarthrosis	Blood removal
Inflammatory versus noninflammatory arthritis	Effusion-induced joint pain
	Effusion-induced functional impairment
	Corticosteroid injection

*The primary consideration for performing any jont tap is to rule out infection as a cause of arthritis. An undiagnosed septic arthritis can lead to rapid (2–14 days), irreversible joint destruction and also provide a reservoir for dissemination of systemic infection in critically ill patients.

(7- or 5-o'clock) is performed with the knee flexed at 90 degrees. The "key to the knee" is placing the needle underneath a "relaxed" patella. General guidelines are as follows:

- Go where the joint capsule appears maximally distended.
- Indent the skin with a retracted ballpoint pen tip to mark the entry site.
- Prepare and maintain a sterile field.
- Use sufficient local anesthetic (e.g., 1% lidocaine without epinephrine).
- Use an 18- or 21-gauge, long needle (larger bore for large or viscous effusions).
- Avoid penetrating abnormal skin (e.g., cellulitis) to tap a joint.
- Correct bleeding diathesis before arthrocentesis, if possible.
- Continuously aspirate from the entry point to the effusion.
- If flow becomes obstructed, pull the syringe back slightly and rotate it 90 degrees.
- Drain the joint dry.

5. **What studies are essential in synovial fluid analysis?**
   The three Cs: culture, cell count, and crystals.
   - **Culture and Gram stains:** Infection is the most important diagnostic issue in acute arthritis. Gram stain and routine culture should be performed on all synovial fluid samples, including those from patients with known rheumatic disease. A positive Gram stain result can direct initial antibiotic selection. Additionally, therapeutic response can be monitored by Gram staining serially obtained synovial fluid specimens. Special stains and cultures (e.g., mycobacteria, fungi, and viruses) are reserved for unusual cases, such as an immunocompromised patient presenting with chronic monoarthritis. The recovery rate of microbes from synovial fluid in nongonococcal bacterial arthritis typically exceeds 95%, in contrast to gonococcal arthritis, for which recovery is only 30%. In "reactive" arthritis, viable organisms are not recovered; the infection (e.g., *Salmonella* enteritis) is extra-articular.
   - **Cell count and differential:** The cell count can reveal the underlying nature of an acute arthritis. Synovial effusions are classified as noninflammatory, inflammatory, or purulent (Table 58-4). In general, large leukocyte counts with polymorphonuclear cell predominance suggest acute infection. However, considerable overlap may exist between "septic" cell counts and those of crystalline arthritis or connective tissue diseases. Likewise, the assumption that low leukocyte counts exclude infection is faulty; trust the culture! As with the Gram stain, serial assessment of leukocyte quantity and type can gauge therapeutic efficacy. A lack of improvement in leukocyte parameters usually indicates treatment failure or a loculated effusion.

TABLE 58-4. CELL COUNT FINDINGS IN NONINFLAMMATORY, INFLAMMATORY, AND PURULENT ARTHRITIS

Feature	Noninflammatory	Inflammatory	Purulent
WBC/mm^2	200–2000	2000–75,000	Often >100,000
PMNs	<25%	>50%	>75%
Prototypic disorder	Osteoarthritis	Rheumatoid arthritis	Septic joint

WBC = white blood cells (leukocytes), PMNs = polymorphonuclear cells.

- **Crystals:** The identification of crystals (e.g., monosodium urate or calcium pyrophosphate) can be diagnostic (i.e., gout or pseudogout); however, crystals do not exclude the possibility of concurrent infection.

Harris ED, Budd RC, Genovese MC, et al (eds): Kelly's Textbook of Rheumatology, 7th ed. Philadelphia, W.B. Saunders, 2005.

6. **Describe the management of acute septic arthritis.**

Acute septic arthritis in the critical care setting occurs primarily in elderly patients with preexisting joint abnormalities (e.g., arthritis, prosthetic joints) and chronic disease (e.g., cancer, cirrhosis, diabetes, renal failure). Extra-articular sources of bacteremia such as the skin (e.g., indwelling catheters, decubitus ulcers), gastrointestinal tract, genitourinary tract, lungs, and IV drug abuse account for most joint infections. On rare occasions, penetrating trauma, arthroscopy, corticosteroid joint injections, and osteomyelitis can cause septic arthritis by direct bacterial inoculation. Acute septic arthritis is best managed by following the three Es: establish, eradicate, and evacuate.

- **Establish the infection:** Diagnostic arthrocentesis is the procedure of choice for identifying the organism(s) responsible for septic arthritis. In most cases, only one joint is affected—usually the knee. However, if polyarticular involvement is apparent, all suspicious joints should be tapped to increase the probability of a positive Gram stain and culture. Recovery of the infectious organism(s) may be enhanced by directly injecting some of the synovial fluid into blood culture bottles. In rare instances, it may be necessary to biopsy the synovium to recover an organism. Blood culture specimens should *always* be obtained as well as specimens for other cultures indicated by the clinical presentation. *Pearl: Staphylococcus aureus* accounts for the majority of nongonococcal joint infections.
- **Eradicate the infection:** Clinical features (e.g., urinary tract infection, pneumonia) and the synovial fluid Gram stain should direct the initial antibiotic choice. Gram-positive organisms are treated with penicillinase-resistant penicillins or first-generation cephalosporins. If methicillin-resistant staphylococci are suspected (e.g., in the setting of IV drug abuse or hemodialysis), vancomycin is indicated. Third-generation cephalosporins or broad-spectrum penicillins with or without aminoglycosides or quinolones are used for gram-negative coverage. With a negative Gram stain result, the preceding antibiotics used in combination provide the best coverage while results of the synovial fluid culture are awaited. The culture and sensitivity results should dictate the final antibiotic regimen. Most nongonococcal septic arthritis infections require at least 2 weeks of IV antibiotics followed by an additional 2–4 weeks of oral therapy. *Pearl:* A negative Gram stain result or the presence of gout crystals in the synovial fluid does not exclude septic arthritis.
- **Evacuate the infection:** The presence of nonviable bacteria or bacterial antigens within a joint may provoke an inflammatory response severe enough to cause irreparable damage. Thus, antibiotics alone are not sufficient treatment for septic arthritis. Bacteria and

inflammatory products should be evacuated from an infected joint by serial arthrocentesis, arthroscopy, or open surgical drainage. Serial arthrocentesis is best performed on a "willing" patient with an accessible, uncomplicated joint (Fig. 58-1).

- **Other measures:** An additional component in the management of septic arthritis is immobilization of the affected joint in a neutral position for a few days. Immobilization should be followed by gentle range-of-motion and strengthening exercises once the joint inflammation subsides. Although nonsteroidal anti-inflammatory drugs (NSAIDs) and corticosteroids have been shown to reduce joint drainage in animal models of septic arthritis, they are not yet recommended in the initial treatment of joint infections in humans. The early administration of anti-inflammatory medications may conceal an ongoing infection. Plain radiographs of the affected joint are usually obtained to rule out osteomyelitis and as a baseline study of joint architecture. Other than effusion, early radiographs of septic joints are usually devoid of diagnostic features.

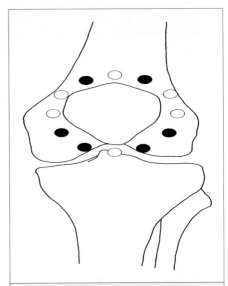

Figure 58-1. Arthrocentesis of the knee. The blackened circles indicate needle insertion sites.

Espinoza LR (ed): Infectious arthritis. Rheum Dis Clin North Am 24:2, 1998.

7. **What is the best procedure for clearing a septic joint?**
   There are three options for evacuating the contents of a septic joint: serial arthrocentesis, arthroscopy, and open surgical drainage. The best method remains controversial and depends on multiple factors, including synovial fluid viscosity, bacterial virulence, joint architecture, patient compliance, and operator performance. Closed-needle aspiration is the traditional procedure for clearing infection from accessible, uncomplicated joints. In general, arthrocentesis and synovial fluid analysis are performed at least once daily for 4–7 days while the patient is taking appropriate antibiotics. Orthopedic consultation is indicated if there is no interim improvement in the physical examination or Gram stain results and cell count of the synovial fluid. Surgical consultation also should be obtained in the following situations:
   - Delayed diagnosis: >1 week
   - Difficult arthrocentesis: viscous, debris-laden synovial fluid
   - Difficult joints: hip, sacroiliac, shoulder, sternoclavicular, wrist
   - Damaged joints: arthritis, prostheses, foreign bodies, trauma
   - Osteomyelitis
   - Patient preference

8. **What clinical features, other than arthritis, are suggestive of connective tissue disease?**
   The diagnosis of connective tissue disorders is largely dependent on the history and physical examination. Laboratory investigations (e.g., antinuclear antibodies) should be

BOX 58-1. CLINICAL FEATURES THAT MAY INDICATE AN UNDERLYING CONNECTIVE TISSUE DISORDER

Cardiac
Dysrhythmias
Pericarditis
Valvular disease
Myocarditis

Cutaneous
Alopecia
Facial rash
Livedo reticularis
Palpable purpura
Calcinosis
Sclerosis
Subcutaneous
  nodules
Erythema nodosum
Psoriasis
Pyoderma

Enteric
Dysphagia/reflux
Malabsorption
Peritonitis
Hepatitis
Pancreatitis
Colitis
Bowel infarction

Genitourinary
Urethritis
Ulceration
Testicular pain
Recurrent fetal
  loss

Hematologic
Anemia
Hemolysis
Leukopenia
Leukocytosis
Thrombocytosis
Thrombocytopenia

Lymphoreticular
Adenopathy
Splenomegaly

Musculoskeletal
Arthralgia
Articular deformity
Tenosynovitis
Myalgia
Muscle weakness

Neurologic
Cognitive dysfunction
Altered behavior
Altered consciousness
Seizure
Stroke
Peripheral
  neuropathy
Aseptic meningitis

Ocular
Xerophthalmia
Episcleritis
Scleritis
Iritis
Visual loss

Oral
Xerostomia
Ulceration
Parotid swelling
Telangiectasia

Pulmonary
Pleuritis
Pneumonitis
Interstitial fibrosis
Hemorrhage
Hypertension
Embolism

Renal
Glomerulonephritis
Tubular acidosis
Nephrolithiasis

Systemic
Fever
Fatigue
Cachexia

Vascular
Acute hypertension
Raynaud's
  phenomenon
Acral cyanosis
Thrombosis

performed to confirm a presumptive diagnosis. Box 58-1 lists clinical features that may indicate an underlying connective tissue disorder, especially when several organ systems are involved simultaneously.

Hochberg MC, Silman AJ, Smolen JS, et al (eds): Rheumatology, 3rd ed. St. Louis, Mosby, 2003.

9. **When does an elevated erythrocyte sedimentation rate (ESR) reflect an underlying connective tissue disorder?**
The ESR is a nonspecific test (Westergren method preferred) for systemic inflammation. ESR elevation typically results from cytokine-induced hepatic synthesis of acute-phase reactants, in particular fibrinogen. However, some noninflammatory factors such as advanced age, female gender, and pregnancy can also cause elevation of the ESR. The ESR can be helpful in the evaluation of numerous rheumatic diseases, but is it not diagnostic. Even when extreme ESR

elevations are encountered (≥ 100 mm/h), infection is more likely (35%) than connective tissue disease (25%). Thus, when an elevated ESR is obtained in a critical care patient, the diagnosis of a connective tissue disorder still depends on the presence of characteristic clinical features (*see* question 8). The ESR is perhaps most useful in serial assessment of ongoing disease severity in disorders such as rheumatoid arthritis, polymyalgia rheumatica, and giant cell arteritis. The "upper limit of normal" ESR value for most patients can be calculated by the following formulas:

- $ESR_{(male)} = age \div 2$
- $ESR_{(female)} = (age + 10) \div 2$

The platelet count (thrombocytosis) can be used as a crude substitute for ESR; platelets act as "acute-phase" reactants.

10. **What laboratory evaluations are useful in the diagnosis of connective tissue disorders?**
There are no screening tests for the diagnosis of connective tissue disease. Because of their lack of specificity, positive serologic test results in the absence of supporting clinical features usually result in misdiagnoses. Serologic evaluation of patients with suspected autoimmune disease should proceed in three stages: systemic inflammation determination, autoantibody identification, and supplemental testing.
1. Systemic inflammation determination: A routine complete blood count and ESR measurement are usually adequate to demonstrate systemic inflammation. Complete blood count abnormalities typically include leukocytosis, a normocytic/normochromic anemia, and thrombocytosis. Additional laboratory indicators of systemic inflammation may include the following:

- ↑ C-reactive protein (more specific, but more expensive than ESR)
- ↑ Fibrinogen
- ↑ Haptoglobin
- ↑ Gamma globulins
- ↑ C3 (third component of complement)
- ↑ Ferritin
- ↓ Albumin
- ↓ Transferrin

2. Autoantibody identification: Serum antibodies (e.g., antinuclear antibody [ANA]) may help confirm a particular connective tissue disorder but should not be used to screen for rheumatic disease. The most frequently used autoantibody tests for suspected rheumatic diseases are rheumatoid factor (anti-immunoglobulin G antibody) and ANA. In autoimmune disease, a positive ANA indicates the presence of specific nuclear antigens, which can usually be identified by an "ANA profile" (Table 58-5). Autoantibodies may also be directed against cellular antigens in the cytoplasm and cell-surface membrane. Common disease associations with specific autoantibodies are listed in Table 58-5. In addition, remember the following:

- A positive ANA test result is suggestive of an autoimmune disorder only if the pretest probability is high.
- A negative ANA test result virtually excludes active systemic lupus erythematosus (SLE).
- Antibody overlap is common (e.g., a patient with lupus erythematosus may simultaneously have double-stranded DNA [dsDNA], Sjögren's syndrome A/RO [SS-A], histone, rheumatoid factor, and phospholipid antibodies).
- Autoantibodies may be seen in persons with nonconnective tissue disorders (e.g., rheumatoid factor in subacute bacterial endocarditis) and in healthy persons.

3. Supplemental testing: Ancillary tests for connective tissue disorders assess disease mechanisms, tissue damage, and disease activity. The investigations listed in Table 58-6 may be useful in the diagnosis and management of some patients with connective tissue disease.

- Hypocomplementemia and high-titer dsDNA antibodies are associated with active SLE; in particular, active lupus nephritis.

Hochberg MC, Silman AJ, Smolen JS, et al (eds): Rheumatology, 3rd ed. St. Louis, Mosby, 2003.

TABLE 58-5. AUTOANTIBODIES AND ASSOCIATED DISORDERS

Autoantibody	Disorder (% Positive)
Rheumatoid factor	Rheumatoid arthritis (85%)
Anticyclic citrulline peptide antibody (Anti-CCP)*	Rheumatoid arthritis (80%)
ANA profile	
■ Anti-dsDNA	Systemic lupus erythematosus (60%)
■ Anti-Sm (Smith antigen)	Systemic lupus erythematosus (30%)
■ Anti-SS-A	Sjögren's syndrome (60%)
■ Anti-SS-B	Sjögren's syndrome (40%)
■ Anti-RNP	Mixed connective tissue disease (95%)
Anti-Scl-70	Diffuse scleroderma (30%)
Anti-centromere	Limited scleroderma (90%)
Anti-histone	Drug-induced lupus erythematosus (90%)
Anti-Jo-1	Polymyositis (20%)
Anti-neutrophilic cytoplasmic antibody	Wegener's granulomatosis (90%)
Anti-phospholipid	Antiphospholipid antibody syndrome (100%)

ANA = antinuclear antibody, dsDNA = double-stranded DNA, Sm = Smith antigen, SS-A = Sjögren's syndrome A/RO, SS-B = Sjögren's syndrome B/La, RNP = ribonucleoprotein, Scl-70 = topoisomerase I, Jo-1 = histodyl-tRNA synthetase.
*Anti-CCP is the most specific test (98% specificity) available for rhematoid arthritis; it probably will replace rheumatoid factor.

TABLE 58-6. DIAGNOSTIC TESTS FOR CONNECTIVE TISSUE DISORDERS

Disorder	Test
Immune complex disease	Complement (C3, C4)
Hemolysis	Coombs' test
Myositis	Creatine kinase
Nephritis	Urinalysis and creatinine
Thrombosis	Lupus anticoagulant or anticardiolipin antibody
Vasculitis	Hepatitis profile or cryoglobulins

11. **When does an elevated serum creatine kinase (CK) level indicate inflammatory muscle disease?**

An increased CK level in conjunction with symmetric muscle weakness is suggestive of an autoimmune, inflammatory myopathy. However, in the critical care setting, the following causes of an elevated CK also merit consideration:

- **Myocardial injury:** Ischemia, infarction, myocarditis, or surgery
- **Muscle trauma:** Ischemia, crush injury, biopsy, or intramuscular injections
- **Drug-induced:** Ethanol, corticosteroids, lipid-lowering agents, cimetidine, cocaine, opiates, benzodiazepines, barbiturates, or zidovudine

- **Infectious myositis:** Bacterial, viral, mycobacterial, fungal, or parasitic
- **Endocrine disorders:** Hypothyroidism or hypoparathyroidism
- **Central nervous system injury:** Ischemia or trauma
- **Miscellaneous disorders:** Seizures, hemolysis, malignant hyperthermia, muscular dystrophy, motor neuron disease, or peripheral neuropathy

Autoimmune muscle inflammation may occur independently (polymyositis), with rash (dermatomyositis), in "overlap" syndromes (e.g., mixed connective tissue disease), or in association with cancer. The core features of polymyositis typically include neck flexor and proximal limb girdle weakness, infrequent myalgias, and elevated serum muscle enzyme levels. Other organ systems may become involved, such as the gastrointestinal tract (dysphagia), the lungs (interstitial lung disease), the heart (myocarditis), the joints (arthritis), and the blood vessels (Raynaud's phenomenon). The diagnosis is established by performing electromyography with subsequent biopsy of the abnormal muscle. Additional serum proteins that can also reflect muscle damage include the aminotransferases, lactate dehydrogenase, aldolase, and myoglobin.

Among muscle proteins, CK is the most sensitive indicator of muscle injury, whereas aspartate aminotransferase is the most specific for actual muscle inflammation.

Bohlmeyer TJ, Wu AHB, Perryman MB: Evaluation of laboratory tests as a guide to diagnosis and therapy of myositis. Rheum Dis Clin North Am 20:845–856, 1994.

12. **What clinical features suggest that a thrombolic event is due to the antiphospholipid syndrome (APS)?**
See Box 58-2. The APS can occur as an independent disorder (primary APS) or in association with another connective tissue disorder (e.g., the "lupus anticoagulant" of SLE). Although most thromboses are focal, a "catastrophic" variant of the APS may occur with rampant vascular occlusion and multiple organ failure.

Phospholipid antibodies are usually detected by one or more of the following investigations:

- False-positive serologic test result for syphilis (Venereal Disease Research Laboratory [VDRL] or rapid plasma reagin [RPR] test)

BOX 58-2. CLINICAL FEATURES OF ANTIPHOSPHOLIPID SYNDROME

Major manifestations
- Recurrent thromboses (venous > arterial; usually lower limb deep venous thrombosis or stroke)
- Multiple miscarriages (third > second > first trimester)
- Low-grade thrombocytopenia (70,000–100,000 platelets/mm^3)
- Anionic phospholipid and/or beta 2 glycoprotein-I or prothrombin antibodies

Other manifestations
- **Cutaneous:** Livedo reticularis, superficial thrombophlebitis, acral ischemic necrosis, or splinter hemorrhages
- **Neurologic:** Seizures, chorea, multi-infarct dementia, transverse myelitis, or migraines
- **Cardiac:** Valvular disease (vegetations), myocardial infarction, or cardiomyopathy
- **Pulmonary:** Embolism, hypertension, or intra-alveolar hemorrhage
- **Skeletal:** Osteonecrosis

- Prolonged activated partial thromboplastin time that *does not* correct with added (1:1 dilution) normal plasma but *does* correct with added phospholipid
- Prolonged Russell viper venom time (lupus anticoagulant)
- Positive anticardiolipin antibody (high-titer immunoglobulin G)
- Beta 2 glycoprotein-1 antibody
  Caution: Some infections or drugs may also induce phospholipid antibodies.

  Hochberg MC, Silman AJ, Smolen JS, et al (eds): Rheumatology, 3rd ed. St. Louis, Mosby, 2003.

13. **How do connective tissue disorders commonly affect the lungs?**
   See Table 58-7.

   Weidemann HP, Matthay RA: Pulmonary manifestations of the collagen vascular diseases. Clin Chest Med 10:677–722, 1989.

TABLE 58-7. EFFECTS OF CONNECTIVE TISSUE DISORDERS ON LUNGS

Disorder	Pleuritis	Pneumonitis	Nodules	Fibrosis	Hemorrhage	↑BP	Emboli
RA	■		■	■			
SLE	■	■		■	■	■	■
DIL	■	■					
SS	■			■			
MCTD	■	■		■	■	■	
PM/DM		■		■			
DSSc		■		■			
LSSc				■		■	
APS					■	?	■
WG	■	■	■	■	■		
CSS	■	■	■	■			

RA = rheumatoid arthritis, SLE = systemic lupus erythematosus, DIL = drug-induced lupus, SS = Sjögren's syndrome, MCTD = mixed connective tissue disease, PM/DM = polymyositis/dermatomyositis, DSSc = diffuse scleroderma, LSSc = limited scleroderma, APS = antiphospholipid syndrome, WG = Wegener's graulomatosis, CSS = Churg-Strauss syndrome, ↑BP = pulmonary hypertension.

14. **How does one differentiate acute lupus pneumonitis from an infectious pneumonia?**
   Acute lupus pneumonitis is characterized by sudden dyspnea, cough with occasional sputum, fever, tachypnea, pleural irritation, infrequent hemoptysis, and hypoxemia. Chest radiographs usually reveal bibasilar infiltrates with pleural effusions; however, unilateral involvement can occur. The white blood cell count is typically normal, although this may be misleading; most patients (>50%) with active SLE have leukopenia. Although acute lupus pneumonitis typically occurs in patients with systemically active disease, it is uncommon overall. A patient with lupus erythematosus with the previously mentioned features is more likely to have a bacterial, viral, mycobacterial, or *Pneumocystis carinii* infection. Furthermore, pharmacologic agents such as NSAIDs, methotrexate, azathioprine, chlorambucil, and

cyclophosphamide may cause a toxic pneumonitis clinically indistinguishable from acute lupus pneumonitis. The diagnosis is one of exclusion and is made after sputum cultures, bronchoalveolar lavage, and lung biopsy offer no evidence of infection. There is no tissue-specific abnormality that can establish the diagnosis. The initial treatment consists of high-dose corticosteroids (1–2 mg/kg prednisone equivalent per day). In addition, IV gamma globulin (1–2 gm/kg given over 1–5 days) may be used as an alternative or as an adjunct to the corticosteroids.

McCune WJ (ed): Systemic lupus erythematosus. Rheum Dis Clin North Am 20:1, 1994.

15. **What special precautions should be taken when intubating a patient with rheumatoid arthritis?**
Cervical spine disease is a common manifestation of rheumatoid arthritis, primarily affecting the C1–C2 articulation. Furthermore, 30% of patients with advanced, erosive arthritis will have radiographic evidence of atlantoaxial subluxation (>3 mm between the C1 arch and the C2 odontoid process). These patients are at risk for spinal cord compression when subjected to manipulative procedures such as endotracheal intubation, even in the absence of symptoms. The following list identifies features on which a preintubation, cervical spine radiograph (with lateral flexion views) should be obtained:
- Physically deforming rheumatoid arthritis
- Rheumatoid arthritis duration > 3 years
- Long-term corticosteroid use
- Osteoporosis risk factors
- Intractable neck pain
- Prior cervical spine subluxation
- Clinical evidence of cervical myelopathy

An anesthesiologist should be present for emergent intubations (without radiographs) or if clinical evidence and/or radiographic findings of atlantoaxial subluxation are present.

Caution: Cricoarytenoid joint arthritis may also complicate endotracheal intubation.

Sorokin R: Management of the patient with rheumatic diseases going to surgery. Med Clin North Am 77:453–464, 1993.

16. **How can acral necrosis be avoided in a patient with Raynaud's phenomenon?**
Raynaud's phenomenon is a stress-induced (e.g., cold temperature) vascular disorder characterized by episodic, reversible ischemia of the extremities. The triphasic color response (white → blue → red) results from vasospastic alterations (ischemia → stasis → hyperemia) of acral blood flow. The following factors may precipitate sustained acral ischemia with resulting necrosis in patients with significant Raynaud's phenomenon:
- Cold stress (including subnormal body core temperature)
- Emotional stress
- Hypoperfusion
- Pharmacologic agents: beta blockers, sympathomimetic drugs (alpha agonists), ergot alkaloids, cocaine

The initial management of Raynaud's phenomenon consists of providing warmth to the extremities, maintaining acral perfusion, and reducing psychological stress. Vasodilators (e.g., nifedipine) and/or sympatholytic agents (e.g., prazosin) are indicated for patients with intolerable symptoms or atrophic, acral skin. Topical 2% nitroglycerin applied for 20 minutes, three times per day to affected digits may improve refractory cases. A daily 325-mg dose of aspirin may be effective for patients with a concurrent, occlusive vasculopathy (e.g., scleroderma).

Harris ED, Budd RC, Genovese MC, et al (eds): Kelly's Textbook of Rheumatology, 7th ed. Philadelphia, W.B. Saunders, 2005.

TABLE 58-8. CARDIAC MANIFESTATIONS OF CONNECTIVE TISSUE DISORDERS

Disorder	Pericarditis	Myocarditis	Valvular Disease	Conduction Defects	CAD
RA	■	■	Nodules		
AS	■		Aoritis/AI	AVB	
Lyme disease				AVB	
ARF	■	■	■		
SLE	■	■	Libman-Sacks endocarditis		■
DIL	■				
NLS				AVB	
MCTD	■	■		AVB	
PM/DM		■		AVB	
DSSc		Fibrosis		SVT/VT	
APS			■	AVB	■
Kawasaki's disease		■			Aneurysms
Takayasu's arteritis		■	AI		■
Marfan's syndrome			MVP/AI/MR		

CAD = coronary artery disease, RA = rheumatoid arthritis, AS = ankylosing spondylitis, AI = aortic insufficiency, AVB = atrioventricular block, ARF = acute rheumatic fever, SLE = systemic lupus erythematosus, DIL = drug-induced lupus, NLS = neonatal lupus syndrome, MCTD = mixed connective tissue disease, PM/DM = polymyositis, dermatomyositis, DSSc = diffuse scleroderma, SVT = supraventricular tachycardia, VT = ventricular tachycardia, APS = antiphospholipid syndrome, MVP = mitral valve prolapse, MR = mitral regurgitation.

17. **Which connective tissue disorders have cardiac manifestations?**
    See Table 58-8.

    Hochberg MC, Silman AJ, Smolen JS, et al (eds): Rheumatology, 3rd ed. St. Louis, Mosby, 2003.

18. **Describe the initial treatment of acute flares of rheumatoid arthritis.**
    See Table 58-9. Disease-modifying agents (e.g., methotrexate) have no role in the management of acute rheumatoid flares, except in the rare instance of severe vasculitis. Physiotherapy is a valuable but often overlooked adjunct to the management of inflammatory arthritis.

    Weisman MH, Weinblatt ME (eds): Treatment of Rheumatic Diseases. Philadelphia, W.B. Saunders, 1995.

19. **How should one manage an acute exacerbation of connective tissue disease?**
    A critical care patient with connective tissue disease is likely to have dysfunction or failure of one or more organ systems. Thus, the traditional approach to the pharmacologic treatment of an acute flare is frequently restricted by the risk of further toxicity. An example is the withholding of NSAIDs in a patient suffering from congestive heart failure, renal insufficiency, hepatic

TABLE 58-9.   INITIAL TREATMENT OF ACUTE FLARES OF RHEUMATOID ARTHRITIS

Manifestation	Initial Treatment*
Keratoconjunctivitis sicca	Hydroxymethylcellulose drops or ointment
Acute synovitis (monoarthritis)	Intra-articular steriod injection
Acute synovitis (polyarthritis)	NSAID (if no risk factors) *and/or* 10–20 mg prednisone equivalent per day
Acute pleuritis	NSAID (if no risk factors) *and/or* ≤15 prednisone equivalent per day
Acute pleuritis (with large pleural effusions)	≤0.5 mg/kg prednisone equivalent per day
Acute pericarditis	NSAID (if no risk factors) *and/or* ≤0.5 mg/kg prednisone equivalent per day

*Only if infection is ruled out or covered with appropriate antibiotics.
NSAID = nonsteroidal anti-inflammatory drug.

dysfunction, gastrointestinal hemorrhage, and/or thrombocytopenia. Other issues that can limit treatment options are limited routes of administration, drug interactions, drug hypersensitivity, pregnancy, wound healing, infection, and level of patient consciousness. In most patients, acute management will involve the administration of some form of corticosteroid. However, corticosteroids are to be avoided in patients with scleroderma, septic arthritis, osteonecrosis, Raynaud's phenomenon, and fibromyalgia. Corticosteroids are not innocuous; they promote impaired wound healing, hyperglycemia, risk of infection, fluid retention, hypokalemia, adrenal insufficiency, and neuropsychiatric disturbances. Life-threatening disease (e.g., systemic vasculitis) will often require the concomitant administration of a cytotoxic agent, such as cyclophosphamide.

20. **When and how are "pulse" corticosteroids used?**
    Pulse corticosteroids are reserved for life-threatening manifestations of rheumatic disease when rapid suppression of systemic inflammation is needed. Acute episodes of systemic vasculitis, lupus cerebritis, and lupus pneumonitis are usually treated with pulse corticosteroids. The pulse typically consists of 1 gm/day of methylprednisolone given intravenously for 3 days. The safest approach to administering such a large dose is to infuse it *slowly* as 250 mg every 6 hours. Adverse reactions may include transient flushing, headache, increased blood pressure, and acute psychosis. It may be prudent to monitor serum electrolyte and blood glucose levels in patients at risk for hypokalemia and hyperglycemia. Patients with concurrent infection should be administered antibiotics before receiving corticosteroids. Arrhythmias, myocardial infarction, and sudden death have been reported in patients with preexisting cardiovascular disease; thus, telemetry is recommended for such patients. In addition, all recipients of pulse therapy are at risk for developing osteonecrosis (avascular necrosis).

21. **Describe the initial treatment of acute flares of SLE.**
    See Table 58-10. In addition, keep in mind the following caveats:
    - Ibuprofen may cause aseptic meningitis in patients with SLE.

TABLE 58-10. INITIAL TREATMENT OF ACUTE FLARES OF SYSTEMIC LUPUS ERYTHEMATOSUS

Manifestation	Initial Treatment*
Fever	NSAID (no risk factors) *and/or* ≤15 mg prednisone equivalent per day
Acute dermatitis (mild)	Topical corticosteroid
Acute dermatitis (moderate)	≤20 mg prednisone equivalent per day
Acute polyarthritis	NSAID (no risk factors) *and/or* 10–15 mg prednisone equivalent per day
Acute myositis	0.5–1 mg/kg prednisone equivalent per day
Acute serositis[†] (mild-moderate)	NSAID (no risk factors) and/or ≤15 mg prednisone equivalent per day
Acute serositis (moderate-severe)	0.5–1 mg/kg prednisone equivalent per day
Acute myocarditis (with congestive heart failure)	1 mg/kg prednisone equivalent per day
Acute nephritis (new onset) (active urine sediment/proteinuria)	1 mg/kg prednisone equivalent per day
Acute cerebritis (with seizures/↓ mental status)	1 gm methylprednisolone per day for 3 days *plus* anticonvulsants *followed by* 1 mg/kg prednisone equivalent per day
Acute thrombosis (with phospholipid antibody)	Anticoagulation (heparin → warfarin, keep INR 3–4)
Acute thrombocytopenia or hemolytic anemia (moderate)	0.5–1 mg/kg prednisone equivalent per day
Acute thrombocytopenia or hemolytic anemia (life-threatening)	1 gm methylprednisolone per day for 3 days *followed by* 1 mg/kg prednisone equivalent per day *and/or* 1–2 mg/kg IV gamma-globulin given over 1–5 days
Acute vasculitis (cutaneous)	≤0.5 mg/kg prednisone equivalent per day
Acute vasculitis (systemic)	1 gm methylprednisolone per day for 3 days *followed by* 1 mg/kg prednisone equivalent per day

*Only if infection is ruled out or covered with appropriate antibiotics.
[†]Acute serositis includes pleuritis, pericarditis, and/or peritonitis.
NSAID = nonsteroidal anti-inflammatory drug, INR = international normalizarion ratio.

- Avoid sulfonamides in patients with SLE; they may induce a disease flare or hypersensitivity reaction.
- Divided, daily doses of corticosteroids are more potent than single daily doses, but the potential for toxicity is also greater.

Wallace DJ, Hahn BH (eds): Dubois' Lupus Erythematosus, 6th ed. Baltimore, Williams & Wilkins, 2001.

22. **How should one manage an acute gout attack?**
    Acute gouty arthritis frequently occurs in hospitalized patients. Predisposing factors include acute illness, preadmission alcohol consumption, trauma, surgery, and medications such as

TABLE 58-11. MANAGEMENT OF AN ACUTE GOUT ATTACK

	Enteral Access	Parenteral Access
Acute monoarthritis (uncomplicated)	NSAID[†] *and/or* colchicine 0.6 mg[‡] *or* intra-articular steroid *or* prednisone 30 mg/day (taper over 2 weeks)	Intra-articular steroid *or* triamcinolone 60 mg IM (single dose) *or* IV methylprednisolone[§]
Acute monoarthritis (complicated*)	Intra-articular steroid *or* prednisone 30 mg/day (taper over 2 weeks)	Intra-articular steroid *or* triamcinolone 60 mg IM (single dose) *or* IV methylprednisolone
Acute polyarthritis (uncomplicated)	NSAID *and/or* colchicine 0.6 mg *or* prednisone 30 mg/day (taper over 2 weeks)	Triamcinolone 60 mg IM (single dose) *or* IV methylprednisolone
Acute polyarthritis (complicated)	Prednisone 30 mg/day (taper over 2 weeks)	Triamcinolone 60 mg IM (single dose) *or* IV methylprednisolone

Complicated is the designation for patients with impaired organ function at risk for nonsteroidal anti-inflammatory drug (NSAID) or colchicine toxicity.
[†]NSAID: prototype is indomethacin 200 mg/day × 2 days, then 150 mg/day tapered according to symptoms.
[‡]Colchicine 0.6 mg is given as one tablet PO twice daily → three times/day to minimize gastrointestinal distress. Intravenous colcichine is not recommended.
[§]IV methylprednisolone is given as 30 mg/day tapered over 2 weeks.
IM = intramuscular.

diuretics, antimycobacterial agents, and low-dose aspirin. Most gout attacks are monoarticular (90%) and commonly affect the first metatarsophalangeal joint (podagra), the mid-foot, or ankle. Occasionally, the arthritis is accompanied by a low-grade fever and/or leukocytosis. Polyarticular gout presentations with systemic features can be confusing and mimic other types of inflammatory arthritis. Thus, the critical component of gout management is arthrocentesis, by which monosodium urate crystals can be detected and infection ruled out. As with other connective tissue disorders, comorbid conditions may complicate the pharmacologic treatment of patients with acute gout. Typical regimens are outlined in Table 58-11.

Note: Allopurinol and probenecid should not be used in acute gout attacks.

Weisman MH, Weinblatt ME (eds): Treatment of Rheumatic Diseases. Philadelphia, W.B. Saunders, 1995.

23. **During an evaluation of back pain, what features are suggestive of a serious disorder?**
In the general population, the etiology of back pain is often idiopathic (85% of all cases) and usually attributed to "mechanical" factors. Regardless, most patients (75%) will have resolution of their symptoms within 1 month of onset. Back pain in a critical care patient may portend a greater problem, however, than that resulting from an uncomfortable bed. The following features are associated with potentially serious causes of back pain:
- Acute, severe pain without obvious cause
- Pain unresponsive to rest or positional change
- Unrelenting nocturnal pain
- Significant trauma

- Constitutional symptoms
- First onset before 30 years of age or after 50 years
- Prolonged morning stiffness
- Peripheral synovitis
- Sensorimotor deficit
- Pain worse with Valsalva maneuvers
- Bowel or bladder dysfunction
- Pain radiation into both lower limbs
- Immunosuppression or prolonged corticosteroid use
- Prior cancer
- Osteoporosis risk factors

Harris ED, Budd RC, Genovese MC, et al (eds): Kelly's Textbook of Rheumatology, 7th ed. Philadelphia, W.B. Saunders, 2005.

BIBLIOGRAPHY

1. Bohlmeyer TJ, Wu AHB, Perryman MB: Evaluation of laboratory tests as a guide to diagnosis and therapy of myositis. Rheum Dis Clin North Am 20:845–856, 1994.

2. Espinoza LR (ed): Infectious arthritis. Rheum Dis Clin North Am 24:2, 1998.

3. Harris ED, Budd RC, Genovese MC, et al (eds): Kelly's Textbook of Rheumatology, 7th ed. Philadelphia, W.B. Saunders, 2005.

4. Hochberg MC, Silman AJ, Smolen JS, et al (eds): Rheumatology, 3rd ed. St. Louis, Mosby, 2003.

5. McCune WJ (ed): Systemic lupus erythematosus. Rheum Dis Clin North Am 20:1, 1994.

6. Polly HF, Hunder GG: Rheumatologic Interviewing and Physical Examination of the Joints, 2nd ed. Philadelphia, W.B. Saunders, 1978.

7. Sorokin R: Management of the patient with rheumatic diseases going to surgery. Med Clin North Am 77:453–464, 1993.

8. Wallace DJ, Hahn BH (eds): Dubois' Lupus Erythematosus, 6th ed. Baltimore, Williams & Wilkins, 2001.

9. Weidemann HP, Matthay RA: Pulmonary manifestations of the collagen vascular diseases. Clin Chest Med 10:677–722, 1989.

10. Weisman MH, Weinblatt ME (eds): Treatment of Rheumatic Diseases. Philadelphia, W.B. Saunders, 1995.

XI. NEUROLOGY

CHAPTER 59

COMA

David C. Bonovich, MD

1. **Define *coma*.**
   Coma is a pathologic condition in which the patient is unconscious and appears to be asleep. The patient cannot be roused and is aware of neither external stimuli nor inner needs. A patient in a coma is unable to interact with his or her environment.

2. **Which anatomic structures must be malfunctioning to produce coma?**
   Coma is caused by dysfunction of the reticular activating system (RAS) in the brain stem or both cerebral hemispheres.

3. **What can we determine about the cause of coma through localizing it anatomically?**
   Cerebral hemispheric or brain stem RAS dysfunction may result from structural or metabolic lesions. Structural lesions of the RAS are usually associated with focal neurologic signs that localize to the brain stem; thus, cranial nerves and ascending and descending nerve tracts between the brain and spinal cord are usually involved and show signs of dysfunction.
   A structural lesion must be large to affect both cerebral hemispheres and produce coma. In the absence of focal neurologic signs, coma is usually the result of a global toxic or metabolic suppression of the cerebral hemispheres, the RAS, or both.

4. **What are the initial steps in managing a patient with coma?**
   As always, the ABCs (i.e., airway, breathing, and circulation) should be addressed first. Oxygen should be administered via face mask, and vascular access should be obtained. If the patient does not have a secure airway, intubation should be performed. If, after a history is obtained and a physical and neurologic examination performed, the cause of coma is uncertain, empiric therapy for reversible causes such as Wernicke's encephalopathy and narcotic overdose should be initiated using thiamine and naloxone. The blood glucose level should be measured, and if hypoglycemia is present, $D_{50}W$ should be administered.

   Mercer WN, Childa NL: Coma, vegetative state, and the minimally conscious state: Diagnosis and management. Neurologist 5:186–193, 1999.

5. **Describe the diagnostic approach appropriate for comatose patients.**
   It is important to have a systematic approach to coma. The history may be obtained from relatives, friends, or paramedics and may suggest an obvious cause such as drug or alcohol overdose, sepsis, or abnormalities of glucose metabolism.
   The general physical examination, beginning with vital signs and proceeding in a systematic manner to include the head, eyes, ears, nose, and throat as well as the lungs, heart, abdomen, extremities, and skin, may help to identify infectious causes, respiratory or cardiac disorders, or liver failure, especially in patients with chronic liver disease. Careful attention should be paid to evaluation of the skin and mucous membranes for needle marks or signs of emboli and to the ocular fundi for evidence of papilledema, which suggests increased intracranial pressure.
   Assessment of the vital signs may suggest an infectious cause or respiratory disorder. The neck should be examined for nuchal rigidity, which suggests the possibility of meningeal irritation.

A rectal examination should be carried out to assess the stool for blood. Although a full neurologic exam might not be possible, one can test brain stem reflexes and look for evidence of focal motor abnormalities as well as reflex asymmetry, including plantar response. A description of the respiratory pattern should be noted.

Imaging studies such as computed tomography (CT) of the brain can be helpful in ruling out structural causes of coma. An electroencephalogram (EEG) can be helpful in ruling out seizures or other EEG patterns suggestive of toxic metabolic abnormalities resulting in coma.

Liao YJ, So YT: An approach to critically ill patients in coma. West J Med 176:184–187, 2002.

6. **How does the finding of a new focal abnormality on neurologic examination affect the management of a comatose patient?**
   Focal neurologic abnormalities generally indicate a structural central nervous system (CNS) lesion such as tumor, abscess, infarct, or hemorrhage. Focal metabolic failure may be seen in hypoglycemia, hyperglycemia, or Wernicke's encephalopathy. Imaging with head CT or magnetic resonance imaging (MRI) should be considered early in the management of such patients to exclude lesions that may require aggressive medical or surgical intervention and to assess prognosis.

7. **Does a nonfocal neurologic exam exclude a mass as the cause of coma?**
   No. Although most cases of coma with a nonfocal neurologic exam are due to toxic-metabolic causes, bilateral subdural hematomas, subarachnoid hemorrhage, hydrocephalus (communicating or noncommunicating), trauma with diffuse axonal injury, or lesions involving the bilateral frontal lobes may not show any gross focal abnormalities on neurologic testing.

8. **What initial laboratory evaluations should be performed in the case of coma of uncertain etiology?**
   A drug screen (both urine and blood), blood alcohol level test, complete blood count, and measurements of serum electrolyte, glucose, calcium, phosphate, magnesium, creatinine, blood urea nitrogen, and liver and thyroid levels should be ordered. An arterial blood gas analysis to asses the pH of the blood as well as the PaO_2 should be performed. Blood, urine, and sputum cultures should be performed if infection is suspected. An initial electrocardiogram should be obtained. A CT scan of the head should be performed if the cause is not obvious or if focal signs are present on neurologic examination. A lumbar puncture should be performed if a primary CNS infection is likely, but only after the presence of a CNS mass has been excluded by CT or MRI.

   Kleeman CR: Metabolic coma. Kidney Int 36:1142–1158, 1989.

9. **Describe the approach to treatment of a comatose trauma patient.**
   Although the general approach is similar, the likelihood of a structural cause of coma is high in patients who have experienced trauma. Traumatic causes of coma include subdural or epidural hematomas, focal intracerebral hemorrhage with mass effect and midline shift, bilateral contusions, direct injury to the brain stem, and diffuse axonal injury. Consideration also must be given to other causes, such as brain stem infarction, hypertensive hemorrhage, hypoxia, hypo- or hyperglycemia, drug or alcohol ingestion, or a primary CNS mass lesion, such as abscess or tumor. If the patient has focal signs on examination, such as a third-nerve palsy involving the pupil, immediate neuroimaging with a CT scan and neurologic critical care or neurosurgical consultation are indicated.

10. **What are the common causes of coma in a medical intensive care unit (ICU)?**
    Most cases of coma in a medical–surgical (nontrauma) ICU are toxic-metabolic and are often multifactorial. Once the effects of sedative and paralytic agents have been considered, sepsis, hypotension, hypoxia, hypothermia, acid–base disorders, glucose and electrolyte abnormalities,

and the adverse effects of medications are common causes. Hepatic and uremic failure often contribute to coma. Primary CNS infections such as meningitis or encephalitis are less common but need to be considered in the appropriate setting. If a severe coagulopathy is present, intracranial hemorrhage and subdural hematomas should be excluded. Focal signs on examination suggest a structural lesion such as a CNS infarction, tumor, or abscess and should be evaluated with a CT or MRI scan. If no obvious cause for coma is apparent, an EEG is indicated to exclude nonconvulsive status epilepticus.

Liao YJ, So YT: An approach to critically ill patients in coma. West J Med 176:184–187, 2002.

11. **What other conditions may mimic coma?**
- **"Locked-in" syndrome:** This syndrome is caused by extensive pontine damage. Patients are conscious but are quadriparetic and can move their eyes vertically and are thus incapable of any other movement or response.
- **Guillain-Barré syndrome:** An acute peripheral nerve disorder characterized by ascending weakness, this syndrome, when extensive, can cause a state of de-efferentation in which the patient is not in a coma but cannot move.
- **Botulism:** Botulism is an acute intoxication with the toxin of *Clostridium botulinum*, characterized by a descending pattern of weakness. Patients initially experience extraocular and pharyngeal muscle weakness (with diplopia, dysarthria, and dysphagia) that quickly progresses to diffuse weakness and respiratory failure.
- **Critical illness neuromyopathies and acute tetraplegic myopathy:** These entities are seen in the critical care setting. If extensive, they can induce profound weakness and numbness.
- **Catatonia:** A rare psychiatric manifestation of severe depression, catatonia is characterized by the finding of waxy flexibility on physical examination and no history of anatomic, toxic, or metabolic brain insult. The condition may improve with electroconvulsive therapy.
- **Psychogenic:** On rare occasions, a coma-like state can be part of a psychosomatic disorder. It can be diagnosed by careful history and physical examination, including oculocaloric testing.

KEY POINTS: COMA

1. Coma is a result of bihemispheric or brain stem dysfunction that causes the patient to be unarousable.

2. Coma resulting from brain stem dysfunction is usually associated with cranial nerve abnormalities.

3. Bilateral subdural hematomas, subarachnoid hemorrhage, and hydrocephalus are examples of lesions that may present as coma without any focal neurologic deficits on neurologic examination.

4. Coma resulting from metabolic derangements such as hypoglycemia or hyperglycemia may present with focal neurologic findings.

5. Several conditions such as "locked-in" syndrome, in which the patient is fully conscious but unable to interact with the environment, may mimic coma.

BIBLIOGRAPHY

1. Alguire PC: Rapid evaluation of comatose patients. Postgrad Med 87:223–228, 1990.
2. Casado J, Serrano A: Coma in Pediatrics: Diagnosis and Treatment. Madrid, Ediciones D'az de Santos SA, 1997.
3. Goetz CG, Pappert EJ: Textbook of Clinical Neurology. Philadelphia, W.B. Saunders, 1999.
4. Kelly BJ: Clinical assessment of the nervous system. In Tobin MJ (ed): Principles and Practice of Intensive Care Monitoring. New York, McGraw-Hill, 1998, pp 977–994.
5. Plum F, Posner J: The Diagnosis of Stupor and Coma, 3rd ed. Philadelphia, F.A. Davis, 1980.

CHAPTER 60

BRAIN DEATH

David C. Bonovich, MD

1. **What is brain death?**

   Brain death was first described by Mollaret and Goulon in 1959 as "coma dépassé."
   Technologic advancements in medicine have enabled physicians to keep the body functioning
   despite a nonfunctioning brain. The advent of successful organ transplantation in the early
   1960s and the necessity of donor organs resulted in the need to define brain death both
   medically and legally. This need led to the publication of the Harvard criteria in 1968.
   Subsequent modifications included more stringent guidelines for the determination of apnea,
   recognition of persistent spinal reflexes in brain death, and additional tests to confirm the
   absence of brain function. The President's Commission for the Study of Ethical Problems in
   Medicine, Biomedical, and Behavioral Research (1981) introduced the Uniform Determination of
   Death Act, which defines death as follows:

   1. The irreversible cessation of circulatory and respiratory functions, *or*
   2. The irreversible cessation of all functions of the entire brain, including the brain stem.

   Mallaret P, Goulon M: Coma dépassé. Rev Neurol 101:3–15, 1959.
   Report of the Medical Consultants on the Diagnosis of Death to the President's Commission for the
   Study of Ethical Problems in Medicine and Biomedical and Behavioral Research. Guidelines for the
   determination of death. JAMA 246:2184–2186, 1981.

2. **What are the current guidelines for the determination of brain death?**

   The diagnosis of brain death is clinical; it is based on certain prerequisites (establishing the
   cause and excluding reversible causes) and clinical signs. It requires the written documentation
   of two licensed physicians. The current concept of brain death is referred to as the *whole-brain
   formulation* of brain death.

   - **Cessation of cerebral function:** This diagnosis requires clinical evidence of a state of deep
     coma (Glasgow Coma Scale score of 3). The patient must be unreceptive and unresponsive to
     noxious stimuli. True decerebrate or decorticate posturing is not consistent with the
     diagnosis of brain death. In some circumstances it is preferable to perform one or more
     confirmatory tests.
   - **Cessation of brain stem function:** This diagnosis requires the lack of brain stem reflexes,
     including the absence of pupillary, corneal, jaw, gag, cough, swallowing, grimacing, and
     yawning reflexes and any kind of spontaneous or inducible extraocular movements
     combined with the persistence of apnea despite adequate stimulus to breathe ($PCO_2 > 60$).
     If brain stem reflexes cannot be clinically evaluated with certainty (as in severe facial trauma),
     confirmatory tests are recommended. In the absence of confirmatory tests, the patient should
     be observed continuously in an intensive care setting for 12 hours. If anoxic damage is
     suspected, observation for 24 hours is recommended. The absence of cerebral blood flow as
     confirmed by cerebral angiography is the only measure of cerebral function that does not
     require additional clinical observation and laboratory evaluation to confirm the diagnosis of
     brain death.

   Benzel EC, Gross CD, Hadden TA, et al: The apnea test for the determination of brain death. J Neurosurg
   71:191–194, 1989.

3. **When can a patient be declared brain dead?**
   Concise reviews by Pitts (1984) and Wijdicks (2001) and the Consensus Statement by the American Academy of Neurology (1995) summarized the current criteria for brain death as follows:
   - **The cause of brain injury must be known.** The cause of brain injury can be determined clinically through careful history and physical examination. Laboratory studies, such as blood counts, coagulation studies, electrolytes, blood gases, serum and urine toxicology, and cerebrospinal fluid analysis, help to establish the cause. In general, however, diagnostic imaging studies are used to produce convincing evidence of irreversible brain damage. CT, MRI, and, in some cases, cerebral angiography are performed to confirm the cause of brain injury.
   - **Metabolic and toxic central nervous system (CNS) depression must be excluded.** Reversible causes of apparent brain death must be ruled out and documented in the chart. These include pharmacologic agents such as barbiturates, benzodiazepines, and neuromuscular blockade; endogenous metabolic disorders, such as severe hepatic encephalopathy, hyperosmolar coma, hyponatremia, and uremia; severe systemic hypotension with a concomitant decrease in cerebral blood flow; and hypothermia. Loss of thermoregulation is often associated with brain death. Normothermia ($>32°C$) must be restored before the determination of brain death.
   - **There must be no demonstrable brain function.** The diagnosis of brain death requires that there be no evidence of brain function. The patient must be unresponsive without spontaneous movement, response to pain, or brain stem function. The possibility of neuromuscular blockade by pharmacologic agents must be ruled out by history and/or the application of a peripheral nerve stimulator. The possibility of the locked-in state should be ruled out by instructing the patient, while the eyelids are open, to move the eyes up, down, and to the sides.

   Pitts LH: Determination of brain death. West J Med 140:628–631, 1984.
   Quality Standards Subcommittee of the American Academy of Neurology: Practice parameters for determining brain death in adults (summary statement). Neurology 45:1012–1014, 1995.
   Wijdicks EF: The diagnosis of brain death. N Engl J Med 344:1215–1221, 2001.

4. **How is the cessation of brain stem function demonstrated?**
   The absence of brain stem function is demonstrated by the absence of brain stem reflexes and the presence of apnea. Tests for brain stem function include the following:
   1. **Pupillary response to light:** The pupils in brain death are fixed and midposition to dilated (5–8 mm in size), without response to light. Pupillary findings in critically ill or comatose patients include the following:
      - **Small, reactive:** Metabolic or sedative drugs (e.g., atropinic agents, adrenergic agents)
      - **Unilateral fixed, dilated:** Cranial nerve III palsy (transtentorial herniation)
   2. **Doll's eyes, or oculocephalic reflex:** Checking this reflex tests midbrain, pontine, and medullary function. In a comatose patient with an intact brain stem, the eyes lag behind when the head is turned suddenly to one side. This lag in eye movement is not present in brain stem injury. The reflex is not present in conscious patients. This maneuver is to be done only when stability of the cervical spine is ensured.
   3. **Cold calorics, or the oculovestibular reflex:** Checking this reflex tests midbrain, pontine, and medullary function. This reflex persists even after the oculocephalic reflex has disappeared; thus, it is important in patients who lack an oculocephalic response. The test is performed by irrigating intact and unobstructed external ear canals (one at a time, 5 minutes between each side) with 50 mL of iced water while both eyes are held open. The normal reflex results in nystagmus, with the fast component away from the side of stimulation. If the communication of the intact brain stem with the telencephalon has been lost, the eyes will deviate tonically toward the irrigated side, without the production

of nystagmus. Extensive brain stem injury, or brain death, results in the absence of all eye movements.

4. **Medullary function:** Lack of medullary function is demonstrated by the absence of the cough and gag reflexes, but the most reliable marker of medullary death is the cessation of spontaneous respirations as demonstrated by the performance of an apnea test.

Pallis C: ABC of brain stem death. From brain death to brainstem death. Br Med J (Clin Res Ed) 285:1487–1490, 1982.
Pallis C: ABC of brain stem death. Part II. Br Med J (Clin Res Ed) 285:1641–1644, 1982.

5. **How is an apnea test performed?**
To demonstrate apnea, one must provide the injured brain stem with an adequate stimulus to breathe. In the apnea test, the arterial tension of carbon dioxide provides the stimulus. The minimum level of PCO_2 required to demonstrate apnea in the severely injured or "dead" brain is a matter of debate in the literature, but minimal levels of 44–60 mmHg have been recommended. Guidelines for apnea testing are outlined in Box 60-1.

Belsh JM, Blatt R, Schiffman PL: Apnea testing in brain death. Arch Intern Med 146:2385–2388, 1986.

6. **Do movements of the limbs in patients who have met all brain death criteria rule out the diagnosis of brain death?**
No. Two types of movements have been described in brain-dead patients:

- **Brain death–associated reflexes:** These have been found in approximately 75% of brain-dead patients, and current guidelines recognize the persistence of these reflexes. They include muscle stretch reflexes, plantar flexor and withdrawal responses, and abdominal reflexes.

- **Brain death–associated automatisms:** These movements include undulating toe flexion movements, eyelid opening, respiratory-like movements, head turning, eyelid and tongue myoclonus movements of the upper and lower face, and the "Lazarus sign." The Lazarus sign refers to complex movements of the upper extremities and may include extension and pronation of the arms, a drawing up of the arms toward the chest in a "praying" posture, or other complex movements. It is thought to be localized to the cervical spinal cord and represents hypoxia to neurons in these areas that have been functionally isolated from the brain.

Jain S, DeGeorgia M: Brain-death associated reflexes and automatisms. Neurocrit Care 3:122–126, 2005.

BOX 60-1.   GUIDELINES FOR APNEA TESTING

1. Ventilate for at least 20 minutes to produce a normal PCO_2 (37–40 mmHg) and hyperoxia with an FIO_2 of 1.00 before disconnection from the ventilator.

2. After disconnection from mechanical evaluation, maintain 100% O_2 flow to endotracheal tube by T-piece. The American Academy of Neurology also suggests using a cannual through the endotracheal tube at the level of the carina with 10 L/min of oxygen for the duration of the test.

3. Continue apnea for 5–10 minutes or until hypoxia, hypotension, or ventricular arrhythmias results. The carbon dioxide level in the blood will rise at a rate of 2–4 mmHg/min.

4. Monitor PCO_2 by arterial blood gas measurements to document a final PCO_2 >60 mmHg, an increase in PCO_2 >20 mmHg, or a pH <7.24.

7. **What are the indications for the use of confirmatory tests in brain death?**
Confirmatory tests are not required in brain death and do not supersede clinical criteria. They can be considered in patients with an indeterminate apnea test results, hypercapnia, severe obesity (which makes detection of respiratory movement difficult), severe congestive heart failure and/or hemodynamic instability, and severe facial trauma (which makes examination of the face and eyes difficult or impossible), or in cases where long-acting barbiturates have been used in medical management. Confirmatory test results may also aid in the transplantation of organs.

8. **What are the accepted confirmatory tests for brain death?**
There are two types of confirmatory tests: those that document loss of bioelectrical activity (e.g., electroencephalogram [EEG], sensory-evoked potential, brain stem auditory-evoked response [BAER]) and those that document loss of blood flow (e.g., pancerebral angiography, scintigraphy, transcranial Doppler).

- **Contrast angiography:** This invasive technique requires catheterization via the femoral or axillary arteries. A definitive test result requires visualization of both extracranial carotid and vertebrobasilar systems. A positive test result is one in which "no flow" is identified within the cranial vault. Typically, the dye column tapers symmetrically with nonfilling of the cervical carotids (pseudo-occlusion) or an abrupt block at the cranial base. This is in marked contrast to the bilateral filling of the external carotid system. The vertebral vessels disappear at the atlanto-occipital junction. Occasionally, the basilar can be seen against the clivus. There is no visualization of the venous phase. This test requires transport to the angiography suite and administration of contrast.
- **Radionucleotide cerebral imaging:** This is a noninvasive, simple, and safe method of measuring cerebral blood flow. Portable gamma cameras allow bedside examinations to be completed in 15 minutes. The test requires an IV bolus of sodium pertechnetate technetium-99m (15–21 mCi/adult) or technetium-99m–labeled hexamethyl propylene amine oxime, followed by anterior images recorded every 3 seconds for a total of 60 seconds. Counts attributable to the external carotid system are eliminated by subtraction techniques or a tourniquet placed around the forehead to eliminate scalp flow. With normal cerebral blood flow, sequential images show activity over the common carotid arteries, anterior and middle cerebral arteries, capillaries, sagittal sinus vein, and internal jugular bilaterally. Occasionally, the scalp veins drain into the sagittal sinus, resulting in minimal late sagittal sinus activity in the absence of identifiable arterial activity.
- **Transcranial Doppler:** This emerging technology is the easiest and fastest test to perform and does not require transport of the patient from the intensive care unit. Documentation of oscillating flow or systolic spikes is typical of brain death. These findings need to be demonstrated on two different occasions 30 minutes apart. There are no reports of clinically brain-dead children or adults who "survive" after demonstration of such transcranial patterns. The examination includes bilateral extracranial vessels (common carotid arteries, internal carotid arteries, and vertebral arteries) and any bilateral intracranial arteries and is repeated in 30 minutes. In approximately 15% of patients this test cannot be done, particularly in older patients. Ventricular drains or skull defects (e.g., craniectomies, neonatal status) that preclude an increase in intracranial pressure interfere with the reliability of the test.

9. **What is the role of EEG in the diagnosis of brain death?**
The EEG is an accepted confirmatory test for brain death. Published guidelines include such factors as electrode positions, time of recording, and impedance settings. Factors that may result in an isoelectric EEG that is indistinguishable from brain death include hypothermia that produces a transient, reversible electroencephalographic silence (ECS). Therefore, a central temperature of at least 32°C (90°F) is required before determination of brain death by EEG. Cardiovascular shock may result in reversible ECS. In this case, loss of electrical activity

results from decreased cerebral perfusion resulting from systemic hypotension. Electrical activity may be restored by increasing systemic blood pressure. Therefore, a systemic blood pressure of at least 80 mmHg is prerequisite to the diagnosis of brain death by EEG. Barbiturate coma or toxic levels of other CNS depressant drugs (e.g., benzodiazepines, trichloroethylene) may also result in ECS; therefore, the possibility of drug overdose must be ruled out by careful history and/or appropriate toxicology screen if the EEG is to reliably diagnose brain death. Most CNS depressant drugs do not produce the clinical criteria necessary for the diagnosis of brain death because of their effect on pupil size (most produce small pupils). Exceptions include scopolamine and glutethimide, which produce large pupils.

American Encephalography Society: Guideline three: Minimum technical standards for EEG recording in suspected cerebral death. J Clin Neurophysiol 11:10–13, 1994.

10. **Discuss the role of BAER in the diagnosis of brain death.**
In brain death, the brain stem and auditory short-latency responses are absent. The observation that all BAER components after wave I or II are absent in brain death but preserved in toxic and metabolic disorders suggests that BAER may be useful in evaluating patients in whom coma of toxic etiology is suspected (in particular, barbiturate coma is known to produce an isoelectric EEG).

KEY POINTS: BRAIN DEATH

1. Brain death is the irreversible cessation of all brain function, including that of the brain stem.

2. Loss of all brain stem reflexes including respiration on two separate examinations >24 hours apart and after ruling out toxic and metabolic causes of coma may be considered clinical evidence of brain death.

3. A patient may be considered to have passed the apnea test if there are no respiratory efforts despite a $PCO_2 > 60$ mmHg and/or a PCO_2 rise > 20 mmHg in the setting of relative hemodynamic stability.

4. Spinal reflexes and automatisms may be present after brain death.

5. Cardiac and baroceptor responses are often lost in the hours and days after brain death.

11. **What are the cardiac manifestations of brain death?**
Despite aggressive cardiovascular support, patients determined to be brain dead progress to cardiovascular collapse within 1 week. In fact, most die within 2 days after the diagnosis of brain death. Heart rate variability is lost (loss of vagal function) as well as heart rate response to atropine-like drugs. The electrocardiographic changes associated with the initial stage of brain death include widening of the QRS complex (i.e., Osborn waves), prolongation of the QT segment, and nonspecific ST-segment changes.
More advanced stages of brain death are marked by bradycardia, followed by conduction abnormalities, including atrioventricular block and interventricular conduction delays. Atrial fibrillation is relatively common in the terminal stages of brain death, with atrial activity often continuing after the cessation of ventricular complexes.

12. **Is it possible to predict which comatose patients will progress to brain death?**
It is not possible to determine with confidence which comatose patients will progress to brain death, even though several studies have identified clinical parameters associated with poor

neurologic outcome. The best predictors of neurologic outcome are the Glasgow Coma Scale score at presentation and the level of brain stem function observed within the first 24 hours after presentation. The lack of pupillary response to light or corneal reflexes on initial examination is a very poor prognostic sign. By 72 hours after cerebral insult, the motor response to pain increases in predictive value; absent or posturing response to pain is associated with poor neurologic recovery.

Conci F, DiRienzo M, Castiglioni P: Blood pressure and heart rate variability and baroreflex sensitivity before and after brain death. Neurol Neurosurg Psychiatry 71:621–631, 2001.

CHAPTER 61

STATUS EPILEPTICUS

David C. Bonovich, MD

1. **Define *status epilepticus* (SE).**

   The World Health Organization defines SE as "a condition characterized by an epileptic seizure that is sufficiently prolonged or repeated at sufficiently brief intervals so as to produce an unvarying and enduring epileptic condition." In the clinical setting, SE may be defined as seizure activity lasting 30 minutes or intermittent seizure activity for 30 minutes or more during which consciousness is not regained. More recently, Chen and Westerlain have advocated defining SE as seizures lasting for more than 5 minutes.

   Chen JW, Westerlain CG: Status epilepticus: Pathophysiology and management in adults. Lancet Neurol 246–256, 2006.

2. **What are the different types of SE? How do they present?**

   SE is best divided into three categories:
   - Convulsive status epilepticus (CSE)
   - Nonconvulsive status epilepticus (NCSE)
   - Partial status epilepticus (PSE)

   Although CSE is the most common form and is life threatening, NCSE may account for up to one-fourth of all cases. All forms of SE may result in serious disability. SE also can be divided into seizures that involve the whole brain (CSE and NCSE) and seizures that involve only part of the brain (PSE). Seizures involving the whole brain can be subdivided into those associated with obvious motor movement (CSE) and those not associated with obvious motor involvement (NCSE).

   CSE is the most serious type of SE. It is characterized by rhythmic shaking of the limbs and body, tongue biting, and loss of consciousness. As the duration of the seizures increases, the movements may become reduced, sometimes to eye fluttering, although generalized electrical activity continues in the brain. Although the diagnosis of CSE is obvious in most cases, the differential diagnosis includes rigors associated with fever and sepsis, myoclonic jerks, and pseudo-SE (i.e., seizures of psychogenic origin not associated with electrical discharges from the brain).

   NCSE may be more difficult to diagnose and may be more common in the elderly population. Although there is no generally accepted classification of NCSE, two major types are recognized: partial complex—which can be then subdivided based on whether the patient has underlying epilepsy or illness or is in a coma—and petit mal. In partial complex SE, alteration of consciousness lasts more than 30 minutes because of abnormal cortical electrical activity. Generalized tonic-clonic motor activity is absent, but stereotypical movements such as lip smacking, chewing, or picking at one's clothes may occur. The patient may be misdiagnosed as intoxicated or as having a psychiatric disorder. Petit mal SE is often difficult to distinguish from partial complex SE, except with electroencephalographic (EEG) recordings. Patients appear lethargic but may be able to answer simple questions slowly. Eye blinking may be present, but automatisms are less common than in partial complex SE.

   Continuous PSE consists merely of persistent focal motor seizures that last longer than 30 minutes and do not impair consciousness.

   Treiman DM, Walker MC: Treatment of seizure emergencies: Convulsive and non-convulsive status epilepticus. Epilepsy Res 68(Suppl 1):S77–S82, 2006.

3. **What are the most common causes of CSE?**
Like other types of seizures, CSE can be divided into symptomatic, idiopathic, and cryptogenic types. Cessation of antiepileptic drugs, withdrawal from alcohol, drug overdose, and cerebrovascular disease are the most common causes of CSE. In the adult population, stroke may account for as much as 50% of SE and is probably the most common cause of CSE in the elderly population. Approximately 50% of adults with CSE have no previous history of epilepsy. Many of these presentations occur in the setting of acute neurologic illnesses such as stroke. Other causes include electrolyte imbalances, head injury, toxic effects of drugs, hypoxic-ischemic insults, brain tumors, central nervous system (CNS) infection, and renal failure. In about 15% of patients, no cause can be found.

Gaitanis JN, Drislane FW: Status epilepticus: A review of different syndromes, their current evaluation, and treatment. Neurologist 9:61–76, 2003.

4. **Why is urgent treatment of CSE a medical necessity?**
Early in the course of CSE, increased metabolic demand is met with increased cerebral blood flow as a result of autoregulation. However, when seizures last longer than 30 minutes, autoregulation becomes impaired and blood flow is unable to keep up with metabolic demand. As a result, lactic acid starts to accumulate in the brain systemically, and glucose and bicarbonate levels fall.

Sound experimental data suggest that permanent cell damage occurs in several cortical and subcortical locations after 60 minutes of convulsive status. In addition, clinical studies have shown that the longer CSE continues, the more difficult it is to control and the greater the incidence of neurologic sequelae. Thus, it is important to recognize and treat CSE early and aggressively before such complications develop.

Prolonged CSE is also associated with other systemic disturbances. An initial increase in minute ventilation gives way to hypoventilation and apnea. Pulmonary vascular resistance may become elevated, and in some cases pulmonary edema may develop. Aspiration is common. Arrhythmias may be seen in up to 60% of patients with prolonged SE. Hyperthermia may result from catecholamine release and prolonged vigorous muscle activity. In addition, lactic acidosis and other metabolic disturbances may develop.

Gaitanis JN, Drislane FW: Status epilepticus: A review of different syndromes, their current evaluation, and treatment. Neurologist 9:61–76, 2003.

5. **What are the most important initial steps when faced with a patient with CSE?**
As always, the ABCs (i.e., airways, breathing, and circulation) must be addressed immediately. Supplemental oxygen should be applied, and a secure IV line should be started. If an adequate airway and ventilation are not present, an endotracheal tube should be inserted, and ventilation should be assisted. If neuromuscular blockade is to be used for intubation, a short-acting agent is recommended to avoid obscuring clinical seizure activity. A 0.9% sodium chloride solution should be the initial IV fluid infused because it can be used to treat hypotension if it occurs and is compatible with IV phenytoin or fosphenytoin. Liberal hydration with normal saline (200 mL/h) should be started to minimize the risk of renal failure from rhabdomyolysis and to prevent dehydration. The following tests should be ordered immediately: complete blood count, drug screen, arterial blood gas analysis, and measurement of glucose concentration, serum osmolarity, and levels of anticonvulsants, serum electrolytes, blood urea nitrogen, creatinine, calcium, magnesium, phosphate, and blood alcohol.

Chen JW, Wasterlain CG: Status epilepticus: Pathophysiology and management in adults. Lancet Neurol 5:246–256, 2006.

6. **Once the ABCs have been addressed, what are the next steps in managing the care of a patient with CSE?**
The following approach is intended only as a guideline. Individual circumstances may dictate different therapies. Although seizures must persist for 30 minutes to be classified as

SE, one should not wait until 30 minutes have passed before initiating therapy. Once IV access has been secured, thiamine (100 mg IV) should be administered, followed by 50 mL of 50% dextrose solution if bedside glucose testing revealed hypoglycemia. Lorazepam, 0.10 mg/kg, should be given at a rate no faster than 2 mg/min and in 4-mg doses to a maximum adult dose of 10 mg. Simultaneously, a loading dose of fosphenytoin should be administered at a rate of 100 mg/min. Fosphenytoin is a water-soluble form of phenytoin and lacks the propylene glycol vehicle that has been implicated in the hypotension and cardiac arrhythmias sometimes seen during traditional IV phenytoin loading. Fosphenytoin is expressed as phenytoin equivalents; thus, the loading dose is the same as for phenytoin (18 mg/kg). If fosphenytoin is unavailable, phenytoin (18–20 mg/kg) given at a rate no faster than 50 mg/min or 25 mg/min in the elderly) should be infused. More than 80% of cases of CSE are controlled by the combination of lorazepam and a phenytoin preparation.

If seizures persist after initial fosphenytoin loading, an additional 5 mg/kg of fosphenytoin (or phenytoin, if it is the only form available) should be given. If this dose is ineffective, tracheal intubation is indicated, if not already secured, because the cardiorespiratory depressant effects of barbiturates (the next drug to be added) and benzodiazepines are additive. In addition, many of patients experience hypotension because barbiturates or further benzodiazepines are administered and require IV hydration and blood pressure support with inotropes such as dopamine.

The optimal treatment of refractory cases of CSE not responsive to phenytoin and lorazepam is an area of ongoing debate. If not already involved, a neurologist who is an expert in SE should be consulted.

Traditionally, phenobarbital (15- to 20-mg/kg loading dose) has been recommended as the next medication, given at a rate no faster than 50–100 mg/min until the full dose was given or the seizures stopped. Phenobarbital loading is followed by a maintenance dose of 1–4 mg/kg/day. If phenobarbital load fails to stop the seizures, many physicians now recommend pentobarbital or midazolam. Pentobarbital is administered as a loading dose of 2–8 mg/kg over 2 minutes, followed by a maintenance dose of 0.5–5 mg/kg/h until the seizures stop clinically or burst suppression is reached on the EEG.

Alternatively, a loading dose of midazolam (10 mg over 3–5 minutes), followed by a maintenance dose of 0.05–0.4 mg/kg/h, can be used until the EEG is free of seizures.

If these steps are unsuccessful, lidocaine, 2 mg/kg over 5 minutes followed by a drip of 3 mg/kg/h for no more than 12 hours, can be used. Lidocaine should not be used in patients with heart or liver failure or patients with cardiac arrhythmias or bundle-branch blocks. General anesthesia with an inhalational agent such as isoflurane can also be considered if the previously mentioned measures are unsuccessful. Propofol recently has been used in the treatment of refractory CSE. Its mechanism of action is still unclear. The loading dose of 1 mg/kg is repeated every 5 minutes until seizure activity is suppressed. A maintenance dose of 2–10 mg/kg/h is then used. An IV preparation of valproic acid has been developed, and animal data suggest that it may be effective in CSE, although this has not been approved by the U.S. Food and Drug Administration.

7. **Are there other agents that can be used in the initial treatment of SE besides fosphenytoin and phenytoin?**
Phenobarbital can be used as a first-line treatment after lorazepam; however, due to its sedating effects and its potential respiratory effects, it is not generally used. An injectable, IV form of valproic acid has been developed and has shown efficacy in the treatment of SE. The usual dose is 20–40 mg/kg as a loading dose.

Peters CN, Pohlmann-Eden B: Intravenous valproate as an innovative therapy in seizure emergency situations including status epilepticus: Experience in 102 adult patients. Seizure 14:164–169, 2005.

8. **What factors should be taken into account in determining which neuromuscular blockers (NMBs) should be administered to a patient with CSE if these agents are necessary?**
   NMBs at times may be desirable to help reduce the metabolic derangements and hyperthermia resulting from prolonged vigorous muscle contraction. All NMBs cause profound muscle weakness, but agents vary greatly in duration of action. If neuromuscular blockade is necessary and continuous EEG recording is *not* being performed, a single dose of a short-acting, nondepolarizing agent should be administered; it is impossible to ascertain clinically whether seizure activity is continuing in the presence of neuromuscular blockade. Anticonvulsant treatment should continue as outlined earlier, and EEG monitoring should be strongly considered. If a long-acting agent is used or if multiple doses of a short-acting agent are given, continuous EEG monitoring is mandatory to prevent unrecognized SE. All patients receiving NMBs should be intubated.

9. **What steps are appropriate after the seizures are controlled?**
   Once the seizures are controlled, it is important to establish the cause of the SE. Appropriate blood work and cultures should be ordered. Imaging with computed tomography or magnetic resonance should be done as soon as possible to rule out structural CNS causes. Lumbar puncture may help to rule out CNS infections and subarachnoid hemorrhage. The administration of empiric antibiotics should be started if an infectious etiology is suspected, and maintenance doses of anticonvulsants should be administered and adjusted based on serum levels.

KEY POINTS: STATUS EPILEPTICUS

1. Status epilepticus is a life-threatening condition that needs to be treated aggressively.

2. Nonconvulsive status is often an underdiagnosed cause of altered mental status in the intensive care setting.

3. In addition to fosphenytoin and phenytoin, valproic acid can be used after benzodiazepines for the prevention of further seizures.

4. Searching for the underlying cause of the seizures is important and involves ruling out metabolic and structural causes.

5. Neuromuscular blockade should only be used under special circumstances and only in the setting of continual EEG monitoring.

10. **Does fever or cerebrospinal fluid (CSF) pleocytosis always indicate an infectious etiology of CSE?**
    Most patients with CSE exhibit an increase in body temperature, which in rare cases may progress to extremes (up to 107°F) even in the absence of an infectious etiology. In addition, mild pleocytosis of peripheral blood and CSF may occur in such patients. Although fever and pleocytosis of the blood and CSF may be the result of CSE, it is imperative not to attribute these findings to the effect of repeated seizures until all other possibilities have been excluded. In general, empiric coverage for infectious etiologies (until all cultures have negative results) is preferable to undertreatment of a serious infection.

11. **What is the significance of postanoxic myoclonus and SE?**
    Stimulus-induced myoclonic status is a poor prognostic indicator after cardiopulmonary resuscitation, suggesting severe neocortical damage. Generalized myoclonic jerks associated

with anoxic coma are stimulus sensitive (i.e., brought on by touch or sound) and associated with burst-suppression on EEG. Myoclonic activity usually lasts 1 or 2 days and can be quite disconcerting to families and medical personnel. Myoclonic status is difficult to treat and is resistant to drugs such as phenobarbital, phenytoin, and benzodiazepines. Some anecdotal data suggest that valproate may be effective in treating this syndrome. However, it must be kept in mind that treatment of myoclonic status does not affect outcome, although it may ease the distress of family and medical staff.

Fahn S: Post-anoxic myoclonus: Improvement with valproic acid. N Engl J Med 299:313–314, 1978.

BIBLIOGRAPHY

1. Aminoff MJ, Simon RP: Status epilepticus: Causes, clinical features and consequences in 98 patients. Am J Med 69:657–666, 1980.
2. Chapman MG, Smith M, Hirsch NP: Status epilepticus. Anaesthesia 56:648–659, 2001.
3. Crawford TO, Mitchell WG, Snodgrass SR: Lorazepam in childhood status epilepticus and serial seizures: Effectiveness and tachyphylaxis. Neurology 37:190–195, 1987.
4. Leppik IE: Status epilepticus. Neurol Clin 4:633–643, 1986.
5. Provencio JJ, Bleck TP, Conners AF: Critical care neurology. Am J Respir Crit Care Med 164:341–345, 2001.
6. Uthman BM, Wilder BJ: Emergency management of seizures: An overview. Epilepsia 30(Suppl 2):S33–S37, 1989.
7. Wijdicks EFM: The Clinical Practice of Critical Care Neurology. Philadelphia, Lippincott-Raven, 1997.
8. Wilder BJ: The use of parenteral antiepileptic drugs and the role of fosphenytoin. Neurology 46(Suppl 1):S1–S28, 1996.

CHAPTER 62

STROKE AND CEREBRAL ANEURYSMS

David C. Bonovich, MD

STROKE

1. **Define *ischemic stroke*.**

   A stroke results from a disruption in blood flow to the brain. *Ischemia* is defined as hypoxemia, a decrease in the delivery of oxygen and glucose to a target organ—in this case, the brain. In the brain, ischemia may be characterized as global (as in cardiac arrest) or focal (involving a specific vessel or a specific group of vessels in the brain); embolic or thrombotic; and large-vessel (involving one of the major blood vessels of the brain) or small-vessel (involving one of the small penetrating vessels of the brain).

2. **Define *intraparenchymal hemorrhage* (ICH).**

   ICH occurs as a result of the rupture of a blood vessel in the brain; usually small penetrating blood vessels. The clinical expression and prognosis of ICH relates to the location of the ruptured blood vessel and the injury to the brain as a result of the rupture. ICH represents 10–15% of all strokes. In the Asian population, ICH appears to represent a higher percentage.

   Jiang B, Wang WZ, Chen H, et al: Incidence and trends of stroke and its subtypes in China: Results from 3 large cities. Stroke 37:63–68, 2006.

   Klatsky AL, Friedman GD, Sidney S, et al: Risk of hemorrhagic stroke in Asian American ethnic groups. Neuroepidemiology 25:26–31, 2005.

   Nguyen-Huynh MN, Johnston SC: Regional variation in hospitalization for stroke among Asians/Pacific islanders in the United States. BMC Neurology 5:21–28, 2005.

3. **What are the major risk factors for thrombotic cerebral infarction?**

   Hypertension is by far the most significant factor. The increased risk is proportional to the degree of hypertension. Age is also a risk factor; the incidence of cerebral infarction increases with age and is 1.3 times higher in men than in women. Other risk factors include diabetes, coronary artery disease, congestive heart failure, atrial fibrillation, and left ventricular hypertrophy. Obesity, hypercholesterolemia, and hyperlipidemia are risk factors in as much as they are risk factors for atherosclerotic disease.

   Mas JL: Atherothrombosis: Management of patients at risk. Int J Clin Pract 59:407–414, 2005.

4. **What are the major risk factors for embolic cerebral infarction?**

   Embolic cerebral events are usually of cardiac origin. Major risk factors include ischemic heart disease with mural thrombus; cardiac arrhythmia, especially atrial fibrillation; prosthetic cardiac valves; rheumatic heart disease; structural valvular abnormalities, such as mitral stenosis; and bacterial endocarditis. Atrial fibrillation alone, without evidence of rheumatic heart disease, increases the risk of stroke by approximately fivefold. Elderly patients incur the greatest risk from atrial fibrillation, as the proportion of strokes due to this arrhythmia increases with age. Atheroscloroses of the aortic arch, carotid arteries, and vertebral arteries are also risk factors.

5. **What are the major risk factors for ICH?**

   Chronic hypertension accounts for about 70% of all ICH. The typical locations for ICH related to hypertension are the basal ganglia, thalamus, pons, and cerebellum. Cerebral amyloid angiopathy results from deposition of amyloid in the media and intima of small to medium-sized blood vessels resulting in lobar hemorrhages. Cerebral amyloid angiopathy is typically seen in the older population. Underlying vascular malformations are also associated with ICH. Other factors to be considered would be acquired or congenital coagulopathies and bleeding into brain tumors.

6. **Does drug abuse predispose patients to stroke?**
   Drug abuse has emerged as a significant risk factor leading to stroke in young patients. Sympathomimetic drugs such as cocaine and amphetamines, in particular, have been associated more frequently with ICH but also with ischemic stroke. Several studies have shown drug abuse to be a commonly identified risk factor among stroke patients under the age of 35 years.

   Riggs JE, Gutman L: Crack cocaine use and stroke in young patients. Neurology 49:1473–1474, 1997.
   Sloan MA, Kittner SJ, Freeser BR, et al: Illicit drug-associated ischemic stroke in the Baltimore-Washington young stroke study. Neurology 50:1688–1693, 1998.

7. **What is the normal value for cerebral blood flow?**
   In normal adults, cerebral blood flow is approximately 55 mL/100 gm of brain tissue per minute, or 15% of normal cardiac output. When blood flow decreases to <20 mL/100 mg/min, evoked potentials are lost and the electroencephalogram becomes isoelectric. When blood flow decreases to <15 mL/100 mg/min and is not quickly restored, irreversible brain injury occurs. In the brain, autoregulation occurs (i.e., over a wide range of blood pressure, cerebral blood flow remains the same). In patients with chronic hypertension, it is possible for the autoregulation curve to shift to the right so that autoregulation occurs over higher pressure ranges than in those without hypertension.

8. **Describe the blood supply to the brain.**
   Four arteries carry blood to the brain. They are the two internal carotid arteries anteriorly and the two vertebral arteries posteriorly. The internal carotid arteries arise from the common carotid arteries. The left common carotid artery is a branch of the left subclavian artery; the right carotid artery arises from the right brachiocephalic trunk. Each common carotid artery bifurcates at the angle of the jaw into external and internal branches. The internal carotid arteries supply the optic nerves, the retina, and the majority of the cerebral hemispheres (the frontal, parietal, and anterior temporal lobes). Branches of the carotid artery include the following:
   - Ophthalmic artery
   - Posterior communicating artery
   - Anterior choroidal artery
   - Anterior cerebral artery
   - Middle cerebral artery

   The posterior circulation is fed by two vertebral arteries. The right and left vertebral arteries arise from the subclavian arteries bilaterally and enter the posterior fossa through the foramen magnum. They give rise to the posterior inferior cerebellar artery and the anterior and posterior spinal arteries before merging to form the basilar artery at the level of the pontomedullary junction. The vertebrobasilar system supplies the cervical cord, brain stem, medial and posterior temporal lobes, and occipital lobes.

   The posterior cerebral artery supplies the occipital lobes. In a majority of patients (70%), this artery originates from the bifurcation of the basilar artery. In 95% of the cases, one or both posterior cerebral arteries arise from the basilar artery, whereas in the remaining 5% the posterior cerebral arteries arise from the internal carotid artery bilaterally. Major branches of the basilar artery include the following:
   - Labyrinthine artery to the middle ear
   - Superior cerebellar artery
   - Posterior cerebral artery
   - Anterior inferior cerebellar artery

9. **Describe the circle of Willis.**
The vertebrobasilar system is joined to the carotid system by an anastomotic ring.
The anterior and posterior communicating arteries link the anterior/posterior and the left/right
hemispheric circulations. Four arteries comprise the circle: posterior communicating artery,
posterior cerebral artery bilaterally, anterior communicating artery, and anterior cerebral
artery bilaterally.

10. **Describe the clinical presentation of a large vascular ischemic stroke.**
The neurologic presentation of a patient experiencing an ischemic cerebral event depends on
the location and size of the infarct. Carotid artery infarction generally results in unilateral
symptoms; vertebrobasilar system infarction may result in bilateral symptoms.
- **Carotid artery occlusion:** This event results in contralateral hemiparesis, hemihypesthesia,
homonymous hemianopia, agnosia, and, if the dominant hemisphere is affected,
global aphasia. Some patients (15%) exhibit ipsilateral Horner's syndrome. Often, the
size of the infarct results in marked cerebral edema, and the patient may become obtunded
or may lapse into a coma. Most carotid occlusions are thrombotic. Transient ischemic
episodes precede major carotid artery occlusions approximately 50% of the time. Some
patients with complete carotid occlusion may have few, if any, neurologic deficits because
collateral blood flow via the circle of Willis may allow sufficient blood flow to prevent
ischemia.
- **Middle cerebral artery ischemia:** This may result in a clinical picture similar to that of carotid
artery occlusion. In acute carotid stenosis (e.g., an atherosclerotic blood vessel that
progresses to complete closure) and carotid artery dissection, emboli may travel to the
middle cerebral artery, leading to ischemia in the middle cerebral artery territory. Such
ischemia typically results in motor dysfunction that affects the face and upper extremity
but spares the leg. Branch occlusions result in fewer deficits. Speech and language function
may be affected because the middle cerebral artery supplies the speech and language
centers of the brain (in the left hemisphere in the vast majority of people).
- **Anterior cerebral artery ischemia:** Much less common in occurrence, anterior cerebral
artery ischemia results in contralateral motor dysfunction that affects the leg more than the
arm and face.
- **Basilar artery occlusion:** Basilar artery occlusion results in bilateral cranial nerve palsies
and quadriparesis. If the infarction includes the reticular activating system in the brain
stem, the patient presents in a coma. It is possible, however, for the high midbrain level
reticular activating system to be spared while motor pathways are affected. This
complete loss of motor function in an awake patient is commonly referred to as
locked-in syndrome. Other symptoms of ischemia to the basilar artery include vertigo,
ataxia, and diplopia.
- **Unilateral vertebral artery occlusion:** This event may result in ischemia of the lateral
medulla (if the posterior inferior cerebellar artery is involved). Ischemia of the spinothalamic
tracts results in ipsilateral ataxia, facial hypesthesia, and contralateral loss of pain and
temperature below the face. Loss of function of the ninth and tenth cranial nerves results
in dysphagia and hoarseness. Horner's syndrome may also occur ipsilateral to the lesion.
This syndrome is commonly referred to as the *lateral medullary syndrome* or *Wallenberg's
syndrome.*

11. **What is a lacunar infarct?**
Lacuna is Latin for a small pit or hollow cavity. Cerebral lacunes are multiple small infarcts
resulting from occlusion of the small penetrating branches (50–150 μm in diameter) of the
major cerebral vessel. The infarcted brain tissue softens and decays, leaving small cavities
(1–3 mm in diameter) that are evident at autopsy. Lacunes produce a variety of sensory and
motor symptoms, depending on their location. Multiple lacunes may result in loss of intellectual

capacity with impairment of recent memory. In some cases, severe dementia may result. There are four classic lunar syndromes:

- **Pure motor hemiparesis:** Weakness that equally affects the face, arm, and leg on one side of the body, with preservation of sensory, intellectual, and speech function
- **Pure hemisensory loss:** Loss of sensation on one side of the body, with preservation of motor, intellectual, and speech function
- **Dysarthria–clumsy hand syndrome:** Weakness predominantly of the hand and dysarthric (slurred) speech
- **Ataxia-hemiparesis:** Ataxia and weakness involving the face, arm, and leg on one side of the body, with a superimposed ataxia; coordination difficulties in excess of what would be expected in pure motor hemiparesis

12. **What is a watershed or border-zone infarct?**
A watershed or border-zone infarct is an area of focal cerebral ischemia resulting from decreased perfusion pressure. Watershed infarcts typically occur bilaterally in boundary zones between major vascular beds such as the middle cerebral artery and the posterior cerebral artery. Bilateral watershed infarcts usually are due to systemic hypotension. Unilateral border-zone infarcts may be associated with ipsilateral large vessel stenosis.

13. **What is an arterial dissection? How does it manifest neurologically?**
An arterial dissection occurs when blood extends into the wall of an artery. When the artery is one that feeds the brain, the manifestation is related to the vascular territory involved and can be the result of embolism from the area of the dissection distally, complete occlusion of the dissected blood vessel with or without embolism, or subarachnoid hemorrhage (SAH). SAH is more common when blood vessels dissect intracranially, whereas in dissection of the neck arteries, embolism or ischemia resulting from complete vessel occlusion is more common.

Both aspirin and heparin are recommended for medical management. Most practitioners prefer heparin, but there are no clear standard of care guidelines regarding its use. More recently, endovascular approaches to both traumatic and nontraumatic dissections have been considered.

Cohen JE, Ben Hur T, Rajz G, et al: Endovascular stent-assisted angioplasty in the management of traumatic internal carotid artery dissections. Stroke 36:e45–e47, 2005.
Edgell RC, Abou-Chebl A, Yadav JS: Endovascular management of spontaneous carotid artery dissection. J Vasc Surg 42:854–860; discussion, 860, 2005.

14. **What is the significance of carotid artery stenosis?**
Carotid stenosis may result in cerebral ischemia, presenting as transient ischemic attacks or, in more severe cases, as stroke. Ischemia is most often the result of atherosclerotic microembolism rather than distal infarction resulting from stenosis. Current recommendations are that symptomatic carotid stenosis >70% should be opened either by surgery or by endovascular techniques.

Gasecki AP, Eliasziw M, Ferguson GG, et al: Long-term prognosis and effect of endarterectomy in patients with symptomatic severe carotid stenosis and contralateral carotid stenosis or occlusion: results from NASCET. North American Symptomatic Carotid Endarterectomy Trial (NASCET) Group. J Neurosurg 83:778–782, 1995.
Higashida RT, Meyers PM, Phatouros CC, et al: Reporting standards for carotid artery angioplasty and stent placement. Stroke 35:e112–e134, 2004.

KEY POINTS: STROKE

1. Effective treatment for ischemic stroke exists and can improve the outcome if administered within specified time limits; remember the adage, "Time is brain." Treatment includes systemic/IV and intraarterial thrombolysis and, in the future, mechanical clot extraction.

2. Systolic blood pressure should be lowered to below 185 mmHg and diastolic blood pressure should be below 110 mmHg before the administration of IV rt-PA for acute ischemic stroke.

3. In a nonthrombolytic candidate with ischemic stroke, blood pressure guidelines should be liberalized to ensure adequate circulation to the zone of tissue at risk (i.e., ischemic penumbra). Systolic blood pressures may be as high as 210 mmHg and diastolic blood pressure as high as 110 mmHg.

4. Patients with symptomatic carotid stenosis ($\geq$70%) are at high risk for stroke and should be treated surgically or endovascularly.

5. Management of intracerebral hemorrhage is largely supportive. The recently completed Surgical Trial in Intracerebral Hemorrhage trial showed that there is no benefit to early surgery in patients with intracerebral hemorrhage.

15. **What is subclavian steal syndrome?**
This syndrome refers to symptoms of vertebrobasilar insufficiency that arise in association with exercise, particularly of the arms. It reflects the diversion (or steal) of blood from the vertebral artery to the brachial artery. When the vasodilation that accompanies exercise is coupled with a proximal subclavian or innominate artery stenosis, blood may flow retrograde through the vertebral artery to fill the dilated vascular pool in the arm. This syndrome is confirmed when symptoms are associated with a decreased blood pressure in one arm and an ipsilateral supraclavicular bruit. It is more common on the left than on the right.

16. **Describe hypertensive encephalopathy.**
This term refers to an encephalopathy characterized by headache, nausea, vomiting, visual disturbances, seizures, confusion, and coma in the setting of severe hypertension. One theory suggests that the rapid rise in blood pressure is accompanied by loss of cerebral autoregulation, producing areas of focal vasospasm and ischemia together with areas of cerebral vasodilation and increased flow. Cerebral edema is a common but not constant feature. Causes are related to age and include (1) acute glomerulonephritis (in children and adolescents), (2) chronic glomerulonephritis (in young adults), (3) eclampsia (in childbearing women), and (4) malignant hypertension (in patients older than 30–40 years). The only consistent sign is systemic hypertension. Papilledema is almost always present, and its absence should cast some doubt on the diagnosis.

17. **Discuss the treatment of acute ischemic stroke.**
Stroke prevention through risk factor modification, antiplatelet agents, and warfarin anticoagulation in atrial fibrillation has favorably affected the incidence of new events. However, effective treatment of stroke in the acute setting has proved a more difficult task.
  In 1995, the use of IV thrombolytic therapy with recombinant tissue plasminogen activator (rt-PA) was shown to improve outcome in patients experiencing acute stroke if therapy could be initiated within 3 hours of onset of symptoms. Other trials using IV rt-PA have not proved successful, mainly because of the time windows (up to 5 hours from symptom onset).

The use of intra-arterial prourokinase has shown benefit in treating middle cerebral artery occlusion if treatment can be initiated within 6 hours of symptom onset. Studies are underway to investigate combination therapy with IV rt-PA followed by intra-arterial rt-PT to determine whether additional benefit over the use of either therapy alone is possible. The goal is to reestablish blood flow before tissue death. The major complication of thrombolytic therapy is intracerebral hemorrhage. In the 1995 study, rates of hemorrhage in patients receiving rt-PA were in the range of 6%, whereas patients not receiving rt-PA had a hemorrhage rate of 0.6%.

In 2004, the results of the Mechanical Embolus Removal in Cerebral Ischemia trial demonstrated that recanalization with a device to mechanically remove the clot from intracerebral vessels could be safely performed and of benefit in patients with ischemic stroke.

The use of antiplatelet agents in the acute setting has been shown to give a small but statistically significant benefit, and the combination of aspirin with rt-PA also has shown benefit in terms of reperfusion, although the risk of hemorrhage may be increased.

The use of heparin in the setting of acute stroke has been a topic of debate for many years. Its use is based on the concept of clot propagation or recurrent embolism from a cardiac or vascular source as a cause of neurologic deterioration in stroke. Anticoagulation has shown benefit in lowering the incidence of stroke in patients with atrial fibrillation. However, its use in the treatment of acute ischemic stroke remains controversial.

Other treatment considerations include the avoidance of acute reductions in blood pressure. Because the blood flow around areas of infarcted brain is already low, further reducing the blood flow by lowering blood pressure can result in an extension of the area of infarction. As a result, higher blood pressures are generally desirable in the setting of acute stroke, and vigorous attempts to lower blood pressure should be avoided. The use of sedative medications in the setting of acute stroke should also be minimized because their use may interfere with the clinician's ability to follow up with serial neurologic examinations.

Finally, routine care considerations—such as range-of-motion exercises for limbs rendered immobile or weak as a result of the stroke; prevention of aspiration, pulmonary emboli, and skin breakdown; and nutritional support—are also important.

Clark WM, Wissman S, Albers GW, et al: Recombinant tissue-type plasminogen activator (Alteplase) for ischemic stroke 3 to 5 hours after symptom onset. The ATLANTIS Study: A randomized controlled trial. Alteplase Thrombolysis for Acute Noninterventional Therapy in Ischemic Stroke. JAMA 282:2019–2026, 1999.

Furlan A, Higashida R, Wechsler L, et al: Intra-arterial prourokinase for acute ischemic stroke. The PROACT II study: A randomized controlled trial. Prolyse in Acute Cerebral Thromboembolism. JAMA 282:2003–2011, 1999.

Gobin YP, Starkman S, Duckwiler GR, et al: MERCI 1: A phase 1 study of Mechanical Embolus Removal in Cerebral Ischemia. Stroke 35:2848–2854, 2004.

National Institute of Neurological Disorders and Stroke rt-PA Stroke Study Group: Tissue plasminogen activator for acute ischemic stroke. N Engl J Med 333:1581–1587, 1995.

18. **Discuss the treatment of ICH.**

Currently the appropriate management of ICH is supportive, although a phase II trial using recombinant factor VII for the treatment of ICH has shown benefit in terms of hematoma expansion and possibly outcome. A phase III trial is currently underway. Otherwise, there are no clear evidence-based guidelines on the management of ICH.

In the past it was recommended to treat blood pressure only if mean arterial pressure was $\geq$130 mmHg. This was based on the idea that there might be an ischemic region surrounding the hematoma. However, recent studies increasingly suggest that there probably is not an ischemic area around the hematoma and that it might be prudent to lower blood pressure more aggressively in the acute setting. Nitroprusside is a very effective antihypertensive agent; however, it may cause intracranial pressure (ICP) problems resulting from venous dilation in the intracranial compartment. More recently, many have begun using nicardipine, a calcium channel blocker, because it has no effect on ICP or cerebral autoregulation.

The use of intraventricular drains might be beneficial in patients with intraventricular extension of their ICH with hydrocephalus. The recently completed Surgical Trial in Intracerebral Hemorrhage trial failed to demonstrate any surgical benefit in patients with intracerebral hemorrhage.

Mayer SA, Brun NC, Begtrup K, et al: Recombinant activated factor VII for acute intracerebral hemorrhage. N Engl J Med 352:777–785, 2005.

Powers WJ, Zalzulia AR, Videen TO, et al: Autoregulation of cerebral blood flow surrounding acute (6 to 22 hours) intracerebral hemorrhage. Neurology 57:18–24, 2001.

CEREBRAL ANEURYSMS

19. **What is the incidence of SAH from ruptured intracranial aneurysms?**
    The incidence is estimated at 10 per 100,000 persons, accounting for 1–2% of all emergency department admissions.

    Edlow JA: Diagnosis of subarachnoid hemorrhage. Neurocrit Care 2:99–109, 2005.

    Mitchell P, Jakubowski J: Estimate of the maximum time interval between formation of cerebral aneurysm and rupture. J Neurol Neurosurg Psychiatry 69:760–767, 2000.

20. **What is the incidence of asymptomatic intracranial aneurysm?**
    Autopsy and angiographic studies have shown that between 3.5% and 6% of the general population have unruptured aneurysms. The risk of hemorrhage from a previously unruptured aneurysm was believed to be about 1% annually; however, more recent data suggest that the risk of rupture of intracranial aneurysms <10 mm in diameter is <0.05% per year.

    International Study of Unruptured Aneurysm Investigators: Unruptured intracranial aneurysms—Risks of rupture and risks of surgical intervention. N Engl J Med 339:1725–1733, 1998.

    Wardlow JM, White PM: The detection and management of unruptured intracranial aneurysms. Brain 123:205–221, 2000.

21. **What are the major types of intracranial aneurysms?**
    - **Saccular aneurysms:** This is by far the most common aneurysmal type and cause of SAH.
    - **Mycotic aneurysms:** One to two percent of intracerebral aneurysms result from septic embolization due to valvular vegetations in patients with bacterial endocarditis, and 10% of patients with endocarditis will develop mycotic intracerebral aneurysms. Mycotic aneurysms typically appear about 4–5 weeks after an acute embolic event. They usually are found in the distal middle cerebral artery circulation, although 10% are found more proximally. Mycotic aneurysms usually resolve with adequate antibiotic therapy but occasionally require endovascular or surgical correction. Streptococci are the most common pathogen.
    - **Traumatic aneurysms:** Although true traumatic aneurysms are rare, false aneurysms are more common. False or pseudoaneurysms result from the disruption of the vessel wall with resulting clot formation. Traumatic aneurysms may be found in association with skull fractures.
    - **Fusiform aneurysms:** Fusiform aneurysms are caused by dilated tortuous vessels that may rupture, dissect, or form thrombi that embolize distally. The pathology of fusiform aneurysms appears to be distinct from the pathology of both atherosclerosis and saccular aneurysms.

    Erdogan HB, Erentug V, Bozbuga N, et al: Endovascular treatment of intracerebral mycotic aneurysm before surgical treatment of infective endocarditis. Tex Heart Inst J 31:165–167, 2004.

    Oohara K, Yamakazi T, Kanou H, Kobayashi A: Infective endocarditis complicated by mycotic cerebral aneurysm: Two case reports of women in the peripartum period. Eur J Cardiothorac Surg 14:533–535, 1998.

22. **What are the risk factors for developing saccular aneurysms?**
    Both congenital and acquired factors are involved. Approximately 4–5% of all familial cerebral aneurysms occur in first-degree relatives; familial aneurysms typically present earlier than

nonfamilial aneurysms. Aneurysms also are associated with arteriovenous malformations (AVMs) and have been noted on the feeding vessels in approximately 7% of patients. Other nonmodifiable risk factors include autosomal dominant polycystic kidney disease, neurofibromatosis type I, and connective tissue disorders such as Ehlers-Danlos type IV, fibromuscular dysplasia, and Marfan's syndrome. Approximately 4–10% of patients with polycystic kidney disease develop intracranial aneurysms, as opposed to 1% in the general population. The exact pathologic cause of saccular aneurysms has not been clearly elucidated, but they tend to occur at bifurcations of major cerebral vessels where flow pressures are highest.

Schrier W, Belz MM, Kaehny WD, et al: Repeat imaging for intracranial aneurysms in patients with autosomal dominant polycystic kidney disease with initially negative studies: A prospective ten-year follow-up. J Am Cos Nephrol 15:1023–1028, 2004.

Wang MC, Rubinstein D, Kindt GW, Breeze RE: Prevalence of intracranial aneurysms in first-degree relatives of patients with aneurysms. Neurosurg Focus 13:2, 2002.

3. **What are the risk factors for intracranial aneurysmal rupture?**
The overall incidence of aneurysmal SAH is about 5–10 per 100,000 person years with an increasing incidence of rupture with advancing age. Family history of SAH is an important predisposing factor; 5–10% of patients have a positive family history. Recent reports indicate that the generally accepted view that aneurysmal SAH is more common in women than in men may not be universally true when ethnicity and geographic location are considered. Size of the aneurysm is also important; larger aneurysms are more likely to rupture than smaller ones. The reported incidence of rupture of aneurysms <10 mm was <0.05% per year, whereas the incidence for rupture of aneurysms >10 mm was 0.5% per year. For aneurysms ≥25 mm in diameter, the risk of rupture was 6% in the first year after discovery.

Ingall T, Asplund K, Mahonen M, Bonita R: A multinational comparison of subarachnoid hemorrhage epidemiology in the WHO MONICA stroke study. Stroke 31:1054–1061, 2000.

International Study of Unruptured Aneurysm Investigators: Unruptured intracranial aneurysms: Risks of rupture and risks of surgical intervention. N Engl J Med 1998 339:1725–1733, 1998.

Sedat J, Dib M, Rasendrarijao D, Lonjon M, Paquis P: Ruptured intracranial aneurysms in the elderly: Epidemiology, diagnosis, and management. Neurocrit Care 2:119–123, 2005.

4. **In addition to aneurysms, what are the other causes of SAH?**
- **Arterial dissection:** Dissections are disruptions of the arterial wall in which blood flows into the intima, creating a false lumen. When they involve the vertebral arteries, they may present with SAH or embolic stroke and often are associated with lower cranial nerve palsies and brain stem infarctions. Anterior circulation dissections also may occur, but SAH associated with anterior circulation dissections is decidedly rare.
- **Cerebral AVMs:** Occasionally, SAH is seen without the normal pattern of intracerebral hemorrhage. In such cases, a concomitant saccular aneurysm must be excluded.
- **Pituitary apoplexy:** Patients usually present with a sudden headache along with deterioration of visual acuity. Eye movement abnormalities and deterioration in level of consciousness also may be seen. Magnetic resonance imaging or computed tomography (CT) usually indicates the pituitary as the source.
- **Perimesencephalic SAH** (so-called *angionegative SAH*): The subarachnoid blood is isolated anterior to the pons. The diagnosis is confirmed by excluding an aneurysm with angiography or CT angiography. The risk for rebleeding is low, and prognosis is good. Patients do not develop the dangerous sequelae seen in aneurysmal SAH.
- **Head trauma:** SAH is common in head trauma. Overall, head trauma is the most common cause of SAH.

25. **What are the signs and symptoms of intracranial aneurysmal rupture?**
The most common presentation is headache. The major characteristics of headache caused by SAH are as follows:

- **Abrupt/sudden onset of headache:** A headache that reaches maximum intensity in a matter of seconds is perhaps the single most important aspect of the headache history.
- **Severity:** Patients with SAH often complain that the headache is the "worst headache of my life."
- **Distinct quality:** The headache in SAH is usually different than other headaches experienced by the patient.
- **Associated symptoms:** The patient experiences nausea, vomiting, neck stiffness, and photophobia, possibly associated with loss of consciousness.

Focal neurologic deficits are sometimes evident at presentation; one of the most common is a third nerve palsy in association with posterior communicating artery aneurysms. Abducens palsies are also seen and thought to be related to increased ICP and possibly to brain stem herniation as a result of traction on the nerve. Depending on location, other neurologic deficits are also seen, including motor and sensory deficits, visual loss, and loss of brain stem reflexes. On the other hand, at least one study has reported that approximately 12% of patients presenting with severe headache, as previously described, are neurologically normal.

Edlow JA: Diagnosis of subarachnoid hemorrhage. Neurocrit Care 2:99–109, 2005.

Edlow JA, Caplan LR: Avoiding pitfalls in the diagnosis of subarachnoid hemorrhage. N Engl J Med 342:29–36, 2000.

26. **What is a sentinel bleed? Why is it significant?**
A sentinel or warning bleed has traditionally been interpreted as an initial minor bleed or "leak" from a cerebral aneurysm. Other possibilities, however, include simple recall bias in patients knowing they have a serious brain illness when asked the question, or an acute expansion, thrombosis, or dissection of the aneurysm without leak or rupture. It is considered a minor bleed because, although it results in a severe headache, it may go unrecognized or may be misdiagnosed (as a migraine headache, for instance). In any case, it is important to have a low threshold for evaluating patients presenting with severe headache as previously described because some studies suggest that those presenting with sentinel or warning symptoms may have worse outcomes.

Leblanc R: The minor leak preceding subarachnoid hemorrhage. J Neurosurg 66:35–39, 1987.

27. **How is SAH diagnosed?**
Noncontrast CT scan of the brain is usually the first test performed. If performed within 24 hours of rupture, CT of the brain has a sensitivity of >90%. However, by day 3 only 85% of patients have abnormal CT scan results, and by 1 week, only 50%. Thus, in addition to CT scanning, lumbar puncture (LP) should also be considered, especially in cases where the CT scan is reported as normal or nondiagnostic. The LP can also help diagnose those patients with atypical presentations of meningitis or other intracranial abnormalities. In addition to diagnosing SAH, the CT scan may also help identify patients with hydrocephalus and give some suggestion as to the location of the aneurysm based on the distribution of the subarachnoid blood.

The presence of xanthochromia, a yellowish discoloration of the spinal fluid that appears by 4 hours after SAH, is the most distinguishing characteristic and will help differentiate patients with a traumatic LP from those with SAH. Xanthochromia can last up to 3 weeks after SAH. To determine xanthochromia, it is important to centrifuge the spinal fluid as soon as possible after the LP so that the red blood cells are at the bottom of the tube. Another way to distinguish between SAH and a traumatic LP is the red blood cell count in sequential tubes: In a traumatic LP, the red blood cells will decrease steadily in sequential tubes. An opening pressure measured at the time of LP will help identify patients with increased opening pressure.

Edlow JA: Diagnosis of subarachnoid hemorrhage. Neurocrit Care 2:99–109, 2005.

28. **What factors are associated with poor prognosis after rupture of an intracranial aneurysm?**
    The amount of blood, older age, posterior circulation aneurysms, early development of hydrocephalus, and decreased consciousness at presentation are all associated with worse outcome. The degree of meningeal irritation, level of consciousness, and presence of focal motor deficits can be used to identify patients who are at increased risk. In 1968, the Hunt and Hess scale was proposed. The scale was an attempt to determine the surgical risk of patients undergoing surgery for SAH and has five different categories or grades:
    - **Grade I:** Asymptomatic or minimal headache and slight nuchal rigidity
    - **Grade II:** Moderate to severe headache, no nuchal rigidity other than cranial nerve palsy
    - **Grade III:** Drowsiness, confusion, or mild focal deficit
    - **Grade IV:** Stupor, moderate to severe hemiparesis, possible early decerebrate rigidity and vegetative disturbances
    - **Grade V:** Deep coma, decerebrate rigidity, moribund appearance

    According to this scale, those patients who have grade III SAH and higher (decreased level of consciousness) have a worse prognosis than those with grades I and II.

    Rosen DS, Macdonald RL: Subarachnoid hemorrhage grading scales. Neurocrit Care 2:110–118, 2005.

29. **What are the major complications of ruptured intracranial aneurysms?**
    Global cerebral ischemia, rebleeding, acute hydrocephalus, vasospasm, and hyponatremia are the major complications after SAH.
    - **Global cerebral ischemia:** When an aneurysm ruptures, there is abrupt increase in ICP that may cause global cerebral ischemia. As ICP rises toward mean arterial pressure, there may be a decrease in the forward flow of blood, and ischemia can result. If the ICP rises above mean arterial pressure, there is no effective forward flow of blood into the intracranial compartment.
    - **Rebleeding:** The incidence of rebleeding in the first 24 hours after initial SAH ranges from 10% to 15%. Rebleeding is associated with an increase in both morbidity and mortality.
    - **Hydrocephalus:** Hydrocephalus occurs as a result of subarachnoid blood interfering with the normal drainage of cerebrospinal fluid from the ventricles of the brain and can sometimes be relieved by urgent ventricular drain placement. Patients who have normal ventricular size as exhibited on initial CT scan should be monitored closely for gradual obtundation, slow pupillary responses to light, and downward deviation of the eyes because any of these might suggest the development of hydrocephalus. A ventricular drain is usually placed urgently in patients who present with a grade III or greater hemorrhage because the decreased level of consciousness may be the result of hydrocephalus.
    - **Hyponatremia:** In the past, hyponatremia has been attributed to the syndrome of inappropriate antidiuretic hormone (SIADH); recently, however, it has been associated more with natriuresis and hypovolemia, referred to as *cerebral salt wasting* (CSW). Both conditions present with hyponatremia, decreased plasma osmolarity, and inappropriately high urine osmolarity. The distinguishing features are that CSW is a state of decreased effective arterial blood volume, whereas SIADH is a state of normal effective arterial blood volume. CSW is treated by volume and sodium replacement and SIADH by fluid restriction.

    The exact cause of CSW has not been determined, although several natriuretic factors have been studied. Treatment involves maintaining adequate volume and supplementing sodium by mouth and/or intravenously. The hyponatremia is usually mild to moderate; only rarely does the sodium level drop below 120 mmol/L. Patients whose serum sodium level is below 133 mmol/L are usually managed with 3% NaCl administered intravenously with close monitoring of serum sodium. The rate of infusion is determined by the serum sodium level, which is generally measured every 4–6 hours depending on the severity of the hyponatremia.

30. **What extracerebral organ dysfunction is associated with aneurysmal rupture?**
The major extracerebral complications include pulmonary and cardiac dysfunction. Pulmonary dysfunction is the most common extracerebral complication and usually involves aspiration, pneumonia, or pulmonary edema. Oxygenation problems can be seen in up to 90% of patients with SAH.

    Aspiration is common after SAH and other types of neurologic events, and the lung damage from aspiration may evolve into pneumonia. Pulmonary edema can be seen acutely in SAH and is believed to be the result of stress failure with raised pulmonary capillary hydrostatic pressure causing disruption of capillary or alveolar endothelium with the subsequent development of high-permeability–type pulmonary edema. Pulmonary edema can also be the result of aggressive fluid administration after the aneurysm is secured. This is especially true in patients with left ventricular dysfunction at baseline or resulting from SAH.

    Cardiac dysfunction is most likely the result of excessive catecholamine release (and thus is linked to stress pulmonary edema [previously described]). Electrocardiographic changes, hypotension, and pulmonary edema are associated findings in patients with cardiac dysfunction. This "neurogenic pump failure" is associated with contraction band necrosis in the heart muscle caused by a dramatic increase in cardiac sympathetic drive and has been referred to as *stunned myocardium,* a condition defined as reversible wall motion abnormalities or reduced left ventricular function. The cardiac dysfunction typically does not correlate with the coronary vascular distribution on electrocardiogram.

    Ohkuma H, Tsurutani H, Suzuki S: Incidence and significance of early aneurismal rebleeding before neurosurgical or neurological management. Stroke 32:1176–1180, 2001.

    Schuiling WJ, Dennesen PJ, Rinkel GJ: Extracerebral organ dysfunction in the acute stage after aneurysmal subarachnoid hemorrhage. Neurocrit Care 2005 3:1–10, 2005.

KEY POINTS: CEREBRAL ANEURYSMS

1. Traumatic brain injury is the most common cause of subarachnoid hemorrhage. However, outside of trauma, aneurysmal rupture is the major cause of subarachnoid hemorrhage.

2. Aneurysmal rupture is associated with both neurologic and systemic complications—specifically, pulmonary and cardiac abnormalities.

3. The major complications after securing of an aneurysm are hyponatremia, vasospasm, and pulmonary edema.

4. Nimodipine administration early in the course of treatment has been associated with improved outcome but not with a decreased incidence of vasospasm.

5. Caution should be used in using aggressive fluid administration to treat vasospasm (i.e., hypervolemic therapy) because it can result in pulmonary edema, especially in patients with poor left ventricular function.

31. **Describe the operative repair of cerebral aneurysms.**
Several different surgical methods are used to repair cerebral aneurysms:
    - **Clipping:** The most effective of all the surgical techniques, clipping involves the dissection of the neck of the aneurysmal sac and the placement of a clip at the origin of the neck from the feeder vessel.
    - **Trapping:** This technique involves permanently occluding the vessel proximally and distally to the aneurysm and relies on the presence of adequate collateral blood flow to the affected area.

- **Proximal ligation:** This technique involves ligation of the feeder artery to reduce blood flow through the aneurysm. The subsequent decrease in blood flow and transmural pressure results in thrombosis or obliteration of the aneurysmal sac. As with trapping, this technique is restricted to specific cases in which collateral blood flow is sufficient to prevent subsequent ischemic damage.
- **Wrapping:** Reinforcement of the aneurysmal wall with synthetic material (e.g., Gelfoam) prevents further enlargement of the sac.
- **Endovascular coiling:** Endovascular coiling is performed by an interventional radiologist. With the use of detachable coils placed in the aneurysmal lumen, intraluminal thrombosis rates >85% have been reported. In 2002, the results of the International Subarachnoid Aneurysm Trial comparing surgical clipping to endovascular coiling reported that endovascular coiling was significantly better in terms of survival free of disability at 1 year.

Molyneux A, Kerr R, Stratton I, Sandercock P, et al: International Subarachnoid Aneurysm Trial of neurosurgical clipping versus endovascular coiling in 2143 patients with ruptured intracranial aneurysms: A randomized trial. Lancet 360:1267–1274, 2002.

32. **When does cerebral vasospasm develop? What are its consequences?**
    Vasospasm may occur in as many as 60–75% of patients after SAH. It occurs between days 4 and 21, with the peak incidence between days 5 and 9. Vasospasm rarely starts after day 12. It may result in further neurologic devastation due to ischemic strokes.
    Vasospasm may be diagnosed clinically by the appearance of neurologic deficits that cannot be explained by other causes such as hydrocephalus, rebleeding, or metabolic derangements. Transcranial Doppler is a useful noninvasive tool for the diagnosis of vasospasm. Spasm is indicated by elevated flow velocities on transcranial Doppler. Angiographically, vasospasm can be demonstrated by the narrowing of large arteries passing through the subarachnoid space. About 30% of angiographically apparent vasospasm is clinically significant.

33. **Describe the treatment of cerebral vasospasm.**
    Treatment involves the prevention or reversal of arterial spasm and minimization of the ischemia that results from the spasm. Strategies include the following:
    - **Calcium channel blockers:** Because of their effect on smooth muscle relaxation, calcium channel blockers have been investigated in multiple clinical trials as a means of preventing vasospasm. Oral nimodipine has been shown to reduce poor outcome after SAH but not to protect against secondary ischemia. This finding implies another effect of the drug— potentially a neuroprotective effect. As a result, nimodipine has become the standard of care in many centers because of its effect on outcome. Other calcium channel blockers have shown a reduction in secondary ischemia but no change in outcome. IV nicardipine is an effective blood pressure control agent and has been shown to reduce the incidence of vasospasm, but it has not yet been shown to improve outcome. As a result, it has been increasingly used as an agent to control blood pressure before the securing of aneurysms.
    - **Hemodynamic therapy:** So-called *triple-H therapy* (i.e., hypervolemia, hemodilution, and hypertension) has been the cornerstone of vasospasm management. Hypervolemic therapy is often used in an attempt to augment cerebral blood flow, but recent reviews and studies have found little evidence to support this practice. Arterial hypertension is believed to have its effect by maximizing cerebral perfusion pressure, thereby increasing blood flow to the brain.
    - **Percutaneous transluminal angioplasty and papaverine therapy:** These strategies are used in an attempt to open narrowed vessels. Although their efficacy has not been demonstrated in randomized, controlled trials, several large observational series have demonstrated marked clinical improvement as well as angiographically sustained dilation of cerebral blood vessels after angioplasty. However, balloon angioplasty is mainly of benefit in dilating more proximal areas of vasospasm. Papaverine is a potent vasodilator that has also shown benefit. Its major limitation is that its effect is transient; treatment may have to be repeated as frequently as every 24 hours.

- **Intra-arterial administration of calcium channel blockers:** Calcium channel blockers have increasingly replaced papaverine therapy in the treatment of patients not amenable to angioplasty. Verapamil at a dose of approximately 3 mg per vessel has demonstrated efficacy in reversing vasospasm without a significant effect on ICP or heart rate. Nicardipine 0.5–6 mg per vessel has demonstrated an immediate and prolonged effect on vasospasm without a significant effect on ICP.

Feng L, Fitzsimmons BF, Young WL, et al: Intraarterially administered verapamil as adjunct therapy for cerebral vasospasm: safety and two year experience. Am J Neuroradiol 23:1284–1290, 2002.

Haley EC Jr, Kassell NF, Torner JC, et al: A randomized trial of two doses of nicardipine in aneurysmal subarachnoid hemorrhage: A report of the cooperative aneurysm study. J Neurosurg 80:788–796, 1994.

CHAPTER 63

LANDRY-GUILLAIN-BARRÉ SYNDROME

David C. Bonovich, MD

1. What is the Landry-Guillain-Barré syndrome (LGBS)?

LGBS is an acute or subacute polyradiculoneuropathy characterized by immune-mediated demyelination. LGBS affects all ages.

2. What factors may predispose a patient to LGBS?

LGBS recently has been associated with cytomegalovirus, Epstein-Barr virus, and bacterial infections with *Campylobacter jejuni*. Up to 50% of patients have experienced a recent respiratory or gastrointestinal infection. An additional 15% have had a recent vaccination. Of all the vaccinations studied, only the 1976–1977 swine flu vaccine was associated with a statistically significant increase in incidence of LGBS, possibly resulting from contamination of the vaccine with the P2-myelin protein from the chick embryos from which the vaccine was made.

Godschalk PC, Bergman MP, Gorkink RF, et al: Identification of DNA sequence variation in Campylobacter strains associated with the Guillain-Barré syndrome by high-throughput AFLP analysis. BMC Microbiol 6:1–34, 2006.

Winer JB: Guillain-Barré syndrome. Mol Pathol 54:381–385, 2001.

3. Describe the pathology of LGBS. How does it explain the typical clinical features of the syndrome?

There are two forms: a demyelinating form (more common) and an axonal form. The prognosis is better for the former. The primary pathologic process in the demyelinating form is segmental demyelination of the peripheral nerves due to an autoimmune process that is both humorally and cell mediated. Because the primary process is a loss of myelin, the peripheral nerves that are most heavily myelinated (i.e., motor and joint-position sensory nerves) are more severely affected than unmyelinated or lightly myelinated nerves (i.e., nerves that mediate pain and temperature sensation).

The axonal form is associated with wallerian degeneration, minimal lymphocytic response, and no demyelination or inflammation. The node of Ranvier appears to be the target of attack in the axonal form, and antibodies to GM1, GM1b, GD1a, and Ga1NacGD1a are implicated in acute motor axonal neuropathy and infections with *C. jejuni*.

Hughes RA, Cornblath DR: Guillain-Barré syndrome. Lancet 366:1653–1666, 2005.

4. What are the typical features of LGBS?

The initial symptoms of LGBS are usually paresthesias in the distal extremities and pain or stiffness in the proximal limbs, followed quickly by progressive weakness of the limbs, trunk, and cranial muscles. The weakness most frequently begins in the legs and spreads in an ascending fashion, although other patterns of disease progression have been described. Patients lose their reflexes early in the course of the disease. It is usually symmetric but does not have to be so.

Respiratory function is often compromised by involvement of the phrenic and intercostal nerves. Patients may develop autonomic dysfunction characterized by wide fluctuations in heart rate and blood pressure. There have been reports of cardiac arrest as a result of autonomic instability. Cranial nerve deficits occur and may affect speech or swallowing. Vibratory sensation and proprioception are usually severely impaired, whereas pinprick and temperature sensation are often normal.

5. **What is the differential diagnosis of subacutely evolving, generalized motor weakness?**
See Box 63-1.

BOX 63-1.   DIFFERENTIAL DIAGNOSIS OF SUBACUTELY EVOLVING, GENERALIZED MOTOR WEAKNESS

Spinal cord injury

Toxins (hexacarbon, lead, thallium, or organophosphate intoxication)

Poliomyelitis

Botulism

Porphyria

Myasthenia gravis

Periodic paralysis

Tick paralysis

Diphtheritic polyneuropathy

Vasculitic polyneuropathy

Lambert-Eaton myasthenic syndrome

Dermatomyositis

Carcinomatous meningitis

Saxitoxin poisoning

---

6. **What are the confirmatory tests for LGBS?**
The diagnosis is usually made predominantly on clinical grounds. LGBS typically presents as an ascending weakness with absent reflexes. Lumbar puncture also may be helpful in the diagnosis. The typical pattern is an acellular spinal fluid with greatly increased protein and normal glucose. In some cases, however, the increase in protein may not begin until well into the course of the illness. Electromyography can be helpful in distinguishing between the axonal and demyelinating forms of LGBS.

7. **What is the typical clinical time course for LGBS?**
The usual course is divided into four phases:
- **Preceding phase:** The relatively asymptomatic period between the preceding illness and the onset of symptoms
- **Initial period:** Characterized by deterioration of strength; lasts less than 4 weeks
- **Plateau phase:** Characterized by a stable or minimally changing examination; lasts from several days to several weeks
- **Recovery phase:** The beginning of remyelination, characterized by slowly improving strength; lasts from several weeks to several months (as long as it takes for remyelination of damaged nerves)

8. **What are the incidence, mortality, and morbidity rates of LGBS?**
The incidence of LGBS ranges between 0.4 and 4/100,000. The major complication of LGBS is respiratory failure; between 10% and 23% of patients with LGBS eventually require mechanical ventilation. Less common than respiratory failure but still to be always considered is autonomic dysfunction. The mortality rate may be as high as 5% (studies quote rates of 2–5%), although it may be higher in patients requiring mechanical ventilation. Most deaths result from secondary complications, such as sepsis resulting from pulmonary and urinary infections; pulmonary emboli; delayed treatment of respiratory failure; and dysautonomias. These complications can be minimized by excellent medical and nursing care in the intensive care unit (ICU).

Chio A, Cocita D, Leone M, et al, for the Register for Guillain-Barré Syndrome: Guillain-Barré syndrome: A prospective population based incidence and outcome survey. Neurol 60:1146–1150, 2003.

Orlikowski D, Prigent H, Sharhar T, et al: Respiratory dysfunction in Guillain-Barré syndrome. Neurocrit Care 1:415–422, 2004.

9. **Which patients with LGBS require ICU observation?**

Any patient with evidence of respiratory muscle or bulbar muscle weakness should be transferred to the ICU for observation. Similarly, patients who show evidence of significant autonomic dysfunction or rapidly progressive generalized weakness should be followed closely in the ICU.

Orlikowski D, Prigent H, Sharhar T, et al: Respiratory dysfunction in Guillain-Barré syndrome. Neurocrit Care 1:415–422, 2004.

10. **What is the best way to monitor respiratory function in a patient with a neuromuscular disease such as LGBS?**

The cause of respiratory failure in LGBS is from progressive mechanical weakness of the respiratory muscles; thus, bedside pulmonary function testing is the best method of assessing and monitoring respiratory function. Measurements of vital capacity and maximum inspiratory and expiratory pressures give good indications of developing weakness in the respiratory muscles. Observation of respiratory patterns—whether the patient uses accessory muscles to breathe, respiratory rate, and how high the patient can count during one inspiration—also may be helpful. Arterial blood gas determinations frequently remain normal until respiratory failure is severe; therefore, such measurements lead to a false sense of security regarding respiratory status.

Orlikowski D, Prigent H, Sharhar T, et al: Respiratory dysfunction in Guillain-Barré syndrome. Neurocrit Care 1:415–422, 2004.

11. **When should patients with LGBS be intubated?**

This issue is controversial, and several factors need to be taken into account. Respiratory failure is due to a combination of respiratory muscle insufficiency, which leads to hypercapnic respiratory failure and pneumonia resulting from an inability to cough adequately or protect the airway. Clinically, neuromuscular respiratory failure is characterized by rapid, shallow breathing, restlessness, sweating, staccato speech, increased accessory muscle use, tachycardia, and the presence of an abdominal paradox. The following are general guidelines for intubation:
- When the vital capacity becomes less than 15 mL/kg of body weight
- When the maximum inspiratory pressure is less than -25 to -30 cm H_2O
- When a patient has such severe bulbar weakness that he or she cannot handle secretions or protect the airway
- When a patient can no longer maintain normal PCO_2 and pH on arterial blood gas determination (often a very late sign)

The rapidity of disease progression also should be considered. The more rapidly evolving the motor weakness, the more aggressive the clinician should be regarding early intubation.

Yavagal DR, Mayer SA: Respiratory complications of rapidly progressive neuromuscular syndromes: Guillain-Barré and myasthenia gravis. Semin Respir Crit Care Med 23:221–229, 2002.

12. **What considerations regarding neuromuscular blockade should be kept in mind when intubating a patient with LGBS?**

Succinylcholine has been associated with hyperkalemia-induced cardiac arrest due to the massive release of potassium from denervated muscle cells in paralyzed patients. This risk is greatest in patients with long-standing paralysis, but its use should be considered contraindicated in all patients with LGBS. Therefore, a nondepolarizing muscle relaxant such as vecuronium, atracurium, or cisatracurium should be used whenever possible.

Roppolo LP, Walters K: Airway management in neurological emergencies. Neurocrit Care 1:405–414, 2004.

13. **Which patients with LGBS experience dysautonomia?**

Autonomic nervous system dysfunction is usually present if the disease is severe enough to require mechanical ventilation and is more commonly seen with the demyelinating form of

LGBS as opposed to the axonal form. Dysautonomia results from either excessive or insufficient sympathetic and parasympathetic activity. In addition, a wide variety of arrhythmias can occur and may be a major cause of mortality. Treatment of dysautonomia consists of hydration and other supportive measures, such as avoiding changes in position and using stool softeners to prevent straining-induced vagal stimulation. If drugs are necessary to treat dysautonomia or arrhythmias, small doses of short-acting, titratable agents are recommended.

Asahima M, Kuwabara S, Suzuki A, Hattori T: Autonomic function in demyelinating and axonal subtypes of Guillain-Barré syndrome. Acta Neurol Scand 105:44–50, 2002.

KEY POINTS: LANDRY-GUILLAIN-BARRÉ SYNDROME (LGBS)

1. LGBS is an autoimmune syndrome characterized by immune-mediated demyelination. There is also an axonal autoimmune form.

2. LGBS is characterized by weakness that ascends from the feet toward the head, as opposed to botulism, which progresses from the head toward the feet.

3. Respiratory failure and autonomic dysfunction are the major risks of LBGS.

4. Diagnosis is confirmed by clinical history and a cerebrospinal fluid profile showing elevated protein levels and no cells.

5. Intravenous immunoglobulin and plasmapheresis are the mainstays of treatment.

14. **Are there any effective treatments for the neurologic injury associated with LGBS?**
   Until 1978, treatment of LGBS was largely supportive. Since then it has been demonstrated that plasma exchange (i.e., removing 50 mL/kg of plasma in each of five sessions on alternating days and replacing it with 5% albumin) is effective in shortening the course of the disease. The beneficial effects of plasma exchange are greatest when it is begun within 2 weeks of disease onset. In addition, high-dose intravenous immunoglobulin (IVIG) (0.4 gm/kg/day for 5 days) has been shown to be equally effective in reducing the number of ventilator days and length of time until the patient can walk.
   IVIG is easier to administer and less costly than plasma exchange, but several small series have suggested that its use is associated with a higher relapse rate than plasma exchange. A large study, however, found IVIG and plasma exchange to be equally effective with no difference in outcome at 48 weeks. Given the potential for serious complications associated with plasma exchange (many related to central line placement and line complications), IVIG is recommended as the initial treatment for LGBS. IVIG is contraindicated in patients with immunoglobulin A deficiency and known anaphylaxis to blood products. Such patients should be treated with plasma exchange. More recently, a review of the Cochrane database concluded that there are no adequate placebo-controlled comparisons with IVIG, but the evidence from randomized trails suggests that when started within 2 weeks from onset, IVIG is as efficacious as plasma exchange and is more likely to be completed than plasma exchange. In the pediatric population, IVIG probably hastens recovery compared with supportive care.

Hughs RA, Raphael JC, Swan AV, Doorn PA: Intravenous immunoglobulin for Guillain-Barré syndrome. Cochrane Database Syst Rev 1:CD002063, 2006.

15. **What is the prognosis in acute LGBS?**

Most patients experience excellent recovery in muscle function with time, often returning to normal. A small percentage of patients are left with various degrees of persistent weakness. In other patients, reflexes remain absent.

16. **Are there any ICU issues unique to LGBS?**

In addition to the obvious need for meticulous pulmonary and nutritional support, special care should be taken to avoid pressure palsies of the arms and the legs. All patients require deep venous thrombosis prophylaxis with intermittent pneumatic compression devices or subcutaneous heparin, in addition to adequate pain control. Also, patients with LGBS are usually completely alert yet often cannot communicate because of intubation and paralysis. Therefore, patients should be allowed to communicate their needs and concerns whenever possible. They may require tremendous emotional support and judicious use of anxiolytic agents.

Kehoe M: Guillain-Barré syndrome: A patient guide and nursing resource. Axone 22:16–24, 2001.

CHAPTER 64

MYASTHENIA GRAVIS

David C. Bonovich, MD

1. **Define *myasthenia gravis* (MG).**

   MG was first described in 1672 by Thomas Willis, who described cases of a "spurious palsy." MG is an autoimmune disorder of neuromuscular transmission manifested by weakness and fatigability of voluntary skeletal muscle. The major characteristic is fatiguing of the skeletal muscle with repeated or continuous activity. There are two forms: ocular MG, in which the weakness is confined to the extraocular muscles, and a generalized form that affects ocular and facial muscles as well as muscles of the trunk.

2. **What are the ages of peak incidence of MG?**

   The incidence of MG is 0.25–2.0/100,000 persons. MG may begin at any age, but it is more prevalent in women in the younger age category (female-to-male ratio, 4:1). The peak incidence for women is between 10 and 40 years of age; for men, between 50 and 70 years of age. Recently, there seems to have been a trend toward an increased incidence in men older than 60 years of age.

   Vincent A, Palace J, Hilton-Jones D: Myasthenia gravis. Lancet 357:2122–2128, 2001.

3. **What are the usual clinical features of MG?**

   MG is characterized clinically by fluctuating weakness of specific muscles. It has a predilection for the extraocular and bulbar muscles. Sixty-five percent of patients will have ocular symptoms, typically double vision and ptosis; one-fourth will have bulbar involvement with slurred or nasal speech and voice changes.

   Scherer K, Bedlak RS, Simel L: Does this patient have myasthenia gravis? JAMA 293:1906–1914, 2005.

4. **Describe the pathophysiology of MG.**

   MG is an autoimmune disease. The target antigen is the nicotinic acetylcholine receptor (AchR) in the postsynaptic membrane of the neuromuscular junction. AchR antibodies may be identifiable in the serum of about 85% of patients, resulting in a marked decrease in the number of functional AchRs, causing faulty neuromuscular transmission. There is a subset of patients that are seronegative to the antibody; however, in these patients MG is still thought to be an antibody-mediated disease. Antibodies to muscle-specific kinase (MuSK) have now been described. MuSK is an essential component in the neuromuscular junction, where it is thought to be involved in maintaining the density of acetylcholine receptors in the junction. Antibody interference with MuSK may cause complement-mediated damage to the neuromuscular junction.

   The thymus may be necessary for removing autoreactive T cells. Disorders of the thymus are common in patients with MG, and the thymus seems to have a role in the pathogenesis of MG. Up to 70% of persons with myasthenia have evidence of lymphoid follicle hyperplasia in the thymus, and up to 15% harbor a thymoma. Other types of autoimmune disorders associated with MG include thyroid disorders, pernicious anemia, Addison's disease, diabetes mellitus, lupus erythematosus, rheumatoid arthritis, and polymyositis.

   Hoch W, McConville J, Helms S, et al: Auto-antibodies to the receptor tyrosine kinase MuSK in patients with myasthenia gravis without acetylcholine receptor antibodies. Nat Med 7:365–368, 2001.

Mossman S, Vincent A, Newsom-Davis J: Myasthenia gravis without acetylcholine-receptor antibody: A distinct disease entity. Lancet 1:116–119, 1986.

Vincent A, Palace J, Hilton-Jones D: Myasthenia gravis. Lancet 357:2122–2128, 2001.

5. **How is the diagnosis of MG confirmed?**
   - **Clinical findings:** Clinical findings of fluctuating weakness with a predilection for the extraocular and bulbar muscles strongly suggest the diagnosis. In some patients, however, the diagnosis may not be clear from the history and clinical examination alone, especially early in the course of the disease.
   - **Response to edrophonium:** The response to edrophonium (Tensilon), a short-acting acetylcholinesterase inhibitor, may be especially helpful in diagnosing MG. Administration of edrophonium increases the concentration of acetylcholine in the neuromuscular junction. The Tensilon test should not be performed unless the clinician is clear about the specific muscles to be tested. The standard dose is 10 mg, but a test dose of 1–2 mg (0.1–0.2 mL) should be given first because, rarely, some patients are sensitive to Tensilon and may develop marked bradycardia or bronchospasm. If the test dose is tolerated, the remaining 8 mg may be given.
   - **Ice-pack test:** The ice-pack test can be helpful in patients with ptosis. In this test, ice packs applied to the eyelids improved ptosis in up to 80% of patients with MG. The improvement is believed to be the result of cooling causing slower kinetics at the acetylcholine receptor site.
   - **Electrophysiologic testing:** Finally, electrophysiologic testing can be quite helpful in diagnosing MG. The use of repetitive-stimulation electromyography is especially useful for patients whose test results are negative for AchR antibodies.

   Kubis KC, Danesh-Meyer HC, Savino PJ, Sergott RC: The ice test versus the rest test in myasthenia gravis. Ophthalmology 107:1995–1998, 2000.

6. **What is the differential diagnosis for MG?**
   Lambert-Eaton myasthenic syndrome (LEMS) is a rare condition in which antibodies are formed against voltage-gated calcium channels, resulting in impaired ability of the presynaptic cells to release acetylcholine. Although MG and LEMS have some common clinical features, LEMS does not involve extraocular muscles; thus, ptosis and diplopia, which are very common in MG, do not occur. In addition, repetitive nerve stimulation (particularly at high frequencies) in LEMS demonstrates an increase in the size of the muscle response. Botulism causes a descending weakness that may involve the extraocular and bulbar muscles and the skeletal muscles but does not have a waxing and waning quality like MG. Hyperthyroidism may cause diplopia but is easily ruled out by thyroid function tests.

   Thavni BR, Lo TC: Update on myasthenia gravis. Postgrad Med J 80:690–700, 2004.

7. **What is the most serious complication of MG?**
   Fatal respiratory failure can result from severe involvement of the respiratory muscles. Respiratory failure can also result from pulmonary aspiration due to difficulty in swallowing and protecting the upper airway secondary to bulbar weakness.

8. **What is the best way to assess respiratory function in patients with MG?**
   As with other neuromuscular diseases, respiratory failure results from muscle weakness; thus, rapid, shallow breathing and paradoxical abdominal movement suggest impending respiratory failure. Hypoxia, hypercapnia, and respiratory acidosis may not occur until late in the course of the disease. Thus, frequent evaluation of respiratory function using vital capacity and mean inspiratory force is the best way to monitor at-risk patients with MG and other neuromuscular diseases that affect the respiratory muscles.

9. **How is MG managed?**
   - **Medical management:** Medical management usually involves the use of long-acting acetylcholinesterase inhibitors such as pyridostigmine (Mestinon). Mestinon significantly improves neuromuscular function in patients with MG. Steroids and other immunosuppressive agents also may be helpful. Azathioprine, methotrexate, cyclosporine, and mycophenolate are believed to be effective.
   - **Thymectomy:** This procedure is often beneficial, with clinical improvement in about 80% of patients. It should be considered especially in patients with generalized MG. Plasma exchange and intravenous immunoglobulin (IVIG) are often used in patients with severe exacerbations and can be highly effective in these settings. Immunoadsorption, a new therapy in which plasma exchange is used in conjunction with a resin that adsorbs acetylcholine receptor antibodies, should be considered in patients with severe myasthenic crisis.

     Scherer K, Bedlack RS, Simel DL: Does this patient have myasthenia gravis? JAMA 293:1906–1914, 2005.
     Thanvi BR, Lo TC: Update on myasthenia gravis. Postgrad Med J 80:690–700, 2004.

10. **What is myasthenic crisis?**
    Myasthenic crisis is a severe, life-threatening worsening of MG. It is defined as weakness resulting from MG severe enough to require mechanical ventilation. Approximately 10–30% of patients with MG will experience myasthenic crises, usually within the first year or two after diagnosis. It occurs more commonly in patients with severe bulbar weakness and thymoma and after physical stress, such as upper respiratory infection or surgery, and is characterized by profound weakness and respiratory failure. It is usually associated with prolonged hospitalization and carries a mortality of about 5%.

    The evaluation of myasthenic crisis in patients with known MG includes ruling out nonmyasthenic causes of respiratory failure, such as pulmonary embolism. Then the search begins for the precipitant of myasthenic crisis. These would include respiratory infection, surgery (especially thymectomy), medication changes, and severe emotional stress.

    Precipitating drugs include some antiarrhythmic agents, neuromuscular blockers, aminoglycosides, quinolones, calcium channel blockers, and beta blockers.

    Lacomis D: Myasthenic crises. Neurocrit Care 3:189–184, 2005.

KEY POINTS: MYASTHENIA GRAVIS (MG)

1. MG is an autoimmune disease in which antibodies are directed against the neuromuscular junction.

2. Most antibodies are directed against muscarinic acetylcholine receptors in the neuromuscular junction. In addition, antibodies directed against muscle-specific kinase (MuSK) have been described recently.

3. MG has a bimodal incidence with a first peak between 10 and 40 years, when it affects predominantly women, and a second peak between 50 and 70 years, when it is more common in men.

4. Seventy percent of patients have evidence of thymic hyperplasia, and 15% have thymoma.

5. Treatment of MG involves the use of steroids and cholinesterase inhibitors and, in selected patients, thymectomy.

6. Myasthenic crisis is characterized by respiratory failure that often requires mechanical ventilation and can be treated with steroids, anticholinesterase medications, plasmapheresis, and IV immunoglobulin.

11. **How should a patient in myasthenic crisis be treated?**
Myasthenic crisis is defined by the need for respiratory assistance. When a patient is believed to be at risk for developing respiratory embarrassment and begins to have difficulty in swallowing (placing the patient at risk for aspiration), he or she should be moved to the intensive care unit. In patients without hypercarbia, a trial of noninvasive ventilation may be tried. A study reviewing the use of noninvasive ventilation in patients with bulbar weakness and respiratory failure in nine patients experiencing 11 episodes of respiratory failure prevented intubation in seven. The others improved despite vital capacities <10 mL/kg.
    When vital capacity falls below 15 mL/kg of body weight or when the patient cannot handle secretions, he or she should be intubated and supported with mechanical ventilation. The goals of therapy should be to reduce the work of breathing, to determine the underlying reason for development of myasthenic crisis, and to restore adequate respiratory and bulbar function. Guidelines are outlined in Box 64-1.

Lacomis D: Myasthenic crisis. Neurocrit Care 3:189–194, 2005.

Rabinstein A, Wijdicks EF: BIPAP in acute respiratory failure due to myasthenic crises may prevent intubation. Neurology 59:1647–1649, 2002.

BOX 64-1.   GUIDELINES FOR TREATMENT OF MYASTHENIC CRISIS

1. During the initial 24–48 hours after intubation, settings for mechanical ventilation should be focused on allowing the ventilator to assume most of the control of breathing; thus, a volume control mode with continuous mandatory ventilation should be considered.

2. A vigorous search for any underlying infection should be initiated, and careful attention should be given to proper suctioning.

3. Careful attention also should be given to the prevention of venous thrombosis. Measures should include the application of sequential compression devices and/or the use of subcutaneous heparin or low-molecular-weight heparin.

4. All anticholinesterase medications should be stopped for 48–72 hours. Often, a drug holiday restores responsiveness to medications later and may help with secretion management.

5. Either plasma exchange or IVIG therapy should be initiated as soon as possible after intubation to hasten neuromuscular recovery. Mestinon may be restarted after several days of plasma exchange, with the dose gradually increased based on clinical response.

6. If there is no response to plasma exchange or IVIG after 5 days, consider adding prednisone (1 mg/kg/day).

IVIG = intravenous immunoglobulin.

---

12. **What is cholinergic crisis?**
Cholinergic crisis results from an overdose of acetylcholinesterase inhibitors causing profound weakness due to continuous depolarization of the postsynaptic membrane, which in turn results in a depolarizing type of neuromuscular blockade. In general, cholinergic crisis causes other symptoms, such as excessive salivation, cramps, diarrhea, and blurred vision. There is also a history of a marked increase in pyridostigmine use. A small dose of edrophonium often differentiates the two conditions because it usually causes significant improvement in myasthenic crisis but worsens cholinergic crisis. This test should be performed only when emergency airway management is available because it can cause severe respiratory failure in patients with cholinergic crisis.

Kothari MJ: Myasthenia gravis. J Am Osteopath Assoc 104:374–384, 2004.

13. **What factors should be considered perioperatively in a patient with myasthenia who is undergoing thymectomy?**

The most important goal is to optimize respiratory muscle function preoperatively. Plasma exchange or IVIG, and sometimes steroids, are used to accomplish this goal. The dose of Mestinon should be reduced as much as possible without compromising respiratory function because patients may become more sensitive to its effects postoperatively. Some recommend withholding the anticholinesterase medication on the morning of surgery to decrease the need for muscle relaxants. If the patient was taking steroids preoperatively, stress doses of steroids should be given in the perioperative period. Extubation should not be considered until all of the effects of the inhalational agents used for anesthesia have fully dissipated and it is clear that respiratory function is adequate. It is better to be conservative in the decision to extubate the patient. After extubation, respiratory function should be monitored closely, and the patient should be observed for signs of fatigue.

Abel M, Eisenkraft JB: Anesthetic implications of myasthenia gravis. Mt Sinai J Med 69:31–37, 2002.

CHAPTER 65

ALCOHOL WITHDRAWAL

Jill A. Rebuck, PharmD, BCPS, and Bruce Crookes, MD

1. **Which patients in the intensive care unit (ICU) are most at risk for alcohol withdrawal?**
Any patient with a history of significant, heavy, or prolonged alcohol intake who has recently stopped or reduced alcohol intake is at risk. Alcohol withdrawal is often observed after elective surgery or emergent hospital admissions, with a substantial portion of all hospitalized trauma patients under the influence of alcohol at the time of injury. Increased morbidity is associated with chronic alcoholism leading to additional surgical procedures, prolonged hospital length of stay, and worse 3-month postoperative outcomes. In addition to alcohol withdrawal, infection, bleeding, and cardiopulmonary insufficiency are the common complications reported in patients with a significant alcohol intake history.

2. **What are the potential signs and symptoms of alcohol withdrawal in an at-risk ICU patient?**
When alcohol intake is abruptly stopped, central nervous system (CNS) excitation may result within a few hours, and tachycardia, hypertension, hyperreflexia, tremor, anxiety, irritability, sweating, nausea, or vomiting may be present, typically peaking with 24–48 hours. Neuronal excitation occurs within 12–24 hours of abstinence and may result in epileptiform seizures in severe cases. Delirium tremens, characterized by visual and auditory hallucinations, disorientation, confusion, altered consciousness, inattention, and profound autonomic hyperactivity may result after the prodromal signs and symptoms of alcohol withdrawal occur, followed by the possibility of death if alcohol withdrawal is unrecognized. The individual response to alcohol withdrawal varies, and patients may exhibit only a few signs and symptoms, although alcohol withdrawal should be considered when a history of long-standing or heavy alcohol consumption is present.

3. **What is the time course for development and the incidence of delirium tremens?**
Delirium tremens is a life-threatening syndrome that is marked by severe neuronal hyperexcitation that usually presents 3–5 days after cessation of alcohol intake with a typical duration of less than 1 week, although the syndrome may present much later (after 1–2 weeks of hospitalization). Delirium tremens occurs in approximately 5% of hospitalized alcoholics and has an associated mortality rate ranging from 1% to 15%.

4. **How often do seizures occur related to withdrawal of alcohol use?**
Between 2% and 5% of alcoholics experience withdrawal seizures, which are usually generalized. These seizures typically occur within 48 hours of the last drink but may occur at any time within the first week of withdrawal. Patients who have a history of previous detoxifications or non–alcohol-related admissions in the past are at an increased risk for the development of withdrawal seizures, known as the "kindling effect." The kindling hypothesis states that every withdrawal episode acts as an irritative phenomenon to the brain, and the accumulation of several alcohol withdrawal episodes tends to lower the seizure threshold.

5. **Does a reliable questionnaire exist to assess the risk of alcohol withdrawal in ICU patients?**
   The CAGE questionnaire consists of four questions:
   - **Cut down:** Have you felt you should cut down on your alcohol consumption?
   - **Annoyed:** Have people annoyed you by criticizing your drinking?
   - **Guilt:** Have you felt guilty about your drinking?
   - **Eye opener:** Have you ever had a drink first thing in the morning (i.e., had an eye opener) to steady your nerves or to get rid of a hangover?

   Patients who respond with any "yes" response should be monitored, and those with three "yes" responses are at high risk of alcohol withdrawal. Unfortunately, in the ICU patient population, most patients are unable to respond due to multiple factors (e.g., mechanical ventilation, sedative and analgesic requirements, extent of injury or critical disease states), and family members may not be reliable sources of pertinent alcohol history.

6. **Which medication class represents the treatment of choice for alcohol withdrawal?**
   Benzodiazepines are the most effective therapy for the prevention and treatment of alcohol withdrawal because they produce a reduction in withdrawal severity, a decreased incidence of delirium tremens, and the ability to reduce seizure risk. Benzodiazepines are effective, in part, because of the cross-tolerance with ethanol at the type A γ-aminobutyric acid (GABA) receptor.

7. **Why is lorazepam the preferred benzodiazepine for the prevention and treatment of alcohol withdrawal in the ICU?**
   Lorazepam represents the preferred benzodiazepine within the intensive care setting for acute prevention or treatment of alcohol withdrawal because of its relatively short half-life, lack of active metabolites, decreased rate of oversedation, ease of titration, absence of a need to adjust therapy in renal failure, and IV availability for either bolus dosing or continuous infusion administration. Although accumulation can still occur and oversedation must constantly be reassessed, lorazepam's metabolism is less dependent on patient age and hepatic function. On transfer to a step-down unit within the hospital, longer-acting benzodiazepines such as diazepam or chlordiazepoxide may be preferred because of their sustained therapeutic effect; however, the risk of oversedation must not be disregarded.

   Peppers MP: Benzodiazepines for alcohol withdrawal in the elderly and in patients with liver disease. Pharmacotherapy 16:49–58, 1996.

8. **Should propofol be considered for refractory delirium tremens?**
   Propofol's mechanism of action is similar to that of ethanol, affecting both glutamate and GABA receptors within the CNS. If symptoms are not well controlled with high-dose benzodiazepines (e.g., greater than lorazepam 20–30 mg/h), a propofol infusion may be considered for an intubated patient as an alternative strategy to control severe delirium tremens. Chronic alcoholism results in only minor alterations in propofol pharmacokinetics. Doses greater than 83 μg/kg/min should be avoided to prevent the development of propofol-infusion syndrome, a rare but potentially fatal complication associated with severe metabolic acidosis, rhabdomyolysis, cardiac dysrhythmias, and cardiovascular collapse.

   McCowan C, Marik P: Refractory delirium tremens treated with propofol: A case series. Crit Care Med 28:1781–1784, 2000.

9. **Are adjunctive therapies available for the prevention and treatment of alcohol withdrawal?**
   Beta blockers, clonidine, carbamazepine, and valproic acid are adjunctive therapies that decrease withdrawal severity. However, their effect on seizures and delirium are less well studied. Beta

blockers reduce autonomic manifestations of acute alcohol withdrawal but possess no anticonvulsant activity, and delirium is an adverse event associated with therapy. The alpha agonist clonidine may be beneficial to decrease withdrawal symptoms in patients exhibiting hypertension and tachycardia. The anticonvulsant carbamazepine does not result in potentiation of the CNS depression caused by alcohol, but it manifests a high frequency of adverse effects (e.g., dizziness, nausea, vomiting). Similar to carbamazepine, valproic acid raises GABA levels in the CNS and has also demonstrated reduced withdrawal symptoms. None of these adjunctive agents should be used in place of benzodiazepine therapy, but rather as additional add-on therapy when symptoms necessitate this action.

Kosten TR, O'Connor PG: Management of drug and alcohol withdrawal. N Engl J Med 348:1786–1795, 2003.

KEY POINTS: PHARMACOLOGIC THERAPIES FOR ALCOHOL WITHDRAWAL

1. Benzodiazepines are the drug of choice for all patients.

2. Lorazepam is the most appropriate benzodiazepine for patients in intensive care.

3. Beta blockers and clonidine are useful adjunctive therapy for hypertension/tachycardia.

4. Carbamazepine or valproic acid, but not phenytoin, also reduce withdrawal symptoms.

10. **In patients at risk for alcohol withdrawal, should treatment be initiated on a symptom-triggered or fixed-schedule basis?**
The literature suggests that symptom-triggered therapy is preferred due to lower total benzodiazepine requirements and shorter duration of treatment compared with fixed-schedule therapy for alcohol withdrawal. However, the majority of data are derived from patients in non-ICU settings, such as inpatient detoxification units. Thus, as-needed versus scheduled benzodiazepine therapy is controversial when applied to an ICU patient because multiple signs and symptoms may be masked due to the increased severity of illness and unresponsiveness of many critically ill patients.

Spies CD, Otter HE, Hüske B, et al: Alcohol withdrawal severity is decreased by symptom-oriented adjusted bolus therapy in the ICU. Intensive Care Med 29:2230–2238, 2003.

11. **Is there a role for supplemental ethanol during alcohol withdrawal in the ICU?**
The use of supplemental ethanol in critically ill patients with a secondary diagnosis of alcohol withdrawal is quite controversial. Proponents of ethanol administration state that patients are less sedated and the risk of respiratory depression is decreased compared with benzodiazepine therapy, with a resultant "smoother" management of alcohol withdrawal. Disadvantages of this approach are related in part to IV ethanol exhibiting zero-order elimination leading to unpredictable pharmacokinetics as well as a narrow therapeutic index. Controlled clinical trials have not demonstrated enhanced efficacy with IV ethanol compared with standard treatment, with reports of continued progression of alcohol withdrawal despite IV ethanol and no decreased effect on the development of symptoms, length of ICU stay, or major complications. Of note, the available literature consists only of clinical studies that used IV ethanol infusions. Enteral administration forms of alcohol have not been studied and may represent some benefit in complicated patient conditions or when a contraindication to a benzodiazepine exists for secondary alcohol withdrawal management in the ICU.

Hodges B, Mazur JE: Intravenous ethanol for the treatment of alcohol withdrawal syndrome in critically ill patients. Pharmacotherapy 24:1578–1585, 2004.

12. **Do alcohol withdrawal clinical pathways improve care?**

Alcohol pathways are useful within the inpatient hospital setting to screen and identify patients who are at risk of developing withdrawal symptoms and to treat the symptoms appropriately. They are often used for patients in whom alcohol withdrawal is a secondary diagnosis that is revealed upon use of a risk screening tool, such as a substance abuse assessment questionnaire. Pathways also have the advantage of facilitating intervention for the underlying alcoholism after discharge. The Clinical Institute Withdrawal Assessment for Alcohol revised scale is a validated, reliable measure of the current severity of alcohol withdrawal composed of 10 items: nausea and vomiting; tremor; autonomic hyperactivity; anxiety; agitation; tactile, auditory, and visual disturbances, headache-related problems; and disorientation. Although this scale is useful for communicative patients who can answer questions, ICU patients with multiple comorbidities may not be able to answer questions because of sedation, mechanical ventilation and related issues. Whatever method is chosen, all patients at risk must be closely monitored for symptoms of alcohol withdrawal.

Sullivan JT, Sykora K, Schneiderman J, et al: Assessment of alcohol withdrawal: The revised Clinical Institute Withdrawal Assessment for Alcohol scale (CIWA-Ar). Br J Addict 84:1353–1357, 1989.

CHAPTER 66

HEAD TRAUMA

David C. Bonovich, MD

1. **What is the epidemiology of traumatic brain injury (TBI) in the United States?**
   TBI ranks second to stroke as a cause of death from neurologic disorders. In the United States alone, approximately 1.4 million people experience head injuries each year; 270,000 require hospitalization; 52,000 die; and 80,000–90,000 incur long-term neurologic disability. The adjusted annual incidence as of 2002 was listed at 79 per 100,000 persons. A report covering the incidence of head trauma in 12 states found that persons older than 75 years of age had the highest incidence (265 per 100,000) followed by persons aged 15–24 years (103 per 100,000). Men were hospitalized approximately twice as often as women. The overall morality rate is listed at 24 per 100,000.

   Centers for Disease Control and Prevention: Incidence rates of hospitalization related to traumatic brain injury—12 states, 2002. MMWR 55:201–204, 2006.

2. **What are the leading causes of head trauma?**
   Motor vehicle crashes, 49%; falls, 28%; all others, 23%. Worldwide, motor vehicle crashes are the leading cause of TBI-related death in young people, and falls are the leading cause in persons older than 65 years of age. A recent paper citing a report from West Virginia reported an average death rate of 23.6 per 100,000 persons. Firearms are responsible for 39% of deaths; motor vehicles, 34%; and falls, 10%. Among firearm-related deaths, the majority result from suicide.

   Leon-Carrion J, Dominguez-Morales R, Barroso Y, et al: Epidemiology of traumatic brain injury and subarachnoid hemorrhage. Pituitary 8:197–202, 2005.

3. **What is the mortality rate associated with severe head trauma?**
   Mortality and morbidity rates are related to increased intracranial pressure (ICP). For patients with severe TBI and ICP < 20 mmHg, the mortality rate is about 20%; for those with ICP > 20 mmHg, the mortality rate is close to 50%. For patients with severe TBI and ICP > 40 mmHg, the mortality rate approaches 75%; for patients with ICP > 60 mmHg, the mortality rate approaches 100%.

4. **What factors are important in predicting outcome from severe head trauma?**
   Factors associated with a poor neurologic outcome include:
   - Intracranial hematoma
   - Impaired or absent pupillary response to light on initial examination
   - Increasing age
   - Early systemic insults: hypotension, hypercarbia, and/or hypoxemia
   - Abnormal motor response

5. **What is the Glasgow Coma Scale? Why is it important?**
   Developed in 1974 by the neurosurgical department at the University of Glasgow, the scale was an attempt to standardize the assessment of the depth and duration of impaired consciousness and coma, particularly in the setting of trauma. The scale is based on eye opening, verbal responses, and motor responses (Table 66-1). Of these, motor response is the most sensitive and correlates best with neurologic outcome. A score of 15 is possible in a completely awake and oriented patient. A score < 8 indicates significant brain injury and the possible need for airway protection.

TABLE 66-1. GLASGOW COMA SCALE

Eye Opening		Motor Response		Best Verbal Response	
Spontaneous	4	Obeys command	6	Oriented	5
To speech	3	Localizes pain	5	Confused	4
To pain	2	Withdraws from pain	4	Inappropriate	3
None	1	Flexes to pain	3	Incomprehensible	2
		Extends to pain	1	None	1
		None	0		

6. **What is the significance of primary versus secondary head injury?**
   - **Primary injury:** Primary injury occurs at the time of impact and can be separated into two phases: (1) the phase resulting from the inciting event and giving rise to contusions, lacerations, and/or axonal injury; (2) evolution of the primary injury. Primary injury cannot be treated directly because there is no treatment for the sudden mechanical disruption of brain tissue.
   - **Secondary brain injury:** This term refers to additional injury and may occur in the hours and days after the primary injury. Secondary injury is the leading cause of hospital death. Hypoxia and hypotension are the most common causes of secondary brain injury. *Hypotension,* defined as a single systolic blood pressure measurement below 90 mmHg, may be associated with a doubling of the mortality rate and an increase in morbidity of patients with TBI. Other causes of secondary injury include intracranial hematomas (e.g., subdural, epidural, and parenchymal) and generalized cerebral edema, resulting in elevated ICP. Seizures are also a cause of secondary brain injury.

     Because primary brain injury cannot be treated directly, the brain must be protected from secondary injury and elevated ICP to provide an optimal environment for spontaneous recovery.

     Cernak I: Animal models of head trauma. NeuroRx 2:410–422, 2005.

7. **What are the important considerations for intubating patients with head trauma?**
   - Associated cervical spine fractures occur in 5–10% of patients with head injury. This often depends on the mechanism of injury (e.g., motor vehicle crashes, fall > gunshot wound). Care should be taken to avoid hyperextension of the neck at the time of intubation. Awake intubation, axial traction, and cricothyrotomy are appropriate options in head-injured patients.
   - Patients are considered to have "full stomachs" and should undergo awake intubation or rapid-sequence induction to avoid possible aspiration of stomach contents.
   - Patients with associated traumatic injuries are often hypovolemic, and care should be taken in administering induction drugs to avoid hypotension.
   - Care should be taken to avoid coughing and straining on the endotracheal tube, both of which result in a marked increase in ICP.
   - Associated maxillofacial and neck injuries should be noted because they may increase the difficulty of intubation.
   - Nasal intubations are contraindicated in patients with basilar skull or LeFort fractures.

8. **What clues suggest the presence of a basilar skull fracture?**
   Basilar skull fractures result in hemotympanum, ecchymosis over the mastoid area (i.e., Battle's sign), or periorbital ecchymosis (i.e., raccoon's eyes).

9. **What percentage of adult patients with head injury experience intracranial hematoma?**
About 40% of head-injured patients experience intracranial hematoma as a result of head injuries. Of these, an estimated 40% are intracerebral, 20% are subdural, and another 20% are epidural.

10. **Why is intracranial hematoma significant?**
Immediate surgical intervention is imperative if patients are to survive. Types of intracranial hemorrhage include subdural and epidural hematoma as well as hematomas associated with brain contusions. In a review of 82 severely head-injured patients with significant subdural hematoma (>5 mm midline shift or hemorrhagic contusion > 2 cm on computed tomography [CT] scan), early surgical evacuation was shown to have a remarkable impact on survival. Patients taken to surgery more than 4 hours after injury had a 90% mortality rate. Evacuation of subdural hematomas within 2 hours after injury may decrease mortality rates by up to 70%.

Seelig JM, Becker DP, Miller JD, et al: Traumatic acute subdural hematoma: Major mortality reduction in comatose patients treated within 4 hours. N Engl J Med 304:1511–1518, 1981.

11. **Describe the physiology of ICP and how ICP is affected by head trauma.**
According to the Monro-Kellie hypothesis, the skull can be considered a closed container inside of which there are three volumes: brain, blood, and cerebrospinal fluid (CSF). Each of these volumes exerts a pressure, and for the pressure inside the skull to remain constant, an increase in the volume of one component must be offset by a decrease in one of the others. Because the brain is considered an unchanging volume, the ICP reflects a reciprocal relationship between the volumes of blood and CSF inside the intracranial compartment. Head trauma can result in increased ICP. An increase in mass due to cerebral edema or hematoma must be accompanied by an increase in venous outflow or CSF volume, or both, to maintain normal ICP.
  Physiologic compensatory mechanisms include the displacement and absorption of CSF together with spontaneous hyperventilation causing a decrease in the $PaCO_2$ and vasoconstriction at the arteriolar level, which in turn decreases cerebral blood volume. If these mechanisms do not provide adequate compensation, the ICP will rise. This fact is demonstrated by the intracranial compliance curve shown in Fig. 66-1. This pressure-volume curve demonstrates a "critical" volume (the knee in the curve), above which compensatory mechanisms are not effective in the noncompliant cranium.

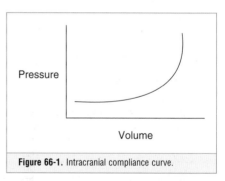

Figure 66-1. Intracranial compliance curve.

12. **How is ICP monitored?**
The three commonly used methods to monitor ICP are the intraventricular catheter, the subarachnoid screw, and the epidural transducer. See a review by Miller and colleagues for further details. Most authorities now believe that, whenever feasible, an intraventricular catheter should be placed so that ICP can be monitored; at the same time, CSF may be removed to treat elevations in ICP.

Miller JD, Butterworth JF, Gudeman SK, et al: Further experience in the management of severe head injury. J Neurosurg 54:288–299, 1981.

13. **What are the mechanisms by which head injury elevates ICP?**
  ■ Increased mass resulting from intracranial hematoma formation
  ■ Cerebral edema resulting from disruption of cell membranes and blood–brain barrier

- Increased blood volume resulting from loss of autoregulation
- Increased CSF volume resulting from an obstruction to flow by edema or clot formation

14. **How does elevated ICP worsen outcome?**

The elevation in ICP without an equivalent rise in systemic mean arterial pressure (MAP) results in a decrease in the cerebral perfusion pressure (CPP) and the risk of brain ischemia. To understand this, one must first understand the concepts of CPP and autoregulation. The ICP can be viewed as the resistive force that blood going into the skull must overcome; therefore, the pressure of the blood inside the skull is the difference between the MAP and the ICP. Thus,

$$CPP = MAP - ICP$$

Blood flow to the brain is autoregulated both from a pressure standpoint and a metabolic standpoint. *Pressure autoregulation* means that within a range of pressures (usually given as a MAP between 50 and 150 mmHg), the blood flow remains the same. In metabolic autoregulation, blood flow is directed toward the area of greatest metabolic need. ICP seems to have a greater impact on pressure autoregulation because an ICP that would decrease intracranial MAP (or CPP) below the threshold for pressure autoregulation would create a situation called *pressure dependency* in which the blood flow to the brain is directly related to the CPP.

Ideally, to obtain a continuous measure of CPP, an arterial line should be placed at the time of ICP monitor placement. This allows accurate moment-to-moment measurement of the systemic MAP and calculation of CPP. The calculation of CPP requires that both transducers be placed at the level of the external auditory canal. A normal ICP is <10 mmHg. An elevation in ICP > 20 mmHg in a resting patient for more than a few minutes may be associated with a significant increase in morbidity. An ICP > 40 mmHg is considered life threatening. A normal CPP is approximately 80–90 mmHg. Previously, a CPP > 60 mmHg was considered adequate to prevent brain ischemia. Currently, however, the minimal CPP in patients with TBI is controversial.

15. **What are plateau waves?**

In 1960, Lundberg published observations of variations in ICP in 143 patients. He demonstrated that ICP may rise to very high levels and that increased ICP cannot be reliably predicted on clinical grounds alone. He also demonstrated the variability of ICP waves over time and described three specific patterns of variation:

- **A waves:** These periods of extremely elevated ICP (50–100 mmHg) last 5–20 minutes. They may be superimposed on an elevated baseline and also may be associated with a marked decrease in CPP. A waves are also called *plateau waves*.
- **B waves:** These high-frequency oscillations (0.5–2/min) result in pressures between 0 and 50 mmHg. Although they are not always pathologic, they often progress to A waves.
- **C waves:** These are small rhythmic oscillations in pressure at a frequency of 4–8/min. They are associated with ICP measurements of 0–20 mmHg and are considered normal.

The presence of plateau waves suggests that pressure autoregulation is intact but that the CPP is on the on the right edge of the autoregulation, explaining the observation that an increase in blood pressure—and therefore, CPP—can abort a plateau wave in some cases.

Lundberg N: Continuous recording and control of ventricular fluid pressure in neurosurgical practice. Acta Psychiatr Neurol Scand 36(Suppl 149):1–193, 1960.

Rosner MJ Daughton S: Cerebral perfusion pressure management in head injury. J Trauma 30:933–941, 1990.

16. **Which patients should be monitored for increased ICP?**

A review of 207 head-injured patients by Narayan and colleagues in 1982 suggested that two groups of patients should be routinely monitored:

1. Patients with abnormal CT scans on admission (high-density lesion consistent with hemorrhage or low-density lesion consistent with contusion)
2. Patients with normal CT scans who demonstrate two or more of the following adverse features on admission:
   - Systolic blood pressure < 90 mmHg
   - Age > 40 years
   - Unilateral or bilateral motor posturing
   Patients who are not routinely monitored should have a repeat CT head scan at 12–24 hours. This study showed that 96% of patients with normal CT scans and fewer than two adverse features had normal ICPs throughout their ICU course, whereas 53–63% of patients with abnormal CT scans developed elevated ICP.

Narayan R, Kishore P, Becker DP, et al: Intracranial pressure: To monitor or not to monitor? J Neurosurg 56:650–659, 1982.

17. **What are the overall targets for treatment in patients with head injury?**
    1. Management and protection of the airway
    2. Controlled ventilation to maintain normal or slightly lower PCO_2
    3. Appropriate triage to early surgery (<4 hours after injury)
    4. Maintenance of cerebral blood flow
    5. Treatment of elevated ICP
    6. Evaluation and treatment of secondary systemic disorders:
       - Gastrointestinal bleeding
       - Disseminated intravascular coagulopathy
       - Neurogenic pulmonary edema
       - Endocrine abnormalities (e.g., diabetes insipidus, syndrome of inappropriate antidiuretic hormone)
       - Hypotension resulting from hemorrhagic or spinal shock
       - Hypoxemia resulting from chest trauma or aspiration

18. **Describe specific treatment for the prevention of secondary brain injury in patients with head injury.**
    Concepts in the treatment of TBI have been evolving over recent years. Previously, ICP-directed therapies and maintenance of adequate CPP through manipulation of blood pressure combined with aggressive treatment of elevations in ICP have been the focus of treatment, and indeed especially CPP-driven therapies still remain at the core of treatment. However, new approaches are being attempted as we gain more understanding of brain physiology through the use of existing methods of neuromonitoring and newer methods that are being developed and validated.
    ICP-directed therapies aim specifically at the treatment of increased ICP. There are several means by which this is accomplished:
    - Elevation of the head of the bed to > 20 degrees to enhance venous drainage
    - Hyperventilation to a PCO_2 of 25–30 mmHg for short periods in the acute setting
    - Mannitol, 0.5–1.0 gm/kg emergently, then every 1–3 hours to maintain a serum osmolarity between 295 and 315 mOsm
    - Furosemide, 0.5 mg/kg, to reduce CSF production, but caution is necessary to avoid dehydration
    - Drainage of CSF from ventriculostomy catheter (most effective in obstructive hydrocephalus, least effective in diffuse edema with narrowed ventricles)
    - Surgical decompression to remove hematoma or necrotic injured brain
    - Attention to head positioning to avoid jugular venous compression and obstruction to the cranial venous outflow tract
    - Pentobarbital coma in hemodynamically stable patients with refractory intracranial hypertension
    - Seizure prophylaxis to prevent the increase in ICP associated with seizures

CPP-guided therapy is based on the idea of (1) manipulating blood pressure to ensure adequate perfusion to areas that are either presumed to be ischemic or thought to be at risk for the development of ischemia and (2) treating elevations in ICP with drainage of spinal fluid, osmotic agents, and sedation. The recommended threshold for CPP is 70 mmHg. More recently, the use of specific CPP thresholds has been questioned. Recent data suggest that lower CPP thresholds might be better tolerated, and individualizing thresholds for CPP might have some benefit.

The "Lund concept" has been advocated more recently. The Lund concept differs considerably from the CPP concept. The former attempts to lower ICP by minimizing or preventing cerebral edema and decreasing intracerebral blood volume via metabolic suppression and by using agents that cause venoconstriction. According to this concept, a lower CPP will limit the development of cerebral edema.

It may turn out that all of these concepts might be applicable in a given patient such that therapy in TBI may eventually become individualized and targeted depending on the mechanism of injury and individual patient response.

Brain Trauma Foundation, American Association of Neurological Surgeons, Joint Section on Neurotrauma and Critical Care: Guidelines for cerebral perfusion pressure. J Neurotrauma 17:507–511, 2000.

Diringer M: What do we really understand about head injury? Neurocrit Car 2:3–4, 2005.

Nordstrom L: Physiological and biochemical principles underlying volume-targeted therapy—The "Lund concept." Neurocrit Care 2:83–96, 2005.

19. **Discuss some of the neuromonitoring devices currently used in the treatment of TBI.**

    The goal of neuromonitoring is to provide a means of early detection of insults and events that might trigger secondary brain injury so that interventions can be made in a timely manner.

    - **ICP monitors:** The use of ICP monitors is important in monitoring ICP so that therapy can be instituted when ICP is elevated to pathologic levels. The types of ICP monitors have been described elsewhere.
    - **Jugular venous oxygen saturation monitors:** One of the first technologies for determining metabolic needs in the brain was jugular venous oxygen saturation monitors ($SjvO_2$). $SjvO_2$ allows an assessment to be made of the delivery and use of oxygen in the brain via the measurement of arteriovenous O_2 saturation differences ($AVDO_2$). The use of $SjvO_2$ requires an assessment of blood hemoglobin and a calculation of the $AVDO_2$ and can be used to determine oxygen extraction in the brain.
    - **Brain tissue oximetry** (BtO_2): BtO_2 is a newer technology that is sensitive to focal ischemic changes that might be missed using $SjvO_2$ monitors. Oxygen moves by passive diffusion from red blood cells to the brain parenchyma. Thus, the O_2 tension in the tissues is reflective of regional cerebral blood flow. As experience with this technology grows, investigators are starting to determine ischemic thresholds for cerebral oxygen tension.
    - **Continuous cerebral blood flow monitors:** These monitors have been introduced using laser Doppler or thermal diffusion technologies. The use of this modality is limited due to its recent introduction, but it is hoped it will allow better assessment and understanding of cerebral blood flow in the future.

    Brigham and Women's Hospital Neurosurgery Group: Principles of cerebral oxygenation and blood flow in the neurological critical care unit. Neurocrit Care 4:77–92, 2006.

20. **How does hyperventilation decrease ICP?**

    Hyperventilation decreases ICP by producing cerebral vasoconstriction and a resultant decrease in cerebral blood flow. There is a relatively linear relationship between PCO_2 of 20–80 mmHg and cerebral blood flow (Fig. 66-2).

    This effect is mediated through acute alterations in cerebral interstitial fluid pH; therefore, it generally becomes less effective after 48–72 hours. Currently, hyperventilation is used to bring

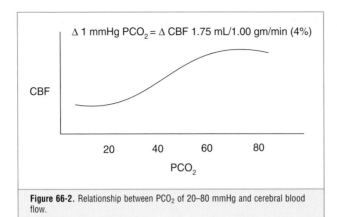

Figure 66-2. Relationship between PCO_2 of 20–80 mmHg and cerebral blood flow.

ICP under control in the acute setting before other decreasing measures can be introduced. If used prophylactically and for long periods, the vasoconstrictive effects of hyperventilation may cause ischemia and worsen outcome. Thus, most authorities recommend that hyperventilation be used only for the acute short-term management of increased ICP.

KEY POINTS: HEAD TRAUMA

1. Traumatic brain injury ranks second behind stroke as a neurologic cause of mortality.

2. The leading cause of morbidity in hospitalized patients with traumatic brain injury is secondary brain injury.

3. For every decrease in systolic blood pressure below 90 mmHg, there is a doubling of mortality and an increase in morbidity.

4. Treatment strategies are aimed at the prevention of secondary brain injury through maintenance of adequate cerebral perfusion and control of ICP.

21. **How does mannitol decrease ICP?**
    Brain tissue has slightly higher osmolarity than blood, with a gradient of approximately 3 mOsm/L maintained by the blood–brain barrier. Mannitol is an osmotically active agent that reverses this osmotic gradient and shifts water from the brain to the blood. An increase in blood osmolarity by 10mOsm/L removes 100–150 mL of water from the brain.

    Hyperosmolar treatment of elevated ICP increases the normal serum osmolarity of 290 to 300–315 mOsm/L. An osmolarity < 300 mOsm/L is not so effective; > 315 mOsm/L results in renal and neurologic dysfunction.

    Over the past several years, the use of hypertonic saline has become used increasingly for osmolar treatment of increased ICP. Hypertonic saline appears to have at least equal efficacy in lowering ICP, and the effect appears to be more prolonged than that of mannitol.

    Qureshi AI, Suarez JI: Use of hypertonic solutions in treatment of cerebral edema and intracranial hypertension. Crit Care Med 28:3301–3313, 2000.

22. **Discuss the role of barbiturates in the treatment of head injury.**
    Barbiturates result in a decrease in the cerebral metabolic rate that may result in a decrease in cerebral blood flow requirements and theoretically should work to lower ICP. They may be effective in lowering ICP and decreasing mortality in the setting of refractory elevation of ICP. However, no data support the prophylactic use of barbiturates. If used, barbiturates must be titrated with caution in patients with head injury because they result in systemic hypotension that, if not adequately treated, results in a detrimental decrease in CPP.

23. **Is there a role for steroids in the treatment of head injury?**
    Steroids are not useful in the treatment of head injury. No data indicate an improved outcome or suggest that they lower ICP in the setting of head injury.

XII. SURGERY AND TRAUMA

BURNS

James C. Jeng, MD, and Mark W. Bowyer, MD, DMCC, COL, USAF, MC

CHAPTER 67

1. **What amount of heat is required to cause contact burn injury?**
   The severity of a contact thermal injury is related to temperature and duration of contact. A heat source less than 45°C (113°F) will result in no injury, regardless of exposure. As the heat intensity increases, the duration of exposure necessary to cause a significant burn decreases. Exposure to water at 54°C (129.2°F) for 30 seconds causes a partial-thickness burn.

2. **What are the initial priorities in the management of burns?**
   1. Stop the burning process.
   2. Attend to the ABCs of standard trauma resuscitation (i.e., airway, breathing, and circulation).
   3. Assume carbon monoxide poisoning for any patient burned in a closed space, and administer 100% oxygen by a nonrebreather mask.
   4. For very small burns, provide rapid but brief rinsing under cool water; this may reduce the amount of tissue destruction. Do *not* use for large burns because hypothermia will result.
   5. Cover the patient with a clean sheet for comfort and to conserve body heat.
   6. Transport promptly to a hospital or burn unit.
      Overzealous fluid resuscitation is the most common mistake in pre–burn unit care.

3. **How is the depth of a burn categorized?**
   The depth of burns are classified as first-, second-, or third-degree. Unusually deep thermal injuries that extend into soft tissues beneath the skin are called *fourth-degree injuries*.
   - **First-degree:** First-degree burns are the most superficial type and involve only the epidermis. This is exemplified by a sunburn. Healing occurs in less than 1 week.
   - **Second-degree:** Second-degree burns or partial-thickness burns are subcategorized into *superficial* and *deep*. Superficial dermal injuries are produced by brief exposures to hot liquids or flames. The skin is bright red and moist with blisters and is extremely hypersensitive. Healing occurs in 10–21 days. Deep dermal injuries, caused by more prolonged exposure to hot liquids or flames, are characterized by dark red or yellow-white skin with large bullae. Healing is very slow, taking longer than 3 weeks, and often results in marked hypertrophic scar formation.
   - **Third-degree:** In third-degree or full-thickness burns, the entire dermis is destroyed, and the burn has a pearly white, charred, or parchment-like appearance. The burn is dry and leathery with thrombosed vessels visible through the eschar. It is hypalgesic because the cutaneous nerves are destroyed. Reepithelialization will never occur, and closure by skin grafting or plastic surgery is required.

   Shakespeare P: Burn wound healing and skin substitutes. Burns 27:517–522, 2001.

4. **How is the extent of burn injury estimated?**
   - In determining the extent of burns, first-degree burns are ignored.
   - For adults, the portion of the body involved with second- and third-degree burns can be estimated using the "rule of nines." This rule divides the body into segments, each of which represents roughly 9% of the total body surface area: 9% for the head and neck and each upper extremity; 18% for each lower extremity, the anterior trunk, and the posterior trunk; and 1% for the genitalia and perineum.

- In pediatric patients, the head and neck comprise a greater percentage and the lower extremities a lesser. Therefore, for an accurate estimate, a burn chart is needed.
- Small burns and irregularly shaped burns can be estimated using the surface of a patient's hand as representative of 1% of the total body surface.

Oliver RI, Spain D: Burns, resuscitation and early management: www.emedicine.com/plastic/topic159.htm

5. **What are the indications for referral to a burn center?**
The following are American Burn Association–sanctioned guidelines for transfer to a burn center:
- Full-thickness burns > 5% total body surface area
- Burns > 20% total body surface area (TBSA) in patients 10–50 years of age
- Burns > 10% TBSA in patients younger than 10 or older than 50 years
- Significant burns involving the face, hands, feet, genitalia, or joints
- Significant electrical, chemical, or inhalation injury
- Preexisting illness or concomitant trauma that could complicate management and increase mortality rates

6. **How do you resuscitate burn shock?**
The two most common formulae for burn shock resuscitation are the Parkland formula and the modified Brooke formula. Both formulae estimate the patient's fluid requirements for the first 24 hours after a burn. One-half of the estimate is given over the first 8 hours, and the second half is administered over the next 16 hours. The Parkland formula estimates the fluid needs as 4 mL/kg body weight/% TBSA burns (lactated Ringer's solution); the modified Brooke formula estimates the fluid requirement as 2 mL/kg/% (also lactated Ringer's solution). These formulae serve only to determine an initial fluid rate, which is then continuously adjusted to achieve an hourly urine output between 30 and 50 mL in a 70-kg adult.

Yowler CJ, Fratianne RB: Current status of burn resuscitation. Clin Plast Surg 27:1–10, 2000.

7. **What factors determine a burn patient's prognosis?**
The three major factors influencing a burn patient's survival are the extent of the burn, age, and presence or absence of inhalation injury. Larger burns, extremes of age, and patients with inhalation injury fare worse. The standard statistic for assessing the patient's mortality is the LA50: the TBSA of the burn associated with death in 50% of patients (i.e., lethal area) having burns of that extent. For young adults (15–40 years of age), the LA50 is approximately 70%.

8. **What is the overarching principle of burn wound care?**
Contemporary burn wound (deep second- and third-degree) care revolves around the basic concept of early excision and grafting. All wounds should be closed by 21 days, either by self-healing or by skin grafting.

9. **What is the role of systemic antibiotics in burn care?**
There is no role for prophylactic systemic antibiotics in burn injury. Major burns are constantly bacteremic. Systemic antibiotics are reserved only for *bona fide* infection or septicemia.

10. **What about topical antibacterial treatments?**
In the United States, two topical agents are most commonly used: mafenide acetate (Sulfamylon) and silver sulfadiazine (Silvadene).
- **Sulfamylon cream:** This agent has the advantages of excellent gram-negative coverage and good eschar penetration. Its disadvantages are pain when it is applied to partial-thickness burns and metabolic acidosis resulting from inhibition of carbonic anhydrase.

- **Silvadene cream:** This agent has enhanced yeast coverage and is painless on application; however, it has decreased eschar penetration and decreased gram-negative coverage. Furthermore, it may cause myeloid toxicity manifested by granulocytopenia.

Several other topical agents are beginning to become more widely accepted (e.g., Acticoat, Aquacel Ag). Most of these agents contain elemental silver as the active antibacterial ingredient. Cerium nitrate added to Silvadene is commonly used outside the United States; it significantly enhances the ability to prevent burn wound sepsis.

Dunn K, Edwards-Jones V: The role of Acticoat with nanocrystalline silver in the management of burns. Burns 30(Suppl 1):S1–S9, 2004.

Sheridan RL, Tompkins RG: What's new in burns and metabolism. J Am Coll Surg 198:243–263, 2004.

11. **How is an invasive burn wound infection treated?**
Immediate excision is the fundamental, compulsory therapy. Topical and systemic antibiotics (after excision) are important adjuvant treatments.

12. **When should you suspect, then diagnose inhalation injury?**
Inhalation injury is common in patients with an impaired mental status (e.g., with alcohol or drug use), in trauma patients, and in patients who have been burned in a closed space. Definitive diagnosis is made by bronchoscopic confirmation of soot or erythema in the trachea. The occurrence of a burn in an open area does not preclude inhalation injury. In patients diagnosed with inhalation injuries, up to 30% sustained their burns in an open area.

- The most sensitive physical finding indicative of inhalation injury is facial burns. Ninety percent of patients who have inhalation injury have facial burns. This finding, however, is not highly specific, as only 50% of patients with facial burns have inhalation injury.
- Other physical findings suggestive of inhalation injury are inflammation of the oropharyngeal mucosa, singed nasal hair, hoarseness, stridor, wheezing, and rales. Carbonaceous sputum, although pathognomonic for inhalation injury, is present less than half of the time.

13. **How are inhalation injuries managed?**
- The flexible fiberoptic bronchoscope is used for diagnosing and managing airway injury. The patient can be examined with an endotracheal tube threaded over the bronchoscope. Significant supraglottic edema mandates immediate intubation.
- Lesser degrees of airway edema are managed with humidified air, elevation of the head of the bed, and maintenance of intubation preparations and precautions.
- Management of lower airway injury is entirely supportive (ventilator) and involves treating the chemical pneumonitis-derived pulmonary edema and pneumonia, the two major consequences of lower airway injury.
- Prophylactic antibiotics and steroids are not beneficial.

McCall JE, Cahill TJ: Respiratory care of the burn patient. J Burn Care Rehabil 26:200–206, 2005.

14. **How is carbon monoxide poisoning diagnosed and managed?**
Carbon monoxide avidly binds to hemoglobin with an affinity 200 times greater than that of oxygen. This reduces the oxygen-delivering capacity of blood and causes tissue hypoxia. The clinical manifestations of carbon monoxide poisoning relate to the central nervous system and to the heart. Confusion, agitation, loss of consciousness, and myocardial depression can be seen. The classic cherry-red lips are seen infrequently. Diagnosis is confirmed by directly measuring carboxyhemoglobin levels.

Optimal therapy for carbon monoxide poisoning is 100% oxygen. Hyperbaric oxygen clearly accelerates carbon monoxide elimination. However, its superiority to normobaric 100% oxygen remains controversial.

15. **When should escharotomy be done?**
    Escharotomy should be considered in all circumferential burns that can impair circulation and or respiratory effort (as in burns to the chest).

KEY POINTS: BURNS

1. The burning process should be stopped as soon as possible.

2. Burn center care improves survival.

3. Common sense should be used in fluid resuscitation of burns, with urine output guiding ultimate amount.

4. Early excision and grafting are the keys to survival.

5. There is no role for prophylactic systemic antibiotic use in burn patients.

6. Inhalation injury and infection are the major causes of mortality.

7. If inhalation injury is suspected, intubate first and ask questions later.

16. **How are chemical burns managed?**
    - Chemical powders should be brushed away before skin lavage.
    - Acids can usually be removed by 30–60 minutes of water irrigation.
    - Alkalis, because of their greater tissue avidity, cause more severe damage and may require hours of lavage.
    - White phosphorus burns can be hazardous because the retained phosphorus particles ignite on exposure to air. These burns can be bathed with copper sulfate, which forms a cupric phosphide coating over the particles and impedes ignition. However, the absorbed copper may cause hemolysis and renal failure. Therefore, the safer approach is the continuous application of water-soaked dressings until the particles are removed. They can be identified under ultraviolet light in the operating room.
    - Hydrofluoric acid is a special case of acid injury and *does* require neutralization with calcium ions delivered topically or via direct tissue injection.

    Burd A: Hydrofluoric acid-revisited. Burns 30:720–722, 2004.
    Dunser MW, Ohlbauer M, Rieder J, et al: Critical care management of major hydrofluoric acid burns: A case report, review of the literature, and recommendations for therapy. Burns 30:391–398, 2004.

17. **How are electrical burns managed?**
    Patients with electrical injury frequently have considerably less cutaneous damage than deeper injury, which may lead to an underestimation of their fluid needs. Under-resuscitation coupled with rhabdomyolysis leads to renal failure. It is therefore important to maintain a brisk hourly urine output ($\sim$ 70–100 mL/h in a full-sized adult) in electrically injured patients and to consider alkalinizing the urine to prevent myoglobin precipitation in the renal tubules.
    - Deep muscle injury and the resultant edema commonly cause a compartment syndrome, necessitating fasciotomy.
    - Spinal compression fractures may occur due to tetanic muscle contractions and cataracts may develop, particularly in patients with a contact point on the head.

18. **What is the role of cardiac monitoring after electrical injury?**
    If a patient has a normal rhythm on cardiac monitoring in the trauma bay or emergency department and a normal 12-lead electrocardiogram, further rhythm monitoring is not routinely required.

19. **What are the systemic consequences of burn injury?**
    The systemic response to burn injury involves all organ systems; a biphasic pattern of early hypofunction and later hyperfunction characterizes the multisystem response to any injury.
    - As with any major injury, the body increases secretion of catecholamines, cortisol, glucagon, renin-angiotensin, antidiuretic hormone, and aldosterone. The consequence is a tendency toward retention of sodium and water and excretion of potassium by the kidney.
    - Profound hypermetabolism occurs after the burn, with an increase in metabolic rate and oxygen consumption, which remain elevated until the wound is covered.
    - The evaporative water loss from the wound may reach 300 mL/m^2/h, which markedly increases heat loss.
    - Immunologic abnormalities in patients with burns may predispose them to infection.

    Arturson G: Forty years in burns research—the postburn inflammatory response. Burns 26:599–604, 2000.
    Pereira CT, Murphy KD, Herndon DN: Altering metabolism. J Burn Care Rehabil 26:194–199, 2005.

20. **What are the nutritional requirements of patients with burns?**
    Burn patients demonstrate marked hypermetabolism and increased catabolism of lean body mass. Nutritional management is aimed at supplying total caloric and nitrogen needs to spare the body tissue mass as much as possible.
    - Total caloric requirements can be calculated with the formula:

    $$25 \text{ kcal} \times \text{body weight (kg)} + 40 \text{ kcal} \times \% \text{ TBSA burn}$$

    - Of the total calories, 20–25% should be protein.
    - Vitamins and minerals are supplied at two to three times the recommended daily allowance.
    - The preferred route is via the intestinal tract, with parenteral nutrition reserved only for patients unable to tolerate enteral nutrition.

21. **What are the major complications associated with burns?**
    Smoke inhalation remains the greatest overall cause of mortality in victims of fires in closed spaces. Infection remains the most frequent cause of morbidity and mortality resulting from burn wounds. With the advent of topical antimicrobials and early excision and grafting, pneumonia has emerged as the most common cause of life-threatening sepsis. Gastrointestinal complications include Curling's ulcers (stress ulceration of the stomach and duodenum in burn patients) and acalculous cholecystitis.

CHAPTER 68

THE ACUTE ABDOMEN

Jennifer Y. Wang, MD, and Madhulika G. Varma, MD

1. **What is an acute abdomen?**
   The term *acute abdomen* refers to the extreme end of the spectrum of abdominal pain. It is
   characterized by the sudden or gradual onset of moderate to severe abdominal pain that persists
   over several hours. The presentation can vary from pain and tenderness in one specific area
   of the abdomen to diffuse pain associated with septic shock.

2. **Name some nonsurgical causes of acute abdominal pain.**
   Numerous medical conditions can cause abdominal pain, obscuring one's ability to diagnose
   truly surgical conditions. These include myocardial infarction, pneumonia, sickle cell pain
   crisis, spontaneous bacterial peritonitis, infectious gastroenteritis, typhlitis, leukemia,
   pancreatitis, inflammatory bowel disease without perforation, hepatitis, and pelvic
   inflammatory disease.

3. **How can a thorough history to evaluate abdominal pain be obtained?**
   A thorough history includes location and time of onset of pain, change in location or severity
   of pain, quality of the pain (i.e., sharp, stabbing, dull aching, or burning), and radiation of pain
   to areas separate from the primary site. Factors exacerbating pain such as oral intake or
   movement should be elicited. Associated symptoms such as vomiting, anorexia, change in
   bowel habits, urinary complaints, or gynecologic symptoms should be elicited but are
   nonspecific and therefore nondiagnostic. Blood in the vomit or stool or a history of melena is
   useful information.

4. **What things should be looked for in a physical examination of someone with
   acute abdominal pain?**
   First, observe the patient's position in bed and his or her voluntary movement. The writhing of
   a patient with visceral pain (e.g., intestinal or ureteral colic) contrasts sharply with the
   motionless appearance of the patient with parietal pain (e.g., appendicitis or peritonitis). Note
   whether the abdomen is flat or distended. Palpate from the least tender to the most tender area
   of the abdomen. Peritoneal signs, when present, can be elicited by gentle percussion of
   the abdomen or by asking the patient to cough. Deep palpation to produce rebound creates
   unnecessary discomfort. A digital rectal examination may reveal tumor or gastrointestinal
   bleeding and can provide an assessment of pelvic peritoneal irritation or inflammation.

5. **What types of stimulation cause abdominal pain?**
   Visceral sensation is mediated by autonomic afferents found in the walls of hollow viscera and in
   the capsules of solid organs. Spasm, distention, inflammation, and ischemia are the primary
   causes of pain in these organs. In contrast, the parietal peritoneum, abdominal wall, and
   diaphragm receive somatic sensory innervation. Direct injury to these structures by cutting,
   crushing, or chemical irritation produces significant abdominal pain. When the parietal
   peritoneum is irritated by blood, stool, or pus, peritonitis results.

   Diethelm ARS, Robbin M: The acute abdomen. In Townsend CM, Beauchamp RD, Evers BM, Mattox K
   (eds): Sabiston Textbook of Surgery: The Biological Basis of Modern Surgical Practice, 17th ed. Philadelphia,
   W.B. Saunders, 2004, pp 825–846.

6. **What signs in a person with acute abdominal pain may indicate the need for an operation?**
Not all cases of acute abdominal pain require surgery, but early surgical consultation can be critical in the evaluation of a patient with suspected intestinal obstruction or peritonitis. Peritonitis can occur due to a perforated viscus, intra-abdominal hemorrhage, or bowel necrosis. Other concerning signs of abdominal catastrophe include tachycardia, hypotension, and worsening acidosis.

7. **Define *referred pain*. To what sites do various abdominal organs refer pain?**
The term *referred pain* denotes a noxious sensation perceived at a place separate from the primary organ involved. Referred pain occurs because afferent nerves from abdominal viscera may enter the spinal cord at levels remote from the site of irritation. The initial pain symptoms may be located at a referred site. For example, in appendicitis, the onset of pain is experienced in the periumbilical region (appendiceal afferents enter the spinal cord at T10) before migrating to the right lower quadrant. Inflammation of the gallbladder may be perceived as scapular or shoulder pain, obstruction of the ureter as testicular pain, and an incarcerated obturator hernia as medial thigh pain.

8. **Which blood tests are helpful in diagnosing the cause of abdominal pain?**
A complete blood count can be informative with infection and gastrointestinal bleeding. Serum electrolyte, blood urea nitrogen, creatinine, and arterial blood gas analyses (to evaluate metabolic acidosis) may indicate the chronicity of illness and help to guide resuscitation. Serum amylase levels, although used primarily as an indicator of acute pancreatitis, can also be abnormally elevated with strangulated or ischemic bowel and perforated ulcer. Although a measurement of lactate level is frequently ordered, in clinical practice it does not typically alter the course of management.

9. **What additional laboratory test can be informative for patients with abdominal pain?**
Urinalysis should be included in any work-up of abdominal pain and may diagnose nephrolithiasis, urinary tract infection, or other renal pathology. Blood cultures should be performed in the case of fever because the presence of gram-negative enteric bacteria or multiple gastrointestinal flora would increase suspicion of an abdominal process.

10. **What type of abdominal imaging is most useful?**
Plain radiographs are only useful to identify dilated small or large bowel with or without air–fluid levels and the presence of free air from a perforation. Ultrasound can accurately identify gallstones, determine the presence of cholecystitis, evaluate the size of the biliary ducts, and evaluate for acute appendicitis, although computed tomography (CT) is more sensitive for the latter. It is also useful in evaluating the size of an abdominal aortic aneurysm (AAA) but does not detect aneurysmal leaks. CT scan with IV and oral contrast is one of the most useful tests in depicting the cause of intra-abdominal pathology. Appendicitis, diverticulitis, masses, aneurysms, bowel obstruction, and many other causes of abdominal pathology can be observed.

Terasawa T, Blackmore CC, Bent S, Kohlwes RJ: Systematic review: Computed tomography and ultrasonography to detect acute appendicitis in adults and adolescents. Ann Intern Med 141:537–546, 2004.

11. **Can an enhanced CT scan (with IV contrast) be obtained in the setting of renal insufficiency?**
The lack of IV contrast results in limitations in interpreting the CT scan. However, the administration of IV contrast can result in a contrast nephropathy, and patients who are ill may already have some degree of renal insufficiency. For patients with mild renal insufficiency, the

administration of either oral N-acetylcysteine or an IV infusion of bicarbonate before and after receiving IV contrast may decrease the risk of contrast nephropathy.

Weisbord SD, Palevsky PM: Radiocontrast-induced acute renal failure. J Intens Care Med 20:63–75, 2005.

12. **Is the differential diagnosis of abdominal pain in the intensive care unit (ICU) different from that in the emergency department?**
The specific illnesses that cause abdominal pain in patients presenting for treatment in the emergency department are also seen in the ICU. Common causes of abdominal pathology in the ICU include peptic ulcer disease with bleeding or perforation, mesenteric ischemia, acalculous cholecystitis, and acute pancreatitis, all of which can be exacerbated by malnutrition and ICU-related physiologic stress. However, many nonabdominal conditions that cause a patient to become critically ill, such as malnutrition, sepsis, acute respiratory distress syndrome, and myocardial infarction, can also cause abdominal pain, making the recognition of symptoms caused by real abdominal pathology difficult.

13. **Does the differential diagnosis of abdominal pain vary by age?**
Yes. In infants and children, the most common diagnoses are intussusception, intestinal volvulus, and incarcerated inguinal hernias. In adolescents, trauma, appendicitis, and mesenteric adenitis are common. In young adults, appendicitis, inflammatory bowel disease, and gynecologic conditions are the leading causes. In adults and elderly patients, the differential diagnosis reflects age and underlying comorbidities. Malignancy, diverticulosis, gallbladder disease, and peptic ulcer disease are frequently diagnosed. Given its bimodal distribution by age, appendicitis must be considered early in the evaluation of elderly patients because the consequences of rupture in elderly patients can be catastrophic.

KEY POINTS: DIFFERENTIAL DIAGNOSIS OF ABDOMINAL PAIN BY AGE

1. Infants and children carry a differential diagnosis of intussusception, intestinal volvulus, and incarcerated inguinal hernias.

2. In adolescents, trauma, appendicitis, and mesenteric adenitis are possible diagnoses.

3. The differential diagnosis in young adults includes appendicitis, inflammatory bowel disease, and gynecologic conditions.

4. Malignancy, diverticulosis, gallbladder disease, peptic ulcer disease, and appendicitis are considerations in adults and elderly patients.

5. Less common but important differential diagnoses in adults are mesenteric ischemia and cecal or sigmoid volvulus.

14. **How does immunocompetence affect the diagnosis of abdominal pain?**
Heightened awareness of atypical causes or presentations of abdominal diseases is necessary for early intervention in potentially treatable conditions. Immunocompromised patients are not only those with HIV infection or those taking immunosuppressive drugs, but also those who are elderly, malnourished, or diabetic. These patients may have a blunted response to disease processes, altering the typical or timely presentation of abdominal illness. Suggestive symptoms and signs, such as fever or an elevated white blood cell count, may not be present. These patients are more susceptible to opportunistic infections or rare neoplasms, requiring a broader

differential diagnosis including intestinal lymphoma, neutropenic enterocolitis, cytomegalovirus infection, tubercular disease, and other less commonly encountered pathologies.

Scott-Conner CEH, Fabreage AJ: Gastrointestinal problems in the immunocompromised host. Surg Endosc 10:959–964, 1996.

15. **Describe the typical presentation of a patient with a small or large bowel obstruction.**
    - **Small bowel obstruction (SBO):** SBO generally begins with the sudden onset of sharp, colicky, diffuse abdominal pain. Nausea and emesis can follow the onset of pain and may relieve it in some cases. Emesis tends to be bilious, gradually becoming more feculent as the process continues. Tachycardia is common; hypotension and dehydration develop as fluid is lost due to vomiting and increasing bowel edema, and fever may be present. Typically, patients report a history of prior surgery, as adhesions are the most common cause of SBO. However, hernias and malignancies should also be considered as a possible cause.
    - **Large bowel obstruction (LBO):** LBO occurs in older patients and tends to have a gradual onset. Patients complain of constipation and abdominal distention; nausea and vomiting are late findings. The patient may give a history of pencil-thin or blood-streaked stools. Colorectal cancer, inflammatory bowel disease, diverticulitis, and volvulus can all cause LBO.

16. **What does the work-up of a patient with bowel obstruction reveal?**
    Laboratory data reveal an increase in hematocrit levels caused by dehydration. The white blood cell count may be elevated if the duration of obstruction has been several hours or more. Plain radiographs of the abdomen with SBO characteristically show bowel dilatation, air–fluid levels, and a nonobstructed colon with air and feces. If the obstruction in very proximal, the plain films may be unremarkable. With colonic obstruction there can be marked dilation of the proximal colon up to the point of obstruction. CT scan is highly sensitive for diagnosis of bowel obstruction, showing a clear transition point from dilated to decompressed intestine. The use of rectal contrast during CT may reveal diverticulitis or malignancy as the source of distal obstruction.

17. **What steps are taken in the management of bowel obstruction?**
    With SBO, a nasogastric tube should be placed, particularly when the stomach appears dilated on imaging studies or if the patient has bilious emesis. The patient should stop oral intake and be given continuous IV fluids. If a prolonged period of bowel rest is anticipated, total parenteral nutrition should be started early, particularly for patients whose nutritional status is already suboptimal. Patients with no systemic indicators of inflammation or peritoneal signs may be managed conservatively at first. However, if no improvement has occurred by 48 hours, the patient should be reassessed for the need for operation. In the setting of LBO, cecal or sigmoid volvulus are a part of the differential diagnosis and are likely to require early surgical intervention.

18. **Compare the presentation of a ruptured AAA with an aortic dissection.**
    - **Ruptured AAA:** Ruptured AAA presents with sudden onset of abdominal pain or intense back pain due to dissection of blood through the retroperitoneal tissue. Patients may be diaphoretic, light-headed, and hypotensive with a pulsatile, midepigastric mass. Prompt aggressive resuscitation with IV fluids and blood is essential to improve outcomes. CT scan may be useful in stable patients, but if the diagnosis is strongly suspected, surgical intervention should not be delayed.
    - **Acute aortic dissection:** This condition usually presents with sudden onset of tearing pain beneath the sternum or between the scapulae; however, abdominal pain can occur when the false lumen occludes renal or mesenteric arteries (5–17% of dissections). Patients may experience numbness or tingling of the extremities from loss of circulation. Because the

pathophysiology is based on medial degeneration, it generally occurs in patients younger than those with advanced atherosclerotic disease.

Hallett JW, Rasmussen TE: Ruptured abdominal aortic aneurysm. In Cameron JL (ed): Current Surgical Therapy, 8th ed. St. Louis, Mosby, 2004, pp 713–718.

Williams CM: Acute aortic dissection and its complications. In Cameron JL (ed): Current Surgical Therapy, 8th ed. St. Louis, Mosby, 2004, pp 729–731.

19. **When should one suspect bowel ischemia as the cause of acute abdominal pain? What should be done?**

A patient with acute mesenteric ischemia, a compromise of blood flow to the small or large intestine, may present with pain out of proportion to the physical examination. The cause can be embolic, thrombotic, or nonocclusive. It should be suspected in patients with atrial fibrillation, hypercoagulable states, congestive heart failure, recent myocardial infarction, or low-flow hemodynamic states (i.e., prolonged hypotension from sepsis). Thrombosis or emboli are more common in the well-vascularized small bowel. When suspected, immediate intervention is required by angiography or surgery. In contrast, low-flow states, which more commonly result in ischemic colitis, can often be managed conservatively with resuscitation, IV antibiotics to treat translocation of bacteria, and maintenance of normal blood pressures. Operative treatment is avoided unless the patient exhibits evidence of transmural necrosis or has systemic signs of illness.

Yashuara H: Acute mesenteric ischemia: The challenge of gastroenterology. Surg Today 35:185–195, 2005.

20. **What is Ogilvie's syndrome?**

Ogilvie's syndrome, or pseudo-obstruction of the colon, is massive dilation of the colon without mechanical obstruction. It is most common in elderly, debilitated patients and patients immobilized by orthopedic procedures or neurologic disorders such as Parkinson's disease. It is also seen in the presence of electrolyte derangements. If dilation of the cecum exceeds 9–12 cm (estimated on plain films), the risk of perforation is significant. Treatment begins with colonoscopic or rectal tube decompression of the colon. Medical therapy includes administration of neostigmine (2.5 mg IV over 3 minutes); treatment should be monitored because of the risk of bradycardia. If these maneuvers fail, surgical decompression with cecotomy may be required.

Vernava AM, DeBarrus J: Ogilvie's syndrome (colonic pseudo-obstruction). In Cameron JL (ed): Current Surgical Therapy, 8th ed. St. Louis, Mosby, 2004, pp 176–178.

ACKNOWLEDGMENT

Special thanks to Dr. Kim Rhoads for her contribution to this chapter in the prior edition.

WEBSITES

1. Abdominal emergencies
   www.merck.com/mmhe/sec09/ch132/ch132a.html

2. Mesenteric artery ischemia
   www.emedicine.com/med/topic2726.htm

CHAPTER 69

PNEUMOTHORAX

Michael E. Hanley, MD

1. **What are the major etiologic classifications of pneumothoraces?**
   Pneumothoraces are classified as spontaneous or traumatic:
   - **Spontaneous:** Spontaneous pneumothoraces occur without antecedent trauma or other obvious cause. A primary spontaneous pneumothorax occurs in a person without underlying lung disease. Secondary spontaneous pneumothoraces occur as a complication of underlying lung disease.
   - **Traumatic:** Traumatic pneumothoraces result from direct or indirect trauma to the chest and are further classified as iatrogenic or noniatrogenic.

   Baumann MH: Pneumothorax. Semin Respir Crit Care Med 22:647–656, 2001.

2. **What are the common causes of pneumothorax in critically ill patients?**
   Most pneumothoraces that develop in the intensive care unit are due to either antecedent noniatrogenic chest trauma or iatrogenic causes. Box 69-1 lists the common causes of iatrogenic pneumothorax. Secondary spontaneous pneumothorax also occasionally develops in critically ill patients, especially those with chronic obstructive pulmonary disease, asthma, interstitial lung disease, necrotizing lung infections, adult respiratory distress syndrome, and *Pneumocystis jiroveci* pneumonia.

   Chen KY, Jerng JS, Liao WY, et al: Pneumothorax in the ICU: Patient outcomes and prognostic factors. Chest 122:678–683, 2002.

   de Lassence A, Timsit JF, Tafflet M, et al: Pneumothorax in the intensive care unit: Incidence, risk factors, and outcome. Anesthesiology 104:5–13, 2006.

BOX 69-1.   COMMON CAUSES OF IATROGENIC PNEUMOTHORAX

Positive-pressure ventilation
Central venous catheter placement
Thoracentesis
Tracheostomy
Nasogastric tube placement*
Bronchoscopy[†]
Pericardiocentesis
Transthoracic needle aspiration
Cardiopulmonary resuscitation

*Due to inadvertent insertion of the nasogastric tube into the tracheobronchial tree.
[†]Especially if transbronchial biopsy is performed.

---

3. **What measures reduce the risk of iatrogenic pneumothorax in patients receiving positive-pressure ventilation?**
End-inspiratory plateau pressure should be kept < 35 cm H_2O, and both positive end-expiratory pressure (PEEP) and auto-PEEP levels should be minimized. Approaches that may help to achieve these goals include using smaller tidal volumes (5–10 mL/kg) in patients with underlying lung disease, using permissive hypercapnia when high minute ventilation is required, and using high inspiratory flow rates. In addition, thoracentesis and subclavian/internal jugular venous line insertion should be performed with utmost care in high-risk patients.

Boussarsar M, Thierry G, Jaber S, et al: Relationship between ventilatory settings and barotrauma in the acute respiratory distress syndrome. Intens Care Med 28:406–413, 2002.

Mayo PH, Goltz HR, Tafreshi M, et al: Safety of ultrasound-guided thoracentesis in patients receiving mechanical ventilation. Chest 125:1059–1062, 2004.

4. **Describe the clinical manifestations of pneumothoraces.**
Dyspnea and chest pain (usually localized to the side of the pneumothorax) are the most common symptoms in primary spontaneous pneumothorax. The most common physical signs are tachycardia and abnormal results of chest examination. The latter includes ipsilateral expansion of the chest and decreased or absent tactile fremitus. Chest percussion and auscultation reveal ipsilateral hyper-resonance and decreased or absent breath sounds. The trachea may be deviated toward the contralateral side.

The symptoms in secondary spontaneous pneumothoraces are more severe than for primary pneumothoraces because pulmonary reserve is already compromised by underlying lung pathology. Dyspnea occurs in virtually all patients and is commonly out of proportion to the size of the pneumothorax. Cyanosis and hypotension are common. Side-to-side differences in the examination of the chest may not be as apparent because many of the physical signs associated with the underlying lung disease are similar to those associated with pneumothoraces.

5. **What subtle signs or symptoms should prompt consideration of pneumothorax in mechanically ventilated patients?**
The sudden onset of any of the following should raise the possibility of a pneumothorax in mechanically ventilated patients:
- Decline in oxygen saturation
- Agitation
- Respiratory distress
- "Fighting the ventilator"
- Sudden increase in peak inspiratory and/or static airway pressure
- Hypotension
- Cardiovascular collapse
- Pulseless electrical activity

6. **How is the diagnosis of pneumothorax established in critically ill patients?**
The diagnosis is established by demonstrating typical chest roentgenographic findings, including a thin pleural line and the absence of lung parenchymal markings between the pleural line and chest wall. However, when chest roentgenography is performed with the patient in the supine position, free pleural air will collect anteriorly and may not be readily apparent. Evidence of an increase in the size of the ipsilateral hemithorax, including contralateral shift of the mediastinum and heart, as well as depression of the ipsilateral hemidiaphragm may be the only roentgenographic clues to the presence of a pneumothorax in such cases. Chest roentgenograms obtained at expiration, with the patient in the lateral decubitus position, or from the cross-table lateral view may be useful in confirming the

presence of free pleural air. If chest roentgenograms are nondiagnostic and the patient is sufficiently stable for transport, computed tomography of the chest may be required to prove the diagnosis.

Rankine JJ, Thomas AN, Fluechter D: Diagnosis of pneumothorax in critically ill adults. Postgrad Med J 76:399–404, 2000.

7. **Describe the treatment of a pneumothorax in critically ill patients.**
Tube thoracostomy should be performed in almost all secondary spontaneous or noniatrogenic, traumatic pneumothoraces, especially if mechanical ventilation is required. Proper positioning of the thoracostomy tube is important in obtaining complete evacuation of pleural air. The tube should be directed to an anterior/apical position. Tube thoracostomy should also be performed for all iatrogenic pneumothoraces due to positive-pressure ventilation. Other forms of iatrogenic pneumothorax require tube thoracostomy only if the pneumothorax (1) is large (>40%), (2) is associated with significant symptoms or arterial blood gas abnormalities, (3) progressively enlarges, (4) does not respond to simple aspiration, or (5) occurs in a patient requiring positive-pressure ventilation.

Baumann MH: What size chest tube? What drainage system is ideal? And other chest tube management questions. Curr Opin Pulm Med 9:276–281, 2003.
Baumann MH, Strange C, Heffner JF, et al: Management of spontaneous pneumothorax: An American College of Chest Physicians Delphi Consensus Statement. Chest 119:590–602, 2001.

8. **Does the development of a pneumothorax portend a worse prognosis for patients with acute respiratory distress syndrome (ARDS)?**
No. The association of pneumothorax and other air leaks (i.e., extrusion of any air outside the tracheobronchial tree) with mortality was studied in 725 patients with ARDS. The 30-day mortality rate for patients who developed a pneumothorax was 46% compared to 40% in patients without pneumothorax ($P = 0.35$). Similarly, the 30-day mortality rate for patients with any type of air leak was 45.5% compared to 39.0% for patients without air leaks ($P = 0.28$).

Weg J, Anzueto S, Balk RA, et al: The relationship of pneumothorax and other air leaks to mortality in the acute respiratory distress syndrome. N Engl J Med 338:341–346, 1998.

9. **What are the potential physiologic consequences of a bronchopleural fistula (BPF) in mechanically ventilated patients?**
See Box 69-2.

BOX 69-2. PHYSIOLOGIC CONSEQUENCES OF A BRONCHOPLEURAL FISTULA IN MECHANICALLY VENTILATED PATIENTS

Inability to maintain adequate alveolar ventilation through loss of effective tidal volume
Inappropriate cycling of the ventilator
Incomplete lung reexpansion
Inability to apply PEEP

PEEP = positive end-expiratory pressure.

10. **Describe the management of a BPF.**

    Management focuses on minimizing air flow through the fistula while maintaining complete evacuation of the pleural space. This is primarily accomplished in patients breathing spontaneously (negative-pressure ventilation) by altering the level of suction applied to the pleural space. The optimal amount of suction must be determined on an individual basis, as the level of suction at which gas flow through the fistula is minimized varies.

    Gas flow across a BPF in mechanically ventilated patients is also influenced by peak inspiratory and mean airway pressures. Management in this setting includes measures that minimize airway pressures while maintaining adequate ventilation. This is accomplished by minimizing PEEP, tidal volume, the number of mechanically delivered breaths per minute, and inspiratory time. Mechanical ventilation should be discontinued as soon as possible.

    Powner DJ, Cline CD, Rodman GH: Effect of chest tube suction on gas flow through a bronchopleural fistula. Crit Care Med 13:99–101, 1985.

11. **How is a persistent BPF managed?**

    If a BPF does not close after 5–7 days of chest tube drainage, or if adequate ventilation cannot be maintained because of the size of the air leak, suturing or resection of the fistula with scarification of the pleura by either thoracoscopy or open thoracotomy should be considered. The decision to perform this procedure should include a consideration of the operative risk to the patient. Prolonged chest tube drainage, intrabronchial bronchoscopic instillation of materials (e.g., Gelfoam or tissue adhesives such as cyanoacrylate-based or fibrin glues) designed to occlude the fistula, differential lung ventilation, or synchronized chest tube occlusion should be considered in patients whose operative risk is increased by significant underlying lung disease or other medical problems.

    Kempainen RR, Pierson DJ: Persistent air leaks in patients receiving mechanical ventilation. Semin Respir Crit Care Med 22:675–684, 2001.

12. **What is reexpansion pulmonary edema?**

    Reexpansion pulmonary edema involves the development of unilateral pulmonary edema after reexpansion of a collapsed lung. The risk and severity of reexpansion pulmonary edema appear to be related to the duration of the pneumothorax as well as the magnitude of negative pressure applied to the pleural space to reexpand the lung. The exact incidence of reexpansion pulmonary edema after treatment of pneumothoraces in humans is unknown, but it is rare. However, the associated mortality is between 10% and 20%.

13. **How can the risk of reexpansion pulmonary edema be minimized?**

    The risk can be minimized by withholding pleural suction during the immediate treatment of pneumothoraces of either unknown duration or duration greater than 3 days. If the pneumothorax is not completely evacuated after 24–48 hours of water seal, or if significant respiratory compromise requires more rapid evacuation, low levels of negative pressure (<20 cm H_2O) should be applied to the pleural space. Nonetheless, reexpansion pulmonary edema has been reported even under these conditions.

    Beng ST, Mahadevan M: An uncommon life-threatening complication after chest tube drainage of pneumothorax in the ED. Am J Emerg Med 22:615–619, 2004.

14. **What is a tension pneumothorax?**

    A tension pneumothorax occurs when the pleural pressure within a pneumothorax is greater than atmospheric pressure throughout expiration and often during inspiration. Tension pneumothoraces generally result from a one-way valve phenomenon and most frequently occur in patients receiving positive-pressure ventilation.

    Barton ED: Tension pneumothorax. Curr Opin Pulm Med 5:269–274, 1999.

KEY POINTS: CLINICAL MANIFESTATIONS OF TENSION PNEUMOTHORAX

1. Sudden deterioration often occurs in patients with tension pneumothorax.

2. Respiratory distress is another manifestation.

3. Cyanosis may occur.

4. Diaphoresis is often present.

5. Cardiovascular instability, including tachycardia and hypotension, sometimes occur.

6. Another manifestation of tension pneumothorax is ipsilateral hyperresonance.

7. Ipsilateral diminished breath sounds also occur.

8. Tension pneumothorax is sometimes accompanied by an increase in the size of the ipsilateral hemithorax.

9. Contralateral shift of the trachea may be present.

15. **Describe the treatment for a tension pneumothorax.**
Time should not be wasted pursuing roentgenographic confirmation if the diagnosis of tension pneumothorax is suspected and the patient exhibits significant hemodynamic instability. High levels (FiO$_2$ = 100%) of supplemental oxygen should be administered and the pneumothorax evacuated. This is best accomplished by emergent placement of a tube thoracostomy. If the diagnosis is in question, or if a tube thoracostomy is not readily available, an alternate approach includes insertion of a large-bore needle attached to a three-way stopcock with a 50-mL syringe partially filled with sterile saline into the pleural space. The needle is inserted under sterile conditions through the second anterior intercostal space in the midclavicular line while the patient is supine. After the needle has been inserted, the plunger is withdrawn from the syringe. The presence of a pneumothorax is confirmed if air bubbles up through the saline. If a pneumothorax is present, the needle should be left in place until air ceases to bubble through the saline and a tube thoracostomy is performed. If air does not bubble up into the syringe, a pneumothorax is not present and the needle may be removed.

Leigh-Smith S, Harris T: Tension pneumothorax—time for a re-think?. Emerg Med J 22:8–16, 2005.

CONTROVERSY

16. **Should a tube thoracostomy be removed immediately in patients receiving positive-pressure ventilation once the air leak has resolved and the lung is completely reexpanded?**
Pro:
1. The tube thoracostomy is no longer required to evacuate air after the BPF has closed and all air has been evacuated. At this point, the chest tube is only a potential source of infection, both at its insertion site and in the pleural space.
2. Patients can be closely monitored and chest tubes reinserted if a pneumothorax recurs.
3. Routine insertion of a prophylactic tube thoracostomy is not indicated in mechanically ventilated patients.

Con:

1. Risk of a recurrent pneumothorax remains high in mechanically ventilated patients, especially if they have ARDS or a necrotic lung process.

2. Most pneumothoraces in mechanically ventilated patients present under tension. Tension pneumothoraces are associated with a higher mortality, especially if there is delay in diagnosis or treatment.

Heffner JE, McDonald J, Barbieri C: Recurrent pneumothoraces in ventilated patients despite ipsilateral chest tubes. Chest 108:1053–1058, 1995.

CHAPTER 70

FLAIL CHEST AND PULMONARY CONTUSION

Rosemary A. Kozar, MD, PhD, James B. Haenel, RRT, and Frederick A. Moore, MD

1. **What is a flail chest? How is it diagnosed?**

   Anatomically, a flail chest may occur with when three or more consecutive ribs or costal cartilages are fractured in two or more places (Fig. 70-1). These circumscribed segments, having lost continuity with the rigid thorax, move inward with inspiration and push outward with exhalation, thus moving paradoxically. Presenting symptoms of pain, tachypnea, dyspnea, and thoracic splinting, along with chest wall contusions, tenderness, crepitance, and palpable rib fractures, are suggestive, but clinical detection of paradoxical chest wall motion is the diagnostic *sine qua non*. Detection often requires careful inspection of the two hemithoraces throughout the respiratory cycle to appreciate subtle paradoxical movement.

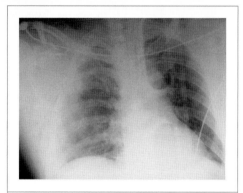

Figure 70-1. Radiograph of a patient with a flail chest.

2. **How does age affect outcome in patients with multiple rib fractures/flail chest?**

   A linear relationship between age, increasing number of rib fractures, and complications, including mortality, has been identified. Age older than 45 years, rather than the previously identified high-risk group of over 65 years, has been shown to be associated with worsening morbidity in patients with more than four rib fractures.

   Bulger EM, Arneson MA, Mock CN, et al: Rib fractures in the elderly. J Trauma 48:1040–1047, 2000.
   Holcomb JB, McMullin NR, Kozar RA, et al: Morbidity from rib fractures increases after age 45. J Am Coll Surg 196:549–555, 2003.

3. **What is the most common intrathoracic injury found in patients sustaining blunt chest trauma?**

   Pulmonary contusion is the most common type of intrathoracic injury in nonpenetrating trauma.

4. **What is a pulmonary contusion?**

   The spectrum of lung parenchymal injury after a blunt chest impact ranges from simple contusion to frank laceration. Pulmonary contusion, by far the most frequent variant, is a bruise or contusion of the lung followed by alveolar hemorrhage and edema. Direct injury causes pulmonary vascular damage with secondary alveolar hemorrhage. In the early phase, these flooded alveoli are poorly perfused; consequently, little shunt exists. However, tissue inflammation develops rapidly, and the resultant surrounding pulmonary edema produces regional alterations in compliance and airway resistance, leading to localized ventilation–perfusion mismatch.

5. **How is a pulmonary contusion diagnosed?**
   The diagnosis is radiologic. The classic finding is a nonsegmental pulmonary infiltrate that occurs within 12–24 hours of injury. The infiltrate may consist of irregular nodular densities that are discrete

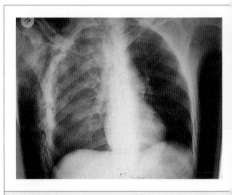

Figure 70-2. Radiograph of a patient with a pulmonary contusion.

or confluent, a homogeneous consolidation, or a diffuse patchy pattern (Fig. 70-2). Aspiration and reexpansion of collapsed right upper lobe (such as due to right mainstem intubation) are causes of early chest x-ray findings that are frequently misdiagnosed as a pulmonary contusion. In most cases, pulmonary contusions do not become apparent until after fluid resuscitation; thus, if seen on early chest radiograph, a more severe contusion is likely. Contusions also tend to worsen over 24–48 hours and then slowly resolve unless complicated by infection, acute respiratory distress syndrome (ARDS), or cavitation.

6. **Which type of intrathoracic injury is a known risk factor for ARDS?**
   Pulmonary contusion has been identified as a risk factor for pneumonia and ARDS. Patients with severe pulmonary contusions, defined as >20% on chest computed tomographic scan, were found to have a significantly higher incidence of ARDS than those patients with moderate (<20%) pulmonary contusions.

   Miller PR, Croce MA, Bee TK, et al: ARDS after pulmonary contusion: Accurate measurement of contusion volume identifies high risk patients. J Trauma 51:223–230, 2001.

   Miller PR, Croce MA, Kilgo PD, et al: Acute respiratory distress syndrome in blunt trauma: Identification of independent risk factors. Am Surg 68:845–850, 2002.

7. **What are the basic treatment strategies for flail chest/pulmonary contusions?**
   The tenets of management center around five principles: close observation of respiratory status, ample pain control, aggressive lung physiotherapy, early mobilization, and adequate nutrition.

8. **In their severe forms, flail chest and pulmonary contusion often coexist. What is the incidence of other concomitant injuries?**
   More than 90% of patients have associated intrathoracic injuries, including pulmonary contusion, hemothorax, pneumothorax, or a combination of these. Three of four patients require tube thoracostomy for hemopneumothorax. Extrathoracic injuries are also common: head injuries occur in 40%, major fractures in 40%, and intra-abdominal injuries in 30%.

   Ciraulo DL, Elliott D, Mitchell KA, et al: Flail chest as a marker for significant injuries. J Am Coll Surg 178:466–470, 1994.

9. **What is the mortality rate and cause of death in combined flail chest/pulmonary contusion injuries?**
   Despite tremendous advances in trauma and critical care, the current mortality rate for these patients is approximately 25%. Improved prehospital care no doubt contributes to this

persistently high mortality by delivering more severely injured patients to the reporting trauma centers. Early deaths are due to extrathoracic hemorrhage (e.g., pelvic fracture, liver injuries) and head injury; late mortality relates to sepsis and multiple organ failure. Factors that portend a poor outcome include presence of shock (blood pressure < 90 mmHg), high injury severity score (>25), associated head injury (Glasgow Coma Scale score < 7), falls from great heights (>20 feet), preexisting disease (e.g., atherosclerotic heart disease, chronic obstructive pulmonary disease, Laënnec's cirrhosis), and advanced age (older than 65 years).

10. **What are the initial priorities in the management of patients with severe blunt chest trauma?**
   Patient management is prioritized according to the physiologic need for survival. The initial ABCs (i.e., airway, breathing, circulation) of advance trauma life support are directed at establishing peripheral oxygen delivery before a specific diagnosis is made. Prophylactic tube thoracostomy for suspected hemopneumothorax, empiric tracheal intubation, and mechanical ventilation are clearly warranted in an unstable, multisystem-injured patient with chest injuries.

11. **What are the pitfalls in pain management of nonintubated patients with blunt chest trauma?**
   Inadequate pain control is a common pitfall in the management of these patients. Sufficient pain control is the vital adjunct that permits patient mobilization, deep breathing, and secretion clearance. However, intermittent dosing of IV narcotics can oversedate if large doses are administered and can depress respiratory efforts and cough reflex, and long intervals allow the patients to experience cycles of significant pain and anxiety. The patient-controlled analgesia device can be an invaluable adjunct in achieving pain control.

12. **Does the type of pain control influence the rate of pneumonia in patients with multiple rib fractures?**
   Epidural analgesia, compared with IV opioids, has been shown to decrease the rate of nosocomial pneumonia and the number of days of ventilation in patients with multiple rib fractures. Although intercostal and intrapleural catheter infusions of anesthetics have also been used in pain control, the most convincingly successful application of regional anesthesia in chest trauma is continuous epidural infusion of local anesthetics or narcotics or, more recently described, continuous intercostal nerve blockade with local anesthetic.

   Bulger EM, Edwards T, Klotz P, Jurkovich GJ: Epidural analgesia improves outcome after multiple rib fractures. Surgery 136:426–430, 2004.
   Haenel JB, Moore FA, Moore EE, et al: Continuous intercostal nerve block for amelioration of multiple rib fracture pain. J Trauma 38:22–29, 1995.

13. **Which respiratory therapy procedure(s) should be used for patients with significant blunt chest trauma?**
   Vigorous ambulation, when possible, remains the best method of restoring normal respiratory physiology. All patients should have pain assessed and receive maximal lung expansion therapy using an incentive spirometer on an hourly basis. Patients not meeting predicted goals with the incentive spirometer should be initiated on either intermittent mouth piece (EZ-PAP) or continuous positive airway pressure (CPAP) therapy via a face mask. Chest physical therapy consists of postural drainage, enhanced coughing maneuvers, chest vibration, and percussion. Prospective studies are lacking for efficacy, and chest percussion is obviously not well tolerated in patients sustaining thoracic trauma. Nasotracheal suctioning is reserved for patients not able to effectively mobilize their secretions.

14. **Do all patients with flail chest require mechanical ventilation? Why or why not?**
   No. Only selected patients with flail chest require mechanical ventilation. Recent studies have shown that patients who are not intubated but are treated with aggressive pulmonary care have

less pneumonia, reduced mortality, and significantly shorter stays in the intensive care unit. Noninvasive CPAP is particularly attractive for patients who do not require emergent intubation initially. CPAP restores functional residual capacity, improves compliance, and stabilizes the flail segment until the underlying pulmonary contusion resolves. CPAP, compared with intermittent positive pressure ventilation, has also been shown to lower the incidence of mortality and nosocomial infections in patients who required mechanical ventilation.

Bolliger CT, Van Eden SF: Treatment of multiple rib-fractures randomized controlled trial comparing ventilatory with nonventilatory management. Chest 97:943–948, 1990.

Gunduz M, Unlungenc H, Ozalevli M, et al: A comparative study of continuous positive airway pressure (CPAP) and intermittent positive pressure ventilation (IPPV) in patients with flail chest. Emerg Med J 22:325–329, 2005.

15. **What is the optimal mode of ventilation for patients with flail chest or pulmonary contusion?**

Because a high percentage of patients sustaining significant pulmonary contusions will develop ARDS, the need for mechanical ventilation is fairly common. The optimal mode of ventilation continues to be debated. In patients with ARDS, lung protective ventilation (LPV) strategies employing a volume- and pressure-limited approach have resulted in a 22% reduction in mortality (i.e., for every 10 patients ventilated with an LPV approach, one life will be saved) in patients with ARDS. Limiting tidal volume to 6 mL/kg of ideal body weight and plateau pressures to <30 cm H_2O reduces lung overstretch and prevents derecruitment injury. Many of the newer modes of ventilation are consistent with an LPV strategy and have shown promising results, but data are lacking as far as showing superiority.

Acute Respiratory Distress Syndrome Network: Ventilation with lower tidal volumes as compared with traditional tidal volumes for acute lung injury and the acute respiratory distress syndrome. N Engl J Med 342:1301–1308, 2000.

Wanek S, Mayberry JC: Blunt thoracic trauma: Flail chest, pulmonary contusion, and blast injury. Crit Care Clin 20:71–81, 2004.

KEY POINTS: FLAIL CHEST AND PULMONARY CONTUSION

1. Increasing age places patients with multiple rib fractures at high risk for pulmonary complications.

2. Pulmonary contusions place patients at increased risk for pneumonia and acute respiratory distress syndrome (ARDS).

3. Twenty-four hours of a prophylactic first-generation antibiotic treatment is indicated for the placement of chest tubes for traumatic hemopneumothoracies.

4. The management of flail chest/pulmonary contusion includes observation of respiratory status, pain control, lung physiotherapy, early mobilization, and adequate nutrition.

5. Lung protective strategies (e.g., tidal volume < 6 mL/kg and plateau pressures < 30 cm H_2O) should be used when patients with a flail chest or pulmonary contusion require mechanical ventilation as a result of ARDS.

16. **What is the role of positive end-expiratory pressure (PEEP) in the management of blunt chest trauma?**

Severe parenchymal injury sets the stage for alveolar collapse, and as a result, PEEP has been an invaluable adjunct to ventilator management. PEEP results in an elevation of transpulmonary pressures at the end of exhalation, thus preventing derecruitment of alveolar units. Identifying optimal PEEP is complex, but in general the goal is to select a PEEP level that prevents derecruitment and allows for FiO_2 reduction. In a recent prospective randomized controlled trial from the Acute Respiratory Distress Syndrome Network, a low-PEEP versus high-PEEP (8.3 ± 3.2 cm H_2O versus 13.2 ± 3.5 cm H_2O) strategy in 549 patients with various degrees of acute lung injury showed no difference in clinical outcomes (24.9% versus 27.5%). When using low tidal volume, PEEP is initially set at 8–10 cm H_2O. If FiO_2 cannot be lowered to 0.60 or if hypoxemia occurs, additional PEEP is used.

MacIntyre NR: Setting the positive expiratory-end pressure—FiO_2 in acute lung injury/acute respiratory distress syndrome. Respir Care Clin 10:301–308, 2004.

National Heart, Lung, and Blood Institute ARDS Clinical Trials Network: Higher *versus* lower positive end-expiratory pressure in patients with the acute respiratory distress syndrome. N Engl J Med 351:327–336, 2004.

17. **What are the indications for surgical stabilization of flail chest injuries?**
The proponents of surgical stabilization claim a reduction in ventilator days, pulmonary complications, pain, and chest wall deformity. A variety of fixation methods have been proposed, including pins, plates, wires, and struts. A prospective study by Tanaka and colleagues randomly assigned patients to receive either surgical fixation within 7 days of injury or mechanical ventilation alone. They demonstrated a reduction in pneumonia, days spent breathing via a ventilator, and days spent in intensive care in those patients undergoing surgery. Despite these reported benefits, stabilizations are seldomly performed. Studies specifically examining this question are few and limited.

Tanaka H, Yukioka T, Yamaguti Y, et al: Surgical stabilization of internal pneumatic stabilization? A prospective randomized study of management of severe flail chest patients. J Trauma 52:727–732, 2002.

18. **What is the long-term morbidity in flail chest injuries?**
Long-term disability has not been well studied. In a recent review of 32 patients with flail chest with a mean follow-up of 5 years, only 12 (38%) had returned to full-time employment. Most complaints were subjective, such as chest tightness, pain, and decreased activity level. Another study reported on 22 patients with isolated flail chest injuries. Follow-up was 2 months to 2 years. Two-thirds of these study participants experienced long-term morbidity. Persistent chest wall pain, dyspnea on exertion, and chest wall deformity were the most frequent complaints. Five (22%) remained disabled. Additional studies are clearly needed.

19. **Are prophylactic antibiotics indicated in patients requiring a tube thoracostomy after chest trauma?**
Prospective randomized trials offer conflicting results, although two meta-analyses suggest that prophylactic antibiotics can reduce empyemas. However, more recently, a level III recommendation by the Eastern Association for the Surgery of Trauma included the use of a first-generation cephalosporin for no longer than 24 hours to reduce the incidence of pneumonia, but not emphyema.

WEBSITES

1. Eastern Association for the Surgery of Trauma, Trauma Practice Guidelines
www.east.org/tpg.html

2. Trauma.org: Pulmonary contusion
www.trauma.org/thoracic/CHESTcontusion.html

3. Trauma.org: Rib fractures and flail chest
www.trauma.org/thoracic/CHESTflail.html

CHAPTER 71

MYOCARDIAL CONTUSION

Joel A. Garcia, MD, and John C. Messenger, MD

1. **What causes cardiac injury in blunt chest trauma or injuries (BCI)?**
   Nonpenetrating cardiac trauma is most often associated with rapid chest deceleration as in motor vehicle accidents, often due to steering wheel trauma or blunt chest trauma experienced by restrained (less likely) and unrestrained passengers. The incidence of myocardial contusion varies depending on the diagnostic modality and criteria used but ranges in the literature from 8% to 71%. Other causes include direct blows to the chest, falls from heights, crush injuries, contact sports and, rarely, a kick from a large animal.

   Hill G, Davies K: Blunt chest trauma: A challenge to accident and emergency nurses. Emerg Nurs 10:197–204, 2002.

2. **What is a myocardial contusion?**
   Myocardial contusion results from direct damage to the myocardium without traumatic involvement of the coronary arteries. Pathologically, there is evidence of myocyte injury with cell necrosis, edema, and interstitial hemorrhage. Often, injury is limited to the subepicardial or subendocardial tissue without evidence of transmural injury. In general, it refers to transient myocardial dysfunction associated with or without laboratory evidence of myocardial necrosis. It is a common injury that may impair ventricular contraction and lead to arrhythmia.

   Bansal MK, Maraj S, Chewaproug D, et al: Myocardial contusion injury: Redefining the myocardial contusion algorithm. Emerg Med J 22:465–469, 2005.

3. **What other myocardial injuries may be associated with blunt chest trauma?**
   Most other injuries of the myocardium associated with blunt chest trauma have accompanying myocardial contusion. These complications include contusion of the right ventricle, laceration or rupture of the atria (more common) or ventricles, perforation of the interventricular septum, and development of ventricular aneurysm or pseudoaneurysm. Direct injury to the coronary arteries with resultant thrombosis or dissection can result in myocardial damage similar to atherosclerotic myocardial infarction. Other rare events include rupture of the aortic isthmus, traumatic occlusion of the subclavian artery, avulsion of the innominate artery, and tear of a competent valve (Fig. 71-1).

   Pretre R, Chilcott M: Blunt trauma to the heart and great vessels. N Engl J Med 336:626–632, 1997.

4. **Are there associated chest injuries that make myocardial contusion more likely after blunt chest trauma?**
   Severe cardiac injury can occur with minimal or absent external signs of chest injury. However, in general, patients with more severe chest trauma, particularly those requiring intensive care, tend to have a higher incidence of myocardial contusion. Associated chest injuries in one large series included rib and clavicle fracture, pulmonary contusion, pneumothorax, hemothorax, flail chest, sternal fracture, and great vessel injury. With any blunt trauma to the chest, the level of suspicion should be high for possible cardiac injury, particularly if faced with arrhythmias or refractory hypotension.

   Sybrandy KC, Cramer MJM, Burgersdijk C: Diagnosing cardiac contusion: Old wisdom and new insights. Heart 89:485–489, 2003.

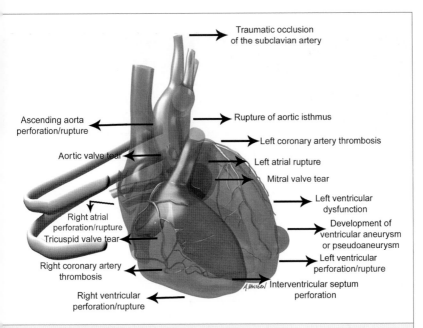

Figure 71-1. Blunt chest trauma injuries.

5. **What clinical features associated with blunt chest trauma suggest myocardial contusion?**
    Myocardial contusion is usually clinically silent. Chest pain is very common in patients with suspected myocardial contusion and is usually related to other thoracic injuries. Patients who present with unexplained sinus tachycardia or hemodynamic instability may have the first manifestations of myocardial dysfunction, but the possibility of pericardial tamponade should always be entertained. The presence of ventricular ectopy in the absence of significant hypoxemia or electrolyte abnormalities may indicate myocardial contusion, especially if seen early in the clinical course.

    Kaye P, O'Sullivan I: Myocardial contusion. Emergency investigation and diagnosis. Emerg Med 19:8–10, 2002.

6. **Which clinical examination findings may be present in myocardial contusion?**
    The finding of a pericardial rub, precordial thrill, and a new murmur suggest myocardial contusion, but these specific findings of cardiac injury are often lacking. The presence of an S_3 heart sound on cardiac examination and rales on auscultation of the lungs suggest myocardial dysfunction and should raise suspicion for contusion. The jugular veins, however, may not be distended in patients who bleed from other lesions, and severe or refractory hypotension may be the only sign of cardiac injury.

    Pretre R, Chilcott M: Blunt trauma to the heart and great vessels. N Engl J Med 336:626–632, 1997.

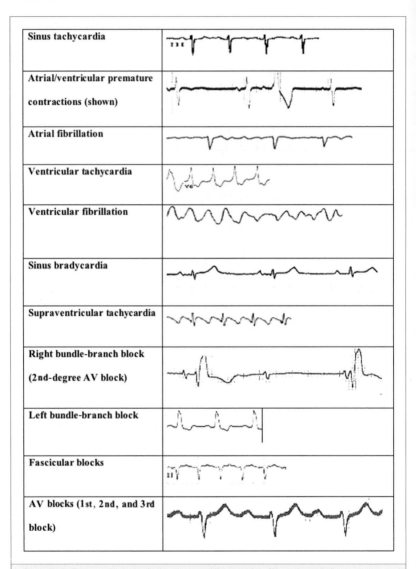

Sinus tachycardia	
Atrial/ventricular premature contractions (shown)	
Atrial fibrillation	
Ventricular tachycardia	
Ventricular fibrillation	
Sinus bradycardia	
Supraventricular tachycardia	
Right bundle-branch block (2nd-degree AV block)	
Left bundle-branch block	
Fascicular blocks	
AV blocks (1st, 2nd, and 3rd block)	

Figure 71-2. Electrocardiographic findings in myocardial contusion. AV = atrioventricular.

7. **What is the role of electrocardiography (ECG) in the diagnosis of myocardial contusion?**

According to recent guidelines, an ECG should be performed at the time of admission for all patients in whom BCI is suspected. ECG findings that are considered abnormal include atrial or ventricular arrhythmias, ST-segment depression or elevation, marked T-wave inversions, interventricular conduction delay, or bundle-branch block. ECG is neither sensitive nor specific in the diagnosis of myocardial contusions. Nonetheless, multiple studies have demonstrated that the presence of a normal ECG in a hemodynamically stable patient identifies a person who is at low risk for complications (Fig. 71-2).

Bansal MK, Maraj S, Chewaproug D, et al: Myocardial contusion injury: Redefining the myocardial contusion algorithm. Emerg Med J 22:465–469, 2005.

8. **What is the role of cardiac enzyme determinations in the diagnosis of myocardial contusion?**

Because myocardial contusion requires myocyte necrosis, one would think that measuring creatine kinase, myocardial bound (CKMB), would be useful. However, it is clear that CKMB is neither sensitive nor specific in the diagnosis of myocardial contusion based on positive echocardiographic and radionuclide imaging studies. In addition, it does not predict cardiac complications in patients with suspected myocardial contusion. Several recent studies have shown no utility to the test, and it should not be used routinely in patients suspected of having myocardial contusion.

Ruppert M, Van Hee R: Creatinine-kinase–MB determination in non-cardiac trauma: Its difference with cardiac infarction and its restricted use in trauma situations. Eur J Emerg Med 8:177–179, 2001.

9. **What is the role of troponin determination in the diagnosis of myocardial contusion?**

Cardiac troponin T and cardiac troponin I are regulatory proteins found exclusively in cardiac tissue. Studies have shown that troponins have a high sensitivity for detecting myocardial injury and a specificity superior to that of CKMB. Nonetheless, several other studies assessing the utility of troponins in BCI have revealed that, despite increased specificity compared with CKMB, they have low sensitivity and low predictive value in diagnosing myocardial contusion and do not affect the management of patients. However, they do serve as a useful screening tool.

Jackson L, Stewart A: Best evidence topic report: Use of troponin for the diagnosis of myocardial contusion after blunt chest trauma. Emerg Med J 22:193–195, 2005.

10. **How is transthoracic echocardiography (TTE) used in the diagnosis and management of myocardial contusion?**

The use of TTE along with Doppler ultrasound is a very useful diagnostic tool in the assessment of myocardial contusion. The presence of segmental wall motion abnormalities suggests contusion, and many investigators are currently using echocardiography as the gold standard. It is also useful for assessing the pericardial space as well as valve structure and integrity. Potential complications of myocardial contusion, such as right or left ventricular mural thrombus, aneurysm, or pseudoaneurysm, can also be recognized. In several studies, however, failure to achieve adequate images occurred in 15–62% of patients studied, limiting the usefulness of this test.

Sybrandy KC, Cramer MJM, Burgersdijk C: Diagnosing cardiac contusion: Old wisdom and new insights. Heart 89:485–489, 2003.

11. **How is transesophageal echocardiography (TEE) used in the diagnosis and management of myocardial contusion?**

It is a more "invasive" test than TTE, but it has a very high success rate and very few complications. In addition, it is a very useful tool for the diagnosis of traumatic aortic rupture and is comparable to computed tomographic scanning or aortography. However, TEE does not appear to be superior to TTE in predicting a subgroup of patients at increased risk for cardiac complications and adds to cost. TEE is recommended in suspected lesions to the great vessels or if the TTE images are suboptimal. Although it is an alternative to TTE when severe chest trauma prevents a complete examination, it is important to recognize the risks because TEE requires the insertion of an esophageal probe with the patient under sedation.

Sybrandy KC, Cramer MJM, Burgersdijk C: Diagnosing cardiac contusion: Old wisdom and new insights. Heart 89:485–489, 2003.

12. **Does imaging of the heart with radioisotopes help in the diagnosis of myocardial contusion?**

   Imaging techniques such as technetium pyrophosphate (infarct scanning), thallium scintigraphy, or radionuclide ventriculography have been studied extensively in the past but have fallen out of favor. In general, these studies are expensive and have failed to predict patients at risk of cardiac complications from cardiac contusions. In particular, they add little if echocardiography is performed. Positron emission tomography has shown advantages in the assessment of myocardial viability, but no data regarding its use in myocardial contusion are available.

   Sybrandy KC, Cramer MJM, Burgersdijk C: Diagnosing cardiac contusion: Old wisdom and new insights. Heart 89:485–489, 2003.

13. **What are the indications for invasive cardiac diagnostic studies in myocardial contusion?**

   Arteriography is indicated with a strong suspicion of coronary involvement with the development of new Q waves, ST-segment elevation in two adjacent leads, or the presence of a continuous cardiac murmur suggesting a possible coronary artery fistula. Right heart catheterization may be useful in patients with hemodynamic instability. The equilibration of intracardiac pressures, particularly with elevated right atrial and pulmonary capillary wedge pressure, is highly suggestive of pericardial tamponade. In addition, right and left ventricular injury, left-to-right shunts, and pulmonary artery hypertension can be diagnosed. All of these conditions are uncommon and can be made noninvasively by TTE.

KEY POINTS: MYOCARDIAL CONTUSION

1. Myocardial contusion is characterized by patchy areas of myocardial necrosis and hemorrhagic infiltrate that can be recognized in surgery or autopsy but not with conventional imaging studies.

2. Due to the anterior location of the right ventricle, it is not surprising that this is the most common site of contusion.

3. Myocardial contusion is usually clinically silent, but sinus tachycardia or hemodynamic instability may be the first manifestations of myocardial dysfunction.

4. Nonspecific electrocardiographic abnormalities are often seen in trauma patients. These may include noncardiac factors such as hypoxia, anemia, abnormal concentrations of serum electrolytes, and changes in vagal or sympathetic tone.

5. It is important to screen all patients with blunt chest trauma to identify those at risk for complications.

14. **What is the optimal approach to the diagnosis of myocardial contusion?**

   As there is no gold standard, investigators have moved away from trying to make the diagnosis of myocardial contusion and have tried to focus on the risk factors that predict cardiac complications in patients who have blunt chest trauma. Upon arrival in the emergency department, a focused physical examination, ECG, and chest radiography should be performed. There is no need to draw cardiac enzyme samples unless the ECG reveals changes suggestive of ischemia or infarction, and serial enzymes should not be drawn routinely. With suspected myocardial contusion and significant arrhythmias or hemodynamic instability, TTE should be performed. If necessary, TEE may be performed if the TTE is nondiagnostic.

15. **Describe the standard treatment of myocardial contusion.**
Asymptomatic patients with no associated injuries may be discharged from the emergency department after short observation if the ECG does not reveal significant abnormalities. Patients who have a prior history of coronary artery disease may be monitored on telemetry for 24 hours and should undergo serial ECGs; however, serial cardiac enzyme measurements should not be ordered routinely. Those patients with cardiac contusions who go on to have complications (e.g., arrhythmias, heart failure) will do so while being monitored in the intensive care unit because they tend to have more associated injuries that require treatment in an intensive care setting.

16. **Is routine hospitalization with ECG monitoring required in all cases of blunt chest trauma with suspected myocardial contusion?**
Some patients will have unrecognized significant myocardial injury that may result in serious ventricular arrhythmias or other cardiac complications. Because myocardial dysfunction has been evident on echocardiograms even in the presence of a normal 12-lead ECG and normal cardiac enzyme levels, all patients with severe injuries should be hospitalized with ECG monitoring for possible adverse cardiac events. On the other hand, in patients with no significant injuries and a normal ECG, a short period of monitoring in the emergency department is sufficient. The prognosis in these patients is excellent, and their clinical course is dictated by noncardiac injuries.

17. **Should all patients with sternal fractures be considered to have myocardial contusions and be admitted for monitoring?**
Sternal and rib fractures (>2) are often an indication of serious intrathoracic injury, usually involving motor vehicle crashes, and are believed to be associated with a high rate of cardiac contusion. Hemodynamically stable patients with a normal chest radiograph and a normal ECG have a very low rate of complications. Such patients can be safely discharged with oral pain medication and instructions to return for outpatient clinical follow-up.

   Limann ST, Kuzucu A, Tastepe Ai, et al: Chest injury due to blunt trauma. Eur J Cardiothorac Surg 23:374–378, 2003.

18. **Which patients requires outpatient follow-up?**
Patients with myocardial contusion require no specific follow-up unless they have a complicated cardiac clinical course. In those with severe wall motion abnormalities noted on echocardiography, a follow-up visit should occur at 4–6 weeks to exclude the rare late complications of aneurysm or pseudoaneurysm. There is no need for a repeat TTE in every patient because wall motion abnormalities resolve in 80–90% of patients with initial abnormal findings.

WEBSITE

Medline Plus: Myocardial contusion
www.nlm.nih.gov/medlineplus/ency/article/000202.htm

XIII. PERIOPERATIVE CARE

LIVER AND HEART TRANSPLANTATION

CHAPTER 72

Claus U. Niemann, MD, and Victor Ng, MD

LIVER TRANSPLANTATION

1. **How many liver transplantations are performed in the United States annually?**
   In the year 2005, 6444 liver transplantations were performed in the United States. This includes a small number from living liver donors. As of May 2006, 17,650 patients were on the waiting list for liver transplantation. Approximately 1751 patients die annually while awaiting liver transplantation. Nationwide, 3-year patient survival after transplant is approximately 76%.

   United Network for Organ Sharing: www.unos.org/

2. **What are the reasons for liver transplantation?**
   The list of diseases treatable by liver transplantation has increased steadily in the last years. The most common causes of end-stage liver disease leading to liver transplantation are chronic viral hepatitis B or C and alcoholic liver disease. The etiology of chronic liver disease can be classified as follows:
   - **Noncholestatic cirrhosis:** Alcohol; hepatitis A, B, C, or D; cryptogenic or autoimmune factors; drug use
   - **Cholestatic cirrhosis:** Primary biliary cirrhosis, secondary biliary cirrhosis, primary sclerosing cholangitis
   - **Acute hepatic necrosis:** Etiology unknown, drug use, acute hepatitis, environmental exposure (e.g., mushrooms)
   - **Metabolic disease:** Wilson's disease, hemochromatosis, primary oxalosis, glycogen storage disease, alpha$_1$-antitrypsin deficiency, tyrosinemia, homozygous hyperlipidemia
   - **Malignant neoplasm:** Hepatocellular carcinoma within the Milan or University of California–San Francisco criteria (most frequently), bile duct carcinoma, hepatoblastoma, hemangiosarcoma (all very rare)
   - **Miscellaneous:** Biliary atresia (in children, the most common indication), cystic fibrosis, polycystic liver disease, Budd-Chiari syndrome, neonatal hepatitis

   The Child-Turcotte-Pugh (CTP) classification has been used widely as an index of disease severity for patients with end-stage liver disease and was used previously for the organ allocation algorithm. However, due to shortcomings of the CTP scores and subsequent limitations in organ allocation, the model for end-stage liver disease (MELD) scoring system has been introduced. The MELD risk score is a mathematical formula that includes creatinine, bilirubin, and international normalized ratio. It does not include the etiology of liver disease.

   Belghiti J: Transplantation for liver tumors. Semin Oncol 32(6 Suppl 8):29–32, 2005.
   Sutcliffe R, Maguire D, Portmann B, et al: Selection of patients with hepatocellular carcinoma for liver transplantation. Br J Surg 93:11–18, 2006.
   Wiesner RH, McDiarmid SV, Kamath PS, et al: MELD and PELD: Application of survival models to liver allocation. Liver Transpl 7:567–580, 2001.

3. **Why might a patient be rejected for liver transplantation?**
   Reasons to deny transplant can vary from center to center. Liver transplantation is an extremely stressful procedure for patients. Significant coronary artery disease, cardiac dysfunction, and

pulmonary hypertension are considered contraindications. Uncontrolled infection or sepsis excludes a patient from transplantation as well. However, a positive human immunodeficiency virus test result, without evidence of acquired immunodeficiency syndrome, is *not* a contraindication. Advanced malignant hepatic disease or metastatic disease is in general considered to be a contraindication, as is uncontrolled and markedly elevated intracerebral pressure in the case of fulminant hepatic failure. Psychosocial factors such as active alcohol abuse or the lack of a good social support system may lead to the exclusion of the patient from transplantation. Hence, it is very important to evaluate the patients adequately in the preoperative phase and order necessary diagnostic tests. Old age *per se* is not a reason to deny liver transplantation. Indeed, patients older than 65 years of age are transplanted with increasing frequency.

Di Benedotto F, De Ruvo N, Berreta M, et al: Don't deny liver transplantation to HIV patients with hepatocellular carcinoma in the highly active antiretroviral therapy era. J Clin Oncol 24:e26–e27, 2006.
Terrault NA, Carter JT, Carlson J, et al: Outcome of patients with hepatitis B virus and human immunodeficiency virus infections referred for liver transplantation. Liver Transpl 12:801–807, 2006.

4. **What is the patient pathophysiology before liver transplantation?**
   It is important to realize that virtually every organ system can be affected by end-stage liver disease. Consequently, global assessment and considerations of all organ systems is of paramount importance:
   - **Central nervous system:** Hepatic encephalopathy and increased intracerebral pressure in acute hepatic failure
   - **Cardiac system:** Hyperdynamic circulation, cirrhotic cardiomyopathy
   - **Respiratory system:** Hepatopulmonary syndrome (i.e., $PaO_2 < 70$ mmHg, or AaO_2 gradient > 20 mmHg, intrapulmonary vascular dilation), portopulmonary hypertension (i.e., precapillary/arteriolar pulmonary hypertension, mean pulmonary arterial pressure >25 mmHg at rest, elevated pulmonary vascular resistance, primary pulmonary hypertension ruled out)
   - **Gastrointestinal system:** Portal hypertension with possible upper gastrointestinal bleeding, ascites
   - **Hematologic system:** Anemia, thrombocytopenia (sequestration into the spleen), prolonged prothrombin time and partial thromboplastin times, and decreased fibrinogen
   - **Renal system:** Hepatorenal syndrome, acute tubular necrosis
   - **Miscellaneous:** Electrolyte disturbances of virtually any kind, immunosuppression, malnutrition with ascites

   Baker K, Nasraway SA: Multiple organ failure during critical illness: How organ failure influences outcome in liver disease and liver transplantation. Liver Transpl 6:S5–S9, 2000.
   Baker J, Yost SC, Niemann CU: Organ transplantation. In Miller RD (ed): Anesthesia, 6th ed. Philadelphia, Churchill Livingstone, 2004, pp 2231–2283.
   Mandell MS: Critical care issues: Portopulmonary hypertension. Liver Transpl 6:S36–S43, 2000.
   Kang Y: Coagulopathies in hepatic disease. Liver Transpl 6:S72–S75, 2000.
   Liver Transplant Anaesthesia and Critical Care Forum: www.litac.net/

5. **What are common complications of patients undergoing liver transplantation?**
   Perioperative complications depend on the medical condition of the recipient (*see* question 4). Hemodynamic instability due to blood loss and massive fluid shifts, severe coagulopathy, electrolyte/glucose abnormalities, renal dysfunction, and respiratory compromise are frequently seen. Ultrasound is warranted if there is doubt about hepatic artery and portal vein patency. Thrombosis of the hepatic artery also requires retransplantation. Biliary leakage or bleeding is also encountered postoperatively.

   In addition, complications can be due to poor organ quality. The organ quality depends on multiple factors including donor age, organ ischemia time, and mechanism of death. Primary nonfunction of the organ, often manifesting immediately after transplantation, requires immediate retransplantation for the patient.

6. **What are indicators of good graft function in the immediate perioperative period?**
Bile production (intraoperatively), correction of negative base excess, normalization of prothrombin time, and decreasing fresh frozen plasma requirements.

7. **Does every patient receiving a liver transplant need to stay intubated and admitted to the intensive care unit (ICU) postoperatively?**
Postoperative intubation is not required, as long as significant respiratory compromise or concern of airway protection is absent. Increasingly, patients are extubated in the operating room. Fluid shifts or blood loss *per se* should not be considered as an indication for postoperative intubation.
   Most centers will admit patients to the ICU for monitoring purposes. However, certain centers, in uncomplicated cases, admit patients to the postanesthesia care unit and subsequently discharge them to the regular patient floor.

   Biancofiore G, Bindi ML, Romanelli AM, et al: Fast track liver transplantation: 5 years' experience. Eur J Anaesthesiol 22:584–590, 2005.
   Mandell MS, Lezotte D, Kam I, et al: Reduced use of intensive care after liver transplantation: Patient attributes that determine early transfer to surgical wards. Liver Transpl 8:682–687, 2002.
   Mandell MS, Lezotte D, Kam I, et al: Reduced use of intensive care after liver transplantation: Influence of early extubation. Liver Transpl 8:676–681, 2002.

8. **How do you manage a patient who has received a liver transplant in the immediate postoperative period?**
The perioperative course of patients undergoing liver transplantation is unpredictable. It can range from uncomplicated to extremely complex. Frequent assessment of cardiac and pulmonary function, serum glucose/electrolyte levels, renal and liver function, as well as coagulation and blood count is of great importance. In most cases, therapy is supportive and follows guidelines established for all intensive care patients. However, certain aspects require special attention:

- **Coagulopathy/bleeding:** Occasionally, patients require postoperative fresh frozen plasma therapy to offset an initially sluggish liver function. Fresh frozen plasma requirements are also considered an indirect measurement of postoperative liver function. In general, the patient can be weaned off fresh frozen plasma infusion over the first few postoperative hours. Aprotinin and aminocaproic acid are administered when severe coagulopathies exist, which are unresponsive to fresh frozen plasma alone. Some centers use these agents routinely in the perioperative phase to minimize blood loss. The need for the administration of platelets or cryoprecipitate is relatively low and reserved for selected cases. Lastly, one should have a low threshold for reexploration. Leakage from vascular anastomosis sites, "bleeders," and diminished flow in the hepatic artery or portal vein should always be the subject of observation.
- **Renal function:** Renal dysfunction is frequently present preoperatively and often worsens during the immediate postoperative period. This is due to temporary renal outflow obstruction during surgery when the inferior vena cava is clamped for insertion of the donor liver. Intraoperatively, venovenous bypass ameliorates the outflow obstruction but is not used at most centers. Postoperative monitoring of renal function and supportive therapy with adequate fluid, Lasix, and dopamine administration is usually sufficient. In some cases, continuous renal replacement therapy (i.e., continuous venovenous hemofiltration) through the immediate postoperative period will help with recovery of renal function.
- **Glucose/electrolytes:** With adequate postoperative liver function and steroid administration, patients tend to be hyperglycemic, which may warrant an insulin drip. Depending on the renal function and diuretic therapy, the potassium level can be either high or low. Calcium homeostasis is usually not a problem in the postoperative period.
- **Immunosuppression:** Allograft rejection can occur at any given point after surgery and is classified as hyperacute, acute, or chronic. The administration of immunosuppressive therapy is usually initiated immediately after surgery. Common drugs, often used in combination,

are cyclosporine, tacrolimus, sirolimus, mycophenolate mofetil, and steroids. These agents can cause a variety of side effects, including undesired drug interactions, hypertension, hyperlipidemia, and osteoporosis.

Baker J, Yost SC, Niemann CU: Organ transplantation. In Miller RD (ed): Anesthesia, 6th ed. Philadelphia Churchill Livingstone, 2004, pp 2231–2283.
Liver Transplant Anaesthesia and Critical Care Forum: www.litac.net/

HEART TRANSPLANTATION

9. **How many heart transplantations are performed in the United States annually?**
    In the year 2005, 2127 heart transplantations were performed in the United States. As of May 2006, 3006 patients were on the waiting list for heart transplantation. Approximately 402 patients die annually while awaiting heart transplantation. Nationwide, 3-year patient survival after transplant is approximately 77%.

    United Network for Organ Sharing: www.unos.org/

10. **What are the reasons for heart transplantation?**
    Cardiac transplantation has become an accepted treatment for selected patients with end-stage heart failure. As with liver transplantation, the number of candidates and the waiting time have increased over the last years. The most common causes of end-stage heart disease leading to heart transplantation are cardiomyopathy and coronary artery disease. The etiology of end-stage heart disease can be classified as follows:
    - **Dilated cardiomyopathy:** Viral, idiopathic, postpartum, and familial factors; Adriamycin; myocarditis; ischemia
    - **Restricted cardiomyopathy:** Sarcoidosis, amyloidosis, endocardial fibrosis, idiopathic factors, secondary radiation, chemotherapy
    - **Retransplantation/graft failure:** Primary failure, hyperacute or acute causes, chronic rejection, restrictive/constrictive factors, accelerated allograft coronary artery disease
    - **Other:** Congenital disease, valvular disease, hypertrophic cardiomyopathy

    It is important to keep in mind that medical treatment of patients with end-stage heart disease continuously improves, the conditions of selected patients can be managed medically, and survival outcomes have become similar to heart transplantation. Hence, heart transplantation should be offered to patients who experience severe disability due to their cardiac disease despite optimal medical treatment and who have no major contraindications for heart transplantation.

    Taylor DO, Edwards LB, Boucek MM, et al: Registry of the International Society for Heart and Lung Transplantation: Twenty-second official adult heart transplant report—2005. J Heart Lung Transpl 24:945–955, 2005.

11. **Why might a patient be rejected for heart transplantation?**
    Contraindications may vary slightly from center to center. Common contraindications include significant/irreversible pulmonary hypertension; renal, hepatic, or cerebrovascular disease; uncontrolled infection or sepsis; and cancer of uncertain status. Other contraindications may be due to the cause of the patient's cardiomyopathy, as in the instance of amyloid or sarcoid disease. In addition, lack of compliance, psychological stability, lack of a supportive social environment, and active drug abuse may exclude a patient from heart transplantation. Old age *per se* is not a reason to deny heart transplantation. Indeed, patients older than 65 years receive transplants with increasing frequency.

    Blanche C, Blanche DA, Kearney B, et al: Heart transplantation in patients seventy years of age and older: A comparative analysis of outcome. J Thorac Cardiovasc Surg 121:532–541, 2001.
    Hunt SA: Who and when to consider for heart transplantation. Cardiol Rev 9:18–20, 2001.

2. What is the physiology after heart transplantation?

Although baseline cardiac function is generally preserved, the cardiac response to demand is significantly altered. Cardiac denervation is nearly always permanent after transplantation. Due to the lack of sympathetic innervation, heart rate can only increase slowly via increased circulating catecholamine levels. Maintaining an adequate stroke volume, therefore, becomes of paramount importance to sustain cardiac output in these patients. Hence, patients who have received heart transplant are very preload dependent. Denervation also affects the pharmacologic therapy in these patients. Drugs that act indirectly on the heart—either through the sympathetic or parasympathetic nervous system—are ineffective. Drugs acting directly on the heart are the agents of choice to modify cardiac physiology. In addition, denervation of the heart prevents the recipient from experiencing chest pain when myocardial ischemia is present.

Ashary N, Kaye AD, Hegazi AR, et al: Anesthetic considerations in the patient with a heart transplant. Heart Dis 4:191–198, 2002.

3. What are common complications seen in patients undergoing heart transplantation?

Long-term survival rates have significantly improved for patients undergoing heart transplantation. However, there are a number of complications that may occur after transplantation. The complications include right or left ventricular failure, pulmonary hypertension, systemic hypertension, heart block, bradyarrhythmias, tachyarrhythmias, early graft failure, allograft rejection, accelerated allograft coronary artery disease, renal dysfunction, infection, and malignancy. The postoperative stability of the patient is also affected by donor characteristics and by the operative technique chosen. The use of the bicaval and total techniques over the biatrial technique has resulted in less atrioventricular valve dysfunction and arrhythmias. Use of these newer techniques has also shown improvements in hemodynamics, exercise capacity, and overall patient survival.

Luckraz H, Goddard M, Charman SC, et al: Early mortality after cardiac transplantation: Should we do better? J Heart Lung Transpl 24:401–405, 2005.

Morgan JA, Edwards NM: Orthotopic cardiac transplantation: Comparison of outcome using biatrial, bicaval, and total techniques. J Card Surg 20:102–106, 2005.

Wagoner LE: Management of the cardiac transplant recipient: Roles of the transplant cardiologist and primary care physician. Am J Med Sci 314:173–184, 1997.

14. How do you manage the treatment of a heart transplant patient in the immediate postoperative period?

Similar to other patients who have undergone cardiac surgery, patients who have received heart transplant require close monitoring via electrocardiography, arterial blood pressure, central venous pressure, pulmonary artery pressure, cardiac output, arterial blood gas measurements, and chest tube output. Most patients will require chronotropic and inotropic support in the form of pacing and/or β-adrenergic agonist infusion (e.g., isoproterenol, epinephrine, dobutamine, dopamine). If cardiac function is still depressed despite pacing and pharmacologic support, mechanical support in the form of intraaortic balloon pumps, ventricular assist devices, or extracorporeal membrane oxygenators can be instituted. Once the hemodynamic state and postoperative bleeding have stabilized, patients may be extubated. Certain aspects warrant special attention:

- **Preload dependence:** As mentioned, patients are very preload dependent due to cardiac denervation. This renders them sensitive to positive-pressure ventilation, bleeding/ tamponade, and pneumothorax.
- **Increased pulmonary vascular resistance (PVR)/right ventricular failure:** Although fixed pulmonary hypertension will have been excluded preoperatively, postoperative increased PVR may still develop. If severe and untreated, it can lead to right ventricular failure in the newly grafted heart. Management of increased PVR includes inhaled vasodilators such as

prostacyclin and nitric oxide. Intravenous vasodilators such as nitroglycerin and nitroprusside are also options. Unfortunately, IV vasodilators are associated with systemic hypotension, and their use may require an additional alpha agonist infusion. If vasodilator therapy is ineffective, right ventricular assist devices or extracorporeal membrane oxygenators may be required.

- **Cardiac arrhythmias:** In addition to bradycardia and heart block, atrial and ventricular tachyarrhythmias are also quite common after heart transplantation. Atrial arrhythmias may be associated with allograft rejection.
- **Rejection/graft failure:** Allograft rejection can occur at any given point after surgery and is classified as hyperacute, acute, or chronic. Diagnosis of rejection of a transplanted heart is difficult and relies mainly on endomyocardial biopsy, particularly in view of vague clinical symptoms and no reliable serologic markers. Serial biopsies are performed postoperatively to detect any sign of rejection.
- **Immunosuppression:** Immunosuppressive therapy is usually initiated immediately after surgery. Common drugs, often used in combination, include cyclosporine, tacrolimus, mycophenolate mofetil, azathioprine, and steroids. These agents can cause a variety of adverse effects and drug interactions (Box 72-1).

Ardehali A, Hughes K, Sadeghi A, et al: Inhaled nitric oxide for pulmonary hypertension after heart transplantation. Transplantation 72:638–641, 2001.

Costanzo MR: New immunosuppressive drugs in heart transplantation. Curr Control Trials Cardiovasc Med 2:45–53, 2001.

Goudarzi BM, Bonvino S: Critical care issues in lung and heart transplantation. Crit Care Clin 19:209–231, 2003.

Miniati DN, Robbins RC: Heart transplantation: A thirty-year perspective. Annu Rev Med 53:189–220, 2002.

BOX 72-1. SIDE EFFECTS OF IMMUNOSUPPRESSIVE DRUGS

Azathioprine: myelosuppression

Cyclosporine: hypertension, $\downarrow$renal function, $\uparrow K^+$, $\downarrow Mg^{++}$, $\downarrow$seizure threshold

Mycophenolate mofetil: myelosuppression, gastrointestinal tract bleeding

Prednisone: hypertension, $\uparrow$glucose, adrenal suppression

Tacrolimus: $\downarrow$renal function, $\downarrow$seizure threshold, $\uparrow$glucose, $\uparrow K^+$, $\downarrow Mg^{++}$

K = potassium, Mg = magnesium.

---

15. **How will the denervated heart respond to medications in the post-transplantation period?**
    - **Indirect cardiac agents:** Drugs such as ephedrine and atropine are mediated via the sympathetic and parasympathetic nervous system. These drugs will have minimal effects. Digitalis will also have no effect on atrioventricular nodal conduction, but it retains its direct inotropic effect.
    - **Direct cardiac agents:** β-Adrenergic agents (e.g., isoproterenol, epinephrine, dobutamine, dopamine, norepinephrine) are unaffected and will improve both chronotropy and inotropy. Phosphodiesterase inhibitors (e.g., amrinone, milrinone) are also unaffected and improve cardiac output as well as cause vasodilation.
    - **Vasodilators:** Nitrates are unaffected and cause both venous and arterial vasodilation. However, due to the denervation, reflex tachycardia is severely depressed.

- **Vasoconstrictors:** Phenylephrine, norepinephrine, and vasopressin are still effective, but less reflex bradycardia is seen.
- **Beta blockers and calcium channel blockers:** These agents retain the ability to decrease heart rate and blood pressure.

Ashary N, Kaye AD, Hegazi AR, et al: Anesthetic considerations in the patient with a heart transplant. Heart Dis 4:191–198, 2002.

Quinlan JJ, Firestone S, Firestone LL: Anesthesia for heart, lung, and heart–lung transplantation. In Kaplan JA (ed): Cardiac Anesthesia, 4th ed. Philadelphia, W.B. Saunders, 1999, pp 991–999.

KEY POINTS: LIVER AND HEART TRANSPLANTATION

1. Postoperative complications of liver transplantation include poor organ function and significant metabolic disturbances (e.g., hyperglycemia).

2. Denervated hearts are preload dependent and respond only to direct-acting cardiac medications. They do not display reflex bradycardia or tachycardia.

XIV. SEDATION AND PAIN MANAGEMENT

USE OF PARALYTIC AGENTS IN THE INTENSIVE CARE UNIT

Michael T. Ganter, MD, and Jean-François Pittet, MD

1. **What are the indications of neuromuscular blocking agents (commonly called *muscle relaxants* or *paralytics*) in the intensive care unit (ICU)?**
   Indications for muscle relaxants in the ICU are summarized in Table 73-1. Neuromuscular blockade always requires adequate sedation and analgesia, otherwise your patient is at risk for awareness (i.e., being awake but paralyzed).

TABLE 73-1. INDICATIONS FOR NEUROMUSCULAR BLOCKADE IN THE INTENSIVE CARE UNIT (ICU)	
Action	**Reason**
Endotracheal intubation	
Mechanical ventilation*	To allow lung-protective ventilation (low tidal volume ventilation, permissive hypercapnia), to increase chest wall compliance and reduce peak airway pressures, to prevent poorly coordinated respiratory efforts
General anesthesia*	To facilitate surgical, pulmonary, gastrointestinal, or radiologic procedures
Transport of intubated ICU patients*	To allow a safe transport
Control of intracranial pressure*	To prevent respiratory or other movements and coughing on tracheal suction in intubated patients with cerebral pathologies
Reduction of muscle oxygen consumption*	
Increased muscle activity*	To facilitate treatment of tetanus, status epilepticus, and neuroleptic malignant syndrome

*Neuromuscular blockade is optional. Consider management with sedation/analgesia alone.

2. **How does the neuromuscular transmission work?**
   Acetylcholine (ACh) is released from storage vesicles in the terminal nerve into the synaptic cleft and binds to *nicotinic* cholinergic receptors on the motor end plate of the skeletal muscle cell.

This initiates ion permeability changes on the muscle cell membrane (depolarization leading to action potential) with subsequent intracellular release of calcium from the sarcoplasmatic reticulum, causing a contraction of the skeletal muscle cell. Depolarization terminates because ACh is rapidly hydrolyzed by the substrate-specific acetylcholinesterase located in the membrane of the motor end plate next to the ACh receptor. Additionally, there is diffusion away from the synaptic cleft as well as reuptake of ACh into the terminal nerve.

3. **What are the two classes of muscle relaxants?**
   Muscle relaxants are classified as *depolarizing* (e.g., succinylcholine) or *nondepolarizing* (e.g., the benzylisochinolines [mivacurium, atracurium, cis-atracurium] and the aminosteroids [vecuronium, rocuronium, pancuronium]), according to their mechanism of action. Both are structurally related to ACh. Basic pharmacology is described in Table 73-2.

TABLE 73-2. PHARMACOLOGY OF COMMON NEUROMUSCULAR-BLOCKING AGENTS IN ADULTS

	Intubation Dose (mg/kg)	Onset of Action (min)	Duration of Action	Continuous Infusion (μg/kg/min)	Primary Elimination
Depolarizing neuromuscular-blocking agents					
Succinylcholine	1.0–1.5	0.5–1.0	Short	N/A	Ester hydrolysis
Nondepolarizing neuromuscular-blocking agents					
Mivacurium	0.2	2–3	Short	8–10	Ester hydrolysis
Atracurium	0.5	1.5–3	Intermediate	5–10	Hofmann, ester hydrolysis
Cis-atracurium	0.15	2–4	Intermediate	0.5–10	Hofmann, ester hydrolysis
Vecuronium	0.1	1.5–3	Intermediate	0.8–1.5	Hepatic
Rocuronium	0.6–0.9	1–2	Intermediate	5–15	Hepatic
Pancuronium	0.1	1.5–4	Long	1–10	Renal, hepatic

4. **Describe the mechanism of action of depolarizing muscle relaxants?**
   They physically resemble ACh and act as an *agonist* by binding to the cholinergic receptors at the motor end plate. The postjunctional membrane is becoming depolarized, and further neuromuscular transmission is blocked. The skeletal muscles are refractory to repeat depolarization because calcium is not being re-sequestered into the sarcoplasmatic reticulum until the muscle relaxant diffuses away from the receptor. This results in the relaxation of skeletal muscles. *Depolarizing* muscle relaxants are not metabolized by acetylcholinesterase in the synaptic cleft, but they are hydrolyzed by the plasma pseudocholinesterase.

5. **Name some esterase enzymes in the body, their localizations, and their functions.**

Acetylcholinesterase (also called *specific* or *true cholinesterase*) is present in the synaptic cleft of the neuromuscular junction and cleaves ACh. Pseudocholinesterase (also called *plasmacholinesterase*) is localized in the plasma and liver and hydrolyses several drugs such as succinylcholine, mivacurium, ester-type local anesthetics, and trimetaphan. Further esterase enzymes include the nonspecific esterases (located in plasma and certain tissues, cleave atracurium and remifentanil) as well as erythrocyte esterase (located in the red blood cells, cleaves esmolol).

6. **When should succinylcholine be used in the ICU?**

Critically ill patients may require emergent intubations. Because many ICU patients are considered to have full stomach or delayed gastric emptying (e.g., not NPO, trauma, ileus, severe illness, comorbidities such as diabetes or renal failure), it is imperative that intubation be done quickly in a well-controlled setting. Succinylcholine has a rapid onset of action (30–60 seconds) and a brief duration of action (typically <10 minutes), making it useful in these situations.

7. **What are the contraindications to the use of succinylcholine?**

Succinylcholine causes the serum potassium concentration to increase by 0.5–1.0 mEq/L in healthy patients. Therefore, it should be avoided in patients with preexisting hyperkalemia. An exaggerated release of potassium after administration of succinylcholine has to be anticipated in conditions such as burn injuries, massive trauma (e.g., crush injuries), prolonged total body immobilization (e.g., long ICU stay), sepsis, and neuromuscular disorders (e.g., upper and lower motor neuron injuries, Duchenne's dystrophy). Furthermore, succinylcholine should not be used in children (because of undiagnosed neuromuscular disorders) and patients susceptible to malignant hyperthermia. Impaired liver function may prolong the neuromuscular blockade.

Malignant Hyperthermia Association of the United States: www.mhaus.org

8. **Is it safe to use succinylcholine in burn patients initially?**

Yes. As with other patients at risk for an exaggerated increase in serum potassium, there is general agreement that it is safe to use succinylcholine in the initial 24 hours after injury. After a burn, extrajunctional ACh receptors start to proliferate outside the neuromuscular junction in proportion to the burn. Rapid elevations of serum potassium levels to >9 mm with cardiac arrest have been documented in this situation after succinylcholine administration. The risk of hyperkalemia appears to peak 7–10 days after injury. However, the exact time and duration of the risk period vary largely.

MacLennan N, Heimbach DM, Cullen BF: Anesthesia for major thermal injury. Anesthesiology 89:749–770, 1998.

9. **Explain the difference in the mechanism of action of *nondepolarizing* compared with *depolarizing* muscle relaxants.**

Nondepolarizing muscle relaxants function as *competitive antagonists* on the cholinergic receptors of the motor endplate. ACh is prevented from binding to its receptors, and no motor end plate potential develops. Depolarizing muscle relaxants function as *agonists* on the cholinergic receptors of the motor end plate. This difference explains their different behavior in various disease states. Upregulation of ACh receptors (e.g., denervation injuries) causes a relative resistance to nondepolarizing muscle relaxants (more ACh receptors are present) but an increased response to depolarizing muscle relaxants because more ACh receptors are present. In a clinical situation with downregulation of ACh receptors (e.g., myasthenia gravis), exactly the opposite happens.

10. **How do you decide which nondepolarizing agent to use?**
   Before prescribing a nondepolarizing muscle relaxant, we have to know a patient's hepatic and renal function, cardiovascular status, and comedications. Basic pharmacology is described in Table 73-2.

   Murray MJ, Cowen J, DeBlock H, et al: Clinical practice guidelines for sustained neuromuscular blockade in the adult critically ill patient. Crit Care Med 30:142–156, 2002.

11. **Which nondepolarizing agent has the shortest duration of action?**
   Mivacurium is the shortest-acting nondepolarizing muscle relaxant (duration of action, 15–30 min after intubation dose). Like succinylcholine, mivacurium is metabolized by pseudocholinesterase. Therefore, the duration of action may be prolonged in patients with low pseudocholinesterase activity—acquired (e.g., renal or hepatic insufficiency, pregnancy, postpartum) or congenital (e.g., defective pseudocholinesterase). One potentially serious side effect is its substantial, dose-dependent histamine release. There are few data about the use of mivacurium in the ICU.

12. **Which nondepolarizing agent is the likely choice for patients with renal or hepatic failure?**
   Atracurium is inactivated in the plasma by Hofmann elimination and ester hydrolysis, so it may be the drug of choice for patients with renal or hepatic failure. However, severe hypothermia and acidosis decrease the rate of the Hofmann elimination, and the dose should be adjusted in these clinical situations. One major adverse effect is histamine release at higher doses. There is some controversy about one active metabolite of the Hofmann elimination, laudanosine. This metabolite has been associated with central nervous system excitation in animals at very high concentrations; however, it seems unlikely to be of clinical significance in humans.

13. **How is cis-atracurium different from atracurium?**
   Cis-atracurium, one of the isomers of atracurium, is 3–4 times more potent than the parent drug. Because less drug is administered, less histamine and laudanosine is released compared with that released with atracurium.

14. **Which nondepolarizing agent is useful in patients with obstructive pulmonary or cardiovascular disease?**
   Vecuronium does not produce histamine release and has no cardiovascular side effects, so it is useful in patients with obstructive pulmonary or cardiovascular disease. The drug is primarily metabolized by the liver. Prolonged neuromuscular blockade may occur in patients with hepatic failure, but there is no difference in half-life in patients with renal failure compared with healthy patients.

15. **Which nondepolarizing agent has the fastest onset of action?**
   Rocuronium is similar to vecuronium but less potent and is the nondepolarizing agent with the fastest onset of action. When given as a bolus of 0.6–0.9 mg/kg, complete neuromuscular blockade is almost always achieved within 2 minutes. In addition to having the same indications as vecuronium, it is the drug of choice for rapid-sequence inductions, if succinylcholine is contraindicated.

16. **What are the distinct features of pancuronium?**
   Pancuronium is a long-acting paralytic agent and does not produce histamine release. Its duration of action is prolonged in hepatic and renal failure: it is metabolized in the liver and then equally eliminated in the bile and urine. Due to a vagal blockade, tachycardia, hypertension, and increased cardiac output may occur.

17. **How can one monitor the level of neuromuscular blockade in the ICU?**
    Neuromuscular monitoring is usually done with a peripheral nerve stimulator. Surface
    electrodes are attached over a peripheral nerve (e.g., ulnar nerve in the forearm) and connected
    to the nerve stimulator. A monophasic, supramaximal current with a square wave form is
    applied and the motor response of the stimulated muscle monitored (e.g., adductor pollicis
    muscle). The duration of each impulse delivered is set to 0.2–0.3 msec. The most widely used
    pattern of nerve stimulation is the train-of-four (TOF) stimulation: four supramaximal stimuli are
    applied over a 2-second period. The observed response can be quantified as TOF count (i.e., the
    number of detectable twitches, 0–4) or as TOF ratio (i.e., the amplitude of the fourth twitch
    divided by the amplitude of the first twitch). TOF count can be measured visually or by tactile
    assessment. However, more sophisticated equipment such as mechanomyography,
    electromyography, or acceleromyography is required to determine the TOF ratio.

    Murphy GS, Szokol JW: Monitoring neuromuscular blockade. Int Anesthesiol Clin 42:25–40, 2004.

18. **How many ACh receptors have to be occupied by a nondepolarizing muscle
    relaxant before the TOF ratio starts to decrease?**
    The TOF ratio is 1.0 in normal subjects in the absence of muscle relaxants. During a partial
    nondepolarizing block, a progressive decrease in the amplitude of each twitch will occur (fade).
    Seventy to seventy-five percent of the ACh receptors have to be occupied before the fourth
    twitch begins to decrease; that is, the TOF ratio starts to decrease to <1.0.

19. **When and how should neuromuscular monitoring be used in the ICU?**
    Neuromuscular monitoring should be used in every patient in the ICU receiving neuromuscular
    blocking agents over a longer period of time. This is how boluses or infusion rates of muscle
    relaxants can be adjusted to optimize the level of neuromuscular blockade. The intended level of
    paralysis depends on the clinical situation. In most situations, it is appropriate to maintain the
    infusion rate of a muscle relaxant at a level that produces partial blockade (e.g., presence of at
    least the first twitch of the TOF).

    Rudis MI, Sikora CA, Angus E, et al: A prospective, randomized, controlled evaluation of peripheral nerve
    stimulation versus standard clinical dosing of neuromuscular blocking agents in critically ill patients. Crit Care
    Med 25:575–583, 1997.

20. **What are the risks related to the use of nondepolarizing muscle relaxants in the
    ICU?**
    Prolonged use is associated with the following risks:
    - Inability to clear pulmonary secretions because of the suppression of cough
    - Atrophy of skeletal muscles
    - Venous thrombosis and pulmonary embolism
    - Osteoporosis with impairment of calcium-phosphorus balance
    - Psychic trauma if the patient is not adequately sedated while paralyzed
    - Skin breakdown
    - Injuries to nerves and limbs resulting from poor positioning

21. **Discuss the interactions between muscle relaxants and other drugs used in the
    ICU.**
    Various drugs either potentiate or inhibit the effect of neuromuscular-blocking agents.
    A summary is given in Table 73-3.

22. **Is prolonged neuromuscular weakness a significant problem in the ICU?**
    Yes. Prolonged paralyses (up to several weeks) after drug discontinuation have been
    documented after the use of nondepolarizing muscle relaxants in the ICU. There are two distinct
    types of prolonged neuromuscular blockade related to muscle relaxants in the ICU. The first type

is a pharmacokinetic problem related to alterations in drug clearance and the formation of active metabolites; the second is a functional neuromuscular problem *not* related to abnormal pharmacokinetics.

TABLE 73-3. INTERACTIONS WITH NEUROMUSCULAR–BLOCKING AGENTS	
Potentiate neuromuscular-blocking effects	
Antibiotics	Aminoglycosides, tetracyclines
	Vancomycin, clindamycin
	Metronidazole
Antiarrhythmics	Quinidine, procainamide, lidocaine
	Beta blockers
	Bretylium
	Calcium channel blockers
Anesthetics	Inhalational anesthetics
	Ketamine
	Local anesthetics
Others	Magnesium
	Lithium
	Dantrolene
	Cyclosporine, cyclophosphamide
	Mineralocorticoids
Inhibit neuromuscular-blocking effects	
Anticonvulsants	Phenytoin
	Carbamazepine
	Sodium valproate
Others	Azathioprine
	Ranitidine
	Theophylline

KEY POINTS: RISKS OF PROLONGED NEUROMUSCULAR BLOCKADE IN THE INTENSIVE CARE UNIT

1. Hypoxia can occur if accidental interruption of the ventilator occurs.

2. No cough reflex can cause retention of pulmonary secretions, occult aspiration, infection, and pneumonia.

3. Thrombosis and pulmonary embolism are other risks of immobilization due to prolonged neuromuscular blockade.

4. Muscle atrophy, acute myopathy, and osteoporosis can occur.

5. Last, the patient is at risk for skin breakdown and decubitus ulcers.

3. **When should an active metabolite be suspected as the cause for prolonged neuromuscular blockade in the ICU?**
An example is 3-desacetylvecuronium, an active metabolite of vecuronium. It has 50% of the pharmacologic activity of the parent compound and a prolonged half-life. This metabolite has caused prolonged weakness in ICU patients receiving vecuronium for longer than 48 hours. Patients at high risk appear to be those who (1) have renal failure, (2) have hypermagnesemia, (3) have metabolic acidosis, or (4) are female.

4. **When should a functional neuromuscular abnormality be suspected as a cause of prolonged weakness?**
A number of drugs can cause neuromuscular weakness (*see* Table 73-3). Other factors, including poor nutrition, infections, atrophy, and demyelination (e.g., chronic inflammatory demyelinating polyneuropathy), may also contribute to prolonged weakness, with or without the use of neuromuscular blocking agents. However, neuromuscular blocking agents may cause an acute myopathy themselves with selective loss of myosin filaments. Most reported cases have occurred after combined treatment with high doses of corticosteroids and muscle relaxants. The risk of this complication is reduced by limiting the administration of neuromuscular blocking agents to ≤48 hours.

5. **How can prolonged neuromuscular blockade be prevented in the ICU?**
Common-sense recommendations seem prudent. First, one should use neuromuscular blocking agents only when indicated, in the lowest effective dose, and for the shortest duration as clinical circumstances allow. Second, one should consider avoiding the use of vecuronium or pancuronium in patients with renal failure. Third, one should consider the avoidance of muscle relaxants in patients receiving corticosteroids. Fourth, one should always monitor the depth of neuromuscular blockade with a peripheral nerve stimulator.

6. **What is the best way to terminate the actions of muscular relaxants?**
The best way is to ventilate the patient and wait until these drugs are metabolized or excreted. The level of neuromuscular blockade should be followed with a peripheral nerve stimulator.

7. **Which drugs can be used to terminate the action of muscle relaxants?**
Nondepolarizing muscle relaxants may be antagonized by cholinesterase inhibitors (anticholinesterases), which block the hydrolysis of ACh. As a result, the concentration of ACh increases at the neuromuscular junction, displacing the nondepolarizing muscle relaxant molecules from the ACh receptor.

8. **What is the usual dosage of cholinesterase inhibitors?**
The following drugs can be administered intravenously:
- Neostigmine, 0.03–0.06 mg/kg
- Pyridostigmine, 0.1–0.4 mg/kg
- Edrophonium, 0.5–1.0 mg/kg

9. **What are the adverse effects of cholinesterase inhibitors? How do we treat them?**
The most common adverse effect is excessive stimulation of muscarinic cholinergic receptors (i.e., parasympathetic stimulation). This results in cardiovascular (e.g., bradycardia, hypotension), pulmonary (e.g., hypersecretion, bronchospasm), gastrointestinal (e.g., increased motility and secretion), and urogenital (e.g., increased bladder tone) symptoms, as well as pupillary constriction (e.g., miosis). To counteract these side effects, it is recommended to administer cholinesterase inhibitors in combination with atropine (0.01–0.02 mg/kg IV) or glycopyrrolate (0.01 mg/kg IV).

PAIN MANAGEMENT IN THE INTENSIVE CARE UNIT

Michael T. Ganter, MD, and Jean-François Pittet, MD

1. **Why do critically ill patients have pain?**
   Pain experienced by patients in the intensive care unit (ICU) may arise from a variety of situations, such as underlying medical disease, trauma, or invasive procedures. Furthermore, monitoring and therapeutic devices (e.g., catheters, tubes and drains, noninvasive ventilation devices, endotracheal tube), routine nursing care (e.g., dressing changes, mobilization, physical therapy, airway suctioning), and prolonged immobility may also cause pain and discomfort in this population.

2. **Is pain relief generally adequate in ICU patients?**
   The degree of analgesia in critically ill patients is often inadequate. One of the reasons is that the level of pain is harder to assess in ICU patients because patients are often confused, unable to communicate, or even paralyzed. Furthermore, practitioners may be overly concerned about the adverse effects of pain treatment.

   Mularski RA: Pain management in the intensive care unit. Crit Care Clin 20:381–401, 2004.

3. **How can one assess pain in critically ill patients?**
   Efforts should be made to objectively quantify and systematically document the patient's level of pain. Pain assessment and response to therapy should be performed regularly by using a scale appropriate to the patient population:
   - In an awake and alert patient, the most reliable and valid indicator of pain is the patient's self report. Several pain assessment tools are available; unidimensional tools are used most frequently (e.g., visual analog scale [VAS], score 0–10; Fig. 74-1).
   - In sedated and noninteractive patients, assessment of pain is more challenging. Physiologic indicators (e.g., heart rate, blood pressure, respiratory rate) and the general presentation/ pain-related behavior of the patient (e.g., posturing, facial expression, movement), as well as the change in these parameters after analgesic therapy, are used to estimate the level of pain.

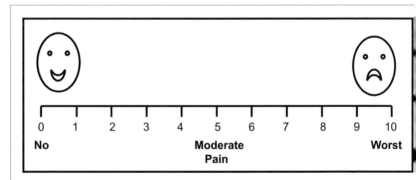

Figure 74-1. Visual analog scale.

4. **What are the therapeutic goals of pain management in the ICU?**
The goal is to adequately manage pain and to provide analgesia to all critically ill patients.
A desirable analgesia is considered, for example, a pain rating ≤3 of 10 using the VAS scale.
Besides the primary goal of optimizing patient comfort, adequate analgesia is crucial to attenuate
potentially deleterious physiologic responses to pain; that is, sympathetic activation with
tachycardia and increased myocardial oxygen consumption, persistent catabolism,
hypercoagulability, and immunosuppression. Other benefits of adequate pain relief are the
prevention of thrombosis and pulmonary embolism by earlier patient mobilization. Furthermore,
epidural anesthesia, for example, may shorten postoperative ileus and lower the morbidity of
cardiovascular and pulmonary complications after thoracic and or abdominal surgeries.

Bonnet F, Marret E: Influence of anaesthetic and analgesic techniques on outcome after surgery. Br J Anaesth 95:52–58, 2005.

KEY POINTS: REASONS FOR ADEQUATE ANALGESIA IN CRITICALLY ILL PATIENTS

1. Patient comfort and ethical aspects are two reasons why adequate analgesia is sanctioned.

2. Attenuation of potentially deleterious physiologic responses to pain is also addressed. This
includes sympathetic activation, increased myocardial consumption, persistent catabolism,
hypercoagulability, and immunosuppression.

5. **Explain the treatment options for a critically ill patient in pain.**
There are nonpharmacologic and pharmacologic options:
- **Nonpharmacologic:** Nonpharmacologic treatment of pain includes proper positioning of
patients, stabilization of fractures, elimination of irritating physical stimulation, and a variety
of therapies to promote patient comfort (e.g., environment modification, music therapy,
relaxation, massage). Because sleep deprivation as well as anxiety and delirium may diminish
the pain threshold, it is important to minimize stimuli that can disturb the normal diurnal sleep
pattern (e.g., noise, artificial light) and to treat anxiety and delirium promptly.
- **Pharmacologic:** Pharmacologic treatment of pain works by inhibition of the release of local
mediators in damaged tissue (e.g., nonsteroidal anti-inflammatory drugs [NSAIDs],
acetaminophen), blocking the nerve conduction (e.g., regional anesthesia), or altering the
perception of pain in the central nervous system (e.g., opioids, acetaminophen, ketamine).

Jacobi J, Fraser GL, Coursin DB, et al: Clinical practice guidelines for the sustained use of sedatives and analgesics in the critically ill adult. Crit Care Med 30:119–141, 2002.

6. **What is the role of opioids in the ICU? How do they act?**
Opioids are the mainstay of analgesic therapy in the ICU. The term *opioids* refers to any agent
with activity at an opioid receptor. There are at least four discreet opioid receptors in the central
and peripheral nervous system; the analgesic effects of opioids are mediated mostly via mu (μ)
or kappa (κ) receptors. Interactions at other receptors may contribute to adverse effects.

7. **Which opioids are recommended for routine administration in ICU patients?**
Morphine, fentanyl, hydromorphone, and sufentanil are the analgesic agents most commonly
used and recommended in the ICU (Table 74-1). Alternatively, the use of other opioids such as
remifentanil and alfentanil may be considered for use in selected patient groups. However, these
drugs are mostly used as adjuncts to anesthesia and for immediate postoperative analgesia
(e.g., rapid onset of action, short elimination half-life), and there are currently few data available
regarding prolonged application in ICU patients.

TABLE 74–1. PHARMACOLOGY OF OPIOID ANALGESICS IN THE ADULT INTENSIVE CARE UNIT (ICU)

	Relative Potency	Bolus Dose*(IV)	Half-Life	Continuous Dose* (mg/h IV)	Comment
Morphine	1	2–5 mg	3–7 h	2–10	Histamine release
					Accumulation of active metabolite (morphin-6-glucuronid), especially in renal insufficiency
Fentanyl	80–100	25–100 µg	1.5–6 h	0.025–0.2	Marked accumulation of parent drug after prolonged infusion
Hydromorphone	5–10	0.25–0.75 mg	2–3 h	0.5–2	
Sufentanil	500–1000	5–20 µg	2–4 h	0.005–0.04	Fast onset/offset and recovery, minimal accumulation
Remifentanil	100	N/A	3–10 min	0.025–0.5	Metabolism through unspecific esterases
					Efficient to treat shivering
Meperidine†	0.1	12.5–50 mg	3–4 h	N/A	Histamine release
					Accumulation of active, neuroexcitatory metabolite (normeperidine), especially in renal insufficiency or high doses
					Interaction with antidepressants

N/A = not applicable.
*Doses are approximate for a 70-kg adult patient; bolus dose may be repeated every 5–15 minutes.
†Not recommended for routine use in ICU patients.

8. **How should one decide which opioid to use? What are their characteristics?**
   Before ordering opioids, we have to determine the goal of analgesia and develop a therapeutic plan. The patient's cardiovascular status, organ functions, and other medications must be known.

   - **Morphine:** Morphine is a naturally occurring, relatively hydrophilic opioid with a long clinical history and therefore excellent physician familiarity with its use. The onset of action is slow (effect site equilibration time, 15–30 minutes), and the duration of action is 2–4 hours. Morphine may reduce preload and systemic blood pressure; thus, it has to be used carefully in hemodynamically unstable or hypovolemic patients. Furthermore, metabolites with analgesic properties and very long half-lives exist and may accumulate in patients with renal failure. Finally, morphine may release a considerable amount of histamine.

   - **Fentanyl:** Fentanyl is a synthetic, highly potent, and highly lipid-soluble opioid. The lipid solubility is responsible for the rapid onset of action (effect site equilibration time, 1–3 minutes). This makes it a preferable analgesic in acutely distressed patients. Fentanyl has a short duration of action (30–45 minutes after one bolus); however, repeated dosing may cause accumulation and prolonged action. Cardiovascular adverse effects are minimal.

   - **Hydromorphone:** Hydromorphone is a semisynthetic opioid that is 5–10 times more potent than morphine and has lipid solubility between that of morphine and fentanyl. The onset and the duration of action are a little shorter compared with morphine (effect site equilibration time, 10–20 minutes; duration of action, 1–3 hours), but hydromorphone is hemodynamically more stable, lacks a clinically significant active metabolite, and does not release histamine.

   - **Sufentanil:** This synthetic, highly lipid-soluble opioid has the highest selectivity for the μ receptor. It has been shown to cause less respiratory depression compared with other opioids, thus it may be preferred in patients with spontaneous ventilation. Sufentanil accumulates less than fentanyl (i.e., it has a shorter context-sensitive half-life).

   - **Remifentanil:** Also a synthetic opioid, remifentanil has a very fast onset and the shortest duration of action. Furthermore, its biotransformation is so rapid and so complete (unspecific esterases, organ independent) that the duration of a remifentanil infusion has little effect on wake-up times. Remifentanil has the shortest context-sensitive half-life among the available opioids (<5 minutes after 4 hours of continuous infusion).

9. **What is the place of meperidine in the ICU?**
   Meperidine is useful in the treatment of postoperative shivering and has been demonstrated to be superior to morphine and fentanyl for this indication. A small IV dose of 10–25 mg is usually efficient. Postoperative shivering can increase oxygen consumption and may be detrimental if it occurs in patients with ischemic heart disease, for example. However, meperidine is not recommended for repetitive use in ICU patients because of its active metabolite (normeperidine, which may cause central nervous system excitation) and its interactions with antidepressants (contraindicated with monoamine oxidase inhibitors, best avoided with selective serotonin reuptake inhibitors).

10. **Which other opioids should be avoided in the ICU for routine analgesia?**
    - **Mixed agonist-antagonists:** Mixed agonist-antagonists (e.g., nalbuphine) may reverse other opioids and may precipitate withdrawal syndrome in patients in whom tolerance or dependence has developed.
    - **Methadone:** Methadone prolongs the QT-interval and induces torsades de pointes ventricular arrhythmia. It is metabolized by the hepatic cytochrom-P450 system, and there is a risk of accumulation after repeated dosing (long half-life, interactions).
    - **Codeine:** Codeine is not useful for most patients because it lacks analgesic potency.

11. **How should opioids preferably be administered for acute pain management in the ICU?**

Parenterally. The IV use is considered superior because regional hypoperfusion due to shock or edema may render the absorption of opioids less reliable via the peroral, subcutaneous, and intramuscular routes. IV opioids can be delivered in three different modes:

- **IV bolus injections:** These injections are often used to treat moderate pain. The doses are titrated to analgesic requirements, avoiding respiratory depression and hemodynamic instability.
- **Continuous IV infusion:** In clinical situations with moderate to severe pain that is only poorly controlled with repeated boluses, a continuous IV infusion may be considered.
- **Patient-controlled analgesia (PCA):** Alternatively, a PCA regimen may be preferable in conscious and alert patients.

12. **Explain the concept of PCA.**

PCA is managed with microprocessor-based pumps that allow the patient to self-administer analgesics according to a predetermined limit set by the physician. The goal of PCA is to produce a relatively stable and effective level of analgesia by allowing the patient to receive multiple small boluses after an initial loading dose. Patients prefer this pain relief technique because they control analgesia administration themselves. The following basic parameters can be set on a PCA pump:

- **Bolus:** The dose administered when the patient pushes the button
- **Lock-out interval:** Minimal length of time between two doses
- **Maximal dose:** The maximum dose to be given
- **Background infusion:** Continuous infusion in addition to the boluses

13. **Why should one avoid routine prescription of background infusions by PCA?**

- PCA continuous infusions (background infusion) bypass the intrinsic safety feature of standard, bolus-only PCA by allowing opioids to be continuously delivered even if sedation is excessive.
- Studies have demonstrated that postoperative patients treated with PCA plus continuous infusion have no improvement in analgesia but have a significantly greater number of adverse effects compared with postoperative patients receiving standard PCA.

14. **What are the adverse effects of opioids?**

Adverse effects of opioids are common and summarized in Table 74-2. Respiratory depression is a concern in spontaneously breathing patients or in those receiving partial ventilatory support. Opioid-induced hypotension in cardiovascularly stable and euvolemic patients is a result of sympatholysis, vagally induced bradycardia, and histamine release (typically after morphine, meperidine, or codeine). Intestinal hypomotility, largely present in critically ill patients, is being enhanced by opioids. To avoid worsening constipation and its complications (e.g., ileus, bacterial translocation), routine prophylactic use of laxatives is crucial.

15. **What is the role of nonopioid analgesics in the ICU? What are their characteristics?**

Acetaminophen and NSAIDs have been shown to decrease the need for opioids and are particularly effective in reducing muscular and skeletal pain. They are often more effective than opioids in reducing pain from pleural or pericardial rubs, a pain that responds poorly to opioids. Basic pharmacology is summarized in Table 74-3.

16. **What are the adverse effects of nonopioid analgesics?**

- **Acetaminophen:** Acetaminophen may be potentially hepatotoxic, especially in patients with depleted glutathione stores. Therefore, acetaminophen should be avoided in the treatment of patients with acute liver failure, and the drug should be maintained at <2 gm/day in patients with a significant history of alcohol intake or poor nutritional status.

TABLE 74-2. SIDE EFFECTS OF OPIOID ANALGESICS

Central nervous system	Miosis
	Euphoria, dysphoria, sedation
	Addiction
Pulmonary	Respiratory depression
	Muscle rigidity (especially highly lipid-soluble opioids)
Cardiovascular	Bradycardia, hypotension
Gastrointestinal	Nausea, emesis
	Constipation, ileus
Urogenital	Urinary retention
	ADH release (water retention)
Other	Histamine release: flushing, tachycardia, hypotension, bronchospasm
	Pruritus

ADH = antidiuretic hormone.

TABLE 74-3. PHARMACOLOGY OF SELECTED NONOPIOID ANALGESICS IN THE ADULT INTENSIVE CARE UNIT

	Dose Recommendations	Half-Life	Comment
Acetaminophen	PO: 325–1000 mg q4–6h IV: 500–1000 mg q6–8h (IV: avoid >2 days use)	2–3 hours	Maximum dose ≤4 gm daily
Diclofenac	PO: 50 mg q6–12h IV: 75 mg (IV: max 150 mg/day, avoid >2 days use)	1–2 hours	Reduce dose if: age >65 years, weight <50 kg, or renal impairment
Ibuprofen	PO: 400 mg q4–6h	1.5–2.5 hours	Reduce dose if: age >65 years, weight <50 kg, or renal impairment
Ketorolac	IV: 15–30 mg q6h (avoid >5 days use)	2.5–8.5 hours	Reduce dose if: age >65 years, weight <50 kg, or renal impairment

PO = per os (by mouth).

- **NSAIDs:** These medications may cause bleeding secondary to platelet function inhibition, gastrointestinal side effects such as ulcers and bleeding, and the development of acute renal failure. Risk factors to development of acute renal failure are patient age, preexisting renal impairment, hypovolemia, and shock. The prolonged use of NSAIDs should be avoided. For example, it has been shown that ketorolac applied for ≥ 5 days has been associated with a twofold increased risk of acute renal failure. Furthermore, NSAIDs should be avoided in patients with asthma and aspirin allergy. The role of the newer NSAIDs in the ICU, the selective cyclo-oxygenase–2 inhibitors, remains unknown so far.

17. **Does ketamine have a role as an analgesic agent in the ICU?**
   Recent guidelines do not recommend the routine use of ketamine, a phencyclidine derivative, in the ICU because of its adverse effects: increases in blood pressure, heart rate, and intracranial pressure, as well as hypersalivation. Moreover, vivid dreams and hallucinations occur in one-third of the patients. To avoid this adverse effect, a hypnotic/anxiolytic agent (e.g., midazolam) should be given before administration of ketamine. However, because of its potent analgesic effect, rapid onset of action, and short duration of action, IV boluses of ketamine (0.5–1.0 mg/kg) have been used in ICU patients to enhance tolerance of limited but painful procedures, such as dressing changes for burns. Furthermore, small doses of ketamine (bolus, followed by 1–2 μg/kg/min) may be a valuable adjunct to routine analgesia to decrease the opioid requirements.

   Guillou N, Tanguy M, Seguin P, et al: The effects of small-dose ketamine on morphine consumption in surgical intensive care unit patients after major abdominal surgery. Anesth Analg 97:843–847, 2003.

18. **What is the role of regional anesthesia in ICU patients?**
   Several regional anesthetic techniques, such as epidural drug applications (mostly local anesthetics, opioids), may provide safe and effective pain control for patients in the ICU while substantially reducing the need for systemic pain medications. In particular, pain relief supplied by regional anesthesia may be superior to that of IV opioids; furthermore, the former provides sufficient analgesia for movement and physical therapy, whereas opioids only eliminate pain at rest. Other advantages include a greater improvement in respiratory function, less constipation, and the provision of analgesia with a minimum of sedation.

19. **What are the limitations to regional anesthesia in the ICU?**
   Regional blocks are time consuming, difficult to perform, and contraindicated in patients who have a congenital or acquired coagulation disorder. Guidelines regarding how to safely provide regional anesthesia have been published by the American Society of Regional Anesthesia. Furthermore, epidural or other catheters used to administer pain medicine may become infected. Also, local anesthetics may have a narrow therapeutic range and may accumulate easily, particularly in patients with renal or hepatic failure.

   American Society of Regional Anesthesia: www.asra.com

20. **Is regional anesthesia safe in the setting of deep vein thromboprophylaxis?**
   Regional anesthesia may be performed in this setting, although practitioners must be vigilant for the development of hematomas (e.g., epidural hematoma). If, for example, IV unfractionated heparin is being used, needle placement or catheter removal should be done ≥ 4 hours after discontinuing heparin, and re-heparinization may be started ≥ 1 hour after an uncomplicated procedure. If low-molecular-weight heparin (LMWH) is being used, the recommendations are based on the dosing regimen. If the single daily dosing regimen is used, a waiting period of ≥ 12 hours for any neuraxial technique should be applied after the last dose of LMWH, and the next LMWH dose should be given ≥ 4 hours after an uncomplicated procedure. In the twice-daily dosing regimen (usually started 24 hours after surgery), the neuraxial catheter should be removed ≥ 2 hours before the first LMWH dose. Detailed guidelines for regional anesthesia in anticoagulated patients have been published from several anesthesia societies and have been summarized recently.

   Krombach JW, Dagtekin O, Kampe S: Regional anesthesia and anticoagulation. Curr Opin Anaesthesiol 17:427–433, 2004.

CHAPTER 75

SEDATION, ANALGESIA, AND DELIRIUM

Brian T. Marden, PharmD, and Jill A. Rebuck, PharmD, BCPS

1. **What is the goal of sedation in most critically ill patients?**
   To decrease anxiety and agitation with production of a calm but communicative state while minimizing patient discomfort. Sedation is necessary to induce amnesia during traumatic experiences.

2. **What is the preferred analgesic for mechanically ventilated patients in the intensive care unit (ICU)?**
   Morphine sulfate and fentanyl are the two most commonly prescribed opioid analgesics. Either can be used to provide analgesia unless there is a compelling indication for which one may be a better option. Morphine sulfate is a more appropriate selection if an intermittent dosing strategy is being used because of fentanyl's shorter duration of action. However, fentanyl is preferred in the setting of hemodynamic instability, renal failure, or patient allergy to morphine sulfate. Both agents undergo hepatic elimination. Fentanyl is extremely lipophilic compared with morphine and thus has a more rapid onset of action. Typical bolus doses of morphine include 2–10 mg every 2–4 hours or infusions of 1–5 mg/h compared with 1–2 µg/kg every hour or infusion of 50–150 µg/h for fentanyl.

3. **Yes, pain is uncomfortable for the patient, but is it really worth being aggressive in treating it when there are so many adverse effects of the agents administered for this purpose?**
   Adverse effects of commonly administered opioids in the ICU include gastric retention, mental status changes, and respiratory depression. However, the consequences of unrelieved pain are significant and justify aggressive pain control. Unrelieved pain inherently results in an endogenous stress response that can lead to tachycardia, increased myocardial oxygen demand, immunosuppression, hypercoagulability, and persistent catabolism. Also, pain may result in a generalized muscle rigidity that can restrict chest wall expansion and worsen pulmonary dysfunction. Perhaps the greatest concern of unrelieved pain is lack of sleep, with increased anxiety and enhanced patient agitation. Figure 75-1 demonstrates how unrelieved pain can create a viscous cycle of undesirable patient conditions. It is always best to adopt the approach that preventing pain is substantially more effective than treating established pain.

4. **Describe the therapeutic effects of benzodiazepines.**
   The therapeutic effects of benzodiazepines are caused by alterations primarily affecting binding to the gamma-aminobutyric acid neurotransmitter. Benzodiazepines have antianxiety, sedative, anticonvulsant, amnestic, hypnotic, and muscle-relaxant properties. Because they have no analgesic activity, an analgesic agent such as morphine should be prescribed.

5. **What is the benzodiazepine of choice for sedation in the ICU?**
   Midazolam is preferred for short-term (<24-hour) therapy, whereas lorazepam is indicated for prolonged treatment (>24 hours) of anxiety. Midazolam is a short-acting agent that rapidly penetrates the central nervous system (CNS), produces onset of sedation within 2–2.5 minutes, and possesses an active metabolite, 1-hydroxymidazolam. Lorazepam is an intermediate-acting benzodiazepine that is less lipophilic than midazolam and thus has a slightly delayed onset of

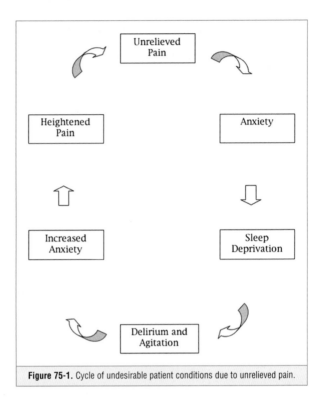

Figure 75-1. Cycle of undesirable patient conditions due to unrelieved pain.

action. Lorazepam has less potential for peripheral accumulation and no active metabolites; moreover, it is associated with more rapid awakening with prolonged administration compared with midazolam.

Jacobi J, Fraser GL, Coursin DB, et al: Clinical practice guidelines for the sustained use of sedatives and analgesics in the critically ill adult. Crit Care Med 30:119–141, 2002.

Pohlman AS, Simpson KP, Hall JB: Continuous intravenous infusions of lorazepam versus midazolam for sedation during mechanical ventilatory support: A prospective, randomized study. Crit Care Med 22:1241–1247, 1994.

6. **What sedative should be chosen for patients who require neurologic monitoring?**
Propofol is preferred for intubated patients who require rapid titration to multiple levels of sedation for neurologic monitoring. Subanesthetic doses produce effects of anxiolysis and amnesia. Propofol has a rapid onset and brief effect due to rapid CNS penetration and redistribution. Elimination is reduced in elderly patients but not in patients with renal or hepatic disease.

7. **How does daily assessment of a patient receiving continuous sedation in the ICU improve outcome?**
Interrupting continuous sedation (e.g., with a benzodiazepine or propofol) until the patient awakens each day shortens the duration of mechanical ventilation as well as the patient's length of stay in the ICU. Thus, it is important to assess each patient daily by performing wake-up examinations and decreasing the infusion rate appropriately, as tolerated by the patient, to eliminate a prolonged recovery period.

Kress JP, Pohlman AS, O'Connor MF, Hall JB: Daily interruption of sedative infusions in critically ill patients undergoing mechanical ventilation. N Engl J Med 342:1471–1477, 2000.

8. **Name various complications that may be seen in agitated adult patients in the ICU.**
   Agitation may be due to pain, anxiety, or delirium. Complications in agitated patients may include self-extubation, removal of arterial lines and venous catheters, increased oxygen requirements, and the negative effect incurred when the patient cannot participate in improving his or her own care. One study concluded that severe agitation and subsequent complications resulted in annual costs exceeding $250,000. Efforts must be made to identify the cause of agitation (e.g., hypoxia, alcohol withdrawal, pain, sleep disturbances) before the administration of pharmacologic agents.

9. **What is the most effective way to decrease the time required to achieve adequate sedation when lorazepam is prescribed for prolonged therapy?**
   Lorazepam is an intermediate-acting benzodiazepine with a slightly delayed onset of action. When administered by continuous infusion for prolonged sedation, dosing during administration influences the time to adequate sedation. Patients should receive a bolus dose (typically 2 mg) before the initiation of continuous infusion. Further infusion rate increases should be accompanied by an additional medication bolus. Otherwise, patients require longer periods to reach steady state and thus may risk oversedation later because of unnecessary increases in infusion rates resulting from inadequate initial sedation.

10. **How do you best control the specific level of sedation for each patient?**
    Several scales are available to improve control of the individual level of sedation for each patient, including the Ramsay, Sedation-Agitation, and Richmond-Agitation-Sedation assessment scales. The sedation level chosen should be reevaluated often because patients' requirements change frequently. Sedation scales are powerful tools because they allow the ICU practitioner to indicate a specific level of sedation to the nursing staff and to decrease the possibility of oversedation. It is important to choose a scale that grades both sedation and agitation.

11. **Sedation scales are all subjective. Is there any way to be more objective?**
    Traditional assessment scales are limited in dependence on motor responsiveness and thus are of limited or no application to patients receiving paralytics or those requiring very high doses of anxiolytics. Computer-processed electroencephalogram (EEG) technology (e.g., such as bispectral index monitoring or patient state analyzer) is used in operating rooms to limit patient recall during surgery. This technology, now approved for use in the ICU, involves placing electrodes to the patient's forehead, where a very complex algorithm turns raw EEG data into a calculated numeric value between 0 (isoelectric EEG) and 100 (maximum awake value). Trials using this technology in critically ill, sedated patients is varied and inconsistent. Bispectral index monitoring or patient state analyzer monitoring is currently not recommended to monitor consciousness levels and guide sedative therapy in the ICU in all patients. However, in situations where patients are either paralyzed or in a state of deep coma, this technology can be considered as an adjuvant to help guide sedation management.

    Fraser GL, Riker RR: Bispectral index monitoring in the intensive care unit provides more signal than noise. Pharmacotherapy 25:19S–27S, 2005.

12. **Which agent—midazolam or propofol—is preferred for short-term sedation in the ICU?**
    Either is acceptable. The two agents are equally effective in providing adequate short-term sedation to critically ill patients. Patients who receive propofol infusions tend to have a shorter time to extubation, although this does not necessarily correlate with decreased length of stay in the ICU. Midazolam may provide less expensive sedation for most patients and may be preferred for short-term use in patients who do not require frequent neurologic monitoring.

    Chamorro C, de Latorre FJ, Montero A, et al: Comparative study of propofol versus midazolam in the sedation of critically ill patients: Results of a prospective, randomized, multicenter trial. Crit Care Med 24:932–939, 1996.

13. **What is the role of dexmedetomidine (Precedex)?**
Potential advantages relate to decreased pain medication requirements and lack of respiratory depression, which may allow faster ventilator weaning either in the immediate postoperative period or in patients with agitation who are having difficulty with ventilator weaning when the current sedative is discontinued. Bradycardia and hypotension, especially in hypovolemic patients, are the most prominent adverse effects. Currently, there are no overwhelming compelling indications supported by clinical data to use dexmedetomidine instead of conventional sedatives, such as propofol, in providing continuous short-term sedation therapy.

14. **What anxiety-related issues must be considered in patients who have an inadequate response to appropriate sedation therapy?**
It is important to assess the level of pain control because most sedatives do not have analgesic properties. In addition, ICU delirium, which may further complicate the clinical picture, should be considered in the differential diagnosis especially because both benzodiazepines and opioids can paradoxically worsen delirium agitation.

15. **Do all patients paralyzed in the ICU require concurrent sedation?**
Yes. All paralyzed patients must receive concurrent analgesia and sedation because neuromuscular-blocking agents reduce neither pain nor anxiety. Patients have been known to suffer long-term psychological consequences, such as posttraumatic stress disorder (PTSD), as a result of being awake during paralysis. It is of critical importance to constantly reassess each patient's condition and discontinue paralytic therapy as early as possible.

16. **Anxiolytic agents make people look comfortable, but is the patient really sleeping?**
Sleep deprivation is a major concern in the ICU and has been associated with depressed cognitive, cardiopulmonary, and immune function. Studies suggest that critically ill patients are limited, on average, to <2 hours of sleep per day. Common medications administered to induce "sleep" actually disrupt natural sleep architecture. Opioids are associated with decreased rapid eye movement sleep, and benzodiazepine infusions completely eliminate stages 3 and 4 of non–rapid eye movement sleep. One proposed advantage of dexmedetomidine is that its pharmacodynamic effects may mimic natural sleep patterns. Whichever agent is selected, it is important to construct a comprehensive approach to promoting sleep and revitalization in the ICU.

    Peruzzi WT: Sleep in the intensive care unit. Pharmacotherapy 25:34S–39S, 2005.

17. **What is propofol infusion syndrome (PRIS)?**
The first published case report in adults of PRIS was published in 2000; since then, >15 cases have been reported, many of them fatal. The syndrome is not well understood but appears to be related to long-term (>48 hours), high-dose (>5 mg/kg/h) propofol infusion. The main features consist of cardiac failure (sudden onset of bradycardia), rhabdomyolysis, severe metabolic acidosis, and renal failure. The hypothesized pathogenetic mechanism involves propofol's impairment of free fatty acid use and mitochondrial activity resulting in cardiac and peripheral muscle necrosis. Patients at greatest risk are those with acute neurologic illnesses, inflammatory conditions, or post-major trauma or those receiving concomitant steroids or catecholamines. To decrease the potential for PRIS, propofol should not exceed doses of 5 mg/kg/h (83 μg/kg/min).

    Vasile, B, Rasulo F, Candiani A, Latronico N: The pathophysiology of propofol infusion syndrome: A simple name for a complex syndrome. Intensive Care Med 29:1417–1425, 2003.

18. **What diluent of lorazepam can cause toxicity if accumulated?**
Intravenous lorazepam contains 830 mg of propylene glycol (PG) per milliliter of solution, a common vehicle used as a drug solubilizer for hydrophobic compounds that, in excess, may

result in significant toxicity. Toxicity effects described include anion-gap metabolic acidosis, hyperosmolality, hemolysis, CNS depression, arrhythmias, and renal failure. Lorazepam dosing thresholds or PG levels do not appear to correlate with toxicity. At a minimum, monitor serum osmolality in patients after receiving ≥48 hours of high-dose lorazepam infusion (>0.1 mg/kg/h). If the calculated osmol gap is elevated in the absence of other causes, a change in sedation therapy to midazolam or propofol (which do not contain PG) should be considered. Patients with decompensated hepatic function will be at a higher risk due to reduced drug clearance.

Arroliga AC, Shehab N, McCarthy K, Gonzales JP: Relationship of continuous infusion lorazepam to serum propylene glycol concentration in critically ill adults. Crit Care Med 32:1709–1714, 2004.

19. **Which medication is useful for the treatment of ICU delirium?**
Haloperidol (Haldol) is the most studied agent for the treatment of delirium in adult ICU patients. It is a neuroleptic agent that binds to postsynaptic dopamine receptors and has strong central antidopaminergic activity. All patients should be monitored closely for extrapyramidal side effects, neuroleptic malignant syndrome, and QT prolongation, which may lead to torsades de pointes. Appropriate Haldol dosing in ICU patients is to administer doubling doses every 15–20 minutes until the patient responds, at which point the total dose administered should be divided and administered in 6-hour intervals. Some anecdotal experience and limited studies suggest that newer second-generation neuroleptics such as olanzapine and quetiapine may be as effective as haloperidol with a more beneficial adverse effect profile.

Jacobi J, Fraser GL, Coursin DB, et al: Clinical practice guidelines for the sustained use of sedatives and analgesics in the critically ill adult. Crit Care Med 30:119–141, 2002.

Riker RR, Fraser GL, Cox PM: Continuous infusion of haloperidol controls agitation in critically ill patients. Crit Care Med 22:433–440, 1995.

Skrobik, YK, Bergeron N, Dumont M, Gottfried SB: Olanzapine vs. haloperidol: Treating delirium in a critical care setting. Intensive Care Med 30:444–449, 2004.

KEY POINTS: FINDING THE BALANCE: KEEPING PATIENTS COMFORTABLE WITHOUT OVERSEDATION

1. Choose the correct anxiolytic agent based on the length of time for which the patient will require therapy.

2. Wake up patients who are receiving continuous sedation daily, if appropriate.

3. Use a sedation scale and titrate sedation therapy to a defined score.

4. Avoid oversedation for the purposes of minimizing patient recall, except when necessary during traumatic events, because delusional memories probably do more long-term psychological harm than factual ones.

20. **Is there any way to diagnose ICU delirium easily?**
Delirium affects up to 80% of mechanically ventilated critically ill patients and has been shown to be an independent predictor of increased mortality and hospital length of stay. ICU delirium is characterized by a fluctuating mental status, inattention, disorganized thinking, and an altered level of consciousness. The Confusion Assessment Method for the ICU has been validated in studies as highly accurate and reliable in diagnosing delirium in critically ill patients. This tool is not labor intensive and can easily be administered in less than 2 minutes. An excellent website and resource for ICU-related delirium is www.icudelirium.org.

Ely EW, Margolin R, Francis J, et al: Evaluation of delirium in critically ill patients: Validation of the Confusion Assessment Method for the Intensive Care Unit (CAM-ICU). Crit Care Med 29:1370–1379, 2001.

Ely EW, Shintani A, Truman B, et al: Delirium as a predictor of mortality in mechanically ventilated patients in the intensive care unit. JAMA 291:1753–1762, 2004.

21. **Why do so many patients in the ICU become delirious?**
The pathophysiology is poorly understood but is thought to be a result of a variety of factors, from neurotransmitter alterations to altered blood flow. The causes are multifactorial and, for understanding purposes, can be divided into four different areas:
    - **Metabolic:** Delirium may result from electrolyte disturbances (e.g., hypernatremia, hypercalcemia), dehydration, serum glucose alterations, liver failure (e.g., hepatic encephalopathy), uremia, or hyperosmolar states.
    - **CNS:** Causes include encephalitis/meningitis, alcohol or drug withdrawal, sleep deprivation, postictal states, and elevated intracranial pressures, associated with head trauma.
    - **Infectious:** Infections such as urinary tract infection, pneumonia, or sepsis often are associated with delirium.
    - **Drugs:** The culprit. Each patient with delirium should be assessed for potential exogenous causes. Common examples include steroids, anticholinergics, opioids, benzodiazepines, and psychotropics. In fact, it was recently demonstrated that the administration of lorazepam was an independent risk factor for the development of delirium in the ICU.

    Pandharipande P, Shintani A, Peterson J, et al: Lorazepam is an independent risk factor for transitioning to delirium in intensive care unit patients. Anesthesiology 104:21–26, 2006.

22. **Do patients ever suffer long-term psychological consequences as a result of their ICU experiences?**
PTSD has been well described in patients after an ICU stay. An earlier study demonstrated that 41% of acute respiratory distress syndrome survivors who could recall two or more traumatic events experienced PTSD. As a result of this and other studies, many clinicians attempted to protect patients from the ICU experience, and thus patients were commonly oversedated. However, a more comprehensive understanding of the etiology of long-term psychological complications considers the important difference between factual and delusional memories. A recent study reported the only predictors of possible acute PTSD-related symptoms were anxiety and the presence of delusional memories without recall of factual events in the ICU. Therefore, instead of oversedating patients, it is best to keep them as alert as possible (with the exception of traumatic experiences requiring paralysis) to allow them to understand and relate to their experience and surroundings.

    Jones C, Griffiths RD, Humphris G, Skirrow PM: Memory, delusions, and the development of acute posttraumatic stress disorder–related symptoms after intensive care. Crit Care Med 29:573–580, 2001.

WEBSITE

ICU Delirium and Cognitive Impairment Study Group
www.icudelirium.org

XV. EMERGENCY MEDICINE

CHAPTER 76

TETANUS

Peter T. Pons, MD

1. **What is tetanus?**
   Tetanus results from acute infection with *Clostridium tetani* (gram-positive anaerobic rod),
   which produces a neurotoxin (exotoxin) that has a primary action of causing profound skeletal
   muscle hypertonicity. In the most severe form, the muscle spasms can cause respiratory failure
   and death.

   Rhee P, Nunley MK, Demetraides D, et al: Tetanus and trauma: A review and recommendations. J Trauma
   58:1082–1088, 2005.

2. **How does the exotoxin/neurotoxin cause the disease?**
   C. tetani manufactures two exotoxins: tetanospasmin and tetanolysin. Most clinical
   manifestations appear to be produced by tetanospasmin. This toxin becomes concentrated in
   the anterior horn of the spinal cord and blocks neurotransmitter release at presynaptic sites of
   inhibitory neurons, thus causing increased muscle tone, hypertonicity, and muscle spasms.
   Tetanolysin is a hemolytic toxin that may cause hemolysis and myocardial injury and
   dysfunction. The toxins spread via lymphatics, blood vessels, and neural pathways to the target
   organ, alpha motor neurons.

   Sheffield JS, Ramin SM: Tetanus in pregnancy. Am J Perinatol 21:173–181, 2004.

3. **Summarize the epidemiology of tetanus.**
   - **Incidence and geographic distribution:** In the United States, there are approximately 40
     cases of tetanus each year. Worldwide, it is estimated that there are between 800,000 and 1
     million deaths. In the United States, the disease occurs most commonly in the Southeast;
     however, the organism is ubiquitous in dirt and dust and is found worldwide. It is less
     common in cold climates.
   - **Incubation period:** The incubation period varies between 2 and 14 days, with a median of 7
     days.
   - **Prognosis:** The mortality rate is 30% in the United States and 40–60% worldwide. The
     mortality is 100% if the disease becomes manifest within 2 days of injury and infection.
     Worldwide, 90% of deaths occur in infants.

   Centers for Disease Control and Prevention: Surveillance summary. MMWR 52:1–8, 2003.
   Dietz V, Milstein JB, van Loon F, et al: Performance and potency of tetanus toxoid: Implications for
   eliminating neonatal tetanus. Bull World Health Organ 74:619–628, 1996.

4. **Who is prone to developing tetanus?**
   - **General:** Most at risk are people who have never been or are inadequately immunized against
     tetanus. It is estimated that 50–90% of patients in the United States are inadequately
     protected (in most cases, these are immigrants or adults older than 60 years). A significant
     percentage (up to 75%) of elderly patients have inadequate serum levels of antibody against
     tetanus in numerous studies that measured actual levels.
   - **Neonates:** Newborns can acquire tetanus after nonsterile transection of the umbilical cord. In
     many countries, local remedies such as cow dung, garlic, coffee, and ashes are applied to the
     umbilical stump to facilitate healing, only to produce tetanus.

- **Drug abusers:** Parenteral drug abusers who administer their drugs by "skin popping" are prone to acquiring tetanus by developing subcutaneous abscesses that support the growth of *C. tetani*.
- **Septic abortion:** Women who have undergone septic abortion are prone to the development of tetanus.
- **Acne:** Cephalic tetanus has been reported as a complication of acne.

Alagappan K, Rennie W, Kwiatkowski T, et al: Seroprevalence of tetanus antibodies among adults older than 65 years. Ann Emerg Med 28:18–21, 1996.

Centers for Disease Control and Prevention: Neonatal tetanus—Montana, 1998. MMWR 47:928–930, 1998.

Centers for Disease Control and Prevention: Surveillance summary. MMWR 52:1–8, 2003.

Sangalli M, Chierchini P, Aylward RB, et al: Tetanus: A rare but preventable cause of mortality among drug users and the elderly. Eur J Epidemiol 12:539–540, 1996.

5. **What sort of wound is prone to infection with *C. tetani*?**
   Most cases result from accidental soft-tissue injury, such as lacerations, puncture wounds, or burns, which may occur indoors or outdoors. The Centers for Disease Control and Prevention reported that almost 50% of wounds resulting in tetanus occurred indoors. Many wounds appear quite minor and sometimes cannot even be found at the time of presentation of clinical tetanus. Some unusual sources include frostbitten parts, poor dentition, denture-induced gum ulcers, and skin infections. *C. tetani* is a strict anaerobe and proliferates only in tissue with low oxygen tension; thus, necrotic tissue, foreign bodies, and associated infection are predisposing factors. Tetanus has also been reported after elective surgery. The organism itself is not invasive; thus, the actual infection is localized. However, once the exotoxin is produced, it is transported systemically.

   Luisto M: Unusual and iatrogenic sources of tetanus. Ann Chir Gynaecol 82:25–29, 1993.

   Rhee P, Nunley MK, Demetraides D, et al: Tetanus and trauma: A review and recommendations. J Trauma 58:1082–1088, 2005.

6. **What are the clinical manifestations of tetanus?**
   The most dramatic and obvious findings in tetanus are in the musculoskeletal system. Initial findings are characterized by increased muscle tone, which is usually first noticed in the face and jaw. Trismus, difficulty swallowing, and facial distortion from the muscle spasms (risus sardonicus) develop. Over the next 24–48 hours, generalized muscle hypertonicity develops and muscle spasms may occur. Spasms of neck and back muscles result in opisthotonic posturing. Other findings are low-grade elevation in temperature and pulse, increased or decreased blood pressure, pain associated with the muscle spasms, rigid abdominal wall (also due to muscle spasms but mimicking an acute abdomen), and clear mentation during these episodes. The disease remains "stable" for the next 5–7 days, followed by recovery over the next 7–10 days. Muscle stiffness may remain for up to 2 months. In neonates, the disease is characterized by irritability, difficulty nursing and swallowing, and hypertonicity of the muscles. If the patient survives, recovery occurs without permanent sequelae. The disease does not confer immunity; therefore, survivors must be immunized to prevent recurrence.

   Attygalle D, Rodrigo N: New trends in the management of tetanus. Expert Rev Anti-Infect Ther 2:73–84, 2004.

   Bunch TJ, Thalji MK, Pellikka PA, Aksamit TR: Respiratory failure in tetanus: Case report and review of a 25-year experience. Chest 122:1488–1492, 2002.

   Cook TM, Protheroe RT, Handel JM: Tetanus: A review of the literature. Br J Anaesth 87:477–487, 2001.

7. **What are the four types of tetanus?**
   - **Generalized:** This is the most common form and is manifested by the full constellation of symptoms and signs. The overall mortality rate is approximately 50%.

KEY POINTS: SYMPTOMS OF TETANUS

1. Trismus is one symptom of tetanus.

2. Difficulty with swallowing may also occur.

3. Patients may experience facial muscle spasms (i.e., risus sardonicus).

4. Generalized muscle hypertonicity and spasms are signs of tetanus.

5. Clear mentation may also be present.

- **Neonatal:** Newborns may acquire tetanus from contamination of the umbilical stump. Immunization of the mother can prevent the disease in neonates. The mortality in infants is 50–60%.
- **Local:** This form is characterized by increased muscle tone near the inoculation site that usually resolves over time. Progression to the generalized form is uncommon but possible.
- **Cephalic:** This rare form presents with trismus and cranial nerve paralysis (cranial nerve VII most commonly, also III, IV, VI, and XII). Generalized tetanus follows in approximately two-thirds of cases.

Jagoda A, Riggio SY, Burguieres T: Cephalic tetanus: A case report and review of the literature. Am J Emerg Med 6:128–130, 1988.

Luisto M: Unusual and iatrogenic sources of tetanus. Ann Chir Gynaecol 82:25–29, 1993.

8. **Are any laboratory studies diagnostic of tetanus?**
Virtually all laboratory studies yield nonspecific, nondiagnostic results. Approximately one-third of patients have mild-to-moderate granulocytosis. Decreased hematocrit may be noted, probably resulting from the hemolysin exotoxin. Electrolyte and calcium levels are generally normal. As the disease progresses, however, 7% of patients develop the electrolyte picture of inappropriate antidiuretic hormone secretion (SIADH), including decreased sodium and serum osmolality. Arterial blood gas levels should be monitored to assess pulmonary function. Of note, cultures for *C. tetani* yielded positive results in only one-third of patients diagnosed with tetanus clinically.

9. **Which diseases are included in the differential diagnosis?**
- **Hypocalcemia:** Decreased serum calcium can produce tetany. Laboratory evaluation is usually diagnostic.
- **Oral infection or abscess:** Infection or abscess in and around the oral cavity (e.g., peritonsillar or dental abscess) can result in trismus or difficulty opening the mouth. Physical examination usually reveals localized swelling and tenderness.
- **Phenothiazine reaction:** Dystonic reactions caused by phenothiazines may cause muscle rigidity or torticollis. The history usually reveals recent drug use; relief of symptoms occurs with IV diphenhydramine.
- **Black widow spider bite:** Pain and muscle spasm are usually acute in onset. Careful physical examination may reveal the telltale spider bite. Administration of calcium intravenously usually relieves the symptoms.
- **Rabies:** Rabies involves the respiratory muscles and muscles of aglutition without causing trismus. As the disease progresses, there is progressive alteration in the level of consciousness and increasing fever.

- **Strychnine poisoning:** Muscle spasms (usually involving the upper extremities) and opisthotonus occur; however, facial muscle involvement develops later in the course. Suicidal ideation or possible homicide attempt may be evident by history.
- **Hyperventilation:** Physical examination reveals carpopedal spasm. Arterial blood gas evaluation shows respiratory alkalosis.

10. **What are the complications of tetanus?**
   Spasm of laryngeal muscles, the diaphragm, and other muscles of respiration may produce hypoxia or respiratory arrest. The compromise in respiratory function may lead to atelectasis and pneumonia. Other complications include vertebral subluxation or compression fracture as a result of the profound muscle contractions (usually in children), dehydration, pulmonary edema, and SIADH.

11. **How is tetanus treated once it becomes manifest?**
   The four primary goals of treatment are as follows:
   1. Relief of muscle spasms
   2. Support of respiratory status and prevention of complications
   3. Treatment of the infection (remove toxin production)
   4. Neutralization of any unbound toxin

   Richardson JP, Knight AL: The management and prevention of tetanus. J Emerg Med 11:737–742, 1993.

12. **How does one go about relieving muscle spams?**
   The patient should be placed in a darkened room with minimal external stimulation. Diazepam, administered intravenously, is useful for relieving muscle spasms. Oral muscle relaxants can be used in mild cases or during convalescence. In severe cases not responding to diazepam, chemical paralysis (with intubation and mechanical ventilation) is indicated. The addition of a sedative is helpful in reducing the effect of external stimulation, but careful monitoring of respiratory status is necessary. Newer work suggests that medications such as dantrolene, baclofen, or magnesium may be beneficial, although evidence from controlled studies is lacking.

   Attygalle D, Rodrigo N: Magnesium as first line therapy in the management of tetanus: A prospective study of 40 patients. Anaesthesia 57:811–816, 2002.
   Attygalle D, Rodrigo N: New trends in the management of tetanus. Expert Rev Anti-Infect Ther 2:73–84, 2004.

13. **What is needed for support of respiratory status and prevention of complications?**
   Close monitoring of the patient's respiratory function is imperative because spasm of laryngeal muscles, the diaphragm, and muscles of respiration can lead to respiratory failure and suffocation. If necessary, endotracheal intubation and mechanical ventilation should be performed. Formal tracheostomy may be needed if intubation cannot be accomplished. Secretions should be suctioned frequently and the patient positioned to minimize aspiration (and decubitus).

14. **What should one do to treat the infection?**
   When a wound or site of infection is identifiable, necrotic tissue or foreign material should be removed and any abscess drained. Antibiotic agents are administered to prevent further proliferation of the organism and therefore decrease toxin production, but there is little evidence that the course of the disease is affected. Penicillin is the drug of choice, and doxycycline or metronidazole may be used in patients who are allergic to penicillin.

15. **Can anything be done to neutralize unbound toxin?**
   Human tetanus immune globulin is the medication of choice for neutralization of free exotoxin. The antiserum will not have any effect on toxin already bound in neurons. Equine antiserum can

be used if human antiserum is not available; however, hypersensitivity, anaphylaxis, and serum sickness are serious complications. After recovery, active immunization is necessary because immunity is not acquired by having the disease.

6. Can tetanus be prevented?
Tetanus is easily prevented by immunization and could be virtually eradicated worldwide by an aggressive immunization campaign. Neonatal tetanus is also preventable if the mother is protected because the antibody can pass through the placental barrier. Part of every routine history should include a review of tetanus immunization; however, the reliability of this information has been questioned in several studies.

Nonimmunized patients or those with unclear histories should undergo active immunization with absorbed tetanus toxoid. The first dose should be given at the time of contact, the second dose 1–2 months later, and the third dose 6–12 months after the second dose. When both toxoid and antitoxin are indicated, they may be given at the same time without concern that one will interfere with the action of the other, but separate injection sites should be used (Table 76-1).

American College of Emergency Physicians: Tetanus immunization recommendations for persons seven years of age and older. Ann Emerg Med 15:1111–1112, 1986.

American College of Emergency Physicians: Tetanus immunization recommendations for persons less than seven years old. Ann Emerg Med 16:1181–1183, 1987.

Gindi M, Oravitz P, Sexton R, et al: Unreliability of reported tetanus vaccination histories. Am J Emerg Med 23:120–122, 2005.

Talan DA, Abrahamian FM, Moran GJ, et al: Tetanus prophylaxis in the emergency department. Ann Emerg Med 43:305–314, 2004.

TABLE 76-1. TETANUS PROPHYLAXIS AFTER INJURY

Immunization History	Toxoid*	Antitoxin	
		Non–Tetanus Prone	Tetanus Prone
None, uncertain, or <3 doses	Yes	No	Yes
3 or more doses	No†	No	No

*If patient is younger than 7 years, administer toxoid as diphtheria-tetanus-pertussis (DPT) vaccine. If patient is older than 7 years, administer toxoid as tetanus-diphtheria (Td) vaccine.
†Yes, if last prior immunization was more than 5 years previous and wound is tetanus prone, or if most recent immunization was more than 10 years previous and wound is not tetanus prone.

CHAPTER 77

ANAPHYLAXIS

Vincent J. Markovchick, MD

1. **Define *anaphylaxis*.**
   Anaphylaxis is a potentially life-threatening systemic immediate hypersensitivity reaction of multiple organ systems to an antigen-induced, immunoglobulin E–mediated immunologic mediator release in previously sensitized persons.

2. **Define *anaphylactoid reaction*.**
   This is a potentially fatal syndrome that is clinically similar to anaphylaxis but is not an immunoglobulin E–mediated response. It may occur after a single first-time exposure to certain agents, such as radiopaque contrast media.

3. **What are the most common causes?**
   Ingestion, inhalation, or parenteral injection of antigens that sensitize predisposed persons. Common antigens include drugs (e.g., penicillin), foods (e.g., shellfish, nuts, eggwhites), insect stings (e.g., hymenoptera) and animal bites (e.g., snakes), diagnostic agents (e.g., ionic contrast media), and physical and environmental agents (e.g., latex, exercise, cold). Idiopathic anaphylaxis is a diagnosis of exclusion that is made when no identifiable cause can be determined.

   Volcheck GW, Li JT: Exercise-induced urticaria and anaphylaxis. Mayo Clin Proc 72:140–147, 1997.

4. **What are the most common "target" organs?**
   The most common organ systems involved are the skin (e.g., urticaria, angioedema), mucous membranes (e.g., edema), upper respiratory tract (e.g., edema, hypersecretions), lower respiratory tract (e.g., bronchoconstriction), and cardiovascular system (e.g., vasodilatation, cardiovascular collapse).

5. **What are the most common signs and symptoms?**
   The clinical presentation ranges from mild to life-threatening. Mild manifestations, which occur in most people, include urticaria and angioedema. Life-threatening manifestations involve the respiratory and cardiovascular systems. Respiratory signs and symptoms include acute upper airway obstruction presenting with stridor or lower airway manifestations of bronchospasm with diffuse wheezing. Cardiovascular collapse presents in the form of syncope, hypotension, tachycardia, and arrhythmias.

6. **What is the role of diagnostic studies?**
   There is no role for diagnostic studies in anaphylaxis because diagnosis and treatment are based solely on clinical signs and symptoms. There is a role for skin testing either before administration of an antigen or in follow-up referral to determine the exact allergens involved. If the diagnosis is in doubt, additional studies may be indicated.

7. **What is the differential diagnosis?**
   Anaphylaxis may be confused with septic and cardiogenic shock, asthma, croup and epiglottitis, vasovagal syncope, hereditary angioedema, carcinoid syndrome, hysterical stridor, myocardial infarction, or any acute cardiovascular or respiratory collapse of unclear etiology.

8. **What is the most common form of anaphylaxis? How is it treated?**
   Urticaria, either simple or confluent, is the most benign and, fortunately, the most common clinical manifestation. This is thought to be due to a capillary leak mediated by histamine release. It may be treated by the administration of antihistamines (orally, intramuscularly, or intravenously) or epinephrine (intramuscularly). H_1 blockers (e.g., diphenhydramine) should be used in all cases, and H_2 blockers (e.g., cimetidine or ranitidine) should be added in refractory cases.

   Runge JW, Martinez JC, Cavavuti EM: Histamine antagonists in the treatment of acute allergic reactions. Ann Emerg Med 21:237–242, 1992.

9. **What is the best route for epinephrine administration?**
   Because the vast majority of patients do not require IV epinephrine, the ideal route for parental administration is intramuscular (IM) rather than subcutaneous. Recent studies have demonstrated that higher and more rapid peak plasma levels are achieved via the IM route.

   Simons FER, Gu X, Simms KJ: Epinephrine absorption in adults: Intramuscular versus subcutaneous injection. J Allergy Clin Immunol 109:871–873, 2001.

10. **Describe the initial treatment for life-threatening forms of anaphylaxis.**
    1. Upper airway obstruction with stridor and edema should be treated with high-flow nebulized oxygen, racemic epinephrine, and IV epinephrine. If airway obstruction is severe or increases, bag-valve-mask–assisted ventilation, endotracheal intubation, or cricothyroidotomy should be performed.
    2. Acute bronchospasm should be treated with epinephrine. Mild to moderate wheezing in patients with a normal blood pressure may be treated with 0.01 mg/kg of 1:1000 epinephrine administered intramuscularly. If the patient is in severe respiratory distress or has a "quiet" chest, IV epinephrine should be administered via a drip infusion: 1 mg epinephrine in 250 mL D_5W at an initial rate of 1 µg/min with titration to desired effect. Bronchospasm refractory to epinephrine may respond to a nebulized beta agonist, such as albuterol sulfate or metaproterenol, in recommended doses.
    3. Cardiovascular collapse presenting with hypotension should be treated with a constant infusion of epinephrine, titrating the rate to attain a systolic blood pressure of 100 mmHg or a mean arterial pressure of 80 mmHg.
    4. For patients in full cardiac arrest, administer 0.1–0.2 mg/kg of 1:10,000 epinephrine via slow IV push or via endotracheal tube. In addition, immediate endotracheal intubation or cricothyroid ostomy should be performed.

11. **What are the adjuncts to initial epinephrine and airway management?**
    If intubation is unsuccessful and cricothyroid ostomy is contraindicated, percutaneous transtracheal jet ventilation via needle cricothyroid ostomy should be considered, especially in small children. Intravenous (IV) diphenhydramine, an H_1 blocker (2 mg/kg), should be administered to all patients. Simultaneous administration of an H_2 blocker such as cimetidine (300 mg IV or ranitidine 50 mg IV) should also be administered. Aerosolized bronchodilators such as metaproterenol are useful if bronchospasm is present. Corticosteroids are usually given but do not have an immediate positive effect. For refractory hypotension, pressors such as norepinephrine or dopamine can be administered. Corticosteroids have limited benefit because of their delayed onset of action, but they may be beneficial in patients with prolonged bronchospasm or hypotension.

12. **What is unique about the treatment of anaphylaxis in patients who are taking beta blockers?**
    Patients who are taking beta blockers may not respond to epinephrine and antihistamines. Glucagon, which has positive inotropic and chronotropic effects mediated independently of α and β receptors, may be efficacious. Glucagon, 1 mg IV, should be administered, followed by 1–5 mg/h if necessary.

    Javeed N, Javeed H, Javeed S, et al: Refractory anaphylactoid shock potentiated by beta-blockers. Cathet Cardiovasc Diag 39:383–384, 1996.

13. **What are the complications of bolus IV epinephrine administration?**
    When epinephrine 1:10,000 is administered via IV push in patients who have an obtainable blood pressure or pulse, there is significant potential for overtreatment and the potentiation of hypertension, tachycardia, ischemic chest pain, acute myocardial infarction, and ventricular arrhythmias. Extreme care must be exercised in elderly patients and in those with underlying coronary artery disease. It is much safer to administer IV epinephrine by a controlled titratable drip infusion with continuous monitoring of cardiac rhythm and blood pressure.

KEY POINTS: ANAPHYLAXIS

1. Life-threatening "target organs" in anaphylaxis include upper airway mucosa (stridor), bronchial smooth muscle (bronchospasm), and the cardiovascular system (shock).

2. The IM route is preferred over the subcutaneous route for epinephrine administration of anaphylaxis.

3. IV epinephrine is indicated in severe respiratory distress and hypotension.

4. If the patient's condition is not responding to antihistamines and epinephrine, consider administering glucagon.

5. Except in cardiac arrest, IV epinephrine should be administered carefully via IV drip infusion to minimize the risk of severe sympathomimetic response effects.

14. **Is there a role for prophylactic treatment in anaphylaxis? How is this performed?**
    When the potential benefits of treatment or diagnosis outweigh the risks (e.g., administration of IV contrast or animal bite antivenom), informed consent should be obtained if the patient is competent. Pretreatment with IV diphenhydramine (Benadryl) and corticosteroids should be carried out. An IV epinephrine infusion should be prepared. The patient should be in an intensive care unit setting with continuous monitoring of blood pressure, cardiac rhythm, and oxygen saturation. Full intubation and cricothyreotomy equipment should be at the bedside. Administration of the antigen (e.g., rattlesnake antivenom) should be started very slowly with a physician at the bedside who is capable of immediately administering IV epinephrine and managing the airway. Nonionic or low-osmolality contrast medium for diagnostic imaging studies should be administered to patients with a history of anaphylaxis to ionic contrast material.

15. **Describe the out-of-Hospital treatment of anaphylaxis.**
    Patients who are known to be at high risk (e.g., previous anaphylactic reaction to hymenoptera) should be prescribed and educated in the self-administration of epinephrine with an autoinjector at the first sign of anaphylactic symptoms. In addition, self-administration of oral diphenhydramine is indicated for the treatment of mild reactions such as urticaria or concomitant with the administration of epinephrine.

BIBLIOGRAPHY

1. Kemp SF, Lockey RF, Wolf BL, Lieberman P: Anaphylaxis: A review of 266 cases. Arch Intern Med 155:1749–1754, 1995.

2. Seyal AM: Anaphylaxis. In Gershwin EM, Naguwa SM (eds): Allergy and Immunology Secrets, 2nd ed. Philadelphia, Elsevier, 2005, pp 167–181.

3. Tran PT, Muellman RL: Allergy, hypersensitivity and anaphylaxis. In Rosen P (ed): Emergency Medicine: Concepts and Clinical Practice, 6th ed. St. Louis, Mosby, 2006, pp 1818–1837.

CHAPTER 78

HYPOTHERMIA

John A. Marx, MD

1. **How is *hypothermia* defined?**

   Specifically, hypothermia is a core temperature of $<35°C$ (95°F). Moderate to severe hypothermia occurs at temperatures below 32.2°C. Physiologically, it is a clinical state of subnormal temperature in which the body is unable to generate sufficient heat to function efficiently. When hypothermia is suspected, it is imperative that thermometers be capable of measuring core temperatures accurately. Many thermometers have a lower limit of 35°C. The rectal temperature is the most practical, although it can lag behind core changes. Ideally, the probe should be inserted to 15 cm and not placed in cold feces.

   Danzl DF: Accidental hypothermia. In Marx JA (ed): Rosen's Emergency Medicine: Concepts and Clinical Practice, 6th ed. St. Louis, Mosby, 2006, p 2244.

2. **What is the function of shivering? When does it occur?**

   Shivering is modulated by the posterior hypothalamus and spinal cord and is limited by fatigue and glycogen depletion. Shivering is an early response to cold stress and is able to increase the basal metabolic rate two- to fivefold. It produces 40–60 kcal/M^2 of body surface area per hour and is operative between 32°C and 37°C. Below 32°C, shivering thermogenesis ceases. There is a progressive depression of the basal metabolic rate down to 24°C. Below 24°C, autonomic and endocrinologic mechanisms for heat conservation are no longer operative.

   Danzl DF, Pozos RS: Accidental hypothermia. N Engl J Med 331:1756–1760, 1994.

3. **What is the J wave?**

   First described in 1938, this electrocardiographic feature is also known as the *Osborn wave* or *hypothermic hump*. It is seen at the junction of the QRS and ST segments and may appear at temperatures below 32°C. It is most often seen in leads II and V_6, but in more severe hypothermia may be seen in V_3 or V_4. Its size increases with temperature depression but is not prognostic. J waves are typically upright in aV_L, aV_F, and the left precordial leads. The J wave is not specific for hypothermia and can be seen in cardiac ischemia, sepsis, certain central nervous system lesions (particularly of the hypothalamus), and occasionally, young normothermic patients.

   Vassallo SU, Delaney KA, Hoffman RS, et al: A prospective evaluation of the electrocardiographic manifestations of hypothermia. Acad Emerg Med 6:1121–1126, 1999.

4. **What are the five causes of heat loss?**

   Radiation, conduction, convection, respiration, and evaporation. Approximately 55–65% of heat loss occurs through radiation. Conduction usually is responsible for only 2–3%, but loss by conduction can increase fivefold in wet clothing and up to 25-fold in cold water. Convection accounts for 10–15% of heat loss and increases markedly with shivering. The heating of inspired air accounts for up to 2–9% of heat loss, and 20–27% is lost via evaporation from the skin and lungs.

5. **In the field, what are the indications to initiate cardiopulmonary resuscitation (CPR) in a patient with suspected hypothermia?**

   Apparent rigor mortis and lividity are not necessarily reliable indicators in severe hypothermia. Pupils can be fixed and nonreactive at temperatures below 22°C. Peripheral pulses are difficult to palpate in patients with profound bradycardia and vasoconstriction. At least 45–60 seconds should be spent in determining whether spontaneous pulse is present because even extreme bradydysrhythmias may be sufficient to meet the very depressed metabolic needs of a hypothermic patient. A Doppler device or ultrasound can assist in determining whether a pulse or cardiac activity, respectively, is present. Moreover, unnecessary handling, including closed chest compressions, is a purported cause of arrhythmias, although definitive evidence for this is lacking. If no evidence of perfusion can be discerned, an arrest rhythm should be presumed and CPR initiated. Respiratory minute volume is also significantly depressed, and careful scrutiny is required to distinguish apnea. A patent airway should always be established, and if the patient is in respiratory arrest, ventilation should be instituted. Endotracheal intubation does not cause dysrhythmias.

CPR in hypothermia is contraindicated under any of the following circumstances: (1) any signs of life are present, (2) lethal (non–hypothermia-related) injuries are obvious, (3) chest wall compression is impossible due to loss of elasticity, (4) "do not resuscitate" status is verified, or (5) the lives of the rescuers are endangered by environmental conditions.

It may be difficult to distinguish primary from secondary hypothermia (e.g., the patient who dies of cardiac arrest in a cold environment). The oft-quoted maxim that a patient is not dead until warm and dead provides an appropriate caution. Physician judgment is needed, however, to help determine when to begin or cease CPR.

Danzl DF, Pozos RS, Auerbach PS, et al: Multicenter hypothermia survey. Ann Emerg Med 16:1042–1055, 1987.

6. **What are the current recommendations for rate and technique in CPR?**
   With regard to duration, it is clear that prolonged closed chest compressions have resuscitated many severely hypothermic patients to normal neurologic status. It is generally recommended that resuscitative measures continue until a core temperature of 35°C has been reached before a patient is declared dead. The lowest recorded temperature in an accidental hypothermia case is 13.7°C (56.7°F). The patient—a physician—after CPR and 3 hours of cardiopulmonary bypass, authored and presented her own case report.

   Optimal guidelines for rate and techniques are evolving. In an animal model of hypothermic cardiac arrest, cardiac output and cerebral and myocardial blood flows of 50%, 55%, and 31%, respectively, of those produced during normothermic closed chest compression were achieved. These compare well with the reduced metabolic demands of a hypothermic patient. Because chest wall elasticity and pulmonary compliance are decreased, more force is needed for chest wall compressions for adequate intrathoracic pressure gradients to be generated.

Gilbert M, Busund R, Skagseth A, et al: Resuscitation from accidental hypothermia of 13.7 degrees C with circulatory arrest. Lancet 355:375–376, 2000.

Maningas PA, DeGuzman LR, Hollenbach SJ, et al: Regional blood flow during hypothermic arrest. Ann Emerg Med 15:390–396, 1986.

7. **What is the preferred mode of therapy for ventricular fibrillation in the setting of hypothermia?**
   Most dysrhythmias of any type will convert spontaneously during rewarming. Ventricular fibrillation occurs at temperatures below 32°C and is most likely to occur at 28°C. The recommended approach to ventricular fibrillation begins with a maximum of three shocks, each at 2 W sec/kg (maximum, 200 W sec). It is unlikely that this will be successful until the core temperature reaches 28–30°C. Bretylium tosylate was the pharmacologic defibrillator of choice for ventricular fibrillation, but it is no longer available. Magnesium sulfate has also been used successfully in this setting. Lidocaine, propranolol, and amiodarone, although not harmful, have little or no efficacy. Procainamide has been reported to increase the incidence of ventricular fibrillation in hypothermia and should not be used. In hypothermia, the fraction of drug bound to protein increases and liver metabolism is decreased. Thus, toxic levels of antiarrhythmics may develop with rewarming. Optimal dosages in this setting are not well established.

Recommendations suggest that intravenous medications should be administered with increased, albeit unspecified, intervals between doses.

Stoner J, Martin G, O'Mara K, et al: Amiodarone and bretylium in the treatment of hypothermic ventricular fibrillation in a canine model. Acad Emerg Med 10:187–191, 2003.

8. **What are the basic types of rewarming?**
See Table 78-1 for a summary of rewarming techniques.
- **Passive external rewarming (PER):** PER minimizes the normal process of heat loss while allowing the body to rewarm spontaneously via shivering thermogenesis. It is indicated for patients with all levels of hypothermia and is sufficient by itself for mild illness. The technique is to cover the patient with an insulating material in an ambient temperature that exceeds 21°C. To be effective, the patient should have a core temperature of 30–32°C (i.e., shivering thermogenesis intact), sufficient glycogen stores, and operative metabolic homeostasis. Advantages of this technique include its noninvasiveness, simplicity, and maintenance of peripheral vasoconstriction.
- **Active rewarming:** Active rewarming, in general, includes techniques that directly transfer heat and is divided into external (AER) or internal core (ACR) methods. Active rewarming should be considered for patients with moderate or severe hypothermia (<32°C), cardiovascular instability, endocrine failure, impaired thermoregulation, mild hypothermia with failure to rewarm with PER, or peripherovasodilatation (traumatic, toxicologic).
  - **AER:** In AER, exogenous heat is transferred to the skin via heating pads, heating blankets, radiant light sources, warm water immersion, hot water bottles, and forced-air warming systems, in which hot forced air is circulated through a blanket (e.g., Bair Hugger). Forced-air warming systems are effective without causing rewarming shock or core temperature afterdrop. Arteriovenous anastomosis techniques have been described, including negative-pressure rewarming. AER is not recommended as the sole method of rewarming for patients with moderate to severe hypothermia, but it may be successful when combined with ACR methods. The heat source should be applied only to the thorax because heat application to the extremities often produces thermal injury to vasoconstricted and hypoperfused skin and increases the metabolic requirements of the periphery, thus increasing cardiovascular demands. The preferred scenario for AER is acute immersion hypothermia in an otherwise healthy patient.
  - **ACR:** ACR techniques minimize pathophysiologic consequences of rewarming. ACR methods include airway rewarming, IV infusion of heated fluid, heated irrigation (e.g., esophageal, gastric, colonic, chest, mediastinal), diathermy, and extracorporeal rewarming (e.g., cardiopulmonary bypass, arteriovenous rewarming, venovenous rewarming, and hemodialysis).

Gregory JS, Bergstein JM, Aprahamian C, et al: Comparison of three methods of rewarming from hypothermia: Advantages of extracorporeal blood warming. J Trauma 31:1247–1252, 1991.

Handrigan MT, Wright RO, Becker BM, et al: Factors and methodology in achieving ideal delivery temperatures for intravenous and lavage fluid in hypothermia. Am J Emerg Med 15:350–353, 1997.

Kornberger E: Forced air surface rewarming in patients with severe accidental hypothermia. Resuscitation 41:1–5, 1999.

9. **What are the preferred methods of ACR?**
A widely used algorithm for ACR in hypothermia is as follows:
Airway rewarming and heated IV fluids can be administered safely and effectively in virtually all patients. Those in extremis should, in addition, be submitted to extracorporeal rewarming (ECR). Other ACR modalities have less efficacy (e.g., heated irrigation), significant complication rates (e.g., peritoneal dialysis), or limited experience in humans (e.g., diathermy).
A rewarming rate of 1–2.5°C/h can be achieved with heated (42–46°C), humidified oxygen delivery. Heat exchange is augmented depending on technique (endotracheal superior to mask)

TABLE 78-1. REWARMING METHODS

External	Internal
Passive external rewarming	**Active core rewarming**
Active external rewarming	Airway
Truncal	Heated IV fluid
Arteriovenous anatomoses	Heated irrigation
	Esophageal
	Gastric
	Colonic
	Chest
	Mediastinal
	Diathermy
	Extracorporeal
	Cardiopulmonary bypass
	Arteriovenous
	Venovenous
	Hemodialysis

and volume of minute ventilation. Advantages include technical ease, avoidance of temperature afterdrop, assured oxygen delivery, decreased viscosity of pulmonary secretions, decreased cold-induced bronchorrhea, and modification of the amplitude of shivering, which in severe cases decreases the metabolic demands of the periphery. An additional method of heat inhalation via face mask is continuous positive airway pressure. Intravenous fluids can be warmed to 43°C (109°F).

ECR, when available, should be instituted in patients with minimal or absent mechanical cardiac activity. ECR can increase core temperature 1–2°C every 5 minutes with a bypass flow rate of 2–3 L/min. Arteriovenous rewarming is appropriate if systolic blood pressure is 60 mmHg or greater. It is accomplished via the connection of percutaneously placed femoral arterial and venous catheters to a fluid warmer. In venovenous rewarming, blood is routed from a central venous pressure catheter through a warmer and returned through a second central line or a peripheral venous catheter. Hemodialysis, although less rapid and effective, will become more practical with the development of two-way flow catheters.

Goheen MSL, Ducharme MB, Kenny GP, et al: Efficacy of forced-air and inhalation rewarming using a human model for severe hypothermia. J Appl Physiol 83:1635–1640, 1997.

Kirkpatrick AW, Garraway N, Brown DR, et al: Use of a centrifugal vortex blood pump and heparin-bonded circuit for extracorporeal rewarming of severe hypothermia in acutely injured and coagulopathic patients. J Trauma 55:407–412, 2003.

Kjaergaard B, Tolboll P, Lyduch S, Trautner S: A mobile system for the treatment of accidental hypothermia with extracorporeal circulation. Perfusion 16:453–459, 2001.

Weinberg AD: The role of inhalation rewarming in the early management of hypothermia. Resuscitation 36:101–104, 1998.

10. **What stabilizing measures should prehospital care providers undertake?**
The patient should be handled as gently and carefully as possible because ventricular fibrillation has been ascribed to excessive mechanical stimulation. In cases of immersion, wet clothing

should be removed. Further heat loss should be limited by provision of a dry and insulated environment. Blankets, sleeping bags, or aluminum-coated foils can be used for this purpose. Ethanol should not be given because it suppresses shivering thermogenesis, promotes peripheral vasodilatation, and can prompt hypoglycemia in these typically glycogen-depleted patients. Massage of the extremities provides unnecessary physical stimulation and, like ethanol, can mitigate both shivering and appropriate peripheral vasoconstriction. If venous access can be acquired, 50 mL of 50% dextrose, 2 mg of naloxone, and 100 mg of thiamine are appropriate. A fluid challenge of 50%-dextrose normal saline, 250–500 mL (preferably heated to 43°C), is indicated because the majority of patients with moderate to severe hypothermia have sustained cold-induced diuresis. Lactated Ringer's solution is a less preferred crystalloid because the hypothermic liver is less able to metabolize lactate.

AER measures are safe in minimally hypothermic patients, but unnecessary. In a patient with moderate to profound hypothermia, only truncal AER should be considered. The only method of ACR appropriate in the field is heated, humidified oxygen. Several portable devices are available for this purpose.

Hypothermia: Guidelines 2000 for CPR and ECC. 102:1–229, 2000.

KEY POINTS: HYPOTHERMIA

1. Endotracheal intubation is a safe and appropriate procedure in patients with hypothermia.

2. Rigor mortis, lividity, and fixed pupils do not necessarily portend death in severe hypothermia.

3. Doppler devices and ultrasound can be used to ascertain the presence of pulse and cardiac activity, respectively.

4. Cardioversion of hypothermia-induced ventricular fibrillation is unlikely to be successful at core temperatures below 28–30°C.

5. External core rewarming is indicated in severe hypothermia when there is little or no cardiac activity.

1. **What procedures are hazardous in the management of a hypothermic patient?**
In patients with moderate and severe hypothermia, cardiac monitoring is indicated and harmless. Central venous pressure catheters can provide useful information and will not precipitate cardiac arrhythmias unless they are inserted into the heart. The placement of pulmonary artery catheters can be quite hazardous in this regard. Transcutaneous pacing is safe. Nasogastric tubes and Foley catheters are frequently required and can be inserted without risk.

Endotracheal intubation was thought to create a higher risk of arrhythmias. However, these reported sequelae were likely coincidental to, rather than caused by, this procedure. Numerous reports have failed to elicit a single case of arrhythmia provoked by endotracheal intubation. Factors that may be responsible for arrhythmias in the immediate post-intubation period include physical stimulation of the patient, acid–base or electrolyte disturbances, and failure to preoxygenate the patient adequately.

Dixon RG, Dougherty JM, White LJ, et al: Transcutaneous pacing in a hypothermic-dog model. Ann Emerg Med 29:602–606, 1997.
Lazar HL: The treatment of hypothermia. N Engl J Med 337:1545–1547, 1997.

12. **Are prophylactic antibiotics indicated for patients with hypothermia?**

Infection, including septicemia (e.g., gram-negative sepsis in adults), may be the cause of, coincident with, or a sequel to hypothermia. Even in the recovery phase of hypothermia, fever and other signs of infection are typically absent. Shaking chills caused by sepsis may unwittingly be ascribed to the shivering of hypothermia. Leukocytosis is often absent due to compromised bone marrow release and circulation of neutrophils.

The incidence of infection in hypothermic neonates is quite high and ranges from 41% to 53% in two series. Pulmonary infections are most commonly found, and bacteriology is likely to reveal the presence of Enterobacteriaceae, *Haemophilus, Staphylococcus,* or *Streptococcus* species. In adults, soft-tissue and pulmonary infections are most likely. Occult central nervous system bacteremia appears to be rare. Gram-negative bacteria, gram-positive cocci, Enterobacteriaceae, and oral anaerobes are likely to be found. Elderly patients with thermoregulatory failure should be considered to have sepsis until proved otherwise.

The key to management is repeated physical examination during and after rewarming. Culture specimens should be secured early in the course of emergency department treatment. Lumbar puncture is indicated in adults with persistent altered mental status after rewarming and should be used more liberally in neonates and elderly patients. Antibiotic prophylaxis is recommended for neonates and elderly patients. Routine prophylaxis does not appear warranted in hypothermic adults who have no obvious manifestations of infection.

Giesbrecht GG: Cold stress, near drowning and accidental hypothermia: A review. Aviat Space Environ Med 71:733–752, 2000.

13. **What is the relationship of alcohol to hypothermia?**

Ethanol has social and pathophysiologic consequences. It is the most frequent associated cause of heat loss in urban hypothermia. Alcoholics are more vulnerable to the hazards of climate because of altered perception due to acute intoxication, inadequate clothing, and insufficient shelter. Heat loss is promoted by peripheral vasodilatation, impaired shivering thermogenesis, and decreased subcutaneous fat caused by malnutrition. There is a strong association between alcohol-induced hypoglycemia and ethanol. An unusual clinical presentation of Wernicke-Korsakoff syndrome is profound hypothermia. This is due to thiamine-depletion–induced hemorrhage in the hypothalamus. The clinical presentation is heralded by hypothermia, bradycardia, hypotension, miosis, and depressed deep tendon reflexes. Therefore, thiamine, 100 mg given intravenously, is indicated in patients with hypothermia. Magnesium, a necessary co-factor for thiamine, is often depleted in a patient with alcoholism, and repletion is required for thiamine administration to be effective.

Reuler JB, Girard DE, Conney TG: Wernicke's encephalopathy. N Engl J Med 312:1035–1039, 1985.

14. **Is AER an effective and safe method of therapy in hypothermia?**

Certain series report excellent success with the use of AER. The preponderance of data, however, indicate that AER, as an isolated measure of rewarming, is associated with high morbidity and mortality rates in patients with severe hypothermia. Candidates for AER are previously healthy patients who develop acute hypothermia (e.g., immersion), in whom minimal pathophysiologic changes have occurred. AER in a patient with minimal hypothermia is probably not harmful. The combination of truncal AER (e.g., using forced-air warming systems) with core rewarming has been successful in patients who have more serious hypothermic conditions.

Pathophysiologic consequences of AER in moderate and severe hypothermia include sudden peripheral vasodilatation accompanied by shock, afterdrop in core temperature, suppressed shivering thermogenesis with decreased overall rate of core rewarming, increased peripheral metabolic demands, and decreased threshold for ventricular fibrillation due to myocardial thermal gradients. AER should not be used alone in a patient with moderate to severe hypothermia. If AER is used, it should be restricted to the torso to prevent core temperature afterdrop and thermal injury to the extremities.

CHAPTER 79

HEAT STROKE

Stephen V. Cantrill, MD

1. What is heat stroke?

Heat stroke is equated with a rectal temperature of approximately 40.5°C (105°F) or greater in a person with a history of exposure to exercise or increased temperature and humidity with accompanying neurologic disturbance, usually in the form of altered mental status. Anhidrosis (i.e., lack of sweating) is not a criterion; sweating may or may not be present.

Bouchama A, Knochel MD: Heat stroke. N Engl J Med 346:1978–1988, 2002.

Vicario S: Heat illness. In Marx JA, Hockenberger RS, Walls RM, et al (eds): Rosen's Emergency Medicine: Concepts and Clinical Practice, 6th ed. St. Louis, Mosby, 2006, pp 2254–2267.

2. Why was a rectal temperature of 40.5°C selected as the threshold?

A rectal temperature of this magnitude or greater implies that the body's mechanisms for dealing with an increased heat load have been overwhelmed and that the pathologic effects of increased temperature may occur.

3. What are the two types of heat stroke? How do they present?

Classic heat stroke is not associated with exercise, but rather with exposure to high heat and humidity over time. This form of heat stroke has a slow onset, often developing over days. It is common in elderly and chronically ill persons, who may present with anorexia, nausea, vomiting, headache, dizziness, confusion, or hypotension. Anhidrosis is common. Exertional heat stroke usually affects young people in good health who are exercising in a hot, humid environment. It is rapid in onset. Nausea, dizziness, and confusion are common. Fatigue, ataxia, coma, and nuchal rigidity or posturing may also occur. Patients often are sweating at the time of presentation.

KEY POINTS: DIAGNOSTIC CRITERIA FOR HEAT STROKE

1. Exposure to increased heat stress due to exercise or increased temperature and humidity is a common factor in heat stroke.

2. Altered mental status is another diagnostic criterion.

3. Patients with heat stroke have a core (rectal) temperature greater than 40.5°C (105°F).

4. Sweating may or may not be present.

4. Which populations are at greater risk for heat stroke?

- **Extremes of age:** Due to relatively poor temperature regulation in young and old persons, especially during heat waves (elevated mean heat index—see further discussion)
- **Chronically ill:** Especially those on drugs that predispose to heat illness
- **Military recruits:** Especially unacclimated northerners training in the south

- **Athletes:** Most commonly, football players and runners
- **Laborers:** Especially if water losses have not been replaced
- **Obese persons:** Heat dissipation is compromised
- **Persons dressed inappropriately for environment or activity level**

Carter R III, Cheuvront SN, Williams JO, et al: Epidemiology of hospitalizations and deaths from heat illness in soldiers. Med Sci Sports Exerc 37:1338–1344, 2005.

Vanhems P, Gambotti L, Fabry J: Excess rate of in-hospital death in Lyons, France during the August 2003 heat wave. N Engl J Med 349:2077–2078, 2003.

5. **Which drugs predispose a person to heat stroke?**
   - **Drugs increasing heat production through increased activity:** Cocaine, amphetamines, ephedrine, phencyclidine, lysergic acid diethylamide
   - **Drugs decreasing thirst:** Haloperidol
   - **Drugs decreasing sweating:** Antihistamines, anticholinergics, phenothiazines, beta blockers

Oh RC, Henning JS: Exertional heatstroke in an infantry soldier taking ephedra-containing dietary supplements. Mil Med 168:429–430, 2003.

6. **What is the most effective measure of the effect of environmental heat in humans?**
   The commonly measured ambient air temperature is a poor gauge because it does not measure the effect of humidity, wind velocity, and radiational heating. Research has shown that an entity known as the wet bulb globe temperature (WBGT) is a much more accurate measure. The WBGT combines the wet bulb temperature (measuring the effect of humidity and wind velocity), the black globe temperature (measuring radiational heating), and the dry bulb temperature (measuring ambient air temperature). Although rarely used in the civilian world, the WBGT is commonly used by the military as a guide to determine the allowable level of activity. The formula for WBGT is as follows:

   $$WGBT = 0.7\,(\text{wet bulb temperature}) + 0.2\,(\text{black globe temperature}) + 0.1\,(\text{dry bulb temperature})$$

National Athletic Trainers Association: Inter-association task force on exertional heat illness consensus statement, 2003: www.nata.org/fpfiles/links/heatillness2.htm

7. **What is the mean heat index? How is it useful?**
   The mean heat index is a recently devised measure developed by the National Weather Service of how hot the environment actually feels to a person over the course of a day. This value is computed from a multiregression analysis equation based on ambient temperature and humidity extremes encountered during a 24-hour period. Values > 29.5°C (85°F) are believed to be dangerous to the population at large. The U.S. National Weather Service has developed methods to create a forecast giving the probability that a specific locale will exceed a certain mean heat index for up to 7 days in the future. These forecasts can be used by local health and emergency officials to prepare the public for times of increased risk from heat and heat stroke.

8. **What is the mortality rate of heat stroke?**
   Mortality rates vary from 0% to 76% in different reports. This high variability is due to the differences in the populations studied. Young, healthy persons with exertional heat stroke usually do quite well, whereas elderly, chronically ill persons with classic heat stroke fare quite poorly.

9. **What differential diagnoses should be considered in patients presenting with a rectal temperature higher than 40.5°C?**
   See Box 79-1.

BOX 79-1.   DIFFERENTIAL DIAGNOSIS OF HEAT STROKE

Meningitis	Neuroleptic malignant syndrome
Typhus	Malignant hyperthermia
Falciparum malaria	Thyroid storm
Rocky Mountain spotted fever	Delirium tremens
Hypothalamic lesion	Anticholinergic overdose

---

10. **What are some of the low-level effects of heat stroke?**
    - Cellular hypoxia
    - Enzyme denaturation and inactivation
    - Cellular membrane disruption

11. **Name some end-organ effects in heat stroke.**
    - **Skeletal muscle:** Rhabdomyolysis
    - **Cardiac:** Hemorrhage, necrosis
    - **Respiratory:** Adult respiratory distress syndrome
    - **Renal:** Acute tubular necrosis
    - **Hepatic:** Centrolobular hepatocellular degeneration
    - **Coagulation:** Thrombocytopenia, disseminated intravascular coagulation
    - **Central nervous system:** Edema, petechial hemorrhages

12. **What is the most important aspect in the treatment of heat stroke?**
    Rapid cooling. Heat stroke is a true medical emergency in which every minute counts. Poor patient outcome is related more to the length of time the temperature remains elevated than to the absolute degree of hyperpyrexia.

13. **What treatment modalities are effective for rapid cooling?**
    Immersion in ice water is effective, although many believe that this must be accompanied by vigorous skin massage to counteract the cutaneous vasoconstriction that may actually impede heat loss. This modality may not be appropriate in comatose or combative patients. Aggressive evaporative cooling, consisting of treatment with tepid water spray (40°C, [104°F]) and a forced air stream from a fan, has proved successful. Ice packs and massage may be used. Techniques such as iced gastric lavage and peritoneal lavage have also been reported. Cooling efforts should be ceased when the patient's temperature falls to 38.5°C (101.3°F) to avoid temperature undershoot and shivering.

    Smith JE: Cooling methods used in the treatment of exertional heat illness. Br J Sports Med 39: 503–507, 2005.

14. **What additional steps should be taken in dealing with heat stroke?**
    - Continuous monitoring of rectal temperature
    - Supplemental oxygen
    - Active airway management, as indicated
    - Cardiac monitor and electrocardiogram
    - Central line or Swan-Ganz catheter placement with central venous pressure/wedge pressure monitoring in patients with hypotension
    - Cautious fluid replacement with normal saline or Ringer's lactate solution
    - Foley catheter and nasogastric tube placement
    - Restraints, as needed

15. **Which laboratory studies are appropriate in a severely ill patient with heat stroke?**
    - Arterial blood gas analyses
    - Serum electrolyte, blood urea nitrogen, creatinine, and glucose measurements
    - Urinalysis
    - Complete blood count with platelet count
    - Prothrombin and partial thromboplastin times, fibrin degradation products
    - Liver function tests, creatine kinase measurement
    - Serum calcium, phosphate, and lactate analyses

16. **What complications may occur in patients with heat stroke?**
    - **Emesis:** Especially in patients who are comatose
    - **Electrolyte disorders:** Hypokalemia, hyperkalemia, hyponatremia
    - **Shivering:** Treat with diazepam, 5 mg IV
    - **Seizures**
    - **Acidosis:** Treat with sodium bicarbonate if severe
    - **Cardiogenic shock:** Treat with isoproterenol; avoid alpha agents
    - **Decreased urinary output:** Treat with mannitol if necessary
    - **Pulmonary edema:** From injudicious fluid replacement
    - **Clotting disorders:** May require fresh frozen plasma, heparin, or platelets
    - **Combative, psychotic behavior:** IV sedation may be necessary

17. **What prognostic signs help to indicate outcome?**
    The longer the duration of the elevated temperature, the poorer the prognosis. Coma, hypotension, hyperkalemia, and an aspartate aminotransferase level >1000 units are associated with a poor prognosis.

18. **What steps can be taken to prevent heat stroke?**
    - Adequate fluid intake during periods of high temperature, high humidity, or increased activity levels
    - Decreased levels of activity as mandated by the WBGT or mean heat index
    - Control of ambient temperature and humidity, if possible
    - Appropriate dress for the weather
    - Prudence during acclimation to a hotter environment
    - Adjustment of dosages of predisposing drugs, if possible, during hot weather
    - Awareness of symptoms of impending heat stroke

19. **Is dantrolene sodium effective in treating heat stroke?**
    Dantrolene sodium uncouples the heat-generating mechanism in muscle and is the drug of choice in treating malignant hyperthermia and neuroleptic malignant syndrome, which cause excessive muscular heat production. The potential benefit of this drug in treating heat stroke has been debated. Many investigators are of the opinion that no benefit would accrue because once treatment has begun, the problem is not heat production but rather heat dissipation. Studies in dogs have confirmed that the administration of dantrolene sodium has no effect on passive cooling rates, pathologic changes, or clinical outcome. Although a human trial demonstrated a significant improvement in cooling rates in patients treated with dantrolene, the trial failed to demonstrate any difference in clinical outcome. In addition, these data have been contradicted by a more recent randomized, double-blind study that showed dantrolene to be ineffective. Routine use of dantrolene sodium in patients with heat stroke is not warranted at this time.

Channa AB, Seraj MA, Saddique AA, et al: Is dantrolene effective in heat stroke patients? Crit Care Med 18:290–292, 1990.

Hadad E, Cohen-Sivan Y, Heled Y, et al: Clinical review: Treatment of heat stroke: Should dantrolene be considered? Crit Care 9:86–91, 2005.

20. **What is the most effective means of inducing rapid cooling?**

Much discussion has centered on use of immersion, iced gastric lavage, or evaporative cooling of a patient with heat stroke, either singly or in combination. Iced peritoneal lavage has also been anecdotally reported. Controlled comparison studies have most commonly used a dog model, which may not adequately represent the human response. At this time, there does not appear to be a "best" method, although many favor evaporative (tepid water spray and forced air) cooling as the best compromise for ease of use, speed of cooling, and patient safety.

Costrini A: Emergency treatment of exertional heatstroke and comparison of whole body cooling techniques. Med Sci Sports Exerc 22:15–18, 1990.

Vicario S: Heat illness. In Marx JA, Hockenberger RS, Walls RM, et al (eds): Rosen's Emergency Medicine, Concepts and Clinical Practice, 6th ed. St. Louis, Mosby, 2006, pp 2254–2267.

White JD, Riccobene E, Nucci R, et al: Evaporation versus iced gastric lavage treatment of heatstroke: Comparative efficacy in a canine model. Crit Care Med 15:748–750, 1987.

GENERAL APPROACH TO POISONINGS

Ken Kulig, MD

CHAPTER 80

1. **What are the most common causes of death from acute poisoning?**
   Table 80-1 lists the categories resulting in the greatest number of deaths, according to the American Association of Poison Control Centers Database.

TABLE 80-1. CATEGORIES OF POISONING RESULTING IN THE GREATEST NUMBER OF DEATHS		
Category	Number	% of All Exposures in Category
Analgesics	658	0.235
Sedatives/hypnotics/antipsychotics	371	0.286
Antidepressants	299	0.290
Stimulants and street drugs	214	0.472
Cardiovascular drugs	162	0.218
Alcohols	114	0.153
Gases and fumes	83	0.206
Anticonvulsants	81	0.202
Chemicals	62	0.133
Muscle relaxants	61	0.261
Antihistamines	55	0.076
Hormones and hormone antagonists	46	0.095
Cough and cold preparations	30	0.028
Automotive products	27	0.185
Cleaning substances	25	0.011

Data from Watson WA, Litovitz TL, Rodgers GC, et al: 2004 Annual Report of the American Association of Poison Control Centers Toxic Exposure Surveillance System. Am J Emerg Med 23:589–666, 2004.

2. **Does syrup of ipecac still have a role in treating acute poisoning?**
   Although syrup of ipecac induces vomiting within 20–30 minutes in most patients who are administered a therapeutic dose, very little poison is removed. It also increases the risk of aspiration after ingestion of drugs, which causes central nervous system depression. Its use has been essentially abandoned, and it is no longer sold over the counter.

   Position paper: Ipecac syrup. J Toxicol Clin Toxicol 42:133–143, 2004.

3. **What is the current role of gastric lavage in treating acute poisonings?**
   Gastric lavage must be performed soon after ingestion to be at all effective in removing drugs from the stomach. For this reason, many clinicians do not lavage patients who have overdosed if more than 1 hour has elapsed since ingestion. Gastric lavage may result in major morbidity (e.g., esophageal perforation). Gastric lavage can be accomplished without prior tracheal intubation in most patients, but it is advised that airway equipment including suction be immediately available at the bedside. Whenever gastric lavage is performed, a large-bore (36 or 40 French tube in adults) should be placed through the mouth, and proper location of the tube in the stomach should be verified clinically or radiographically.

   Position paper: Gastric lavage. J Toxicol Clin Toxicol 42:933–943, 2004.

4. **Is there a role for cathartic agents in treating acute poisoning?**
   The theory behind cathartics is that they will speed up gastrointestinal (GI) transit time, allowing activated charcoal to catch up with pills in the bowel, and perhaps also prevent desorption of drug from activated charcoal. A single dose of a cathartic agent is commonly used, although this practice is of unproven benefit. Multiple-dose cathartics should never be used because life-threatening complications from electrolyte imbalance may result. A single dose of a saline cathartic such as magnesium sulfate or magnesium citrate or a single dose of sorbitol (approximately 1 gm/kg) is unlikely to be harmful but is of unproven benefit.

   Position paper: Cathartics. J Toxicol Clin Toxicol 42:243–253, 2004.

5. **Is there a role for whole-bowel irrigation in the treatment of acute poisoning?**
   Whole-bowel irrigation uses a polyethylene glycol electrolyte solution such as GoLYTELY or Colyte, which are not absorbed. The irrigation fluid is given orally or by nasogastric tube at a dose of 1–2 L/h. This procedure is commonly used when packets of street drugs such as heroin or cocaine have been ingested or when the ingested substance is radiopaque (i.e., iron tablets). The limitations of the procedure include the fact that unless the patient is awake, cooperative, and able to sit on a commode, there is a risk of vomiting and aspiration. This is in addition to the logistical problem of having an unconscious patient in bed with massive diarrhea.

   Position paper: Whole bowel irrigation. J Toxicol Clin Toxicol 42:843–845, 2004.

6. **What is the role of multiple-dose charcoal in the treatment of acute poisoning?**
   Multiple-dose charcoal has been shown to enhance the elimination of many drugs that have already been absorbed from the GI tract or that are given intravenously (Box 80-1). This process has been called *gastrointestinal dialysis* and has been shown to be quite effective for theophylline and perhaps phenobarbital poisoning. For the majority of acute poisonings in which use of multiple-dose charcoal is being contemplated, the primary reason for giving

---

BOX 80-1. DRUGS WITH ALTERED PHARMACOKINETICS IN RESPONSE TO MULTIPLE-DOSE CHARCOAL

Amitriptyline	Dextropropoxyphene	Meprobamate	Piroxicam
Atrazine	Diazepam	Methotrexate	Prophyrins
Carbamazepine	Digitoxin	Nadolol	Proscillaridin
Chlorpropamide	Digoxin	Nortriptyline	Quinine
Cyclosporine	Doxepin	Phenobarbital	Salicylates
Dapsone	Glutethimide	Phenylbutazone	Sotalol
DesmethyldiazepamImipramine		Phenytoin	Theophylline

multiple-dose charcoal is to prevent absorption of drugs from the GI tract, not to enhance their elimination from the blood.

7. **Is forced diuresis of benefit in the treatment of acute poisoning?**
Very few drugs are excreted unchanged in the urine, such that even increasing urine flow significantly above baseline is unlikely to be of benefit. However, by manipulating the pH of the urine by infusions of bicarbonate solution along with enhanced urine flow, in certain cases drug elimination can be increased. This method is most commonly used for salicylates and phenobarbital. By placing 3 ampules of sodium bicarbonate in 1 L of D_5W along with potassium chloride and infusing this solution at rates sufficient to produce at least a normal urine flow and a urine pH of 7.5 or greater, the elimination of salicylate and phenobarbital can be increased. Intake, output, and urine pH should be monitored hourly with a Foley catheter in place.

KEY POINTS: PREVENTION OF FURTHER ABSORPTION IN ADULT ORAL DRUG OVERDOSE

1. Ipecac routinely causes vomiting, but almost no drug is actually removed.

2. Gastric lavage is an invasive procedure that may cause esophageal perforation and rarely removes much drug from the stomach.

3. Whole-bowel irrigation is rarely useful unless there is a way to track movement of drugs through the gastrointestinal tract (e.g., the drug is radiopaque).

4. Activated charcoal adsorbs most drugs but needs to be administered relatively soon after the overdose to have a clinical benefit.

5. Cathartic are generally of little or no benefit.

8. **When are extracorporeal techniques such as hemodialysis or hemoperfusion indicated?**
Drugs can be successfully removed by extracorporeal maneuvers only if they are found in significant quantities in the blood, which is the case for only a few drugs. The rest are rapidly distributed into tissues and not amenable for removal. In practice, the substances most commonly dialyzed after overdose include aspirin, lithium, methanol, ethylene glycol, and rarely, theophylline. Dialysis has the advantage over hemoperfusion in that it is frequently easier and faster to get started and can correct fluid and electrolyte abnormalities. Drugs for which charcoal hemoperfusion is sometimes used include theophylline, phenobarbital, and a handful of other, less-common agents such as paraquat and amatoxin.

9. **How can the diagnosis of a drug overdose be made when the patient is unconscious and history is unavailable?**
Drug overdose in an unconscious patient is sometimes a difficult diagnosis to make and may require some detective work on the part of the physician. All unconscious patients should receive dextrose (unless the Dextrostick glucose test shows euglycemia) and naloxone (Narcan). Whenever possible, examination of the pill bottles available to the patient is important. Discovering which chemical agents were available to the patient, including street drugs and household chemicals such as pesticides, may be important. If track marks are seen, consider street drugs commonly given intravenously such as opiates, cocaine, and amphetamine. The physical examination is extremely useful in narrowing the diagnosis to a class of drug or chemicals. The most common toxic syndromes are listed in Box 80-2.

510 GENERAL APPROACH TO POISONINGS

BOX 80-2. THE MOST COMMON TOXIC SYNDROMES

Anticholinergic

Common signs: Dementia with mumbling speech, tachycardia, dry flushed skin, dilated pupils, myoclonus, slightly elevated temperature, urinary retention, decreased bowel sounds. Seizures and dysrhythmias may occur in severe cases.

Common causes: Antihistamines, antiparkinsonism medication, atropine, scopolamine, amantadine, antipsychotics, antidepressants, antispasmodics, mydriatics, skeletal muscle relaxants, many plants (most notably jimson weed).

Sympathomimetic

Common signs: Delusions, paranoia, tachycardia, hypertension, hyperpyrexia, diaphoresis, piloerection, mydriasis, hyperreflexia. Seizures and dysrhythmias may occur in severe cases.

Common causes: Cocaine, amphetamine, methamphetamine (and derivatives 3,4-methylenedioxyamphetamine [MDA], 3,4-methylenedioxymethamphetamine [MDMA], 3,4-methylenedioxyethylamphetamine [MDEA]), over-the-counter decongestants (e.g., phenylpropanolamine, ephedrine, pseudoephedrine). Caffeine and theophylline overdoses cause similar findings resulting from catecholamine release, except for the organic psychiatric signs.

Opiate/sedative

Common signs: Coma, respiratory depression, miosis, hypotension, bradycardia, hypothermia, pulmonary edema, decreased bowel sounds, hyporeflexia, needle marks.

Common causes: Narcotics, barbiturates, benzodiazepines, ethchlorvynol, glutethimide, methyprylon, methaqualone, meprobamate.

Cholinergic

Common signs: Confusion/CNS depression, weakness, salivation, lacrimation, urinary and fecal incontinence, GI cramping, emesis, diaphoresis, muscle fasciculations, pulmonary edema, miosis, bradycardia (or tachycardia), seizures.

Common causes: Organophosphate and carbamate insecticides, physostigmine, edrophonium, some mushrooms (*Amanita muscaria, Amanita pantherina, Inocybe* species, *Clitocybe* species).

Serotonin syndrome

Common signs: Fever, tremor, uncoordination, agitation, mental status changes, diaphoresis, myoclonus, diarrhea, rigidity.

Common causes: Fluoxetine, sertraline, paroxetine, venlafaxine, clomipramine; also, the preceding drugs in combination with monoamine oxidase inhibitors.

CNS = central nervous system, GI = gastrointestinal.

10. **When is a urine toxicology screen useful in cases of drug overdose?**
Urine toxicology screens have evolved into quick, inexpensive clinical tools that can now be performed at the patient's beside. However, results are often nonspecific. For example, a patient taking an over-the-counter decongestant may test positive for methamphetamine because the

chemical structures of the two drugs are similar. Confirmation by a more specific technique would be indicated in that situation. Many drugs commonly taken in overdose are not found on a typical screening panel. It is therefore important to know what is being screened for in advance and to order more precise tests when indicated. Direct communication with the laboratory is often useful.

11. **What are alternatives to urine toxicology screens?**
Alternatives include testing discrete serum levels of the toxins in question in blood (e.g., for aspirin, acetaminophen, digoxin, iron, lithium) or requesting confirmation of any drugs found in urine (e.g., cocaine metabolite). In some forensic cases (e.g., suspected date rape or attempted homicide by poisoning), it may be valuable to draw blood and urine, communicate with the laboratory about which specific tests might be done, and then label and save other specimens in case further testing is indicated.

12. **What other tests may be useful in an unconscious patient suspected of taking an overdose?**
Electrocardiography can help diagnose overdose of tricyclic antidepressants, cardiac medications, or drugs that prolong the QT interval. The chest radiograph, if demonstrating noncardiogenic pulmonary edema, should make one think of opiates or salicylates. Aspiration pneumonitis may occur whenever central nervous system depression is present; this condition is nonspecific but may hasten the need for intubation. An abdominal radiograph may have positive results for radiopaque material in the gut, which may be a heavy metal such as iron, arsenic, or mercury; a drug such as phenothiazine or potassium; or a chemical such as chlorinated hydrocarbon solvents. Liver function tests may help to diagnose ingestion of hepatotoxins such as acetaminophen or carbon tetrachloride. A urinalysis may demonstrate the presence of calcium oxalate crystals, suggesting ethylene glycol poisoning. Persistent unexplained metabolic acidosis should always prompt the search for other diagnostic clues to aspirin, methanol, or ethylene glycol poisoning. An elevated creatine phosphokinase level in a patient experiencing overdose should prompt hydration, perhaps with a bicarbonate solution.

KEY POINTS: USE OF NALOXONE (NARCAN)

1. Naloxone will reverse most opiate sedation unless the patient has already suffered hypoxic encephalopathy, in which case a partial or no response may be seen.

2. If the patient is sedated but breathing, a small dose of naloxone, such as 0.4 mg, can be given to avoid precipitating withdrawal symptoms.

3. If the patient is not breathing, 2 mg IV should be the starting dose, and occasionally more will need to be given to get a response.

4. Naloxone will not reverse noncardiogenic pulmonary edema.

5. Because of its short half-life (about 1 hour), its ability to reverse opiates may be shorter than the effect of the drug ingested, especially for drugs with long half-lives (e.g., methadone).

13. **What antidotes are commonly used in toxicology?**
The most commonly used antidotes are list in Table 80-2.

TABLE 80-2. ANTIDOTES

Toxin	Antidote	Dose and Comments
Acetaminophen	N-acetylcysteine	140 mg/kg, then 70 mg/kg q4h, p.o. or IV for 17 doses. or less if the transaminase levels remain normal as the acetaminophen level becomes nondetectable. The FDA has approved IV N-acetylcysteine (Acetadote), which involves a 20-hour protocol.
Anticholinergics	Physostigmine	1–2 mg IV adults, 0.5 mg in children, over 2 minutes for anticholinergic delerium, seizures, or dysrhythmias.
Arsenic, lead, and mercury	BAL	3–5 mg/kg, IM only. Injections are painful. Cannot be used in patients with peanut allergy.
	D-Penicillamine	20–40 mg/kg/day p.o.; 500 mg t.i.d. in adults; may cross-react with penicillin in allergic patients.
Benzodiazepines	Flumazenil	0.2 mg, then 0.3 mg, then 0.5 mg, up to 5 mg; not to be used if the patient has also overdosed on tricyclic antidepressants. May precipitate seizures if the patient has also been taking large doses of benzodiazepines chronically. Not approved for use in children, but probably safe.
Beta blockers and calcium channel blockers	Glucagon	5–10 mg IV in adults, then infusion of same dose per hour.
Black widow spider bite	*Latrodectus* antivenin	1 vial, by slow IV infusion, usually curative; may cause anaphylaxis. Generally reserved for severe cases refractory to opiates, calcium, and benzodiazepines.
Calcium channel blockers	Calcium	1 gm calcium chloride IV in adults, 20–30 mg/kg in children, over a few minutes with continuous monitoring.
Calcium channel blockers or beta blockers	Glucagon	5–10 mg in adults, then infusion of same dose per hour.
Cyanide	Sodium thiosulfate	50 mL of 25% (12.5 gm; 1 ampule) in adults; 1.65 mL/kg in children, IV.
Cyanide, H_2S	Sodium nitrite	10 mL of 3% (300 mg; 1 ampule) in adults; 0.33 mL/kg in children, slowly IV.

Continued

Digitalis glycosides	Digoxin-specific FAB fragments	10–20 vials if patient is in ventricular fibrillation; otherwise, the dose is based on serum digoxin concentration or the amount ingested.
Ethylene glycol	Fomepazole	15 mg/kg × 1, then 10 mg/kg q12h × 4, then 15 mg/kg. Dose is increased if patient is receiving dialysis.
	Pyridoxine	100 mg IV daily.
	Thiamine	100 mg IV daily.
Hydrofluoric acid	Calcium gluconate	3.5 gm in 5 oz of KY jelly topical.
Iron	Deferoxamine	15 mg/kg/h IV; higher doses reported to be safe.
Isoniazid, hydrazine, and monomethylhydrazine	Pyridoxine	5 gm in adults, 1 gm in children, if ingested dose unknown; antidote may cause neuropathy if very large doses are administered.
Lead	DMSA, Succimer	Reported useful for arsenic and mercury poisoning as well; one 100-mg capsule per 10 kg body weight t.i.d. for 5 days, then b.i.d. for 2 weeks with chelation breaks between rounds of therapy.
	EDTA	75 mg/kg/day by continuous infusion; watch for nephrotoxicity; best done in hospital.
Methanol	Folate or leucovorin	50 mg IV q4h in adults while patient has serious toxicity.
	Fomepazole	15 mg/kg×1, then 10 mg/kg q12h× 4, then 15 mg/kg. Dose is increased if patient is receiving dialysis.
Methanol and ethylene glycol	Ethanol	Loading dose, 10 mL/kg of 10%; maintenance dose, 0.15 mL/kg/h of 10%; double rate during dialysis. Ethanol levels must be monitored frequently, and hypoglycemia prevented.
Methemoglobin-forming agents	Methylene blue	1–2 mg/kg IV, one 10-mL dose of 10% solution (100 mg; one ampule) is initial adult dose.
Opiates	Nalmefene	2 mg; much longer half-life than naloxone.
	Naloxone	2 mg; less to avoid narcotic withdrawal, more if inadequate response; same dose in children.

Continued

TABLE 80-2. ANTIDOTES—CONT'D

Toxin	Antidote	Dose and Comments
Organophosphates and carbamates	Atropine	Test dose 1–2 mg IV in adults, 0.03 mg/kg in children; titrate to drying of pulmonary secretions
	Protopam (praliidoxime; 2-PAM)	Loading dose 1–2 gm IV in adults; 25–50 mg/kg in children; adult maintenance 500 mg/h or 1–2 gm q4–6h.
Rattlesnake bite	*Crotalidae* antivenin, either CroFab or Wyeth formulation, depending on availability	5 vials minimum dose, by infusion in normal saline, at increasing rate, dependent on patient tolerance; either may cause anaphylaxis, but CroFab appears less likely to do so.
Serotonin syndrome	Cyproheptadine (Periactin)	4 mg p.o. as needed in adults; 2 mg p.o. as needed in children. No parenteral form available; antidote may cause an anticholinergic syndrome if dosing excessive.
Sulfonureas	Octreotide (Sandostatin)	50 μg SC q12h or 5–10 μg/kg/24 hours IV. Dosing can be increased in cases of refractory hyposglyemia.
Tricyclics	Bicarbonate	44–88 mEq in adults; 1–2 mEq/kg in children; best used IV push and not by slow infusion.
Valproic acid	L-carnitine (Carnitor)	For elevated ammonia levels, optimum dose uncertain and unknown if outcome is affected. The Pediatric Neurology Advisory Committee has recommended 100 mg/kg/day up to 2gm/day. May be given IV or p.o.

p.o. = per os (i.e., by mouth), FDA = U.S. Food and Drug Administration, BAL = British anti-Lewisite (dimercaperol), H_2S = hydrogen sulfide, FAB = fragment of antigen binding, DMSA = dimercapto-succinic acid, EDTA = ethylenediamene tetra-acetic acid, t.i.d. = three times per day, b.i.d. = twice per day, 2-PAM = pralidoxime chloride, SC = subcutaneous.

CHAPTER 81

ASPIRIN INTOXICATION

Ken Kulig, MD

1. **Is salicylate intoxication a serious problem in adults?**

   In a classic paper reviewing salicylate deaths in Ontario, 51 cases of salicylate deaths in adults were described. Despite the fact that many of these patients were obviously salicylate toxic in the hospital, unaggressive treatment—particularly, no starting hemodialysis when clearly indicated—resulted in fatal outcomes. Physicians get a false sense of security when seeing salicylate levels slowly decline, without recognizing that the reason for the decline may be that the salicylate is moving into tissues (including the brain) and thereby worsening toxicity. Salicylate intoxication resulting in mental status changes, persistent metabolic acidosis, or pulmonary edema should always be taken seriously and treated aggressively in an intensive care unit (ICU). Aggressive use of hemodialysis can be lifesaving.

   McGuigan MA: A two-year review of salicylate deaths in Ontario. Arch Intern Med 147:510–512, 1987.

2. **What is the cause of death when patients die from salicylate intoxication?**

   Pulmonary edema and cerebral edema are the most common causes of death. Persistent severe metabolic acidosis and hypokalemia may also contribute to the onset of ventricular dysrhythmias. In some patients, precipitous cardiovascular collapse can occur in the absence of obvious pulmonary or cerebral edema. This is generally a later finding seen in the hospital when the patient has been managed with unaggressive treatment for hours as the serum salicylate levels in an acute overdose approaches and exceeds 100 mg/dL.

   Chapman BJ, Proudfoot AT: Adult salicylate poisoning: Deaths and outcome in patients with high plasma salicylate concentrations. Q J Med 72:699–707, 1989.

3. **What are the symptoms and signs of aspirin intoxication?**

   The earliest symptoms are usually nausea, vomiting, tachypnea (which may be perceived by the patient as dyspnea), and tinnitus. These symptoms are self-limited in mild or moderate intoxications. In severe poisonings, persistent vomiting (which may include hematemesis) may occur, and the patient gradually becomes more dyspneic as acidosis worsens and pulmonary edema begins. Concomitant mental status changes including confusion, bizarre behavior, hallucinations, seizures, and coma may occur. Hyperpyrexia, sometimes life-threatening, may occur, requiring drastic cooling measures. Mild coagulopathy and hepatic damage may also be seen.

   Anderson RJ, Potts DE, Gabow PA, et al: Unrecognized adult salicylate intoxication. Ann Intern Med 85:745–748, 1976.

4. **What is the toxic dose of aspirin?**

   A dose of 150–300 mg/kg (or up to approximately 65 regular-strength tablets in an average-sized adult) usually results in moderate toxicity after a single acute ingestion. Greater than this amount frequently results in more serious toxicity. Oil of wintergreen is a more dangerous source of salicylate—1 teaspoon contains the equivalent of 21 regular-strength adult aspirin tablets. Thus, oil of wintergreen intoxications must always be taken seriously. The toxic dose of aspirin during chronic therapy varies from person to person. The maximum recommended dose is 8 regular-strength aspirin tablets per day for a normal-sized adult. Under certain conditions, doses exceeding this may result in drug accumulation and can be life-threatening, especially in elderly persons.

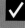

KEY POINTS: DIFFERENCES BETWEEN ACUTE AND CHRONIC SALICYLATE INTOXICATION

1. Chronic intoxication is more likely to occur in the elderly due to overuse (i.e., for the treatment of arthritis) and not intentional overdose.

2. Chronic intoxication causes toxicity at lower serum levels than acute intoxication.

3. Chronic intoxication is more likely to result in pulmonary edema.

4. Chronic intoxication should prompt hemodialysis at lower serum salicylate levels than acute intoxication.

5. **When should salicylate levels be drawn?**
It is common practice to wait 6 hours after an acute overdose to draw an aspirin level in order to plot the level on the Done nomogram. The nomogram has many drawbacks and is no longer commonly used by toxicologists. When the history suggests a very large ingestion, more than one serum salicylate level separated by several hours is needed. If the level is rising, especially when the aspirin preparation is sustained release, the patient should be treated with IV bicarbonate and further samples obtained to recheck levels. It is imperative that the correct units be used when interpreting levels. Therapeutic salicylate levels in patients taking aspirin for arthritis are 15–30 mg/dL. Some laboratories report salicylates in milligrams per milliliters. The conversion is as follows:

$$(\text{milligrams per milliliters}) \times 10 = \text{micrograms per milliliters}$$

6. **What is the Done nomogram? how should it be used?**
The Done nomogram was developed by observing the kinetics of aspirin after overdose in children and in experimental animals. Based on extrapolated half-lives seen, the nomogram was thought to perhaps be predictive of the degree of toxicity after a single acute aspirin overdose. It should not be used when oil of wintergreen, enteric-coated aspirin tablets, or any of the newer variety of slow-release preparations are ingested. It should never be used in the case of chronic aspirin ingestion. The nomogram should not be used to determine expected toxicity in the patient who is already significantly symptomatic. In significantly symptomatic patients, the salicylate level should be measured more than once. The clinical status of the patient is far more important than the salicylate level in guiding therapy.

Kulig K: Salicylate intoxication: Is the Done nomogram reliable? AACT Clin-Toxicol Update 3:1, 1990.

7. **What are the indications for alkaline diuresis to treat aspirin intoxication?**
Alkaline diuresis is generally safe and quite effective at eliminating aspirin from the body. It should be undertaken in patients who are significantly symptomatic and who have significantly elevated salicylate levels (i.e., >40 mg/dL). Adding 3 ampules of sodium bicarbonate to 1 L of D_5W and the appropriate amount of potassium (most aspirin-intoxicated patients are significantly potassium depleted) and running the fluid at a rate fast enough to induce a urine output of at least 2 mL/kg/h will greatly enhance the excretion of salicylate. Contraindications to alkaline diuresis include pulmonary edema, cerebral edema, and renal failure. Urine output and pH should be closely monitored. Failure to achieve an alkaline urine (i.e., pH > 7.5) is often the result of hypokalemia.

Prescott LF, Balali-Mood M, Critchley JA, et al: Diuresis or urinary alkalinization for salicylate poisoning? Br Med J 285:1383–1386, 1982.

KEY POINTS: MOST COMMON TOXICOLOGIC CAUSES OF SEVERE PERSISTENT UNEXPLAINED METABOLIC ACIDOSIS FOR WHICH THERE ARE ANTIDOTES AND SPECIFIC TREATMENTS

1. Salicylate overdose is a common cause of toxicology.

2. Methanol ingestion is another cause.

3. Severe metabolic acidosis can also be caused by ingestion of ethylene glycol.

8. **What other laboratory test result abnormalities commonly occur after salicylate ingestion?**
   The serum bicarbonate level is often low initially as a compensatory mechanism for hyperventilation and later because of a salicylate-induced metabolic acidosis. Hypokalemia, severe and difficult to correct, usually occurs in the sicker patients. Coagulopathy with a mildly elevated prothrombin time and international normalized ratio (INR) is also common.

   Gabow PA, Anderson RJ, Potts DE, et al: Acid-base disturbances in the salicylate-intoxicated adult. Arch Intern Med 138:1481–1484, 1978.

KEY POINTS: MOST COMMON LABORATORY ABNORMALITIES AFTER MAJOR ACUTE SALICYLATE INGESTION

1. Low pCO_2 due to hyperventilation occurs.

2. Low serum bicarbonate, primarily due to metabolic acidosis, is another effect.

3. Major salicylate ingestion also causes hypokalemia due primarily to renal losses.

4. Elevated prothrombin time and INR are present.

5. Hypoglycemia, especially in very young or very old persons, can occur.

9. **Is there a role for multiple-dose charcoal after aspirin ingestion?**
   Aspirin tablets can form concretions in the gastrointestinal tract. Because of their chemical nature, they tend to clump together and slowly release salicylate, which can result in steadily rising levels over long periods. For this reason, multiple-dose charcoal may be useful in significant ingestions. Charcoal also slightly enhances the elimination of salicylate that has already been absorbed, although not enough to use it for this reason only.

   Kirshenbaum LA, Mathews SC, Sitar DS, et al: Does multiple-dose charcoal therapy enhance salicylate excretion? Arch Intern Med 150:1281–1283, 1990.

10. **What are the indications for hemodialysis or hemoperfusion for aspirin poisoning?**
    Hemodialysis is recommended over hemoperfusion because it can, in addition to rapidly removing aspirin, correct electrolyte and acid–base abnormalities. Indications for hemodialysis include cerebral edema, pulmonary edema, oliguric renal failure, or severe acid–base

abnormalities that are not corrected with rehydration and bicarbonate. After acute overdose, dialysis should be considered when serum salicylate levels are >80 mg/dL and probably should be done in most cases with levels that are >100 mg/dL. In patients who are critically ill with lower serum salicylate levels, dialysis should also be considered.

Jacobsen D, Wiik-Larsen E, Bredesen JE: Haemodialysis or haemoperfusion in severe salicylate poisoning. Hum Toxicol 7:161–163, 1988.

KEY POINTS: PRIMARY REASONS TO INSTITUTE HEMODIALYSIS AFTER ACUTE SALICYLATE OVERDOSE

1. If the serum salicylate is rising and approaching 100 mg/dL, hemodialysis should be initiated.

2. Mental status abnormalities possibly due to cerebral edema are another indication.

3. Developing pulmonary edema should prompt the initiation of hemodialysis.

4. Hemodialysis should be begun if the patient experiences renal failure or oliguria.

5. Severe metabolic acidosis is another indication.

11. **When can patients be safely discharged from the ICU after aspirin poisoning?**
    In addition to having a return to baseline mental status and pulmonary function, patients should have serial determinations of aspirin level to document that it is going down and that it has at least reached low therapeutic levels (15–20 mg/dL). Vital signs should be normal with no residual tachypnea, and acid–base status should be normal. Even after having charcoal stools, some patients will continue to absorb aspirin from the gastrointestinal tract, with late intoxication being seen. If the levels are not falling, the patient should be kept in the ICU.

CHAPTER 82

ACETAMINOPHEN OVERDOSE

Ken Kulig, MD

1. **What are common symptoms and signs after acetaminophen overdose?**
   Patients are frequently asymptomatic for the first 8–12 hours after even a massive acetaminophen overdose. However, patients who have taken a large overdose usually experience severe nausea and vomiting at 8–12 hours after ingestion, which can be protracted for the next several days. This may make oral administration of the antidote difficult, and antiemetic agents may need to be given. Patients are frequently very pale and diaphoretic during this period. As the hepatic enzymes rise, generally beginning between 18 and 24 hours after ingestion, the liver may become enlarged and tender. In severe cases resulting in fulminant hepatic failure, encephalopathy occurs after 3–4 days. Hypoglycemia should always be ruled out in patients with altered mental status after acetaminophen poisoning.

2. **When should an acetaminophen level be measured after an overdose?**
   The acetaminophen treatment nomogram should be used only after a single acute overdose when a plasma level is measured between 4 and 24 hours after ingestion. Levels assessed before 4 hours are difficult to interpret; however, if the level is zero, the patient has probably not ingested acetaminophen. Levels that are high before 4 hours after ingestion may actually fall to below the nomogram line by the time the 4-hour level is measured. If the time of ingestion is unknown, the acetaminophen level cannot be plotted on the nomogram line. A regional poison control center can be called for advice in difficult or unusual cases. Chronic overdoses are difficult to correlate with acetaminophen levels, and the nomogram should not be used.
   In general, treatment with the antidote is benign and should be commenced if transaminase levels are elevated after excessive acetaminophen dosing.

3. **Should activated charcoal be given after an acetaminophen overdose?**
   Activated charcoal effectively binds acetaminophen in the gastrointestinal tract and, if given early enough, can help ensure that the patient does not develop a toxic acetaminophen level. Activated charcoal does not prevent the absorption of N-acetylcysteine (Mucomyst) to a significant degree. The dose of oral Mucomyst does not have to be increased after activated charcoal is given.

4. **How does the antidote work?**
   N-acetylcysteine is thought to work by a variety of mechanisms:
   - By acting as a glutathione surrogate that detoxifies the toxic metabolite formed within liver cells
   - By being converted to glutathione itself
   - By blunting the inflammatory response that can contribute to hepatic necrosis
   - By increasing sulfation of acetaminophen, which also prevents the formation of the toxic metabolite

   If the antidote is given within 8 hours of overdose, it is effective even if the overdose has been massive. If given between 8 and 24 hours after ingestion, it is less effective but still works. Even after 24 hours, N-acetylcysteine may be beneficial at preventing worsening liver injury.

   Harrison PM, Keays R, Bray GP, et al: Improved outcome of paracetamol-induced fulminant hepatic failure by late administration of acetylcysteine. Lancet 335:1572–1573, 1990.

5. **How should liver function test results be interpreted after an acetaminophen overdose?**

   It is not uncommon to see hepatic enzyme levels rise into the tens of thousands after an acute acetaminophen overdose without the development of clinically apparent fulminant hepatic failure. When massive hepatic necrosis and hepatic encephalopathy develop, transaminases are usually falling 3–5 days after the overdose, and the bilirubin level and international normalized ratio (INR) continue to rise. Usual treatment for hepatic failure should begin, the liver transplant center should be notified if that has not already occurred, and the administration of N-acetylcysteine should be continued until transaminase levels, the bilirubin level, and the INR are close to normal. Even when transaminase levels have risen to the 5000–10,000 range, full recovery of liver function can occur.

6. **How should N-acetylcysteine be given? when can it be stopped?**

   Currently in the United States there are three options for antidotes for acetaminophen overdose, all of which contain N-acetylcysteine:
   1. The IV formulation acetylcysteine (Acetadote) approved by the U.S. Food and Drug Administration. The package insert recommends a 20-hour protocol, but the maintenance dose of 6.25 mg/kg/h can be continued longer at the discretion of the physician if the transaminase levels are significantly elevated or the acetaminophen level is still detectable.
   2. Oral Mucomyst, given every 4 hours. This has traditionally been given for 72 hours but currently is usually discontinued after 24–36 hours if the transaminase levels have remained normal and the acetaminophen level is zero.
   3. Using oral Mucomyst intravenously through an IV filter according to an every-4-hour protocol, with the same stopping point as for option 2.

   Sivilotti MLA, Yarema MC, Juurlink DN, et al: A risk quantification instrument for acute acetaminophen overdose patients treated with N-acetylcysteine. Ann Emerg Med 46:263–271, 2005.

   Smilkstein MJ, Bronstein AC, Linden CH, et al: Acetaminophen overdose: A 48-hour intravenous N-acetylcysteine protocol. Ann Emerg Med 20:1058–1063, 1991.

   Smilkstein MJ, Knapp GL, Kulig KW, et al: Efficacy of oral N-acetylcysteine in the treatment of acetaminophen overdose. N Engl J Med 319:1557–1562, 1988.

   Woo OF, Mueller PD, Olson KR, et al: Shorter duration of oral N-acetylcysteine therapy for acute acetaminophen overdose. Ann Emerg Med 35:363–368, 2000.

KEY POINTS: ACETAMINOPHEN ANTIDOTES

1. Oral Mucomyst should be given every 4 hours.

2. Intravenous Mucomyst (off-label use) should be given every 4 hours.

3. Intravenous Acetadote, approved by the U.S. Food and Drug Administration for IV use, should be given by infusion over the course of 20 hours.

7. **When should liver transplant be considered after massive acetaminophen overdose?**

   Acetaminophen overdose is currently the most common diagnosis in patients requiring a liver transplant. However, the vast majority of patients who develop even major biochemical evidence of liver damage after acetaminophen overdose do well with antidotal and supportive therapy and recover completely with eventual normal hepatic function. In a subset of patients who have taken a massive overdose and present to the hospital very late, fulminant hepatic necrosis and death from liver failure can occur. In these cases, the local liver transplantation center should be notified about a potential candidate so that a suitable donor can be found, if needed.

Bernal W, Wendon J, Rela M, et al: Use and outcome of liver transplantation in acetaminophen-induced acute liver failure. Hepatology 27:1050–1055, 1998.

Larson AM, Polson J, Fontana RJ, et al: Acetaminophen-induced acute liver failure: Results of a US multicenter, prospective study. Hepatology 42:1364–1372, 2005.

8. **Is there a role for hemodialysis or hemoperfusion after acetaminophen overdose?**

N-acetylcysteine works extremely well at preventing hepatic toxicity if given early enough after an overdose (i.e., within 8 hours). In rare cases where the serum acetaminophen level is extremely high many hours after the overdose (i.e., more than 20 hours), some authors have advocated consideration of hemodialysis or hemoperfusion. The procedure will at best remove only the acetaminophen that is circulating, which may comprise a fraction of the total dose ingested. It is not clear whether removing that amount of drug will improve outcomes. These procedures are not generally recommended for that reason.

9. **How does acute or chronic ethanol ingestion alter the treatment of patients with acetaminophen overdose?**

Chronic ethanol abuse stimulates cytochrome P 450 (CYP 450) in the liver, the pathway responsible for the formation of the toxic metabolite of acetaminophen. However, ethanol itself is partially metabolized by that pathway, which may competitively inhibit the formation of the toxic metabolite. Chronic alcoholics, in addition, are likely to maintain poor nutrition and therefore to be glutathione depleted. It is unlikely that chronic alcoholics who ingest a therapeutic dose of acetaminophen (up to 1 gm/dose and the maximum of 4 gm/day) are at greatly increased risk for hepatic toxicity, although they are likely to be at greater risk if that maximum daily dose is exceeded. Acute alcohol ingestion may be mildly hepatoprotective in alcoholics and nonalcoholics alike.

Schmidt LE, Dalhoff K, Poulsen HE: Acute versus chronic alcohol consumption in acetaminophen-induced hepatotoxicity. Hepatol 35:876–882, 2002.

KEY POINTS: EFFECT OF ETHANOL INGESTION ON ACETAMINOPHEN HEPATOTOXICITY

1. Chronic ethanol ingestion induces CYP 450, which causes more toxic metabolite to be formed.

2. Chronic ethanol ingestion also tends to deplete glutathione due to nutritional deficiencies, which would likely make acetaminophen more toxic.

3. Acute ethanol ingestion may be slightly hepatoprotective.

10. **What effect does chronic consumption of acetaminophen have on liver function?**

Recent data from a small sample studied over 14 days (26 volunteers were given 4 gm/day of acetaminophen, 80 were given 4 gm/day with one of three opiate regimens concurrently, compared with 39 control subjects given placebo) demonstrated that rises in transaminases to levels three times normal occurred in 38% of acetaminophen-treated patients, 39% of patients treated with acetaminophen plus opiate, and no patients in the control group. The maximum recommended dose of acetaminophen (4 gm/day), long thought to be completely safe, appeared to cause rises in transaminase levels, which quickly fell to normal when the administration of acetaminophen was discontinued. The clinical significance of these data is unclear.

Watkins PB, Kaplowitz N, Slattery JJ, et al: Aminotransferase elevations in healthy adults receiving 4 grams of acetaminophen daily—A randomized controlled trial. JAMA 296:87–93, 2006.

11. **What organ systems besides the liver can be affected by acetaminophen overdose?**

After massive ingestions, coma and metabolic acidosis may occur. Renal damage (the renal parenchyma contains CYP 450) and pancreatitis have also been described.

Curry RW, Robinson JD, Sughurre MJ: Acute renal failure after acetaminophen ingestion. JAMA 247:1012–1014, 1982.

Schmidt LE, Dalhoff K: Hyperamylasaemia and acute pancreatitis in paracetamol poisoning. Aliment Pharmacol Ther 20:173–179, 2004.

CARE OF THE CRITICALLY ILL PREGNANT PATIENT

Stephen E. Lapinsky, MB, BCh, MSc

CHAPTER 83

1. **What are normal arterial blood gas findings in pregnancy?**

   Pregnancy results in increased ventilation because of elevated carbon dioxide production as well as an increase in respiratory drive mediated largely by progesterone. These changes cause a low arterial partial pressure of carbon dioxide, at about 30 mmHg by term. Plasma bicarbonate is decreased to 18–21 mEq/L, maintaining the arterial pH in the range of 7.40–7.45. Alveolar to arterial oxygen tension difference is usually unchanged, and the mean arterial PO_2 is generally about 100 mmHg.

2. **How does pregnancy affect hemodynamics?**

   Cardiovascular physiology changes significantly during pregnancy, characterized by an increase in blood volume, an elevation in cardiac output, and a small decrease in blood pressure, resulting in a number of changes in the normal hemodynamic values in the third trimester (Table 83-1). In the supine position, the gravid uterus may produce significant mechanical obstruction of the inferior vena cava, reducing venous return and resulting in a decrease in cardiac output and hypotension. Maternal syncope or fetal distress may result. Supine hypotension syndrome may be avoided by positioning the patient on her left side, or at least with the right hip slightly elevated.

   Clark SL, Cotton DB, Lee W, et al: Central hemodynamic assessment of normal term pregnancy. Am J Obstet Gynecol 161:1439–1442, 1989.

TABLE 83-1. EFFECT OF LATE PREGNANCY ON PULMONARY ARTERY CATHETER MEASUREMENTS

Parameter	Change from Nonpregnant Value
Central venous pressure	No change
Pulmonary capillary wedge pressure	No change
Cardiac output	30–50% increase
Systemic vascular resistance	20–30% decrease
Pulmonary vascular resistance	20–30% decrease
Oxygen consumption	20–40% increase
Oxygen extraction ratio	No change

3. **What factors affect oxygen delivery to the fetus?**

   Oxygen delivery to the fetus is determined by the maternal arterial oxygen content, uterine blood flow, and placental function. A number of factors may adversely affect blood flow to the uteroplacental vasculature, which is normally maximally vasodilated. A decrease in maternal cardiac output reduces fetal oxygenation. The maternal response to hypotension does not favo the uterus, and catecholamines (endogenous or exogenous) may aggravate fetal hypoxia by producing uterine vasoconstriction. Uterine blood flow may also be reduced by maternal alkalosis and during uterine contractions.

4. **Are there any special concerns to be considered when intubating a critically ill pregnant patient?**
   The upper airway in pregnancy may be edematous and friable due to the effects of estrogen and aggravated in the presence of preeclampsia because of excessive edema. The nasal route should be avoided, and a smaller endotracheal tube may be necessary. Due to the reduced functional residual capacity and increased oxygen consumption, a pregnant woman will become hypoxemic more rapidly than nonpregnant critically ill patients during intubation. This procedure should be carried out by the most skilled person available. The incidence of failed intubation is eight times higher in the obstetric population than in nonobstetric patients.

   Munnur U, de Boisblanc B, Suresh MS: Airway problems in pregnancy. Crit Care Med 33:S259–S268, 2005.

5. **Describe the principles of management of severe preeclampsia.**
   The most important aspect of management is the well-timed delivery of the fetus. Supportive treatment involves fluid management, control of hypertension, and prevention of seizures. Preeclamptic patients are usually volume depleted and require volume expansion, but excessive fluid administration may result in pulmonary or cerebral edema. Hypertension is managed to prevent maternal vascular damage and does not alter the pathologic process of preeclampsia. Commonly used regimens include small boluses of hydralazine (5–10 mg IV), boluses or infusion of labetalol, or oral calcium antagonists. Seizure prophylaxis should be undertaken with magnesium sulfate, using a loading IV bolus of 4 gm over 20 minutes followed by an infusion of 2–3 gm/h. Toxic levels (usually >5 mmol/L) can cause respiratory muscle weakness and cardiac conduction defects and are usually seen in a patient with associated renal failure. Hypocalcemia is common and should not be treated unless symptomatic. The effects of magnesium sulfate (toxic as well as therapeutic) can be reversed with IV calcium.

   Lapinsky SE, Kruczynski K, Slutsky AS: State of the art: Critical care in the pregnant patient. Am J Resp Cri Care Med 152:427–455, 1995.

6. **What are the clinical features of the "HELLP syndrome"?**
   The HELLP syndrome (i.e., hemolysis, elevated liver enzyme levels, and low platelet count) is a complication of preeclampsia characterized by multiorgan dysfunction. The diagnostic features are the presence of thrombocytopenia, elevated liver enzymes, and a microangiopathic hemolytic anemia. The patient may present with epigastric or right upper quadrant pain, nausea, and vomiting, with or without other features of preeclampsia. Significant hemorrhage may result from the thrombocytopenia. A rare but catastrophic consequence of HELLP syndrome is hepatic hemorrhage, manifesting with sudden shock or acute abdominal pain.

7. **What is acute fatty liver of pregnancy?**
   This is an uncommon complication of pregnancy manifesting with acute fulminant hepatic failure during the third trimester. Increased awareness of this condition has resulted in earlier diagnosis, with milder liver disease and an improved outcome. The clinical presentation is with malaise, anorexia, and vomiting, followed by abdominal pain and jaundice. The patient deteriorates rapidly with acute liver failure manifested by coagulopathy, hemorrhage, renal

failure, and encephalopathy. Management requires urgent delivery of the fetus and supportive therapy for fulminant hepatic failure.

KEY POINTS: CAUSES OF ADMISSION TO THE INTENSIVE CARE UNIT (ICU) DUE TO PREGNANCY-SPECIFIC CONDITIONS

1. Respiratory failure can take the form of amniotic fluid embolism, tocolytic pulmonary edema, preeclampsia, or peripartum cardiomyopathy.

2. Hepatic dysfunction may occur, including acute fatty liver of pregnancy or HELLP syndrome.

3. Renal failure (e.g., preeclampsia/HELLP syndrome, idiopathic postpartum renal failure) may prompt admission to the ICU.

4. Hypertensive complications in the form of preeclampsia may occur.

5. Pregnant patients might require intensive care because of hemodynamic compromise, such as obstetric hemorrhage or obstetric sepsis.

8. **How does amniotic fluid embolism present?**
Amniotic fluid embolism is a rare but catastrophic obstetric complication usually associated with labor, delivery, or other uterine manipulations. The typical presentation is a sudden onset of severe dyspnea, hypoxemia, and cardiovascular collapse, which may be accompanied by seizures. The maternal presentation is accompanied or preceded by sudden fetal distress. A significant portion of patients die acutely within the first hour. Survivors commonly develop a disseminated intravascular coagulopathy and acute respiratory distress syndrome. Management is supportive, and the prognosis for mother and fetus is poor.

Clark SL, Hankins GDV, Dudley DA, et al: Amniotic fluid embolism: Analysis of the national registry. Am J Obstet Gynecol 172:1158–1167, 1995.

9. **What are the causes of acute respiratory failure in pregnancy?**
Respiratory failure may occur as a result of pregnancy-specific complications or other conditions, some of which may be aggravated by the pregnant state (Box 83-1). The pregnancy-specific diseases include amniotic fluid embolism, pulmonary edema resulting from the use of tocolytic therapy or related to preeclampsia, or peripartum cardiomyopathy. Although pregnant patients may have diseases similar to those in nonpregnant patients, pregnancy may increase the risk of venous thromboembolism, acute asthmatic attacks, and gastric aspiration. Changes in immune function in pregnancy predispose to increased severity of varicella pneumonia as well as *Listeria* and coccidioidomycosis infections. Of interest is an association between the presence of pyelonephritis and the development of acute respiratory distress syndrome in pregnancy.

Lapinsky SE: Cardiopulmonary complications of pregnancy. Crit Care Med 33:1616–1622, 2005.

10. **Does the management of pulmonary embolism differ in pregnant patients?**
Investigation of suspected pulmonary embolism is similar to that in nonpregnant patients, beginning with duplex ultrasound. False-positive results may occur due to venous occlusion by the enlarged uterus. Ventilation-perfusion scanning and chest computed tomography angiogram can be carried out with a low risk of fetal radiation exposure. Unfractionated heparin and

---

BOX 83-1. CAUSES OF RESPIRATORY FAILURE IN PREGNANCY

Pregnancy-specific factors

Amniotic fluid embolism

Tocolytic pulmonary edema

Preeclampsia complicated by pulmonary edema

Pulmonary edema due to peripartum cardiomyopathy

Obstetric sepsis with ARDS

Trophoblastic embolism

Risk increased by pregnancy

Venous thromboembolism

Asthma

Pulmonary edema due to preexisting heart disease

Aspiration

ARDS associated with pyelonephritis

Pneumonia (especially varicella)

ARDS = acute respiratory distress syndrome.

---

low-molecular-weight heparin are safe and effective in pregnancy. Warfarin is usually avoided due to the risk of embryopathy with first-trimester use and central nervous system abnormalities and bleeding risk with second- and third-trimester use. Thrombolysis has been used successfully during pregnancy and the postpartum period but should be limited to life-threatening situations.

Greer IA: Prevention and management of venous thromboembolism in pregnancy. Clin Chest Med 24:123–137, 2003.

11. **What are the risks of radiologic procedures in pregnancy?**

Radiologic investigations are often necessary for management of critically ill pregnant patients. Estimated fetal radiation exposure varies from <0.01 rad (0.1 mGy) for a chest radiograph to about 2–5 rad (20–50 mGy) for pelvic computed tomography (Table 83-2). Techniques such as shielding the abdomen with lead and using a well-collimated x-ray beam can effectively reduce exposure. The potential adverse effects of fetal exposure to radiation are oncogenicity and teratogenicity. A twofold increased risk of childhood leukemia may occur with relatively low-dose radiation (2–5 rad). Teratogenicity is thought not to occur at low-radiation doses; microcephaly and hydrocephaly have been described after exposure of 10–150 rad. Although radiation exposure in pregnancy carries definite risks, the likelihood of any adverse effect is about 0.1% per rad.

Lowe SA: Diagnostic radiography in pregnancy: Risks and reality. Aust N Z J Obstet Gynaecol 44:191–196, 2004.

12. **How do the manifestations of severe trauma differ in pregnant patients?**

Trauma is a common cause of morbidity and mortality in pregnancy. The increased blood volume allows the mother to tolerate moderate blood loss, but this higher volume of hemorrhage necessitates more rapid IV fluid replacement. Fetal or amniotic injury may cause maternal coagulopathy, which can exacerbate hemorrhage. Occult uterine or retroperitoneal hemorrhage always should be considered. In the third trimester, abdominal trauma usually

TABLE 83-2. ESTIMATED FETAL RADIATION EXPOSURE DURING RADIOGRAPHIC STUDIES WITH APPROPRIATE SHIELDING

Radiographic Study	Estimated Fetal Dose (rad)
Chest x-ray	0.001
Ventilation-perfusion scan	0.012–0.050
CT scan of head	0.001
CT scan of chest	0.05–0.1
CT scan of abdomen/pelvis	2–5

CT = computed tomography.

involves the uterus. Other intra-abdominal organs may be compressed in the upper abdomen, and injury in this area may cause significant organ damage. Physical signs of peritonism may be reduced because of stretching of the peritoneum. The bladder is at increased risk of injury as it extends above the pubis, and it should be remembered that some degree of ureteric dilation is normal in pregnancy. The fetus is at risk of morbidity resulting from maternal hypotension, direct injury, fetomaternal hemorrhage, or placental abruption.

Pearlman MD, Tintinalli JE: Evaluation and treatment of the gravida and fetus following trauma during pregnancy. Obstet Gynecol Clin North Am 18:371–381, 1991.

13. **Is management of cardiac arrest different for pregnant patients?**
Management of cardiac arrest in pregnancy follows usual protocols with some modifications. Cardiopulmonary resuscitation administered with the patient in the supine position may cause impaired venous return, so a left lateral tilt position should be used or the uterus manually displaced to the left side. Cardiac compression may be technically difficult due to a highly enlarged uterus or engorged breasts. No change in pharmacologic therapy is necessary, and drugs should not be withheld when clinically indicated. Electrical defibrillation may be performed in pregnancy after removal of any fetal monitoring device. When initial attempts at resuscitation have failed, perimortem cesarean section should be considered if the fetus is at a viable gestation. Ideally, this should be initiated within 4 minutes of cardiac arrest for optimal fetal outcome. Cesarean section has been reported to reverse aortocaval compression and allow successful resuscitation of both the mother and infant.

14. **How is massive obstetric hemorrhage managed?**
Supportive measures include adequate venous access, rapid volume replacement, and blood product support. A dilutional coagulopathy should be anticipated. Ultrasound allows assessment of the uterine cavity for retained placental fragments that necessitate uterine curettage. Uterine massage and intramuscular methylergonovine (which should be avoided in the presence of hypertension) are used for uterine atony. Oxytocin infusion is administered in a dose higher than that used for augmentation of labor (e.g., 20–40 units in 1000 mL normal saline at a rate up to 100 mU/min). Prostaglandin analogs are very effective; carboprost tromethamine is given by intramuscular or intramyometrial injection in a dose of 0.25 mg, which may be repeated.

If pharmacologic methods fail, invasive approaches may be required. These include radiologic embolization and surgical exploration to repair lacerations, to reduce blood flow by arterial ligation or, if necessary, to remove the uterus.

15. **Which cardiac lesions present problems in pregnancy?**

The changes in cardiovascular physiology in pregnancy may result in decompensation in a patient with preexisting heart disease. The cardiac output rises during pregnancy, reaching a peak at about 28 weeks, 40–50% above baseline levels. Cardiac lesions limiting cardiac output (e.g., mitral stenosis, aortic stenosis) therefore present a significant risk of precipitating pulmonary edema or hypotension in the third trimester. This risk is particularly high during labor because of the tachycardia and volume shifts associated with delivery. Pulmonary hypertension is associated with significant morbidity and mortality because of the limitation of cardiac output and the inability to respond to postpartum fluid shifts. Congenital heart abnormalities are generally better tolerated in pregnancy unless complicated by pulmonary hypertension. Pregnancy may predispose the patient to the development of cardiomyopathy.

Siu SC, Colman JM: Heart disease and pregnancy. Heart 85:710–715, 2001.

XVIII. PSYCHIATRY

DELIRIUM

Marshall R. Thomas, MD, and Jonathan Berry, MD

CHAPTER 84

1. **What is delirium?**

   Delirium is an acute confusional state caused by global dysfunction of the central nervous system and associated with impairments in attention, cognition, and perception. It usually develops over a short period of time (hours to days), and the severity of symptoms fluctuate over the course of the day. Disturbances of memory, psychomotor behavior, emotion, and the sleep–wake cycle may be seen. Old terms for delirium included *intensive care unit* (ICU) *psychosis* and *ICU syndrome*. These terms should be abandoned because they imply that the ICU environment itself causes delirium and may prevent clinicians from aggressively searching for underlying causes.

2. **Why is it important to diagnose delirium?**

   Delirium is a common problem in hospitalized medical and surgical patients, with an incidence as high as 20% in hospital patients in general, 20–50% in elderly hospitalized patients, and 60–80% in ICU patients. Delirium is associated with substantial morbidity and mortality. The diagnosis of delirium should prompt a thorough work-up for underlying causes. In particular, prompt evaluation for the seven WHHHIMP etiologies (i.e., Wernicke's encephalopathy, hypoxia, hypoglycemia, hypertensive encephalopathy, intracerebral hemorrhage, meningitis/encephalitis, and poisoning/intoxication) is important because failure to identify and treat these causes of delirium may result in injury or death.

3. **What morbidity and mortality rates are associated with delirium?**

   The presence of delirium is associated with substantial increases in morbidity and mortality. Delirium in elderly patients, for example, has been shown to increase the risk of mortality at 6 and 12 months. Delirium in mechanically ventilated ICU patients increased the duration of mechanical ventilation, use of physical restraints, hospital costs, and 6-month mortality rates. Cognitive deficits, particularly in elderly patients and patients AIDS, may persist for months after hospital discharge. Some patients will never return to their predelirium baseline.

   Ely EW, Shintani A, Truman B, et al: Delirium as a predictor of mortality in mechanically ventilated patients in the intensive care unit. JAMA 291:1753–1762, 2004.

4. **Describe the clinical features of delirium.**

   The clinical features of delirium are variable, may develop rapidly, and often fluctuate over time. Delirious patients exhibit deficits in attention and concentration with a fluctuating level of arousal that is sometimes interspersed with lucid intervals. Emotional lability, memory impairment (especially involving recent events), disorientation, and disorganization of thought and speech may be present. Psychomotor disturbances may manifest as hypoactivity, hyperactivity, or alternations between the two. A delirious patient may be emotionally labile and may experience perceptual disturbances such as illusions and hallucinations (most often visual or auditory). Delusions may occur and may be paranoid in nature.

5. **Describe risk factors for delirium.**

   Many factors increase a patient's risk for developing delirium, and their effect is additive. The risk factors for developing delirium (Box 84-1) include baseline patient characteristics that

---

BOX 84-1.   RISK FACTORS FOR DELIRIUM

Baseline patient characteristics that increase the risk of delirium

- Older age (generally defined as older than 60–65 years; risk continues to increase with age)
- Preexisting cognitive impairment (e.g., dementia, traumatic brain injury)
- Drug or alcohol dependence
- Visual or hearing impairment

Clinical factors that increase the risk of delirium

- Polypharmacy (in particular, psychoactive drugs, anticholinergic drugs, opiates, sedative-hypnotics)
- Severe illness (in particular, cancer)
- Treatment in the intensive care unit, particularly if receiving mechanical ventilation
- Postoperative state (high blood loss, longer duration of surgery, certain types of surgery)
- Poor pain control, inadequate analgesia
- Infection, severe burns
- Hypovolemia, hypoalbuminemia, fever or hypothermia, metabolic disturbances, significant organ dysfunction (e.g., azotemia, hepatic insufficiency)

Environmental factors that increase the risk of delirium

- Isolation
- Immobility (includes restraint)
- Sleep deprivation

---

increase the risk in certain persons and clinical and environmental factors that increase the risk for all patients.

6. **How is delirium diagnosed?**

   Delirium is a clinical diagnosis. The criteria of the *Diagnostic and Statistical Manual of Mental Disorders,* Fourth Edition, Text Revision (DSM-IV-TR) (Box 84-2), are the most widely accepted and guide the assessment and diagnosis of delirium. Standard bedside interviews that do not specifically assess for mental status changes on a medical or surgical unit frequently fail to diagnose many cases of delirium. The patient's mental status should be assessed, and the examination should include an evaluation of level of arousal, attention, concentration, orientation, memory, and thought processes. Because delirium waxes and wanes, serial mental status examinations should be performed. Intermittent lucid intervals may lead to the diagnosis being overlooked or incorrectly thought to be resolved.

7. **How can detection of delirium be improved?**

   Up to 60–80% of cases of delirium go unrecognized, particularly cases of hypoactive delirium. Given the high incidence of delirium on medical and surgical services, a high index of suspicion and a low threshold for more targeted assessments should be maintained. Routine mental status screening should be considered for high-risk patients, such as elderly persons and patients in the ICU. Screening tools can improve the detection of delirium. The Confusion Assessment Method (CAM) is a standardized screening tool for delirium that has a sensitivity of 94–100%, a specificity of 90–95%, and high interobserver reliability. The Confusion Assessment

> **BOX 84-2. DSM-IV-TR CRITERIA FOR DIAGNOSIS OF DELIRIUM DUE TO A GENERAL MEDICAL CONDITION**
>
> A. Disturbance of consciousness (i.e., reduced clarity of awareness of the environment) with reduced ability to focus, sustain, or shift attention.
>
> B. A change in cognition (such as memory deficit, disorientation, language disturbance) or the development of a perceptual disturbance that is not better accounted for by a preexisting, established, or evolving dementia.
>
> C. The disturbance develops over a short period of time (usually hours to days) and tends to fluctuate during the course of the day.
>
> D. There is evidence from the history, physical examination, or laboratory findings that the disturbance is caused by the direct physiologic consequences of a general medical condition.
>
> From American Psychiatric Association: Diagnostic and Statistical Manual of Mental Disorders, 4th Edition, Text Revision. Washington, DC, American Psychiatric Association, 2000, with permission.

Method for the Intensive Care Unit (CAM-ICU) is an adaptation for ICU patients that can be used with patients who are nonverbal.

Ely EW, Margolin R, Francis J, et al: Evaluation of delirium in critically ill patients: Validation of the Confusion Assessment Method for the Intensive Care Unit (CAM-ICU). Crit Care Med 29:1370–1379, 2001.

Inouye SK, van Dyck CH, Alessi CA, et al: Clarifying confusion: The confusion assessment method. A new method for detection of delirium. Ann Intern Med 113:941–948, 1990.

8. **What causes delirium?**

The underlying causes of delirium are broad, and any given case may have multiple etiologies. Many clinicians use the mnemonic "I WATCH DEATH" to help remember the various causes of delirium (Table 84-1). The approach to the work-up for underlying causes is detailed in question 11.

9. **Which drugs are most likely to be associated with delirium?**

Available evidence suggests that medications often play a role in the pathogenesis of delirium. Numerous drugs have been associated with delirium, but this association is based on data from case reports and retrospective studies that lack control groups. Evidence is strongest for use of multiple psychotropic active medications and opiates as risk factors for delirium. Although more studies are needed to better delineate the specific relative risk of delirium associated with different medications, it remains important to minimize the use of drugs that can cause or exacerbate delirium in at-risk patients and to consider the effect of these drugs in the work-up and treatment of delirium (Box 84-3).

Gaudreau JD, Gagnon P, Roy MA, et al: Association between psychoactive medications and delirium in hospitalized patients: A critical review. Psychosomatics 46:302–316, 2005.

10. **What psychiatric diagnoses may be confused with delirium?**

The symptoms of delirium suggest diagnoses such as schizophrenia, depression, mania, anxiety, and dementia. Cognitive impairment may not be obvious on routine clinical examination. The acute onset of symptoms, prominent impairment of attention, and a waxing and waning mental state help distinguish delirium from psychiatric diagnoses. Dementia can be difficult to distinguish from delirium, particularly when information about baseline cognitive functioning is unavailable. An altered level of consciousness, the presence of hallucinations, and psychomotor disturbances are additional features that favor a diagnosis of delirium.

TABLE 84-1.	DIAGNOSIS OF DELIRIUM USING MNEMONIC "I WATCH DEATH"
Infection	Sepsis, meningitis, encephalitis, CNS abscess, syphilis, HIV, any infection (e.g., urinary tract infection or pneumonia, particularly in the elderly)
Withdrawal	Alcohol, benzodiazepines, barbiturates
Acute metabolic	Hyponatremia or hypernatremia, hypocalcemia or hypercalcemia, hyperkalemia, acidosis, alkalosis, hypoglycemia or hyperglycemia, hepatic or renal failure
Trauma	Closed-head injury, postoperative states, heat stroke, severe burns
CNS pathology	Seizures, hemorrhage, stroke, tumor (CNS primary or metastases), vasculitis, hydrocephalus
Hypoxia	Anemia, carbon monoxide poisoning, hypotension, pulmonary or cardiac failure
Deficiencies	Vitamin B_{12}, folate, niacin, thiamine
Endocrinopathies	Hyperadrenocentrism or hypoadrenocorticism, myxedema, thyroid storm, hyperparathyroidism
Acute vascular	Hypertensive encephalopathy, arrhythmia, shock
Toxins or drugs	Medications, illicit drugs, pesticides, solvents
Heavy metals	Lead, mercury, manganese

CNS = central nervous system, HIV = human immunodeficiency virus.
Adapted from Wise MG, Rundell JR: Clinical Manual of Psychosomatic Medicine. Washington, DC, American Psychiatric Publishing, 2005, with permission.

11. **How should the work-up of delirium be pursued?**
   An accurate history is important and can be obtained from the patient, the chart, the hospital staff, and/or the patient's friends and family, as appropriate. This information helps to delineate whether there has been a change from the patient's baseline mental status, what symptoms are present, and whether symptoms are fluctuating and may identify possible etiologies. Vital signs physical and neurologic examinations, mental status examination, and laboratory data should be reviewed. As delirium waxes and wanes, serial mental status exams should be performed. All medications the patient is taking should be reviewed and temporal relationships noted between changes and onset of symptoms.

12. **What laboratory studies are indicated in the work-up of delirium?**
   The routine laboratory work-up of delirium includes the following: measurement of electrolytes (including calcium, magnesium, and phosphorus); complete blood count; measurement of glucose, blood urea nitrogen and creatinine; liver function tests; arterial blood gas analysis; and urinalysis. Chest x-ray and electrocardiogram should also be considered.

13. **What additional studies may be indicated in the work-up of delirium?**
   As clinically indicated, consideration should also be given to the following: Venereal Disease Research Laboratory (i.e., test for syphilis), testing for human immunodeficiency virus, urine culture and sensitivity, urine toxicology screen, vitamin B_{12} and folate levels, heavy metal screen, antinuclear antibody, ammonia level measurement, thyroid-stimulating hormone measurement, analysis of serum medication levels (e.g., digoxin), testing for urinary porphyrins.

BOX 84-3. PARTIAL LIST OF DRUGS THAT MAY CAUSE DELIRIUM

Analgesics: Opiates (particularly meperidine), NSAIDs, tramadol

Anticholinergic medications: Antispasmodics, atropine, benztropine, scopolamine, antihistamines, promethazine

Antidepressants: SSRIs, tricyclic antidepressants

Corticosteroids

Sedative-hypnotics: Barbiturates, benzodiazepines

Sympathomimetics: Cocaine, amphetamines, theophylline, epinephrine

Dopamine agonists: Amantadine, bromocriptine, levodopa, carbidopa, pergolide, pramipexole

Anticonvulsants: Phenobarbital, phenytoin, carbamazepine, valproate

H_2 blockers: Cimetidine, ranitidine, famotidine

Antihypertensives: Beta blockers, diuretics, clonidine

Cardiac: Lidocaine, digitalis, quinidine, procainamide, amiodarone, mexiletine

Antineoplastics: Methotrexate, tamoxifen, vinblastine, vincristine

Antibiotics/antifungals/antivirals: Acyclovir, amphotericin B, cephalosporins, quinolones, chloroquine, gentamicin

Other: Disulfiram, baclofen, donepezil, interferon, oral hypoglycemics, lithium

NSAIDs = nonsteroidal anti-inflammatory drugs, SSRIs = selective serotonin reuptake inhibitors.
Adapted from Wise MG, Rundell JR: Clinical Manual of Psychosomatic Medicine. Washington, DC, American Psychiatric Publishing, 2005, with permission.

blood cultures, lumbar puncture, computed tomography or magnetic resonance imaging of the brain, and electroencephalography.

American Psychiatric Association: Practice Guidelines for the Treatment of Patients with Delirium. Am J Psychiatry 156:1–20, 1999.

14. **How is delirium treated?**

The most important intervention in treating delirium is to identify and correct any and all underlying causes. Patients with delirium should be monitored and supervised closely. They should be reoriented frequently; easily visible calendars and clocks may be helpful in this regard. The presence of family members and familiar objects may help alleviate anxiety and paranoia. Patients should be given their glasses and hearing aids when possible. A normal circadian rhythm (day–night cycle) should be maintained, with as few disturbances as possible during the night. Excessive stimuli (e.g., alarms, another delirious patient in the same room) should be minimized. The use of physical restraint should be minimized while providing for the safety of the patient and others.

15. **Describe the pharmacologic management of delirium.**

Patients with delirium should have their medications reviewed, and medications that may be causing or exacerbating the delirium should be discontinued, changed to a less problematic alternative, or reduced to the lowest effective dose. The American Psychiatric Association guidelines recommend haloperidol as the first-line agent for pharmacologic management of delirium. The use of second-generation antipsychotics is discussed later. Since the guidelines were produced, there have been case reports and open-label trials supporting the efficacy of the second-generation antipsychotics risperidone, olanzapine, ziprasidone, and quetiapine. Benzodiazepines should be avoided except in special circumstances such as delirium from alcohol withdrawal or delirium related to seizure or, at low doses, as an adjunct treatment for patients with agitation refractory to antipsychotic agents.

16. **How is haloperidol used in the treatment of delirium?**
Haloperidol is a high-potency, first-generation neuroleptic agent with minimal anticholinergic adverse effects. Its acute side effects may include dystonia, pseudo-parkinsonism, and akathisia. In addition, haloperidol can prolong the QT interval corrected for heart rate (QTc) and infrequently has been associated with torsades de pointes. It should not be used in patients with a baseline QTc greater than 450 msec. QTc and electrolytes should be monitored during treatment. Haloperidol can be administered orally, intramuscularly (IM), or intravenously. Intravenous use, although common, is not approved by the U.S. Food and Drug Administration. When converting an oral dose to an IM or IV dose, the IM and IV dose is twice as potent as the oral dose (e.g., 5 mg IV = 10 mg oral).

17. **How is haloperidol dosed in the treatment of delirium?**
Haloperidol may be given in doses of 2, 5, or 10 mg for younger patients or 0.5, 1, or 5 mg for older or frail patients with mild, moderate, or severe agitation, respectively. Doses may be repeated (at double the previous dose) at 30-minute intervals until the patient is less agitated. A low dose of lorazepam (0.5–1 mg IV over 1 minute, which may be repeated in 30 minutes if the patient is still agitated) may be added if haloperidol alone is ineffective at controlling agitation. Once the patient is calm, add the total haloperidol dose used over 24 hours and administer the same dose over the next day in divided doses (with a larger dose at night). As the patient's condition improves, the haloperidol may be tapered off over several days (50% per day).

KEY POINTS: DELIRIUM

1. Delirium is a medical emergency, and a prompt and thorough work-up for underlying causes is indicated.

2. Standardized screening instruments such as the CAM and CAM-ICU can help physicians detect delirium.

3. Treatment of delirium should be directed at treating underlying causes, when possible.

4. Haloperidol is a first-line agent for the pharmacologic management of delirium.

5. There is evidence for the use of quetiapine, risperidone, and olanzapine in the treatment of delirium.

6. Benzodiazepines should not be used as monotherapy for delirium except in special circumstances, such as delirium resulting from alcohol withdrawal.

18. **How are second-generation antipsychotic agents used in delirium?**
In recent years, there have been case reports and open-label trials that support the use of some second-generation antipsychotic agents (e.g., risperidone, olanzapine, quetiapine, and ziprasidone) in the treatment of delirium. These newer agents may offer a lower risk of extrapyramidal adverse effects and may be effective in treating cases of delirium poorly

responsive to haloperidol. However, they are also associated with their own liabilities (such as possible increased risk of vascular events in elderly persons). Little is known about dosing these newer agents in delirium. Patients should be started on a standing dose with as-needed doses available. They should be monitored for sedation, hypotension, orthostasis, tachycardia, and extrapyramidal symptoms while the dose is titrated. Electrolyte levels and the QTc should be monitored in at-risk patients. Elderly patients, unstable patients, and patients with central nervous system abnormalities should be given at doses at the low end of the dosing range, monitored closely, and titrated slowly. As for haloperidol, medication should be titrated until an effect is accomplished and tapered after the patient's delirium resolves. There are insufficient data to recommend dosing for ziprasidone.

Schwartz TL, Masand PS: The role of atypical antipsychotics in the treatment of delirium. Psychosomatics 43:171–174, 2002.

WEBSITES

1. American Psychiatric Association Practice Guidelines (including treatment of delirium)
www.psych.org/psych_pract/treatg/pg/prac_guide.cfm

2. ICU Delirium and Cognitive Impairment Study Group
www.icudelirium.org

CHAPTER 85

ANXIETY AND AGITATION IN THE INTENSIVE CARE UNIT

Marshall R. Thomas, MD, and Jonathan Berry, MD

1. **What are anxiety and agitation?**

   Anxiety has both psychological (excessive apprehension, fear) and physiologic (motor tension, autonomic hyperactivity) manifestations. Agitation, on the other hand, is characterized by excessive motor activity that may be associated with underlying contributing factors such as pain or anxiety. Both anxiety and agitation can be caused by a broad array of medical and psychiatric conditions or may reflect a psychological reaction to the circumstances that surround being a patient in the intensive care unit (ICU). For example, ICU agitation may result from fear, pain, discomfort, delirium, drug withdrawal/toxicity, hypoxia, akathisia, or a combination of factors.

2. **Which medical conditions are associated with anxiety and agitation?**

   See Box 85-1.

BOX 85-1. MEDICAL CONDITIONS ASSOCIATED WITH PROMINENT SYMPTOMS OF ANXIETY

Akathisia
Angina
Asthma
Carcinoid syndrome
Cardiac arrhythmias
Cardiomyopathies
Chronic obstructive pulmonary disease
Congestive heart failure
Delirium
Dementia
Drug toxicities (stimulants, xanthines, sympathomimetics, thyroxine, hallucinogens, anticholinergics)
Drug withdrawal (sedative-hypnotic, opiate, tricyclic antidepressant, alcohol)
Encephalopathy
Hypercalcemia

Hypercortisolism
Hyperkalemia
Hyperthermia
Hyperthyroidism and hypothyroidism
Hyperventilation
Hypocalcemia (hypoparathyroidism)
Hypoglycemia
Hyponatremia
Hypovolemia
Hypoxia
Myocardial infarction
Pain
Parkinson's disease
Partial complex seizures

Pheochromocytoma
Pneumonia
Pneumothorax
Porphyria
Postconcussive syndrome
Poststroke syndrome
Pulmonary edema
Pulmonary emboli
Respiratory dependence
Systemic lupus erythematosus
Tumors in the area of the third ventricle
Valvular disease

---

3. **What drugs are associated with anxiety in the medical setting?**
See Box 85-2.

BOX 85-2. DRUGS ASSOCIATED WITH ANXIETY IN THE MEDICAL SETTING			
Anticholinergics	**Stimulants**	**Miscellaneous**	**Miscellaneous—cont'd**
Benztropine	Amphetamine	Anabolic steroids	Nicotinic acid
Diphenhydramine	Caffeine	Baclofen	NSAIDs
Meperidine	Cocaine	Bupropion	Procaine derivatives
Oxybutynin	Methylphenidate	Calcium antagonists	Progestins
Pilocarpine	Phentermine	Corticosteroids	SSRIs
Propantheline	Xanthines	Cycloserine	Sodium lactate
Quinidine	**Sympathomimetics**	Disopyramide	Sumatriptan
Tricyclic antidepressants	Albuterol	Dronabinol	Thyroxine (in excess)
Trihexyphenidyl	Aminophylline	Estrogens	Drug withdrawal
	Ephedrine	Fluoroquinolones	Antidepressants
Dopaminergics	Epinephrine	Hallucinogens	Barbiturates
Amantadine	Isoproterenol	Interferon	Benzodiazepines
Bromocriptine	Metaproterenol	Metrizamide	Narcotics
Carbidopa-levodopa	Phenylephrine	Metronidazole	Sedatives
Metoclopramide	Pseudoephedrine	Mexilitene	
Antipsychotics	Theophylline	Monosodium glutamate	
Pergolide			

NSAIDs = nonsteroidal anti-inflammatory drugs, SSRIs = selective serotonin reuptake inhibitors.
Adapted from Goldberg RJ, Posner DA: Anxiety in the medically ill. In Stoudmire A, Fogel BS, Greenberg DB (eds): Psychiatric Care of the Medical Patient, 2nd. New York, Oxford University Press, 2000, pp 165–180.

4. **Why is the identification of anxiety and agitation important in the ICU?**
Anxiety and agitation often complicate the medical evaluation and management of patients in the ICU. Anxiety can produce agitation and cause physiologic changes such as tachycardia, hypertension, increased catabolism, and oxygen consumption. In patients who have experience myocardial infarction (MI), higher levels of anxiety have been associated with increased in-hospital complications and increased risk of future MI. Agitation can also seriously complicate the management of ICU patients when patients interfere with monitoring devices or remove endotracheal, IV, and nasogastric tubes or urinary, arterial, and central venous catheters.

5. **What is akathisia?**
Akathisia is a movement disorder commonly caused by dopamine-receptor blockers (including antipsychotics and antiemetics such as metoclopramide and promethazine). Affected patients experience feelings of motor restlessness and a strong urge to move. Patients may tap their feet, rock, pace, or cross and uncross their legs. Akathisia is sometimes mistaken as worsening of the underlying agitation or psychosis. Dopamine-blocking medications should be discontinued,

changed to an alternative medication, or tapered to the lowest effective dose. Beta blockers such as propanolol (10 mg four times/day to 40 mg three times/day) are the standard treatment. Benzodiazepines may also be effective.

6. **Describe the signs and symptoms associated with alcohol withdrawal.**
Approximately 25% of hospitalized inpatient adults have an alcohol-related disorder. Alcohol withdrawal should be considered in any patient who develops anxiety within the first several days of admission. In the ICU, other medical conditions or medications (e.g., beta blockers and narcotics) may alter the clinical presentation and obscure the diagnosis. Signs of alcohol withdrawal typically occur within 6–48 hours of cessation or reduction in drinking and include anxiety, irritability, tremor, insomnia, anorexia, nausea, tachycardia, hypertension, and diaphoresis. More severe cases may progress to agitation, delirium, hallucinations, fever, and seizures.

7. **What are the features of alcohol withdrawal delirium (i.e., delirium tremens [DTs])?**
In the past, approximately 5% of patients who were hospitalized with alcohol dependence developed alcohol withdrawal delirium, the most common cause of psychotic symptoms in alcohol-dependent patients. Risk factors include >10 years of heavy drinking, prior history of DTs, alcohol withdrawal seizures, and major medical illness. Signs and symptoms include confusion, disorientation, agitation, fluctuating level of consciousness, delusions, vivid hallucinations (most often visual but may also be tactile or auditory), fever, and marked autonomic arousal. The usual onset is 2–7 days after cessation of drinking. With aggressive treatment, the reported mortality rate of 40% associated with DTs can be reduced to <1%.

8. **What is alcohol-induced psychotic disorder (i.e., alcoholic hallucinosis)?**
Alcohol-induced psychotic disorder is a syndrome in which vivid hallucinations (usually auditory) occur shortly after cessation of alcohol, but they occur in the presence of an otherwise clear sensorium and with a relative paucity of autonomic symptoms. Patients respond to these usually derogatory hallucinations with fear, anxiety, and agitation. In the majority of cases, symptoms recede within a few hours to a few days, but in a small number of cases the symptoms may become chronic. If standard alcohol withdrawal treatment does not provide relief, antipsychotic agents may be added to treat agitation or hallucinations.

9. **How is alcohol withdrawal treated?**
Benzodiazepines are the treatment of choice for moderate to severe alcohol withdrawal. The intermediate half-life benzodiazepines, lorazepam and oxazepam, are preferred in patients prone to excessive accumulation and overdose (e.g., elderly patients and patients with hepatic impairment, delirium, or dementia). They reduce withdrawal symptoms and decrease the likelihood of delirium and seizures. All patients treated for alcohol withdrawal should be given thiamine, 100 mg by mouth (PO)/intramuscularly (IM), immediately then daily; folic acid, 1 mg PO daily; and a multivitamin PO daily. Thiamine (100 mg IV/IM) should be given before any glucose infusion to prevent Wernicke-Korsakoff syndrome. Complicated alcoholic withdrawal may require significantly higher doses of benzodiazepines and use of adjunctive medications.

American Society of Addiction Medicine: Guidelines for treatment of alcohol withdrawal and the Clinical Institute Withdrawal Assessment–Alcohol, revised: www.asam.org

10. **What adjunctive medications may be used to treat alcohol withdrawal?**
Antipsychotic agents such as haloperidol may be used to help control agitation and psychotic symptoms, but these should only be used adjunctively with benzodiazepines. There is increasing evidence that divalproex and carbamazepine are effective for mild to moderate alcohol withdrawal, but benzodiazepines remain the drugs of choice in most cases. Beta blockers and centrally acting alpha agonists such as clonidine reduce the autonomic manifestations of alcohol withdrawal, but there is no evidence that they lower seizure or delirium risk. Barbiturates and

propofol have been used to treat DTs refractory to high-dose benzodiazepines but are usually not first-line choices.

Mayo-Smith MF, Beecher LH, Fischer TL, et al: Management of alcohol withdrawal delirium, an evidence-based guideline. Arch Intern Med 164:1405–1412, 2004.

11. **Describe the syndrome of sedative-hypnotic withdrawal.**
Sedative-hypnotic agents include benzodiazepines, barbiturates, and miscellaneous other central nervous system depressants (e.g., chloral hydrate). Sedative-hypnotic withdrawal is symptomatically similar to alcohol withdrawal. The time of onset and duration of the syndrome vary with the half-life of the agent; symptoms may start several hours after stopping short-acting agents to several days for longer-acting agents. Withdrawal can be life-threatening. Treatment consists of a gradual taper of the agent or an equivalent dose of a longer-acting agent (e.g., diazepam for benzodiazepine withdrawal or phenobarbital for barbiturates).

12. **What is the opiate withdrawal syndrome? How can it be managed?**
Opiate withdrawal occurs in the hospital when opiates are discontinued or tapered too rapidly or when an antagonist such as naloxone is used to treat overdose. Patients switched to treatment with narcotics with mixed agonist-antagonist properties, such as pentazocine, may also experience withdrawal. Symptoms include anxiety, rhinorrhea, lacrimation, piloerection, mydriasis, abdominal pain, nausea, vomiting, diarrhea, tachycardia, and hypertension. Although intensely uncomfortable, opiate withdrawal is rarely life-threatening. Opiate withdrawal can be treated with a more gradual tapering of the opiate or mitigated by adjunctive use of a centrally acting α_2-adrenergic agonist such as clonidine.

13. **What are the symptoms of antidepressant withdrawal?**
Abrupt discontinuation of selective serotonin reuptake inhibitors, serotonin-norepinephrine inhibitors, monoamine oxidase inhibitors, and tricyclic antidepressants can cause withdrawal syndromes. Symptoms begin 1–4 days after cessation of the medication and last up to 2 weeks. They may include paresthesias, anxiety, agitation, anorexia, nausea, vomiting, diarrhea, myalgias, insomnia, nightmares, hyperreflexia, akathisia, and delirium. Reinstitution of the antidepressant therapy with a more gradual taper effectively treats the withdrawal syndrome.

14. **What psychiatric causes of anxiety and agitation can be seen in the ICU?**
Anxiety and substance use disorders are the most common psychiatric disorders in the general population. History is often critical in distinguishing new onset of anxiety or agitation from preexisting psychiatric symptoms. Anxiety disorders (such as those listed in Box 85-3) may be worsened by the stress of being in the ICU. Anxiety is frequently comorbid with mood disorders, and agitation can be seen with depression or mania. Patients with psychotic disorders such as schizophrenia can also become anxious and agitated. Symptoms may worsen if antipsychotic, anxiolytic, mood-stabilizing, or antidepressant medications are discontinued in the ICU.

15. **How is agitation managed in the ICU?**
The first step in treating agitation is to ascertain the underlying cause or causes. Some causes such as hypoxemia, hypoglycemia, or alcohol withdrawal require prompt treatment. Treating reversible causes such as pain, discomfort, or excessive tidal volume in ventilated patients may resolve the agitation. Nonpharmacologic interventions such as reassurance, reducing environmental stimulation, or involving family members should be attempted. Pharmacologic treatment varies according to the underlying cause. Physical restraints should be used only when the risk of harm to the patient or others outweighs the risk of physical or psychological harm from restraint.

Maccioli GA, Dorman T, Brown BR, et al: Clinical practice guidelines for the maintenance of patient physical safety in the intensive care unit: Use of restraining therapies—American College of Critical Care Medicine Task force 2001–2002. Crit Care Med 31:2665–2676, 2003.

BOX 85-3. SELECTED ANXIETY DISORDERS

Generalized anxiety disorder: At least 6 months of excessive anxiety and worry with accompanying symptoms such as restlessness, easy fatigue, irritability, sleep disturbances, or muscle tension. The majority of these patients have at least one additional mental disorder (e.g., panic disorder or a depressive disorder).

Panic attacks: Short-lived episodes of intense fear with accompanying symptoms such as palpitations, diaphoresis, shortness of breath, chest pain, and fear of dying.

Panic disorder: Recurrent unexpected panic attacks accompanied by worry about recurrence, concern about consequences of the attacks, and/or a change in behavior caused by the attacks. Agoraphobia (i.e., fear of places where help might not be available or escape might be hard or embarrassing in the event of a panic attack) may or may not be present.

Acute stress disorder: Exposure to an intense, fear-inducing traumatic event accompanied or followed by feelings of dissociation (e.g., emotional numbing), reexperiencing of the event, avoidance of stimuli that cause reexperiencing, and anxiety or increased arousal. Symptoms begin within 4 weeks of the event and last 2 days to 4 weeks.

Posttraumatic stress disorder: Exposure to an intense, fear-inducing traumatic event followed by persistent reexperiencing, avoidance of stimuli associated with the trauma, emotional numbing, and increased arousal. Symptoms must be present for at least 1 month. Comorbid psychiatric diagnoses such as substance-related disorders and mood disorders are common.

Adjustment disorder with anxiety: Symptoms of anxiety occur within 3 months of an identifiable stressor and seem excessive or cause impairment in social or occupational functioning.

Anxiety due to a general medical condition: Anxiety, panic attacks, obsessions, or compulsions with evidence that the symptoms are the result of a general medical condition.

---

16. **What is the general approach to pharmacologic treatment of agitation in the ICU?**

Pharmacologic management varies according to underlying cause of the agitation. Pain, anxiety and delirium are the most common causes requiring medication. Rating scales such as the numeric (pain) rating scale and the Riker Sedation-Agitation Scale should be used to assess response to treatment. Analgesic agents (usually opiates) should be used for pain, sedatives such as benzodiazepines for anxiety or alcohol and sedative/hypnotic withdrawal, and antipsychotics such as haloperidol for most cases of delirium. Many patients will have more than one etiology for their agitation and will require a combination of drugs to treat the agitation and its underlying causes.

Jacobi J, Fraser GL, Coursin DB, et al: Clinical practice guidelines for the sustained use of sedatives and analgesics in the critically ill adult. Crit Care Med 30:119–141, 2002.

17. **What are nonpharmacologic interventions for anxiety and agitation?**

Normal psychological reactions to being a patient in the ICU can often be managed without anxiolytic medication. An exception may be patients with cardiac issues such as unstable angina or MI, in whom the treatment of anxiety may improve survival rates. Reassurance, frequent contact with staff, and family visits can help alleviate patients' anxiety. Encouraging normal sleep cycles by limiting noise and dimming lights at night and engaging the patient in relaxation exercises such as deep breathing and sequential muscle relaxation, music therapy, and massage also help reduce anxiety. Careful attention to the patient's mental state can help prevent the development of the posttraumatic anxiety symptoms often seen in ICU patients.

18. **What are pharmacologic treatments for anxiety?**
    Benzodiazepines are effective anxiolytics and are the mainstay of pharmacologic treatment of anxiety in the ICU. Antipsychotic agents such as haloperidol or risperidone may be used when respiratory depression is a concern (e.g., anxiety during weaning from a ventilator). Although many antidepressants and buspirone have anxiolytic effects, they take weeks to show effects. Beta-blocking drugs can help with physiologic symptoms such as tremor and tachycardia, but they tend to have little effect on the psychological aspects of anxiety. Stopping outpatient anxiolytics, antidepressants, or antipsychotics on ICU admission may precipitate anxiety, and these agents should be continued when possible.

19. **How should patients who require neuromuscular-blocking agents be treated?**
    It is extremely important that patients treated with sustained neuromuscular-blocking agents (NMBAs) receive adequate sedation and analgesia. NMBAs do not have amnestic or analgesic effects, and untreated patients may have the extremely unpleasant experience of being awake, in discomfort or pain, and unable to move. The effectiveness of analgesia or sedation is difficult to assess once a patient is paralyzed because normal signs and symptoms of fear, anxiety, and pain are likely to be absent. Current guidelines recommend titrating sedative and analgesic drugs to a level at which the patient does not appear to be conscious before initiation of neuromuscular blockade.

KEY POINTS: ANXIETY AND AGITATION IN THE INTENSIVE CARE UNIT (ICU)

1. Adequate treatment of anxiety and agitation reduces morbidity and possibly mortality among patients in the ICU.

2. It is important to assess the adequacy of pain management and the possibility of drug and alcohol withdrawal in an agitated ICU patient.

3. Consider akathisia as a cause of agitation in patients treated with dopamine receptor blockers.

4. Opiate withdrawal is rarely life-threatening, whereas alcohol or benzodiazepine withdrawal may be so.

5. Abrupt discontinuation of treatment with antidepressants may cause a withdrawal syndrome.

6. For patients with a history of alcohol abuse, thiamine should be given before any glucose infusion to prevent Wernicke-Korsakoff syndrome.

7. Aggressive treatment of alcohol withdrawal delirium can reduce mortality to <1%.

8. It is extremely important that patients treated with NMBAs receive adequate sedation and analgesia.

WEBSITES

1. American Society of Addiction Medicine: Guidelines for treatment of alcohol withdrawal and the Clinical Institute Withdrawal Assessment–Alcohol, revised
   www.asam.org

2. Society of Critical Care Medicine: Clinical practice guidelines for sustained use of sedatives and analgesics, use of restraints, and neuromuscular blockade
   www.sccm.org

CHAPTER 86

NEUROLEPTIC MALIGNANT SYNDROME

Ryan P. Peirson, MD, and James L. Jacobson, MD

1. **What is neuroleptic malignant syndrome (NMS)?**
   NMS is a rare, potentially fatal, idiosyncratic complication of antipsychotic medications.
   The usual presentation consists of four primary features:
   - Hyperthermia
   - Extreme generalized rigidity
   - Autonomic instability
   - Altered mental status

2. **What are the specific criteria for diagnosis of NMS?**
   There are no universally accepted criteria for diagnosis of NMS. There must be a recent
   history of exposure to antipsychotic medication. Usually the exposure occurs 24–72 hours
   before onset of the syndrome. However, NMS can occur with chronic usage. For common
   features, see Table 86-1.

TABLE 86-1. FEATURES OF NEUROLEPTIC MALIGNANT SYNDROME	
Primary Features	**Common Features**
Hyperthermia	Laboratory evidence of muscle injury
Extreme generalized rigidity (often called "lead pipe" rigidity)	Leukocytosis
Autonomic instability	Incontinence
■ Labile hypertension (less often, hypotension)	Tremor
■ Tachycardia	Tachypnea
Altered mental status	Mutism
	Dysphagia
	Diaphoresis
	Sialorrhea

3. **Are there specific laboratory findings for NMS?**
   No laboratory findings are pathognomonic for NMS, but certain studies are important both to
   support the diagnosis of NMS and to exclude other systemic illnesses. Common laboratory
   abnormalities include massive elevation of creatine phosphokinase level (muscle fraction) and

leukocytosis. Electrolyte disturbances, such as hypernatremia, hyponatremia, hyperkalemia, hypocalcemia, hypomagnesemia, and hypophosphatemia, may occur secondarily, along with hypoxia and acid–base abnormalities. Urinalysis often reveals proteinuria and myoglobinuria. Blood urea nitrogen and creatinine levels may be elevated, indicating renal compromise resulting from rhabdomyolysis. Cerebrospinal fluid (CSF) values are usually normal, but a nonspecific increase in CSF protein has been reported in 37% of cases.

4. **Are special diagnostic tests or imaging studies useful?**
An electroencephalogram (EEG) may show diffuse slowing without focal abnormalities. Structural imaging studies of the central nervous system should be normal.

5. **What studies should be performed to evaluate for other systemic illnesses?**
Studies should include complete blood count with a differential white blood cell count; measurement of serum electrolytes, creatinine, blood urea nitrogen, and muscle and hepatic enzymes; blood gas analysis; thyroid function tests; urinalysis; electrocardiography; appropriate cultures for infection; and brain imaging, electroencephalography, and CSF studies (when indicated).

6. **What is the differential diagnosis of NMS?**
The differential diagnosis includes several processes that can cause increased temperature due to abnormal thermoregulation (Table 86-2).

TABLE 86-2. DIFFERENTIAL DIAGNOSIS OF NEUROLEPTIC MALIGNANT SYNDROME	
Primary Central Nervous System Disorders	**Systemic Disorders**
Infections (e.g., viral encephalitis, postinfectious encephalitis, HIV)	Infections
Tumors	Metabolic conditions
Cerebrovascular disease	Endocrinopathies (e.g., thyrotoxicosis, pheochromocytoma)
Head trauma	Autoimmune disease (e.g., systemic lupus erythematosus)
Seizures	Heat stroke
Serotonin syndrome	Toxins (e.g., carbon monoxide, phenols, strychnine, tetanus)
Major psychoses (lethal catatonia)	Drugs (e.g., salicylates, dopamine inhibitors and antagonists, stimulants, psychedelics, monoamine oxidase inhibitors, anesthetics, anticholinergics, alcohol or sedative withdrawal)

HIV = human immunodeficiency virus.
Adapted from Caroff SN, Mann SC, Lazarus A, et al: Neuroleptic malignant syndrome: Diagnostic issues. Psychiatr Ann 21:130–147, 1991.

7. **Discuss the cause of NMS.**

   The pathophysiology of NMS is poorly understood. The mechanism thought to be responsible is central dopamine receptor antagonism in the basal ganglia and hypothalamus and peripheral dopamine antagonism in postganglionic sympathetic neurons. The relatively infrequent occurrence of NMS, however, suggests the concurrence of other factors. Speculations have included imbalances with other neurotransmitter systems (e.g., gamma aminobutyric acid, serotonin, and glutamate), abnormalities in second messenger systems, and the presentation of particular risk factors.

8. **Which agents have been implicated in the genesis of NMS?**

   Currently, all of the antipsychotic medications have been reported to cause NMS, including reports implicating atypical antipsychotic medications (e.g., clozapine, olanzapine, risperidone, quetiapine, ziprasidone, and aripiprazole). NMS also has been reported with some antiemetic medications such as prochlorperazine maleate, metoclopramide, trimethobenzamide, and droperidol, all of which share dopamine antagonism. Rare cases have been reported in overdose of tricyclic antidepressants and citalopram. Abrupt cessation of antiparkinsonian drugs can cause a similar syndrome. The hallucinogen phencyclidine and the anesthetic ketamine, both antagonists of the N-methyl-D-aspartate receptor, can cause a similar syndrome.

9. **What risk factors predispose patients to the development of NMS?**

   Suggested risk factors include dehydration, a primary diagnosis of affective disorder (especially bipolar disorder and psychotic depression), catatonia, psychomotor agitation, concurrent presence of delirium or dementia, concurrent use of other neuroactive medications, higher relative doses and parenteral administration of antipsychotics, increased dose of antipsychotics, young age, male sex (may be related to a higher likelihood of high doses of neuroleptics in males), prior history of NMS, electrolyte disturbances, a recent history of substance abuse or dependence, and any co-occurring medical illness. Recent evidence also suggests genetic vulnerability as a potential risk factor.

10. **How common is NMS?**

    Rates as low as 0.02% and as high as 2.5% have been reported, but overall the rate appears to be about 0.2%.

11. **Does NMS have a genetic predisposition?**

    Evidence suggests familial susceptibility for NMS. However, the answer is not clear. Researchers have found TaqI A polymorphisms in the dopamine receptor subtype 2 *(DRD2)* gene in psychiatric patients with NMS as compared with psychiatric patients without NMS. Further research is needed to better understand this relationship.

12. **What is the mortality rate associated with NMS?**

    Mortality from NMS has been declining since its original description in 1968. The earliest reports suggested mortality rates as high as 75%. In the early 1980s, mortality rates declined to 20–30%. Current studies suggest that the mortality rate declined further, probably to less than 15%. Declining mortality rates are most likely due to increased familiarity with the syndrome, which leads to more judicious use of antipsychotics and early recognition and treatment. Death results from cardiac or respiratory arrest stemming from cardiac failure, infarction, or arrhythmia; aspiration pneumonia; pulmonary emboli; myoglobinuric renal failure; or disseminated intravascular coagulation.

13. **Discuss the management of NMS.**

    Early recognition and supportive treatment are crucial. Increased temperature, elevated blood pressure, tachycardia, muscle stiffness not responsive to antiparkinsonian agents, clustering of risk factors, dysphagia, sialorrhea, and severe diaphoresis early in the course of treatment with antipsychotic medication should alert the physician to the possible emergence of NMS. Antipsychotic agents and other potentially neurotoxic medications must be stopped. Supportive measures to lower temperature and to ensure adequate hydration are essential. Electrolyte disturbances must be corrected. The patient should be closely monitored for signs of impending respiratory failure resulting from severe muscle rigidity and an inability to handle oral secretions. Cardiac and renal function should be monitored closely. Although there is no evidence that osmotic diuresis hastens recovery from NMS, it may help to maintain renal function. If renal failure occurs, dialysis may be required.

Bhanushali MJ, Tuite PJ: The evaluation and management of patients with neuroleptic malignant syndrome. Neurol Clin North Am 22:389–411, 2004.
Neuroleptic Malignant Syndrome Information Service: www.nmsis.org

14. **What pharmacologic treatments are useful?**

Pharmacologic intervention is usually reserved for severe cases and has a less clear role because of the lack of controlled prospective data. Dopamine agonists (e.g., bromocriptine and amantadine) and/or direct muscle relaxants (e.g., dantrolene) have been used, and decreased mortality rates have been reported with both types of therapy. Dosages vary widely, but doses of bromocriptine have been documented between 2.5 and 35 mg/day. Bromocriptine can be started at 2.5–5 mg three times daily given orally (or via nasogastric tube in patients with dysphagia or severely compromised mental status). Dopamine agonists, particularly in higher doses, can cause psychosis or vomiting, which clearly can complicate the picture and compromise the patient's health. The only data available for direct-acting muscle relaxants are for dantrolene. Doses of up to 10 mg/kg have been used. The goal is to decrease muscular rigidity to decrease the hypermetabolic state in skeletal muscle, which is partially responsible for the hyperthermia in NMS. Dantrolene can cause hepatoxicity, which can lead to overt hepatitis and death. Combinations of dantrolene and dopamine agonists have been used, although there is no evidence that they further decrease mortality when used in combination. Anticholinergic medications commonly used to treat pseudoparkinsonism have little benefit and may further compromise thermoregulation. Recent studies suggest that benzodiazepines may reduce recovery time in NMS. Benzodiazepines also can be useful in managing an agitated, hyperactive patient once NMS has begun to resolve. Electroconvulsive therapy also may play a role in treating NMS, but further research is needed.

15. **Will NMS recur with subsequent use of neuroleptic medication?**

The risk of recurrence decreases with time. The recurrence rate in patients rechallenged with antipsychotics before 2 weeks after resolution of NMS is high. Patients cautiously rechallenged 2 weeks or more after resolution of NMS often tolerate antipsychotics without difficulty. A low-potency antipsychotic agent is chosen for the rechallenge. Dosing should be conservative and increased gradually. Interest in the concurrent use of the calcium channel blocker nifedipine has also shown promise in prevention of recurrence, although the data are still incomplete. Some persons are prone to NMS; close observation for early symptom recurrence is crucial.

16. **Is there any way to prevent NMS?**

No. Early recognition and, when clinically warranted, lower dosing, avoidance of parenteral antipsychotic agents and rapid increases in dosage, and minimization of other risk factors (e.g., dehydration) may decrease the incidence of NMS. Catatonia may be a strong risk factor for the development of NMS. Thus, antipsychotics should be avoided in catatonic patients if possible.

17. **Are there alternatives to antipsychotic treatment for acutely psychotic patients?**

There are a number of treatment options. Benzodiazepines may help in the management of a hyperactive psychotic patient and may lower the absolute dose of antipsychotic needed. When the primary diagnosis is affective disorder (as in a significant percentage of patients developing NMS), aggressive treatment of the manic or depressive illness with mood stabilizers or antidepressants is indicated. It is usually necessary to administer antipsychotic medications concomitantly when psychotic symptoms are present. Electroconvulsive therapy is a viable alternative for manic psychosis, depressive psychosis, and catatonia.

18. **Are there alternatives to antipsychotic treatment for patients with chronic psychotic illnesses?**
In chronic psychotic disorders (e.g., schizophrenia, schizoaffective disorder, delusional disorder) there may be no alternative to the use of antipsychotic medications. Hence, cautious rechallenging with different classes of antipsychotics (with special attention to atypical antipsychotic agents and treatment of reversible risk factors) is virtually always necessary. Avoidance of polypharmacy, if possible, is also advisable.

19. **Are malignant hyperthermia (MH) and NMS related?**
MH and NMS have similar clinical presentations but different pathophysiologies. MH develops after exposure to inhalation anesthetics, such as halothane, and depolarizing muscle relaxants, such as succinylcholine. MH is characterized by diffuse muscle rigidity, fever, hypermetabolism, elevated serum creatine kinase (muscle fraction), hyperkalemia, tachycardia, hypoxemia, acidosis, and myoglobinuria. It is caused by a genetic defect in a sarcoplasmic reticulum calcium channel protein, which results in excessive calcium release in skeletal muscle after exposure to triggering medications. Susceptibility to MH is diagnosed by the muscle contracture test. In susceptible people, excessive contractions occur in muscle strips exposed to varying concentrations of halothane and caffeine. Family studies and muscle contracture testing indicate that patients with one of the disorders do not appear to be at increased risk for the other.

20. **What is serotonin syndrome?**
Serotonin syndrome is a rare but potentially fatal syndrome characterized by the triad of altered mental status, autonomic dysfunction, and neuromuscular abnormalities, which is thought to result from central and peripheral hyperserotonergic activity. The similarity between serotonin syndrome and NMS often leads to misdiagnosis. Serotonin syndrome can develop after the addition of a serotonergic medication (e.g., monoamine oxidase inhibitor, tricyclic antidepressant, selective serotonin reuptake inhibitor) to a regimen that already includes serotonin-enhancing drugs or after overdoses of serotonergic drugs. The presentation is heterogeneous, but common clinical features include confusion, hypomania, agitation, restlessness, myoclonus, hyperreflexia, diaphoresis, tachycardia, blood pressure fluctuation, shivering, tremor, diarrhea, incoordination, and fever.

Boyer EW, Shannon M: The serotonin syndrome. N Engl J Med 352:1112–1120, 2005.
Brown T, Frian S, Mareth T: Pathophysiology and management of the serotonin syndrome. Ann Pharmacother 30:527–535, 1996.

21. **How is serotonin syndrome differentiated from NMS?**
Serotonin syndrome follows a history of exposure to serotonergic medications. Compared with NMS, in serotonin syndrome tremor and myoclonus are more prominent than muscle rigidity, fever is present less often, and the laboratory test result abnormalities seen in NMS (e.g., elevated creatine phosphokinase level) are usually absent. Discontinuation of the serotonergic medications and supportive treatment are most important. As with NMS, the role of pharmacologic treatment in serotonin syndrome is unclear because of the lack of controlled, prospective studies. Lorazepam, propranolol, and cyproheptadine may be effective in treating symptoms. Propranolol and cyproheptadine have serotonin antagonist properties.

KEY POINTS: NEUROLEPTIC MALIGNANT SYNDROME (NMS)

1. NMS can develop with exposure to any antipsychotic medication—even with chronic use.

2. When considering the differential diagnosis, one should pay particular attention to recent changes in doses and psychotropic polypharmacy.

3. Other agents, such as antiemetic agents, can also cause NMS.

4. Treatment is primarily supportive.

5. In most cases, the most important factors that distinguish NMS from serotonin syndrome are hyperthermia and rigidity.

ACKNOWLEDGMENT

The authors gratefully acknowledge the contribution of Erin Fellner, MD, for revisions to a previous edition.

BIBLIOGRAPHY

1. Addonizio G, Susman VL: Neuroleptic Malignant Syndrome: A Clinical Approach. St. Louis, Mosby, 1991.

2. Pope HG Jr, Keck JR, McElroy SL: Frequency and presentation of neuroleptic malignant syndrome in a large psychiatric hospital. Am J Psychiatry 143:1227–1232, 1986.

3. Rosebush P, Stewart T: A prospective analysis of 24 episodes of neuroleptic malignant syndrome. Am J Psychiatry 146:717–725, 1989.

4. Shalev A, Heresh H, Munitz H: Mortality from neuroleptic malignant syndrome. Clin Psychiatry 50:18–22, 1989.

5. Suzuki A, Kondo T, Otani K, et al: Association of the TaqI A polymorphism of the dopamine D(2) receptor gene with predisposition to neuroleptic malignant syndrome. Am J Psychiatry 158:1714–1746, 2001.

XIX. ETHICS

ETHICS

David Shimabukuro, MDCM

1. **What are the principles on which judicial decisions regarding patients' acceptance or refusal of medical care are based?**

   This issue tends to arise when there is a conflict between the patient, family members, and/or the medical team. There are no legal statutes pertaining to this issue, except in cases of extremis (i.e., brain death and organ transplantation), but the courts' opinions have been expressed via case law. A majority of their decisions are based on two important and distinct principles: (1) autonomy of the individual and (2) informed consent. The concept of *autonomy* can be defined as the fundamental right to choose one's own destiny, regardless of the eventual outcome. Of course, the choice made cannot cause harm to others. As for the principle of informed consent, it is much harder to define because it also includes the concept of competency (*see* question 2). Most would agree, though, that an informed consent is a decision made by a competent person after receiving information about available treatment options along with the risks, benefits, and consequences of these options (including the option of no treatment). Autonomy and informed consent, along with several other minor principles, form the basis for the concept of self-determination.

   Jonsen AR, Siegler M, Winslade WJ: Clinical Ethics, 2nd ed. New York, Macmillan, 1986.

   Wear AN, Brahams D: To treat or not to treat: The legal, ethical and therapeutic implications of treatment refusal. J Med Ethics 17:131–135, 1991.

2. **How does one determine the competency of a patient? What action should be taken if it is suspected that the patient is not competent to make health care decisions?**

   Before determining a patient's competence, one needs to know the definition of competency. In simple terms, it is the capacity to be autonomous. In legal matters, competence is a property of an individual determined by a normative standard based on current moral beliefs of society. As such, it is a value judgment that varies from moment to moment and situation to situation. Thus, there is no universal definition of competence. Practically speaking, a "functional approach" is used to establish a patient's competence. This involves meeting three specific criteria: (1) free action; (2) authenticity; and (3) effective deliberation. In free action, a patient must be capable of action that is intentional and completely voluntary. It cannot be the result of coercion, duress, or undue influence. For authenticity, one must be certain that the patient is acting in character—that is, consistent with his or her values, attitudes, and life plans (i.e., "authentically"). As for effective deliberation, the patient must realize that a decision has to be made. He or she should be aware of the alternatives and their consequences and then be able to make an informed decision based on an informed evaluation. Therefore, a competent patient should be acting freely and within character while also being able to deliberate and express clearly the issues at hand. Given this approach, it is easy to see how determining the competence of a patient can be very difficult. For those times when it is not clear, a physician can request a psychiatric consultation. A psychiatrist, or any other physician, can deem a patient incompetent, but it only becomes legal and binding when argued in front of a judge and determined in a court of law. In most cases, it is not necessary to go to the courts because the patient's family or other concerned persons do not contest the patient's competence (i.e., comatose or heavily sedated patients) and the treating physicians' plans. When a patient is deemed incompetent, it is necessary to appoint a surrogate to make health care decisions. This is usually done informally by simply designating a family member or next of kin to speak on behalf of the patient. When there is no available family, a conservator needs to be appointed by the court.

Jonsen AR, Siegler M, Winslade WJ: Clinical Ethics, 2nd ed. New York, Macmillan, 1986.
Nathanson JA: When does a patient have the right to refuse lifesaving medical treatment? Can Med Assoc J 150:1323–1326, 1994.

KEY POINTS: FUNCTIONAL APPROACH TO DETERMINE THE COMPETENCY OF A PATIENT

1. To be considered competent, a patient must be capable of free action.

2. There must be an authenticity to the patient's actions.

3. Effective deliberation must be present; that is, the patient must realize that a decision has to be made.

3. **Is an "advance directive" a legal document?**
   An advance directive is a document one creates while competent to express future wishes regarding medical care in the event that he or she becomes incompetent or otherwise unable to make his or her preferences known. Living wills are a popular form of an advance directive. Such directives indicate what type of care a person wishes to receive and may also appoint an individual or third party (e.g., durable power of attorney, health care proxy) to be responsible for making decisions should the person become incapacitated. Most readily available advance directive documents are very general in nature and lack specificity in terms of conditions for aggressive treatment or withdrawal of care. However, authoring an advance directive should be encouraged by all physicians to their patients because it designates a health care decision maker. Despite the lack of legal statutes, courts tend to uphold an individual's advance directive unless there is a specific reason to doubt its validity. The Patient Self-Determination Act of 1991 (enacted by U.S. Congress in 1990) now requires all hospitals to discuss advance directives and to have forms available to their patients at the time of admission.

   Greco PJ, Schulman KA, Lavizzo-Mourey R: The Patient Self-determination Act and the future of advance directives. Ann Intern Med 115:639–643, 1991.

4. **What is an ethics committee? What is its role?**
   An ethics committee is an interdisciplinary group (i.e., physicians, nurses, risk managers, and other health care professionals) that assists in resolving ethical problems involving issues that affect the care and treatment of patients currently in the hospital. The committee commonly reviews and makes recommendations on specific cases, helps to further clarify to the patient or the patient's surrogates the options and alternatives, and provides support to the members of the health care team who are involved in a difficult ethical dilemma. The ethics committee does not make decisions but provides consultation and information to guide the actual decision makers.

   American Medical Association: Council on Ethical and Judicial Affairs. Code of Medical Ethics. Chicago, American Medical Association, 1997: www.ama-assn.org

5. **What is the health care provider's recourse when he or she morally disagrees with a patient's plan of care?**
   First, the provider should discuss the disputed plan with other caregivers to determine whether his or her concerns are valid. The provider should then express his or her concerns with the persons proposing the plan. An open, nonconfrontational discussion between the parties allows

each side to see the other's rationales and points of view. In the end, if no resolution can be achieved, a consultation with the ethics committee is an excellent means of reexamining and reapproaching the issue. When these actions fail to reconcile the caregiver to the patient's course of treatment, a request to be removed from the case should be made. The request should be honored and the provider removed as long as others are available to care for the patient.

American Medical Association: Council on Ethical and Judicial Affairs. Code of Medical Ethics. Chicago, American Medical Association, 1997: www.ama-assn.org

KEY POINTS: ROLE OF ETHICS COMMITTEE

1. The ethics committee reviews and makes recommendations on specific cases.

2. Its members help to further clarify to patients and their families the options and alternatives.

3. This multidisciplinary group provides support to all parties involved in difficult ethical dilemmas.

6. **Who is ultimately responsible for determining a patient's "do-not-resuscitate" status?**
The decision to withhold resuscitation attempts from a cardiopulmonary arrest should ideally be a collaborative one, determined by the patient, the patient's family, and the primary physician. On most occasions, the objective medical opinion of the attending physician is the determining factor in a patient's or family's decision not to resuscitate. However, should a conflict arise, a resolution should be obtained through a fair decision-making process, involving the ethics committee. A do-not-resuscitate order must be signed by a physician; all other signatures, if required, are legally irrelevant. A do-not-resuscitate order is not synonymous with an order to withhold standard medical care.

American Medical Association: Council on Ethical and Judicial Affairs. Code of Medical Ethics. Chicago, American Medical Association, 1997: www.ama-assn.org

Bone RC, Rackow EC, Weg JG: Ethical and moral guidelines for the initiation, continuation, and withdrawal of intensive care. Chest 97:949–958, 1990.

7. **What constitutes "extraordinary" measures? What about when they are futile?**
Extraordinary measures are any treatments that impose a greater burden to the patient than provide any benefit. This term is highly variable and can be applied to the same treatment for the same patient but at different time points. Such interventions may cause the patient undue pain and expense for questionable gains. Does this then imply that extraordinary measures are futile? From a legal standpoint, there is no meaningful definition for the term *futility*. However, ethically, physicians are not obligated to deliver care that, in their best judgment, would not have a reasonable chance of benefiting the patient, even if it is demanded by the patient or his or her representative. Conflict can arise between the medical staff, patients, and patients' families as to what is "futile" treatment. Decisions and conflict resolution should follow a due-process approach.

American Medical Association: Council on Ethical and Judicial Affairs. Code of Medical Ethics. Chicago, American Medical Association, 1997: www.ama-assn.org

Bone RC, Rackow EC, Weg JG: Ethical and moral guidelines for the initiation, continuation, and withdrawal of intensive care. Chest 97:949–958, 1990.

8. **Is it ethically appropriate to withhold or terminate life-sustaining medical interventions?**

From a legal and ethical perspective, there is no difference between withholding and terminating life-sustaining medical measures (i.e., any treatment that serves to prolong life without reversing the underlying medical condition). When treatment interventions are "futile" or unable to improve a patient's condition, they often merely prolong life and delay the inevitable death of the patient. Withholding or terminating life support is often a very difficult decision to make and, ideally, should be made preemptively by the patient via an advance directive. More often, though, an advance directive is not available and it falls to the family to make this difficult decision. Regardless of who exactly decides, legally and ethically, the decision should be based on what the patient would have decided (i.e., substituted judgment) or on the best interests of the patient (i.e., what outcome would most likely promote the patient's well-being).

American Medical Association: Council on Ethical and Judicial Affairs. Code of Medical Ethics. Chicago, American Medical Association, 1997: www.ama-assn.org

Bone RC, Rackow EC, Weg JG: Ethical and moral guidelines for the initiation, continuation, and withdrawal of intensive care. Chest 97:949–958, 1990.

Luce JM: Withholding and withdrawal of life support from critically ill patients. West J Med 167:411–416, 1997.

9. **Can a physician legally write an order for a "slow-code"?**

Slow-code usually implies a short resuscitation attempt with disregard to speed and time. The decision to refrain from cardiopulmonary resuscitation should be clear and communicated to all involved parties. The term *slow-code* is a contradiction in terms and conveys a confusing message. There either is a full resuscitation attempt, an attempt with specific limitations, or no attempt at all. It is not legal to write a slow-code order.

American Medical Association: Council on Ethical and Judicial Affairs. Code of Medical Ethics. Chicago, American Medical Association, 1997: www.ama-assn.org

10. **Is it acceptable to provide treatment to patients based on their financial status?**

It is simplistic to believe that the financial situations of the patient and the health care facility do not influence patient care decisions. With that in mind, it is unacceptable to deny emergent medical care to a patient in need; the clinician must always consider the patient's welfare as the primary objective. However, once the patient is in stable condition and out of imminent danger, it is legal to transfer the patient to another institution that is willing to accept the financial burden of the patient.

American Medical Association: Council on Ethical and Judicial Affairs. Code of Medical Ethics. Chicago, American Medical Association, 1997: www.ama-assn.org

11. **What is the difference between euthanasia and assisted suicide? Although illegal, are these methods morally and ethically acceptable?**

To provide a thorough answer to these questions would take several chapters and is beyond the scope of this book. In brief, *euthanasia,* or "good death," can be defined as active or passive, voluntary or involuntary, and performed by commission or omission. From a legal and ethical standpoint, the controversy surrounds active euthanasia or the "administration of a lethal agent by [a physician] to a patient for the purpose of relieving the patient's intolerable and incurable suffering." *Assisted suicide* can be defined to occur when "a physician facilitates a patient's death by providing the necessary means and/or information to enable a patient to perform the life-ending act." The American Medical Association considers both acts to be fundamentally incompatible with the physician's role as a healer. To date, no individual has been convicted for assisted suicide even though it is a felony in many states. However, because euthanasia can be subsumed under homicide, one physician has been found guilty in a court of law (Dr. Jack Kevorkian was convicted of second-degree murder in 1999). Over the past 20 years, several physicians have pleaded guilty to euthanasia and have been sentenced to probation.

As of December 2001, only one state, Oregon, has legalized physician-assisted suicide. This legislation was accepted by voters in 1994 and went into effect in 1997. In November 2001, U.S. Attorney General John Ashcroft ordered the Drug Enforcement Agency to revoke the license for prescribing controlled substances of physicians who have engaged in assisted suicide because it was not consistent with appropriate medical care and the proper use of a controlled substance. In 2004, the U.S. Ninth Circuit Court of Appeals ruled in a two-to-one decision that John Ashcroft had "overstepped" his boundaries and the licenses could not be revoked.

In reference to the morality of active euthanasia and physician-assisted suicide, because morals are based on societal values, one can argue that given its acceptance in the Netherlands and even in the United States (Oregon's Death with Dignity Act), both acts are morally acceptable. On the other hand, given the fact these concepts are not universally accepted, their morality can be questioned. Of course, their ethics have been and continue to be debated today. Interestingly, though, less than 100 years ago, suicide itself was considered an illegal act and punishable according to the penal code.

American Medical Association: Council on Ethical and Judicial Affairs. Code of Medical Ethics. Chicago, American Medical Association, 1997: www.ama-assn.org

Stone TH, Winslade WJ: Physician-assisted suicide and euthanasia in the United States. J Leg Med 16:481–507, 1995.

12. **How does one assess the need for increased analgesia in a dying patient? How does one provide adequate analgesia while avoiding euthanasia?**
In a dying patient, the prolongation of life is no longer the primary goal; rather, the relief of pain and discomfort are foremost. To deny analgesia in such a situation, regardless of the fact that it may depress respiration or blood pressure, would be to deny the patient one of the few interventions that can increase comfort at a time when he or she may need it the most (i.e., concept of secondary effect). If the patient is conscious, attempts should be made to communicate with him or her. If the patient is unresponsive, pain medication should be administered based on physiologic responses such as heart and respiratory rate, blood pressure, and facial expression.

Luce JM: Withholding and withdrawal of life support from critically ill patients. West J Med 167:411–416, 1997.

CHAPTER 88

WITHDRAWAL OF TREATMENT

David Shimabukuro, MDCM

1. **What are the general circumstances in which withdrawal of critical care may be considered?**

   The cessation of life-sustaining medical treatment should be considered when the relative burden of pain or suffering caused by the intervention to the patient outweighs the benefits in quality of life or prolongation of life, or in other cases, when further treatment is medically inappropriate or futile. Quality-of-life considerations are solely those of the patient, the patient's family, and proxy health care decision makers, whereas inappropriate medical management is determined by the physicians. Ideally, when a consensus has been reached among the patient concerned persons, and the medical team that further medical intervention is inappropriate or medically inadvisable, aggressive care should be withdrawn and palliative care instituted.

2. **Why is it important to understand the issues involved in the withdrawal of treatment in the intensive care unit (ICU)?**

   It is important because limiting or withdrawing treatment in the ICU occurs regularly. In fact, a national survey done about 10 years ago has shown that approximately 90% of patients who die in the ICU do so after the decision has been made to limit or withdraw care. In addition, several prior studies have demonstrated that patients' families are often dissatisfied with both patient management and communication with their physicians after the decision to withdraw treatment has been made. Naturally, this decision shifts the goals of treatment from cure or recovery to palliation, which focuses on symptom management and allows the patient to maintain dignity while dying in a comfortable and pain-free state. For most physicians, this is also a difficult transition. According to Truog and colleagues, there is "an emerging perspective that palliative care and intensive care are not mutually exclusive options, but rather should be coexistent."

   Pendergast TJ, JM Luce. Increasing incidences of withholding and withdrawal of life support from the critically ill. Am J Respir Crit Care Med 155:15–20, 1997.

   Society of Critical Care Medicine: www.sccm.org/SCCM/Professional+Development/Critical+Care+Ethics/

   Truog, RD, Cist, AFM, Brackett, SE, et al: Recommendations for end-of-life care in the intensive care unit: The Ethics Committee of the Society of Critical Care Medicine. Crit Care Med 29:2332–2348, 2001.

3. **Who may make the decision to withdraw medical care?**

   A competent patient able to provide informed consent may refuse life-sustaining treatment at any time, regardless of the opinions of the family or the medical team. Psychiatric consultation may help to determine concerns influencing the patient's appreciation of the consequences of the decision or to determine competence, but in most instances this is not necessary. A patient may have also formulated an advance directive that specifies decision-making preferences in the event of incapacitation. An *a priori* designated health care proxy (i.e., durable power of attorney) selected by the patient can consent to the withdrawal of treatment with the understanding of the concept of substituted judgment (knowing the patient's moral values and experiences, what he or she would decide in this specific situation). In the rare event that no individual is identified to make medical decisions, depending on individual state laws, a court order or a court-appointed health care proxy may be necessary.

4. **Are advance directives followed by physicians?**

   Multiple studies indicate that physicians often do not follow the stated wishes of their patients. In the multi-institutional Study to Understand Prognoses and Preferences for Outcomes and Risks of Treatments (SUPPORT), 31% of patients before intervention preferred that cardiopulmonary resuscitation (CPR) be withheld, whereas only 47% of physicians reported this preference at the time of the first interview. Do-not-resuscitate orders were actually written for only 49% of the patients who stated they did not want CPR. Not adhering to an advance directive is disrespectful to the patient and disregards the basic ethical principle of patient autonomy.

   The SUPPORT Principal Investigators: A controlled trial to improve care for seriously ill hospitalized patients: The study to understand prognoses and preferences for outcomes and risks of treatments. JAMA 274:1591–1598, 1995.

5. **Is withdrawal of nutrition and hydration considered the same as withdrawal of other medical treatment?**

   Several state court cases have defined *nutrition* and *hydration* as medical treatments that can be withdrawn when a general decision has been made to terminate all medical therapies. However, at this time, there is no national consensus as to whether nutrition and hydration are considered "treatments."

   A competent patient may decide this matter for him- or herself. Nutrition and hydration for incapacitated patients often entail involved medical procedures such as gastrostomies and parenteral nutrition, which are sometimes painful. Although withdrawal of nutrition and hydration may not ultimately be different on ethical grounds from other medical treatments, it may have a different legal status depending on state statute. This should be explored by the provider in his or her own state before these modalities are discontinued.

6. **What are the ethical and clinical principles of withdrawing life support?**

   There are six principles involved in deciding to terminate aggressive medical care and move toward palliation. First of all, it should always be kept in mind that the goal of withdrawing life-sustaining treatments is to remove all treatments that are not desired or do not provide patient comfort. There should be a shift toward palliation. Second, withholding treatments that prolong life are morally, ethically, and legally no different than withdrawing the treatments. Third, actions with the sole purpose of hastening death are morally and legally incongruous with our society's current values. Fourth, any treatment can be withheld or withdrawn. This can be applied to nutrition and hydration if they are considered "treatments." Unfortunately, this will ultimately be decided in the judicial system. Fifth, the withdrawal of life support is a medical procedure. Finally, when circumstances justify the withholding of medical treatments, very strong consideration should be given to withdrawing current life-sustaining treatments.

   Curtis JR, Rubenfeld GD (eds): Managing Death in the Intensive Care Unit. Oxford, Oxford University Press, 2001.

7. **How should care be withdrawn?**

   One of the clinical principles of withdrawing life support is that it is a clinical procedure. As such, it should be performed like most other procedures in the ICU. A decision is made to stop life-sustaining therapy and informed consent is obtained, in this case, by a health care proxy. A plan is then formulated and the handling of complications anticipated. In most institutions, this is achieved by protocol orders. Once the orders are written, the patient should be moved to an appropriate setting. This could mean the patient is transferred to a general hospital room or a palliative care unit. However, in most instances, the critically ill patient remains in his or her ICU room. The plan is then instituted, ensuring adequate sedation and analgesia at all times. The entire process should be documented in the patient's medical record. The process and outcome of the procedure should be evaluated each time in an attempt to improve the quality of care to the patient and his or her family.

   Curtis JR, Rubenfeld GD (eds): Managing Death in the Intensive Care Unit. Oxford, Oxford University Press, 2001.

8. **Should the administration of neuromuscular-blocking agents be stopped before life-sustaining care is withdrawn?**

   In general, all paralytic agents should be immediately stopped when the decision has been made to withdraw care. Ideally, physicians should wait for the return of sufficient muscle function to detect spontaneous movements and attempts at respiration by the patient before treatment modalities are removed. This allows for the possibility of important interaction between the patient and his or her family. In addition, it provides nurses with additional clinical information as to the adequacy of sedation and analgesia. In rare circumstances, especially when there have been prolonged infusions of neuromuscular-blocking agents, it may not be possible to wait for any return of muscle activity because the burden of continuing with aggressive care contradicts the change in goals to minimize pain and suffering and to ensure dying with dignity.

KEY POINTS: WITHDRAWAL OF CARE

1. The physician alone cannot make the decision to withdraw support. A competent patient or a designated health care proxy should make the decision. If the patient or family is not available to make the decision, the physician must consult with the legally appointed proxy.

2. Withdrawal of nutrition and hydration has proven to be a problem for physicians in that each state decides legally as to the status of these actions. Therefore, physicians must know their state law regarding withdrawal of nutrition and hydration.

3. The administration of neuromuscular-blocking agents should be stopped when the decision to withdraw support has been made, and ideally, withdrawal of support should be done after neuromuscular function has returned.

INTENSIVE CARE UNIT ADMINISTRATION

Antoinette Spevetz, MD, and Carolyn E. Bekes, MD, MHA

1. **What role should the medical director of an intensive care unit (ICU) play in management of the unit?**

   The medical director of an ICU can play a key role in establishing and maintaining the environment in which a critically ill patient can receive high-quality care with optimal resource allocation. Important aspects of medical director involvement include bed triage and efforts to contain costs by increasing efficiency of care and control of resource use. It has been suggested that critical care training programs incorporate a management training component. See Box 89-1 for duties of an ICU director.

   Brilli RJ, Spevetz A, Branson RD, et al: Critical care delivery in the intensive care unit: Defining critical roles and the best practice model. Crit Care Med 29:2007–2019, 2001.

   Shortell SM, Zimmerman JE, Rosseau DM, et al: The performance of intensive care units: Does good management make a difference? Med Care 32:508–525, 1994.

BOX 89-1. RESPONSIBILITIES OF THE MEDICAL DIRECTOR

1. Ensure that care is delivered to the critically ill patient via a multidisciplinary group.
2. Develop clinical and administrative protocols.
3. Coordinate quality-improvement activities.
4. Take responsibility for the delivery of care in the ICU.
5. Oversee patient triage, bed allocation, and discharge planning.
6. Participate in the activities of the critical care committee and establishment of relationships with other ICUs in the hospital.
7. Ensure continuing education for nursing, respiratory therapy, etc.

---

2. **Does an intensivist affect patient outcome or cost of care in the ICU?**

   Evidence indicates that involvement of an intensivist in patient care leads to decreased mortality rates and more effective use of resources.

   Pronovost PL, Kenckes MW, Dorman T, et al: Organizational characteristics of intensive care units related to outcomes of abdominal aortic surgery. JAMA 281:1310–1317, 1999.

3. **What are the roles for a clinical pharmacist and critical care nurse on the critical care team?**

   The complex pharmacologic issues of patients in the ICU warrant inclusion of a clinical pharmacist on the critical care team. Drug–drug interactions and adverse drug reactions dramatically decrease when a pharmacist is part of a multidisciplinary team. An appropriately trained critical care nurse has been shown by Pronovost and colleagues to improve the outcome of patients with abdominal aortic aneurysm when appropriate staffing ratios are maintained.

   Pronovost PJ, Dang D, Dorman T, et al: Intensive care unit nurse staffing and the risk of complications after abdominal aortic surgery. Eff Clin Pract 4:199–205, 2001.

4. **Why is everyone so concerned about cutting the cost of ICU care? Should cost be a factor in decision making in the ICU?**
   On average, ICUs comprise only 5–10% of a hospital's beds, but >20% of the hospital's budget is devoted to the care of patients in these beds. Across the United States, this represents 1.5% of the gross national product. In light of the high cost of critical care, physicians are challenged to document that high-cost/high-tech care results in the desired outcomes. The physician should use available resources in the most cost-effective manner for the maximal benefit of the patient.

   Angood P: Right Care, Right Now™—You can make a difference. Crit Care Med 33:2729–2732, 2005.
   Kirton OC, Civetta JM, Hudson-Civetta J: Cost-effectiveness in the intensive care unit. Surg Clin North Am 76:175–200, 1996.

5. **Does the structure of an ICU affect the quality or cost of care?**
   The multidisciplinary team approach using appropriate protocol and guidelines significantly reduces cost and improves patient outcomes. Several different models for structuring an ICU have been used. Evidence does not support any one model but clearly shows that when a formal structure is implemented, mortality rates and number of ICU days are reduced.

   Zimmerman JE, Shortell SM, Rousseau DM, et al: Improving intensive care. Observations based on organizational studies in nine intensive care units: A prospective multicenter study. Crit Care Med 21:1443–1451, 1993.

6. **What is the role of scoring systems in an ICU?**
   Although it is controversial whether scoring systems can predict outcomes for individual patients, there is little question that they provide an objective description of the acuity of a population of patients. This information is useful when one attempts to compare outcomes of care between units and can be used for performance improvement projects as well as clinical research. It also may benefit the physician during family discussion and can be used to compare an individual case with a group of similar patients for potential outcome.

   Knaus WA, Draper EA, Wagner DP, et al: An evaluation of outcome from intensive care in major medical centers. Ann Intern Med 104:410–418, 1986.
   Kollef MH, Shuster DP: Predicting intensive care unit outcome with scoring systems: Underlying concepts and principles. Crit Care Clin 10:1–18, 1994.
   Shortell SM, Zimmerman JE, Rousseau DM, et al: The performance of intensive care units: Does good management make a difference? Med Care 32:508–525, 1994.

7. **At what stage of the patient's stay in the ICU should the care team start thinking about the patient's discharge planning, both from the ICU and from the hospital?**
   Although in many instances of serious illness it may seem premature, it is probably useful to give thought to the probable length of the ICU stay, hospital discharge status, and needs from the time of admission. In a large number of cases, unnecessary delays later in the patient's hospitalization can be averted by timely consideration of whether it is likely that the patient will ultimately be able to be discharged to home or will require a period of institutional rehabilitation and identification of rehabilitation requirements.

8. **Describe the composition of the critical care committee.**
   The activities of multidisciplinary critical care units should be supervised by a hospital committee composed of representatives of those departments and divisions admitting patients to the unit. In addition, the director of nursing and nursing education for the unit together with the unit physician director and the head of the division, section, or department of critical care medicine should be committee members. It is usually appropriate for one of the latter two members to chair the committee. There should also be members from nursing, pharmacy, respiratory, and dietary, as well as other team members who routinely participate in the care of the critically ill patient. See Box 89-2 for responsibilities of a critical care committee.

KEY POINTS: INTENSIVE CARE UNIT (ICU) ADMINISTRATION

1. Critical care nurses, pharmacists, respiratory therapists, and intensivists working as a team are key to improving the outcome of critical care patients.

2. Intensivists have the responsibility to oversee the environment of care.

3. Hospitals must focus on controlling the cost of care, including care delivered in the ICU.

4. Critical care committees have the responsibilities for oversight of the delivery of care in the ICU.

BOX 89-2. MAJOR DUTIES OF THE CRITICAL CARE COMMITTEE

1. Define the purpose and goals of the unit. These may be incorporated in a brief mission statement.

2. Develop comprehensive policies and procedures outlining the organizational and working systems whereby the unit will achieve its goals. These policies should address, among other issues, the authorities and process for triaging (i.e., admissions and discharges) patients and admission and discharge criteria, as well as the credentialing requirements and regulations for physicians, nurses, and ancillary personnel working in the unit. Policies should be developed for important aspects of patient care peculiar to the unit environment (e.g., intra- and interhospital patient transport, avoidance and control of infection).

3. Define and ensure appropriate levels of education and training for all personnel working in the unit. Ensure adequate initial orientation and ongoing in-servicing for all personnel working in the unit.

4. Recommend to the medical staff the adoption of regulations designed to allow the committee to accomplish the previously discussed tasks in an efficient manner.

5. Develop and maintain an ongoing performance improvement program designed to monitor standards of patient care and identify opportunities to improve outcomes and the efficiency of care delivery. Develop reliable benchmarking measurements permitting the comparison of outcomes achieved in the unit against results reported for similar patients in large databases.

6. Maintain an ongoing database on patient acuity, lengths of stay, use of resources, complications, and markers for patient outcome. Provide a mechanism for reviewing all complications and untoward events so that corrective action can be instituted where appropriate.

7. Approve and submit an annual budget for the unit designed to permit the attainment of the declared goals. The development of the budget will be the joint responsibility of the nursing and physician directorship of the unit.

9. **How should disagreements between physicians and families regarding care goals for incompetent patients be resolved?**
The guiding principle for determining the goals of care for any patient is the determination of the patient's wishes. In those cases in which the patient is incompetent, this may be difficult. When

the patient has an advance directive in place, it is helpful to review this document and attempt to extrapolate the patient's instructions to the situation under review. Often, however, the instructions may be insufficiently detailed to permit a confident decision to be reached. If a health care surrogate has been named, discussions with this person may often provide the necessary insight into the patient's philosophy and wishes to allow the surrogate to reach a decision based on the information regarding prognosis and therapeutic options provided by the care team. In the great majority of cases, the care team will be in agreement with these decisions. Even when no surrogate has been named, discussions with family members and friends often allow a consensus to be reached regarding what the patient would have wanted in this situation.

In a minority of cases, however, there may be disagreement between the family of an incompetent patient and the team providing care regarding which direction the care should take. In situations such as this, a consultation with the ethics committee may be beneficial for both the family and the health care team.

10. **What are the commonly accepted definitions of an *open unit,* a *semiclosed unit,* and a *closed unit?***
    - **Open unit:** In an open unit, patients may be admitted and cared for by all qualified physicians as defined in the hospital's credentialing policies. The patients may remain on the attending physicians' service, and the unit director will only have clinical involvement with patients by consultative request. Triaging of patients will only take place at times of bed shortage and may be carried out by the director or, occasionally, by negotiation between the nursing administration and the attending physicians.
    - **Semiclosed unit:** In a semiclosed unit, the unit director or his or her designee has the authority to approve or reject requests for admission and can request that patients be transferred out when demand exceeds resources. The director's involvement in patient care may vary, ranging from mandatory consultation, co-attending status, or consultation upon request only, to consultation or involvement only in emergency situations or when there are questions regarding the standard of care.
    - **Closed unit:** In a closed unit, the director and his or her team assume responsibility for the management of all patients admitted to the unit. The patient is transferred to the service of the critical care team at the time of admission and transferred back to the original attending at the time of discharge. In most instances a patient's care is managed by the critical care team in collaboration with the admitting attending physician, although in some units (e.g., trauma units) the unit team may be the sole attending.

    Brilli RJ, Spevetz A, Branson RD, et al: Critical care delivery in the intensive care unit: Defining critical roles and the best practice model. Crit Care Med 29:2007–2019, 2001.
    Society of Critical Care Medicine: http://sccm.org/professional_resources/guidelines/index.asp

11. **Does a closed versus open unit offer benefits in terms of patient care?**
    Several studies have shown decreased rates of mortality and complications in closed units compared with open units. This finding may be related to the concentrated attention that the patient receives from a board-certified intensivist in the former.

    Brilli RJ, Spevetz A, Branson RD, et al: Critical care delivery in the intensive care unit: Defining critical roles and the best practice model. Crit Care Med 29:2007–2019, 2001.
    Society of Critical Care Medicine: http://sccm.org/professional_resources/guidelines/index.asp

12. **What are the legal requirements pertaining the interhospital transport of patients? Where are they defined?**
    The legal requirements are contained in the Consolidated Omnibus Reconciliation Act (COBRA) of 1986 and the OBRA amendment of 1990. The principal requirements are as follows:
    - The patient or representative must give informed consent to the transfer, which should be documented. If this is not possible, the reason should be documented.

- The sending physician must contact a physician at the receiving hospital who has the authority to admit the patient to an appropriate unit.
- The sending physician must detail the patient's condition and should receive advice regarding arrangements for stabilization and transport.
- The receiving physician must accept the patient and confirm that appropriate resources are available for the patient's management.
- Agreement must be reached regarding who has responsibility for management during transport if no physician accompanies the patient.
- The method of transportation shall be determined by the sending physician after consultation with the receiving physician.
- The transporting service shall be notified of the impending transfer, the patient's condition, and the support requirements.
- The receiving hospital shall secure a nurse to report on the patient's condition.
- A complete copy of the chart including all laboratory and imaging studies shall be sent with the patient.
- A minimum of two people (excluding the operator of the vehicle) shall accompany the patient and at least one shall be an RN, MD, or advanced EMT capable of rendering advanced cardiac life support (ACLS) and advanced trauma life support (ATLS).
- If no physician accompanies the patient and if there is no means of communicating with a physician during transport, the accompanying personnel should have preauthorization to carry out lifesaving interventions.
- Equipment available during transport shall include all that is necessary to establish and maintain endotracheal ventilation, monitor blood pressure and rhythm, defibrillate, treat arrhythmias, and provide IV fluid and medication support. There shall be equipment permitting communication to both the sending and receiving hospitals during transportation.
- Monitoring during transport shall be of continuous electrocardiography, blood pressure, respiratory rate, and whatever patient-specific parameters require observation. If the patient is being ventilated, the ventilator must have pressure and disconnect alarms, and the airway pressure must be displayed.

Federal Register, Vol 56, No 235, December 6, 1991, p 64175.

CHAPTER 90

QUALITY ASSURANCE IN THE INTENSIVE CARE UNIT

Antoinette Spevetz, MD, and Carolyn E. Bekes, MD, MHA

1. How is quality assessed?

The definition of *quality* encompasses many things but clearly involves meeting the expectations of the consumer. In health care, this standard usually involves the satisfaction of patients, physicians, and payers as well as good clinical outcomes, appropriate resource use, cost containment, and attention to patient safety.

2. What is benchmarking?

To *benchmark* means to compare one's own performance-related data with similar data from another institution. The Joint Commission on Accreditation of Health Care Organizations (JCAHO) requires that hospitals benchmark with other hospitals. This process is most useful when performance-related data are compared in units with a similar patient population.

> Joint Commission for Accreditation of Healthcare Organizations: www.jointcommission.org/NR/rdonlyres/48DFC95A-9C05-4A44-AB05-1769D5253014/0/AComprehensiveReviewofDevelopmentforCoreMeasures.pdf

3. What is the relationship between intensive care unit (ICU) organization and quality of care?

Evidence indicates that the structure and organization of an ICU can influence outcome. A collaborative relationship among members of the health care team appears to be critical. The use of clinical protocols clearly improves patient outcomes. A multidisciplinary approach with the addition of a full-time intensivist greatly improves the quality of patient care in the ICU, as does the presence of critical care nurses with appropriate staffing ratios, clinical pharmacists on the unit, and respiratory therapist–driven protocols in weaning from mechanical ventilation.

> Dimick JB, Pronovost PJ, Heitmiller RF, Lipsett PA: Intensive care unit physician staffing is associated with decreased length of stay, hospital cost, and complications after esophageal resection. Crit Care Med 29:753–758, 2004.
>
> Joint Commission for Accreditation of Healthcare Organizations: www.jointcommission.org/NR/rdonlyres/48DFC95A-9C05-4A44-AB05-1769D5253014/0/AComprehensiveReviewofDevelopmentforCoreMeasures.pdf
>
> Kane SL, Webber RJ, Dasra JF: The impact of critical care pharmacists on enhancing patient outcomes. Intensive Care Med 29:691–698, Epub March 29, 2003.
>
> Pronovost PL, Dang D, Dorman T, et al: Intensive care unit nurse staffing and the risk of complications after abdominal aortic surgery. Eff Clin Pract 4:199–206, 2001.
>
> Pronovost PL, Kenckes MW, Dorman T, et al: Organizational characteristics of intensive care units related to outcomes of abdominal aortic surgery. JAMA 281:1310–1317, 1999.
>
> Rudis MI, Brandl KM: Position paper on critical care pharmacy services. Society of Critical Care Medicine and American College of Clinical Pharmacy Task Force on Critical Care Pharmacy Services. Crit Care Med 28:3746–3750, 2000.

4. List the uses to which severity of illness scoring systems are commonly applied.

- **Stratification:** Stratification of the severity or acuity of illness of a number of patients with the same principal diagnosis, by such classification systems as the Acute Physiology and Chronic Health Evaluation (APACHE) II or III, may allow comparison of outcomes related to differing therapeutic approaches and thus permit identification of the best modes of treatment. Clearly, such conclusions can be reached only if the patient groups being treated are matched for severity of illness.

- **Efficiency of care delivery:** Efficiency can be measured only if objective measures of resource use together with stratification of initial acuity of illness related to likely outcome—derived from the study of results in a large variety of diverse care settings—are available. These may be provided by the APACHE system and the Therapeutic Intervention Scoring System, among others.
- **Decision making in clinical management:** Decision making may be aided by considering the information provided by scoring systems, as may prognostic estimates for individual patients. Although such information should always be interpreted in conjunction with the clinical data pertaining to the specific patient, it may be helpful in presenting data to patients and families attempting to make informed treatment decisions.
- **Economics:** Scoring of patients can assist in appropriate billing and reimbursement code application.

Knaus WA, Draper EA, Wagner DP, et al: An evaluation of outcome from intensive care in major medical centers. Ann Intern Med 104:410–418, 1986.

Kollef MH, Shuster DP: Predicting intensive care unit outcome with scoring systems: Underlying concepts and principles. Crit Care Clin 10:1–18, 1994.

Shortell SM, Zimmerman JE, Rousseau DM, et al: The performance of intensive care units: Does good management make a difference? Med Care 32:508–525, 1994.

5. **What are the three major components of the credentialing process identified by the Society of Critical Care Medicine in its Guidelines for Granting Privileges for the Performance of Procedures in Critically Ill Patients?**
   - **Identification of procedures requiring credentialing:** This includes high-risk, high-volume, and risk-prone procedures.
   - **Delineation of specific standards:** These standards should be defined (on a national level, when possible) by practitioners who commonly perform the procedures for which the privileges are requested.
   - **Credentialing mechanism:** This mechanism should be developed individually by each institution.

Guidelines Committee, Society of Critical Care Medicine: Guidelines for Granting Privileges for the Performance of Procedures in Critically Ill Patients. Crit Care Med 21:292–293, 1993.

Society of Critical Care Medicine: www.sccm.org/professional_resources/guidelines/table_of_contents/Documents/Granting_Privileges.pdf

6. **Who should be responsible for performance improvement activities in the ICU?**
   Although ultimately the board of trustees is responsible for the assurance of the quality of care in the hospital as whole, the actual measurement and tracking of performance improvement is delegated to the staff of the unit. The unit director in collaboration with the nurse manager and other members of the health care team should attempt to identify areas for improvements in care delivery. A formal plan should be developed and implemented using the process of identifying an issue, implementing change, and remeasuring: PDSA process (plan, do, study, act) or PDCA process (plan, do, check, act). Results should be communicated both up and down the hierarchy.

Brilli RJ, Spevetz A, Branson RD, et al: Critical care delivery in the intensive care unit: Defining clinical roles and the best practice model. Crit Care Med 25:1007–2019, 2001.

Curtis JR, Cook DJ, Wall RJ, et al: Intensive care unit quality improvement: A "how-do" guide for the interdisciplinary team. Crit Care Med 34:211–218, 2006.

Shortell SM, Zimmerman JE, Rousseau DM, et al: The performance of intensive care units: Does good management make a difference? Med Care 32:508–525, 1994.

7. **What database should be used for performance improvement activities?**
   The administrative databases available in most hospitals were designed for financial applications and do not contain the types of data usually required for performance improvement. However,

with the increasing use of the electronic medical record, data collection will become more automated. At present, manual data collection is needed for many performance improvement projects. Project Impact™ is a national electronic database designed to assist individual institutions with improvement of clinical outcomes in an effective manner through the use of benchmarking.

Rafkin HS, Hoyt JW: Objective data and quality assurance programs: Current and future trends. Crit Care Clin 10:157–177, 1994.

8. **Over the years, the terminology has changed. What is the chief conceptual difference between *quality assurance* and *performance improvement?***
   The original strategy of quality assurance sought to make a series of observations (i.e., indicators) intended to ensure that the delivery of care was being carried out in compliance with the current highest standards defined at that time. The emphasis tended to be on methodology of care delivery and the avoidance of complications. The more recent term of *performance improvement* seeks to examine the entire care-delivery system with the goal of identifying areas where improvement(s) can be instituted, even though the current system may seem adequate. This process is accomplished by familiarizing groups of personnel who will often be in a position to make valuable suggestions for improvement with an intimate knowledge of the systems under review. The impact of process change can then be examined by following predetermined markers of outcome with regard to both patient outcome and resource use; thus, at present, the emphasis is on outcome rather than simply on process.

9. **List a number of observations on which to base assessment of outcome.**
   Although a variety of indicators can be used to assess outcome, the following usually provide a reasonable database and can be used for benchmarking when similar data are available from other institutions:
   - **Patient satisfaction:** This should include not only the patient's subjective opinions but also some objective observations of outcome such as activities of daily living scores. A significantly understudied aspect of this parameter is the posthospital status of the patient.
   - **Length of stay:** The length of stay both in the hospital and in the ICU for patients who have been stratified by diagnosis, acuity, and comorbidities on admission provides valuable insight into outcomes and an excellent database for benchmarking, if studied consistently over a reasonable period.
   - **Mortality indexed to severity of illness:** Although this information can provide a simple benchmarking tool, the data should be critically reviewed because death cannot always be equated with a bad outcome.
   - **Incidence of unanticipated returns to the ICU during the same hospital stay:** This indicator may yield important information if examined in some detail. In addition to the actual incidence (which can be used for benchmarking), the individual cases should be reviewed. This may reveal a need to review the criteria for transferring patients from the unit or the compliance with the same. Alternatively, it may stimulate consideration of the adequacy of the care capabilities of the environments receiving the patients upon discharge from the unit.
   - **Incidence of complications:** Complications may be linked to procedures (e.g., line placement, endotracheal intubation) or to general management (e.g., nosocomial infection, medication errors). Of major importance are those that have a clear impact on patient welfare. The criteria for identifying these and the methodology for data collection and analysis should be defined and consistently applied.

   Core measures are another tool for compliance, with measures known to improve outcome and to benchmark the results of individual ICUs with the peer group.

Joint Commission for Accreditation of Healthcare Organizations: www.jointcommission.org/NR/rdonlyres/ 48DFC95A-9C05-4A44-AB05-1769D5253014/0/AComprehensiveReviewofDevelopmentforCoreMeasures.pdf

10. **How applicable to the ICU is the "clinical or critical pathway" approach to the maintenance of cost-effective care delivery?**

Although the development of so-called "clinical pathways" has had considerable success in reducing costs while maintaining or improving standards of care and clinical outcomes, this methodology appears to be mainly applicable to patients with diagnoses wherein there is a fairly homogeneous group of patients who run broadly similar courses. Good examples of these diagnoses are acute coronary syndromes and hip fractures. In the case of the patient population in a mixed adult medical-surgical ICU, however, there is no such homogeneity and it is often virtually impossible to describe an average course for a given diagnosis. Such a diversity of progression exists that relates primarily to the individual patient circumstances, that it is of little value to compare the course of an individual patient with the "clinical pathway." A much better approach in the ICU is to write treatment algorithms applicable to discrete segments of the patient's care within the continuum of the entire illness (e.g., weaning using therapist-driven protocols, use of the vent bundle, Center for Disease Control (CDC) line insertion bundle, or sepsis bundle) (*see* Boxes 90-1 and 90-2). The use of this approach maintains all the advantages of getting groups together to discuss and agree on a unified approach toward aspects of care (thus reducing expensive diversity) without wasting time and energy on trying to define nonexistent "average" courses of these illnesses.

BOX 90-1. FIVE COMPONENTS OF THE VENTILATOR BUNDLE

1. Elevation of the head of the bed to at least 30 degrees
2. Daily sedation vacation
3. Daily assessments of readiness to extubate
4. Peptic ulcer disease prophylaxis
5. Deep vein thrombosis prophylaxis

BOX 90-2. FIVE COMPONENTS OF THE CENTRAL LINE BUNDLES

1. Hand hygiene
2. Maximal barrier precautions
3. Chlorhexidine skin antisepsis
4. Appropriate catheter site and administration system care
5. No routine replacement

---

11. **Why is there such a focus on patient safety these days?**

Based upon the Institute of Medicine report released in 2000, there are more than 60,000 preventable deaths in United States hospitals each year. The health care industry needs to reanalyze its processes in the delivery of care to decrease errors. If one compares the airline industry with health care, we see a very different system of delivery. In health care, we have accepted errors as part of doing business. We must now change that thinking and closely examine each of our processes and look at ways to do things differently. The Institute for Healthcare Improvement's 100,000 Lives Campaign (Box 90-3) is focusing on many aspects of health care delivery, including care in the ICU.

Institute for Healthcare Improvement: 100,000 Lives Campaign: www.ihi.org/IHI/Programs/Campaign
Kohn LT, Corrigan JM, Donaldson MS (eds): To Err is Human: Building a Safer Health System. Washington, DC, National Academy Press, 2000.

BOX 90-3. INSTITUTE FOR HEALTHCARE IMPROVEMENT'S 100,000 LIVES CAMPAIGN

1. Deploy rapid response teams.
2. Deliver reliable, evidence-based care for acute myocardial infarction.
3. Prevent adverse drug events.
4. Prevent central line infections.
5. Prevent surgical site infections.
6. Prevent ventilator-associated pneumonia.

KEY POINTS: KEY ELEMENTS OF PERFORMANCE IMPROVEMENT

1. All members of the intensive care team, including physicians, nurses, and respiratory therapists, are responsible for performance improvement activities.
2. Each unit and hospital should develop a standardized process for performance improvement (e.g., plan, do, study, act [PDSA]).
3. Implementation of standardized care "bundles" improves patient safety.
4. The health care industry is critically examining its practices and adopting methods from other industries to ensure a culture of safety.

CHAPTER 91

SCORING SYSTEMS FOR COMPARISON OF DISEASE SEVERITY IN INTENSIVE CARE UNIT PATIENTS

Benoit Misset, MD

1. **What are severity scores?**
   Scoring systems have been developed to compare the severity of disease among patients in intensive care units (ICUs). These scores are established at admission or during the ICU stay. The scores include the assessment of several physiologic parameters that have been documented to play an independent role in predicting hospital death. The scores presented in this chapter are only those used to assess general disease severity. Other scoring systems are used to assess particular organ function (i.e., Acute Lung Injury Score for evaluation of acute respiratory distress syndrome).

SCORES AT ICU ADMISSION

2. **Which scores are used for assessing the general severity of disease at ICU admission?**
   The three most frequently used systems are the Acute Physiology and Chronic Health Evaluation (APACHE), the Simplified Acute Physiology Score (SAPS), and the Mortality Probability Model (MPM). The most recent versions of each system are the APACHE III, the SAPS III, the MPM II0 (at admission), and MPM II24 (at 24 hours).

   Knaus WA, Draper EA, Wagner DP, Zimmerman JE: APACHE II: A severity of disease classification system. Crit Care Med 13:818–829, 1985.
   Knaus WA, Wagner DP, Draper EA, et al: The APACHE III prognostic system: Risk prediction of hospital mortality for critically ill hospitalized adults. Chest 100:1619–1636, 1991.
   Le Gall JR, Lemeshow S, Saulnier F: A new Simplified Acute Physiology Score (SAPS II) based on a European/North American multicenter study. JAMA 270:2957–2963, 1993.
   Lemeshow S, Teres D, Klar J, et al: Mortality Probability Models (MPM II) based on an international cohort of intensive care unit patients. JAMA 270:2478–2486, 1993.
   Moreno RP, Metnitz PG, Almeida E, et al: SAPS 3—From evaluation of the patient to evaluation of the intensive care unit. Part 2: Development of a prognostic model for hospital mortality at ICU admission. Intensive Care Med 31:1345–1355, 2005.

KEY POINTS: MOST COMMON ITEMS OF THE SEVERITY SCORES MEASURED AT INTENSIVE CARE UNIT (ICU) ADMISSION

1. Age
2. Previous health status
3. Acute physiologic imbalance at ICU admission
4. Reason for admission
5. Mode of admission

KEY POINTS: USUAL GOALS OF MEASURING A SEVERITY SCORE AT INTENSIVE CARE UNIT (ICU) ADMISSION

1. Prediction of death is an important goal of measuring severity score at the time of ICU admission.

2. Severity score is determined to enable comparison of ICU populations in scientific studies.

3. Performance and benchmarking are important reasons to measure the severity score, when linked to observed mortality.

3. **Why were scores to assess general disease severity at ICU admission developed?**

   - **To assess performance of the ICU:** The ICU patient is a medical or a surgical patient who presents with either acute failure of one major vital function or a high risk of developing such failure. Because the mortality rate of ICU populations is usually high and varies widely depending on patient admission policies, an objective assessment of the patients' general disease severity is necessary to ensure that the mortality rate in an ICU is consistent with the overall severity of its patient population at admission. The ratio between observed and predicted mortality, called the *standardized mortality ratio*, is the simplest way to assess the performance of an ICU. It allows comparisons among mortality rates of various ICUs or the mortality rates documented in one ICU over time.

   - **To assess the patient's risk of death:** The scores give an objective evaluation that helps the clinician confirm the severity of a patient's illness. However, these scores cannot be used to make decisions about individual patients (e.g., withdrawal of support).

   - **To compare or match populations in clinical studies:** In randomized controlled studies, the scores have been used to confirm that the populations obtained by randomization had a similar disease severity at admission to the ICU. In case-controlled studies, the scores have been used to match the control to the case patients.

4. **How were scores assessing general severity at ICU admission constructed?**
   Scores were constructed in large, multicenter, prospective populations. The variables were selected and weighed by consensus (APACHE II) or through multiple logistic regression analyses (APACHE III, SAPS II and III, and MPM II) to determine whether the parameters were independent predictors of hospital death. The tested variables include age, worst values over the first 24 hours of ICU admission for certain acute physiologic abnormalities (e.g., sodium, potassium, partial arterial oxygen tension, urine output, Glasgow Coma Scale), category at admission (i.e., medical or surgical patient), and several underlying diseases (e.g., metastatic cancer, acquired immunodeficiency syndrome). The MPM system also includes several therapeutic items (e.g., number of venous lines). The SAPS III—by far the most recent one—is based on a more complex methodology. It has the advantage of being based on a worldwide population and of giving a larger place to prior health status and to circumstances of admission in addition to the physiologic imbalance at ICU admission. MPM0 and SAPS III are the only systems for which data are collected entirely at admission to the ICU (i.e., within 1 hour), which reduces the role of a potential suboptimal care in the first day of the ICU in the assessment of severity.

5. **How were scores assessing general disease severity at ICU admission validated?**
   All of these models were validated in the initial studies in a subset of patients that were not used for construction of the scoring system. The performance of a scoring system was considered

adequate if it showed good discrimination in predicting hospital mortality and had a good calibration for the entire population under investigation. *Discrimination* in predicting hospital mortality is assessed with receiver operating characteristics (ROCs): the higher the area under the ROC curve, the more discriminative the test. The *calibration* in the entire population is measured with the goodness-of-fit test: the observed mortality must not be statistically different from the expected mortality in population deciles of equal probability intervals. The lower the H value and the higher the corresponding *P* value, the better the calibration.

6. **Which scores have been validated adequately?**
   The APACHE I and II, SAPS I, and MPM I have not been constructed or validated with the current accepted methodologic standards. The SAPS II, MPM II, and APACHE III scores have been shown to have good discrimination and calibration in large multicenter studies.
   - **SAPS II:** The SAPS II is well validated. The score needs to be updated with more recent ICU populations.
   - **MPM II:** The MPM II is well validated and has the advantage of being the only score available at ICU admission rather than at 24 hours after admission. This advantage is made possible because the score includes some therapeutic items (e.g., venous lines, drainage systems). The MPM II score also needs to be updated with more recent ICU populations.
   - **APACHE III:** The APACHE III is well validated and updated regularly, but its use is limited by the fact that clinicians must pay to know and use its equation for calculating death probability.
   - **SAPS III:** The SAPS III is well validated and updated because it has been published most recently, in 2005—that is, 12 years after the most recent among the other systems. Unlike the APACHE III, its construction details were diffused to the entire scientific community, and its use is free of charge.

SCORES DURING THE ICU STAY

7. **Why were scores assessing disease severity during the ICU stay developed?**
   The scores measuring daily severity were developed to improve the prediction of an individual patient's death (already provided by scores at admission), to assess the activity and the performance of ICUs, and to match patients in clinical investigations. These scores are particularly useful as inclusion criteria in randomized studies in which patients are entered into the investigation several days after admission. These scores are also used as matching criteria in case-control studies addressing the attributable morbidity of ICU-related adverse events, such as nosocomial infections.

8. **Which scores have been developed for assessing severity during the ICU stay?**
   Various scores have been developed using ICU samples of various sizes. The scores developed on the largest ICU populations include the Organ System Failure score (OSF), the Organ Dysfunction and Infection score (ODIN), the Logistic Organ Dysfunction Score (LODS), the Sequential Organ Failure Assessment score (SOFA), and the Multiple Organ Dysfunction Score (MODS).

   Fagon J-Y, Chastre J, Novara A, et al: Characterization of intensive care unit patients using a model based on the presence or absence of organ dysfunctions and/or infection: The ODIN model. Intensive Care Med 19:137–144, 1993.

   Knaus WA, Draper EA, Wagner DP, Zimmerman JE: Prognosis in acute organ-system failure. Ann Surg 202:685, 1985.

   Le Gall JR, Klar J, Lemeshow S, et al: The Logistic Organ Dysfunction system: A new way to assess organ dysfunction in the intensive care unit. JAMA 276:802–810, 1996.

   Marshall JC, Cook DJ, Christou NV, et al: Multiple organ dysfunction score: A reliable descriptor of a complex clinical outcome. Crit Care Med 23:1638–1652, 1995.

   Vincent JL, de Mendonca A, Cantraine F, et al: Use of the SOFA score to assess the incidence of organ dysfunction/failure in intensive care units: Results of a multicenter, prospective study. Crit Care Med 26:1793–1800, 1998.

KEY POINTS: COMMON USES OF THE ORGAN DYSFUNCTION SCORES

1. Organ dysfunction scores are used to match the patients in case-controlled or exposed–unexposed studies.

2. Scores are also useful in adjusting the cohorts in risk-factor multivariate analyses.

9. **How were the scores assessing severity over the course of the ICU stay constructed?**

Sequential scores measure the number and/or the intensity of organ dysfunction. By contrast with the SAPS, MPM, and APACHE scores, they do not take age, category of admission, or underlying diseases into account because these items do not change over the ICU stay. The OSF, ODIN, SOFA, and MODS scores were constructed empirically. The OSF and ODIN assess the number of organ dysfunctions, and the SOFA and MODS also assess the intensity of organ dysfunction. The MODS construction included testing of its validity, reproducibility, and sensitivity of each test item between observers. The choice and the weight of each LODS item are derived from a multiple logistic regression model, using hospital mortality as the dependent variable. The construction was made from the data collected during the first day in the ICU.

10. **How were these scores validated (*see* question 9)?**

Discrimination for predicting mortality is better in multivariate models when the evolution of the score and its initial values are taken into account. This principle was demonstrated with the LODS score.

Metnitz PG, Lang T, Valentin A, et al: Evaluation of the logistic organ dysfunction system for the assessment of organ dysfunction and mortality in critically ill patients. Intensive Care Med 27:992–998, 2001.

Moreno R, Vincent JL, Matos A, et al: The use of maximum SOFA score to quantify organ failure/dysfunction in intensive care: Result of a prospective multicenter study. Intensive Care Med 25:686–696, 1999.

11. **What did these scores add to the description of ICU patients (*see* question 9)?**

1. The use of the OSF score initially showed that a 100% prediction of death could be made in the most severely afflicted patients after several days. However, the same score was eventually used to demonstrate that care in the ICU had improved over years, such that published results were no longer valid 10 years later. These investigations documented that such scores are a method to assess ICU performance.

2. The mean time of occurrence of each organ failure is not the same. The peak of dysfunction for the neurologic system occurs usually before the second day; for the respiratory, cardiovascular, renal, and coagulation systems, around the third day; and for the hepatic system, around the fifth day.

3. The weight of each organ failure in predicting death is not the same: hematologic and hepatic failures have less effect on mortality than respiratory, cardiovascular, renal, and neurologic failures.

4. The weight of each organ failure in predicting death is not the same over time. The same increase in respiratory dysfunction has a worse prognosis after 1 week of ICU stay. Hepatic dysfunction has an effect on mortality only after 3 weeks of ICU stay.

Cook R, Cook D, Tilley J, et al: Multiple organ dysfunction: Baseline and serial component scores. Crit Care Med 29:2046–2050, 2001.

12. At what time of the ICU stay should one use either of these scores (*see* question 9)?
See Fig. 91-1.

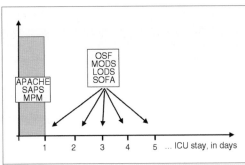

Figure 91-1. When should we measure the severity scores? APACHE = Acute Physiology and Chronic Health Evaluation, SAPS = Simplified Acute Physiology Score, MPM = Mortality Probability Model, OSF = Organ System Failure score, MODS = Multiple Organ Dysfunction Score, LODS = Logistic Organ Dysfunction Score, SOFA = Sequential Organ Failure Assessment score, ICU = Intensive Care Unit.

CHAPTER 92

EVIDENCE-BASED CRITICAL CARE

Michael Young, MD, and Brian T. Marden, PharmD

1. **What is the role of evidence-based medicine in the intensive care unit (ICU)?**
   Thirty years ago, ICU medical decision making was largely driven by anecdote, expert opinion, intuition, and a rudimentary understanding of pathophysiology. Although the scientific gaps remain wide, the recent relative explosion of high-quality ICU clinical trials clearly justifies an evidence-based approach. This allows the physician to more reliably identify the best care available for each ICU patient when selecting diagnostic tests, choosing treatment strategies, and determining prognosis.

2. **How does one ensure that ICU patients receive the evidence-based care that matters the most?**
   Choosing from the growing list of evidence-based strategies defining best ICU care can be daunting. To define the most important evidence-based strategies, we used three criteria:
   - **Strength of the evidence:** The strength of evidence is determined by the hierarchy of study design (randomized controlled trial is the best) and outcome measures (order of priority: reducing morbidity, mortality, adverse events, surrogate outcomes, indirect connection to clinical outcome).
   - **Prevalence of the problem and effect size:** More common ICU issues and larger effect size (e.g., mortality reduction of 10% versus 1%) weighed higher.
   - **Ease of implementation:** Raising the head of the bed up to 45 degrees to prevent pneumonia is probably far easier than the purchase and implementation of an electronic information system. However, judging the ease of implementation is largely subjective.

3. **What is the impact of using the "intensivist model" of ICU care?**
   The Leapfrog Group safety initiative defines the *intensivist-model ICU* as an ICU managed by fellowship trained critical care physicians who provide care exclusively in the ICU during the day and are available within 5 minutes by pager at other times. The relative mortality reduction seen with this model is 15–60%. Substantial mortality reductions were found in medical ICUs, mixed medical/surgical ICUs, and pure surgical ICUs. The mechanism for the improved care has not been well studied. Widespread adoption of the intensivist model is constrained by the limited number of intensivists, the costs involved, and perceived threats to physician autonomy.

   Pronovost PJ, Angus DC Dorman T, et al: Physician staffing patterns and clinical outcomes in critically ill patients. JAMA 288:2151–2162, 2002.

   Young MP, Birkmeyer JD: Potential reductions in mortality rates using an intensivist model to manage intensive care units. Eff Clin Pract 6:284–289, 2000.

4. **Are ICU outcomes changed by emergency response teams that evaluate patients "at risk" on the ward?**
   ICU patient outcomes are strongly influenced by the care provided in the emergency department and on the ward before transfer to the ICU. Emergency response teams composed of intensivists, hospitalists, and nurses are increasingly used to identify ward patients at risk for catastrophic deterioration and to facilitate escalation of care and potential transfer to the ICU. Criteria to urgently evaluate ward patients often include hemodynamic compromise (systolic blood pressure < 85 mmHg; heart rate < 40 and >140), respiratory insufficiency (respiratory

rate > 35 breaths/min; pH < 7.25; PCO_2 > 60 mmHg need or a 100% nonrebreather mask), low urine output, and acute deterioration in level of consciousness.

Bellomo R, Goldsmith D, Uchino S, et al: Prospective controlled trial of effect of medical emergency team on postoperative morbidity and mortality rates. Crit Care Med 32:916–921, 2004.

Young MP, Gooder VJ, McBride K, et al: Inpatient transfers to the intensive care unit: Delays are associated with increased mortality and morbidity. J Gen Intern Med 18:77–83, 2003.

5. **How do ICU clinical pharmacists improve ICU care?**
In a large prospective study, a pharmacist making the rounds in a medical ICU reduced avoidable drug errors by 66%. A number of studies have demonstrated large pharmacoeconomic benefits from having dedicated ICU pharmacists rounding with the ICU team. ICU pharmacists assist physicians in pharmacotherapy decision making by providing drug information, monitoring for adverse effects, and providing pharmacokinetic consultations.

Brilli RJ, Spevetz A, Branson RD, et al: Critical care delivery in the intensive care unit: Defining clinical roles and the best practice model. Crit Care Med 26:2007–2019, 2001.

Leape LL, Cullen DJ, Clapp MD, et al: Pharmacist participation on physician rounds and adverse drug events in the intensive care unit. JAMA 281:267–270, 1999.

6. **What are the implications of the national shortage of ICU nurses?**
The traditional ratio of patients to nurses in adult ICUs is 2:1 or 1:1. Excess mortality has been noted with ratios of 3:1. In addition, worse medical outcomes are associated with nursing inexperience and times of nursing shortage. A nationwide shortage of ICU nurses threatens our ability to provide excellent or even good ICU care. The average age of the current ICU RN workforce is 50 years of age, so the critical shortage of ICU nurses is likely to worsen.

Pronovost PJ, Dang D, Dorman T, et al: Intensive care unit nurse staffing and the risk for complications after abdominal aortic surgery. Eff Clin Pract 4:223–235, 2001.

Tarnow-Mordi WO, Hau C, Warden A, Shearer AJ: Hospital mortality in relation to staff workload: A 4-year study in an adult intensive-care unit. Lancet 356:185–189, 2000.

7. **Is "family-centered" care feasible in the ICU?**
ICUs are arguably set up to fail in providing core family needs. There is a wealth of literature supporting the idea that factors such as consistent communication, spacious and comfortable waiting areas, and unrestricted visiting policies improve family satisfaction and secondarily have a positive effect on patient outcomes. Creating a "family-centered" environment commands resources and, at many times, requires a major shift in local culture; however, results from hospitals that do institute a formalized approach have demonstrated success in reducing family member frustration and contributed to an overall positive feeling of satisfaction.

Berwick DM, Kotagal M: Restricting visiting hours in ICUs. JAMA 292:136–737, 2004.

Lederer MA, Goode T, Dowling J: Origins and development: The Critical Care Family Assistance Program. Chest 128:65S–75S, 2005.

Official Patient and Family Web Site of the Society of Critical Care Medicine: www.icu-usa.com

8. **Multidisciplinary care—fad, fiction, or a new way of life in the ICU?**
Although the Joint Commission on Accreditation of Healthcare Organizations, the Institute for Healthcare Improvement, and the Society of Critical Care all strongly promote the use of multidisciplinary care, there is surprisingly little rigorous study of this area. Evidence that RNs, MDs, RTs, pharmacists, and other ICU clinicians working in a collaborative fashion improve medical outcomes includes studies in the following areas:

- ICU checklists
- Ventilator weaning
- Telemedicine

There is almost no data measuring the prevalence or quality of collaborative care in the ICU.

Pronovost P, Berenholtz S, Dorman T, et al: Improving communication in the ICU using daily goals. J Crit Care 18:71–75, 2003.

Rosenfeld BA, Dorman T, Breslow MJ, et al: Intensive care unit telemedicine: Alternative paradigm for providing continuous intensivist care. Crit Care Med 28:3925–3931, 2000.

Young MP, Gooder VJ, Oltermann MH, et al: The impact of a multidisciplinary approach on caring for ventilator-dependent patients. Int J Qual Health Care 10:15–26, 1998.

9. **Isn't the need for deep vein thrombosis (DVT) prophylaxis old news for ICU patients?**

Studies have demonstrated DVT rates of 13–31% in critically ill patients who were not receiving prophylaxis. Most patients in the ICU have at least one major risk factor for development of a DVT and thus should be receiving an appropriate prophylactic therapy. However, studies have demonstrated that, on average, only 69% of critically ill patients received thromboprophylaxis. Aggressive staff education, computerized support systems, and use of admission order sets have been shown to improve rates of thromboprophylaxis. Every ICU should have a system in place to make sure that each patient is assessed for risk of venous thromboembolism and that appropriate prophylaxis strategies are implemented.

Geerts W, Selby R: Prevention of venous thromboembolism in the ICU. Chest 124:357S–363S, 2003.

10. **Placing patients on mechanical ventilation at 45 degrees—recipe for self-extubation and pressure sores or prevention of pneumonia?**

The incidence of ventilator pneumonia is 10–15 cases per 1000 ventilator days. Aspiration of upper airway secretions in mechanically ventilated patients is common. A randomized trial demonstrated a threefold reduction in the rate of ventilator-associated pneumonia in mechanically ventilated patients who had the head of the bed inclined at 45 degrees compared with patients who were supine. Implementation of raising the head of the bed has been low. Barriers to instituting this practice include concerns of patient comfort, increased pressure ulcers, and self-extubations. However, published data have not validated these concerns, and more study is needed.

Drakulovic MB, Torres A, Bauer TT, et al: Supine body position as a risk factor for nosocomial pneumonia in mechanically ventilated patients: A randomized trial. Lancet 354:1851–1858, 1999.

11. **How do we reduce the risk of gastrointestinal bleeding among critically ill ICU patients?**

Stress-related mucosal disease results in clinically significant bleeding at an average rate of 6% (0.1–39%) in critically ill patients not receiving prophylaxis, with associated mortality rates >50%. A large observational study identified mechanical ventilation ≥48 hours and coagulopathy as independent predictors of stress-induced bleeding. Other risk factors include hepatic or renal disease, sepsis, severe burns, hypotension, or recent gastrointestinal tract bleeding. Critically ill patients without major risk factors should not receive prophylaxis. Studies have demonstrated that both H_2-receptor antagonists and proton pump inhibitors are effective in reducing clinically significant stress ulcer–related bleeding.

12. **Steroids in septic shock—another case of déjà vu all over again?**

The interest in using steroids in the treatment of septic shock has waxed and waned over the past 30 years. Two common ICU situations for which there is solid evidence to support the use of steroids when treating septic patients include the following:

- Stress-dose steroids given to patients with relative adrenal insufficiency and severe sepsis or septic shock
- Steroids given to patients who have recently received chronic steroid treatment (≥5 mg/day of prednisone for 7 or more days)
- Controversial: use of steroids in "late acute respiratory distress syndrome" (ARDS) and among critically ill non-ICU patients with relative adrenal insufficiency but without sepsis

Annane D, Sebille V, Charpentier C, et al: Effect of treatment with low doses of hydrocortisone and fludrocortisone on mortality of patients with septic shock. JAMA 228:862–871, 2002.

Krasner AS: Glucocorticoid-induced adrenal insufficiency. JAMA 282:671–676, 1999.

13. **Using insulin drips on up to 75% of ICU patients sounds like a lot of work. Is the benefit worth the effort?**

Stress hyperglycemia and preexisting diabetes mellitus are common among patients admitted to the ICU. A randomized controlled trial using an insulin infusion to maintain blood glucose levels between 80 and 110 mg/dL versus "regular care" detected a 34% relative reduction in mortality. Aggressive insulin therapy is not an easy task for ICU nurses. However, with multidisciplinary support, education, and data feedback, insulin drip protocols can be implemented successfully in the ICU.

Krinsley JS: Effect of an intensive glucose management protocol on the mortality of critically ill adult patients. Mayo Clin Proc 79:992–1000, 2004.

Van de Berghe G, Wouters PJ, Weekers F, et al: Intensive insulin therapy in critically ill patients. N Engl J Med 345:1359–1367, 2001.

14. **Is the interest in using drotrecogin alfa (activated) for patients with severe sepsis fading?**

Drotrecogin alfa (activated) was approved by the U.S. Food and Drug Administration for the treatment of sepsis-induced organ dysfunction associated with a high risk of death, such as an Acute Physiology and Chronic Health Evaluation (APACHE) II score of $\geq$25. It was the first drug to significantly reduce mortality (absolute reduction of 6.1%) in patients with severe sepsis. A large prospective randomized trial in less-sick patients (one organ dysfunction) found no benefit. A prospective trial involving pediatric patients also found no benefit. Drotrecogin alfa (activated) should be considered for use in any adult patient with sepsis-induced multiple (two or more) organ failure.

Bernard GR, Vincent JL, Laterre PF, et al: Efficacy and safety of recombinant human activated protein C for severe sepsis. N Engl J Med 344:699–709, 2001.

15. **Is the use of low tidal volumes among patients with acute lung injury (ALI)/ARDS widespread?**

Since the publication of the ARDS Net trial results regarding 6 versus 12 mL/kg tidal volumes (predicted body weight), many ICU clinicians have tried to implant the low-tidal-volume strategy. Although the use of the low-tidal-volume strategy was associated with an absolute mortality reduction of 9%, a growing number of studies indicate poor compliance with the ARDS Net protocol. Barriers to use of the low-tidal-volume strategy include use of actual versus predicted body weight, under-recognition of ALI/ARDS, and clinician concern that use of the low-tidal-volume strategy may require more sedation or worsen hypoxia.

Rubenfeld GD, Cooper C, Carter G, et al: Barriers to providing lung-protective ventilation to patients with acute lung injury. Crit Care Med 32:1289–1293, 2004.

Young MP, Manning HL, Wilson DL, et al: Ventilation of patients with acute lung injury: Has new evidence changed clinical practice? Crit Care Med 32:1260–1265, 2004.

16. **Are significant complications inevitable when central lines are used?**

Central line complication rates are highly dependent on operator experience. Complication rates can also be dramatically reduced by use of the following strategies:

- Maximally sterile barriers
- Antibiotic-impregnated catheters
- Avoidance of using femoral venous catheters (subclavian generally preferred)
- Ultrasound guidance when using the internal jugular approach
- "Three stick rule": after two or three attempts to locate the vein with the needle, the procedure is turned over to the most experienced operator available

McGee D, Gould M: Preventing complications of central venous catheterization. N Engl J Med 348:1123–1133, 2003.

17. **Transfusion triggers for transfusion thresholds—a case where less is more?**
Approximately 95% of critically ill patients are anemic by day 3 of their ICU stay. A large randomized trial demonstrated significant reductions in mortality rates when ICU patients received a more restrictive blood transfusion threshold (hemoglobin < 7 gm/dL) versus a more traditional trigger (hemoglobin < 10 gm/dL). Despite these findings, implementation of the more restrictive transfusion threshold has been modest.

Corwin HL, Gettinger A, Pearl RG, et al: The CRIT study: Anemia and blood transfusion in the critically ill—Current clinical practice in the United States. Crit Care Med 32:39–52, 2004.
Hebert PC, Wells G, Blajchman MA, et al: A multicenter, randomized, controlled trial of transfusion requirements in critical care. N Engl J Med 340:409–417, 1999.

18. **What medications should one always consider in patients with acute myocardial infarction?**
Many medications commonly used to treat patients with acute coronary syndromes are not supported by robust data. However, there is powerful evidence supporting the use of the following therapies:

- Aspirin <24 hours after hospital arrival and continued after hospital discharge
- Beta-blocker therapy <24 hours after hospital arrival and at discharge
- Angiotensin-converting enzyme inhibitor or angiotensin receptor blocker at hospital discharge in patients with a left ventricular ejection fraction <40%
- Thrombolytic agents received <30 minutes of hospital arrival and <6 hours after onset of symptoms

Joint Commission on Accreditation of Healthcare Organization: Acute Myocardial Infarction Core Performance Measures: www.jointcommission.org/performancemeasurement/acute+myocardial+infarction

19. **Hand hygiene between patient contacts—would Semmelweis be proud?**
In the 19th century, Dr. Ignaz Semmelweis, a Viennese obstetrician, alienated himself from the medical society with his attempts to persuade clinicians to wash their hands to reduce the spread of disease among patients. Practitioners today still routinely fail to perform adequate hand hygiene > 50% of the time between patient contacts. ICUs are sites of especially low adherence to hand hygiene because of the busy environment and increased caregiver–patient contacts. Hand hygiene compliance in the ICU must dramatically improve to ensure that no patient suffers or dies "at the hands" of his or her caregiver.

Centers for Disease Control and Prevention: Hand hygiene in healthcare settings: www.cdc.gov/handhygiene/
Gawande A: On washing hands. N Engl J Med 350:1283–1286, 2004.

KEY POINTS: EVIDENCE-BASED MEDICINE

1. The science guiding medical treatment in most clinical situations in the ICU is limited, leading to understandable clinician variability. However, even in areas with strong scientific backing, compliance with evidence-based medicine is often poor.

2. To optimize ICU patient outcomes, clinicians must identify and implement the evidence-based therapies that matter the most.

3. Effective implementation of specific evidence-based therapies probably requires an ICU organization that includes intensivists, ICU pharmacists, and an experienced ICU nurse workforce, including 1:2 or 1:1 nurse-to-patient ratio.

4. Evidence-based ICU therapies vary widely in the size of their effect on mortality, morbidity, costs, and ease of implementation.

20. **How does one avoid oversedation among patients who are mechanically ventilated?**

Mechanically ventilated patients often receive continuous sedatives while intubated. Accumulation of sedatives is an independent predictor of increased ventilator days as well as longer ICU and hospital length of stay. A randomized controlled trial demonstrated that daily "sedation vacations" reduced median ventilator days by 2.4 days and ICU length of stay by 3.5 days. Sedation vacations also meant fewer complications related to critical illness and reduced risk of developing posttraumatic stress disorder. Although this intervention does not increase resource use, successful implementation requires multidisciplinary protocol development and implementation.

   Kress JP, Pohlman AS, O'Connor MF, et al: Daily interruption of sedative infusions in critically ill patients undergoing mechanical ventilation. N Engl J Med 342:1471–1477, 2000.

21. **Electronic decision support tools—just another name for "cookbook medicine"?**

In the ICU, complexity, information overload, scientific uncertainty, and human limitations contribute to unwanted variation of care, which is a major contributor to preventable mortality and morbidity. Decision-support tools can reduce unwanted variation. Examples in which decision support tools have improved ICU outcomes include antibiotic prescribing in the ICU, compliance with low-tidal-volume strategies, and tight glucose control. Effective decision-support tools have not supplanted the need for attentive on-site clinicians, nor have they proved to undermine physician education.

   Morris AH: Developing and implementing computerized protocols for standardization of clinical decisions. Ann Intern Med 132:373–383, 2000.

INDEX

Page numbers in **boldface type** indicate complete chapters.

Mechanical ventilation *(Continued)*
 transbronchial biopsies during, 87
 ventilator settings in, 52
 weaning from, **51–56**, 140
  effect of early tracheotomy on, 74
Medullary function, brain death-related absence of, 387
Melanoma, metastatic
 to the brain, 363
 to the pericardium, 363
MELD score, for end-stage liver disease, 459
Melena, 291
Meningitis, **214–223**
 acute, 224
 aseptic, 227–228
 chronic, 224
 contagiousness of, 229
 cryptococcal, 228–229
 endocarditis-related, 220–221
 ibuprofen-related, 377
 meningococcal, 229
 mortality rate in, 226
 pneumococcal, 226
 recurrent, 227
 tuberculous, 226–228
Mental status examination, for delirium diagnosis, 532
Meperidine, 477
 as hypotension cause, 478
Metabolic diseases, as hepatitis cause, 308
Metabolic environment, evaluation of, 11
Methadone, 477
Methemoglobin, effect on pulse oximetry readings, 22
Methicillin-resistant *Staphylococcus aureus*,
  235–238
α-Methyldopa, contraindication in stroke patients,
  262–263
3,4-Methylenedioxymethamphetamine, as
  hyponatremia cause, 288
Methylxanthines, 125
Microcephaly, 526
Midazolam, 481–484
 as status epilepticus treatment, 393
Military recruits, heat stroke in, 501
Minerals, as total parenteral nutrition components, 45
Mineral supplementation, in acute renal failure patients,
  275
Mitral regurgitation, 191, 193
Mitral stenosis, 193–195
 severity classification of, 195
Mitral valve
 anatomy and function of, 191
 in endocarditis, 218–219
Mitral valve prolapse syndrome, 168
Mivacurium, pharmacology of, 468
Mixed agonist-antagonist opioids, 477
Mixed venous oxygen saturation (SvO$_2$), 28
Monitoring
 hemodynamic, **27–30**
  in pericardial tamponade, 202–203

Monitoring *(Continued)*
 neurologic, sedation during, 482
 perfusion,
  global *versus* local, 30
  of tissue beds, 30
Moraxella catarrhalis, as pneumonia cause, 106
Morphine, 475, 477, 481
 as angina treatment, 167
 as hypotension cause, 478
Mortality, indexed to severity of illness, 564
Mortality Probability Model (MPM), 567–570
Mortality rate
 in acute respiratory distress syndrome, 144
 in gastrointestinal hemorrhage, 291–292
 in heat stroke, 502
 in meningitis, 226
 in neuroleptic malignant syndrome, 544
 in untreated malignant hypertension, 261
Motor hemiparesis, lacunar infarct-related, 399
Motor vehicle accidents, as head trauma cause, 423
Motor weakness, subacutely evolving, generalized,
  410
Mouth opening, evaluation of, 66
Mucolytic therapy, for chronic obstructive pulmonary
  disease, 126
Multidisciplinary care, 573–574
Multidrug-resistant bacteria, **230–235**
Multiple-organ dysfunction syndrome, 143,
  205–208
 sickle cell disease-related, 357–358
Muscle disease, inflammatory, 371–373
Muscle relaxants. *See* Neuromuscular-blocking
  agents
Muscle spasms, tetanus-related, 487–490
Muscle weakness, myasthenia gravis-related, 414
Musset's sign, 198
Myasthenia gravis, **409–413**
Myasthenic crisis, 416–417
Mycobacterium, as cellulitis cause, 255
Mycophenolate mofetil, side effects of, 464
Mycoplasma pneumoniae, as cause, 106
Myelinolysis, central pontine, 289
Myocardial infarction
 as abdominal pain cause, 436
 acute, **165–168**
 aortic dissection-related, 186
 biochemical markers for, 171–172
 definition of, 169
 as diabetic ketoacidosis precipitant, 321–322
 differentiated from anaphylaxis, 492
 hypertensive crisis-related, 261
 Killip classes of, 174
 nonatherosclerotic causes of, 170
 pharmacotherapy for, 576
 Q-wave differentiated from non–Q wave, 172
 with ST-segment elevation, 168, 172–173
 without ST-segment elevation, 173
Myocardial ischemia, 170, 191–192

Norepinephrine, as severe sepsis syndrome treatment, 209
Nurses, critical care, 557
  shortage of, 573
Nutritional assessment, of critically ill patients, 39
Nutritional support
  in burn patients, 435
  in critically ill patients, **35–38**
  in pancreatitis patients, 301
  in renal failure patients, 275
  withdrawal of, 555–556

O

Obesity
  as coronary artery disease risk factor, 169
  as heat stroke risk factor, 502
  as thrombotic cerebral infarction risk factor, 396
  as wound infection risk factor, 254
Ocular disorders
  endocarditis-related, 220–221
  myasthenia gravis-related, 414
Oculocephalic reflex, 385
Oculovestibular reflex, 386–387
Ogilvie's syndrome, 440
Ohms' law, 261
Oil of wintergreen intoxication, 515–516
Omega-3 fatty acids, 40
  as pharmaconutrients, 46
Oncologic emergencies, **355–359**. See also specific types of cancer
100 Top Secrets, **1–8**
Opiate-hypnotic withdrawal syndrome,
Opiates, as delirium cause, 531
Opioid analgesia, 478, 475
  adverse effects of, 478, 481
    bronchoconstriction, 116
  contraindicated, 477
  effect on sleep, 484
  mixed agonist-antagonist, 477
  parenteral administration of, 478
Ortner's syndrome, 194
Osborn wave, 495
Osler's nodes, 222–223
Osmolality, of serum, 285, 287, 290
Osmolarity, of serum, 323–324
Osteomyelitis, 257
  candidal, 231
Outcome assessment, 564
Overdampening, 27
Oversedation, during mechanical ventilation, 577
Oximetry. See also Pulse oximetry
  versus arterial blood gas analysis, 34
  brain tissue, 428
Oxygen-carrying solutions, hemoglobin-based, 340
Oxygen consumption, during pregnancy, 523
Oxygen delivery (DO_2)
  determinants of, 10

Oxygen delivery (DO_2) (Continued)
  to fetus, 523–524
  formula for, 30
Oxygen dissociation curve, 33
Oxygen saturation (SaO_2), 10, 30
  calculated versus measured, 32–33
  pulse oximetry determination of, 21, 23–24
Oxygen therapy
  for angina, 167
  arterial blood gas sampling after, 32
  for asthma, 118
  for carbon monoxide poisoning, 433
  for chronic obstructive pulmonary disease, 126
  in comatose patients,
  for cor pulmonale, 134
  for hypoxemic acute respiratory failure, 138
  as postoperative wound infection prophylaxis, 255
  for status epilepticus, 392

P

Pacemakers, **83–88**
  electromagnetic interference with, 94
  failure of, 94
  "R on T" phenomenon of, 94
Packed red blood cell (PRBC) transfusions, 339, 358
Pain
  abdominal
    diabetic ketoacidosis-related, 318
    peritonitis-related, 313
  adverse effects of, 481
  assessment of, 474
  in chest, **159–165**. See also Angina
    aortic dissection-related, 185
    atypical (noncardiac), 165–167
    differential diagnosis of, 165
    endocarditis-related, 222–223
    myocardial contusion-related, 453
  epigastric, pancreatitis-related, 298
Pain management, **467–473**
  in blunt chest trauma, 449
  inadequate, 474
  relationship to sedation, 484
Palliative care, 554
Pancreas, fluid loss from, 37
Pancreatitis
  as abdominal pain cause, 436
  acute, **291–296**
    biliary, 302
    image-guided treatment of, 302
    severe, 297–298, 301–302
    severity and prognosis estimation of, 299–300
  as diabetic ketoacidosis cause, 318, 321–322
  enteral nutrition in, 43–44
Pancuronium, 468, 470
Papaverine, as cerebral vasospasm treatment, 407
Papilledema, 261
Paralytic agents. See Neuromuscular-blocking agents
Parapneumonic effusions, thoracentesis of, 114

Starvation, critical illness-related, 39
Starvation ketosis, 318–319
Statins. *See* 3-Hydroxy-3-methylglutaryl coenzyme A
    reductase inhibitors
Status asthmaticus, 117–118
Status epilepticus, **391–395**
    convulsive, 391–392, 395
    nonconvulsive, 391
    partial, 391
Stenotrophomonas maltophilia, 238
Stereotactic radiosurgery, 363–364
Sternum, fractures of, 452, 457
Steroids. *See also* Corticosteroids
    as acute respiratory distress syndrome treatment,
        146
    as adrenal insufficiency cause, 330
    as adrenal insufficiency treatment, 331–332
    as elevated intracranial pressure treatment, 430
    inhaled, as asthma treatment, 122–123
    as meningitis treatment, 226–227
    as septic shock treatment, 209, 574–575
    stress-dose, as adrenal insufficiency treatment,
        331–332
Stimulants
    as anxiety cause, 537
    poisoning with, 507
Street drugs, overdose with, 507, 509
Streptococcus
    as endocarditis cause, 221–223
    group A, as cellulitis cause, 255–257
Streptococcus agalactiae, as meningitis cause, 226
Streptococcus bovis, as endocarditis cause, 223
Streptococcus pneumoniae
    antibiotic-resistant, 106–107, 237–238
    as endocarditis cause, 220–222
    as meningitis cause, 226
    as pneumonia cause, 105–106, 108–109
    in sickle cell disease, 356
Stress, as coronary artery disease risk factor, 169
Stress-related mucosal disease (SRMD), 294–295, 574
Stress ulcers, 149, 212, 292, 294 *See also* Stress-
    related mucosal disease (SRMD)
Stridor
    anaphylaxis-related, 492
    hysterical, 492
Stroke, 396, 402
    carotid artery stenosis-related, 399–400
    cerebral embolic, 396
    endocarditis-related, 220–221
    hemorrhagic
        embolic, 220
        sickle cell disease-related, 357
    ischemic, 396, 398, 400–401
    thrombotic, sickle cell disease-related, 357
Strychnine poisoning, differentiated from tetanus, 490
Subclavian steal syndrome, 400
Substance abuse disorders, 539 *See also* Alcohol
    abuse; Drug abuse

Succinylcholine
    as cardiac arrest cause, 411
    contraindications to, 469
    as hyperkalemia cause, 283
    indications for use of, 469
    pharmacology of, 468
Sudden cardiac death, hypertrophic cardiomyopathy-
    related, 90
Sufentanil, 475, 477
Suicide, assisted, 552–553
Sulfamylon cream, as burn injury treatment, 432
Sulfonamides, contraindication to, 377
Superior vena cava syndrome, 360, 364
Supine hypotension syndrome, 523
Surviving Sepsis Campaign Guidelines, 208
SvO_2 (mixed venous oxygen saturation), 28
Sweat, fluid loss from, 35–36
Sympathomimetic drugs, as anxiety cause, 537
Syncope
    anaphylaxis-related, 492
    aortic stenosis-related, 197
    neurocardiogenic, 90
Syndrome of inappropriate secretion of antidiuretic
    hormone, 287, 405, 489–490
Synovial fluid analysis, 367–368
Synovitis, rheumatoid arthritis-related, 377
Systemic inflammatory response syndrome (SIRS),
    205–208
Systemic lupus erythematosus
    flares of, 377–378
    myasthenia gravis associated with, 414
Systemic vascular resistance
    as blood pressure determinant, 261
    measurement of, 30
    during pregnancy, 523

T
Tachyarrhythmias, 177
Tachycardia
    alcohol withdrawal-related, 419
    atrial, 177
    atrioventricular nodal reentrant (AVNRT), 177–178
    atrioventricular reentrant (AVRT), 178
    pharmacotherapy for, 177
    pneumothorax-related, 442
    supraventricular, 177
        chemical cardioversion of, 183
        reversible causes of, 180
    torsades de pointes, 179–181
    ventricular, 177
        chemical cardioversion of, 183
        differentiated from supraventricular
            tachyarrhythmia, 178
        reversible causes of, 180
        therapeutic hypothermia for, 183
    Wolff-Parkinson-White syndrome-related, 178–179
Tacrolimus, side effects of, 464
Tagged red blood cell scans, 294

Treatment *(Continued)*
  withdrawal of, **549–554**
    in severe sepsis syndrome patients,
Tricuspid valve, closure of, 27
Tricyclic antidepressants
  as cardiopulmonary arrest cause, 17–18
  as hyponatremia cause, 288
  as neuroleptic malignant syndrome cause, 544
  overdose of, 511
Triiodothyronine
  in euthyroid sick syndrome, 333
  in myxedema coma, 336–337
  in thyroid storm, 335
Triple-H therapy, for cerebral vasospasm, 407
Trismus, 488–489
Troponins, cardiac
  as acute pericarditis indicator, 201
  as myocardial contusion indicator, 455
  as myocardial infarction indicator, 171
Trousseau syndrome, 353–354
Tuberculosis
  as hemoptysis cause, 154
  as meningitis cause, 226–228
  as peritonitis cause, 313
Tumor lysis syndrome, 360–362
Tumor necrosis factor-α, 206
Tunnel infections, 239, 245
Turner's syndrome, 185
Typhlitis, 436
Typhoid fever, as bioterrorism agent, 248, 251

U

Ulcers
  Curling's, 435
  diabetic, 255–257
  duodenal, 292
  hemorrhage from, 293
  stress, 149, 212, 292, 294 *See also* Stress-related
    mucosal disease (SRMD)
  vascular insufficiency, 255–257
Ulnar artery, Allen test of, 27
Ultrafiltration, 273
  slow continuous, 273
Ultrasound, transcranial Doppler, as brain death
  confirmatory test, 388
Unconscious patients, drug overdose diagnosis in, 509,
  511
Upper esophageal sphincter, 147
Uremia, as indication for renal replacement therapy,
  273
Uremic syndrome, 270
Urinalysis, for acute renal failure diagnosis, 267
Urinary output, heat stroke-related decrease in, 504
Urinary tract infections, as diabetic ketoacidosis
  precipitant, 321–322
Urine
  electrolyte concentrations of, in acute renal failure,
    267–268

Urine *(Continued)*
  fluid loss from, 35
  pH of, in forced diuresis, 509
  potassium excretion in, 280
Urine toxicology screen, 510–511
  alternatives to, 511
Urticaria, 493
  anaphylaxis-related, 492
  patient's self-treatment of, 494

V

Vallecula, 65
Valvular heart disease, **191–199**
  aortic regurgitation, 197, 199
  aortic stenosis, 195–197
  connective tissue disease-related, 376
  mitral regurgitation, 191, 193
  mitral stenosis, 193–195
Vancomycin
  as meningitis treatment, 226–227
  as prosthetic valve endocarditis treatment, 222
Vancomycin-resistant *Enterococcus,* 235–238
Varices
  endoscopic treatment of, 293
  as gastrointestinal hemorrhage cause, 292
  hemorrhage from, 293
Variola virus, as smallpox causative agent,
  251–252
Vascular disorders, as disseminated intravascular
  coagulation cause, 350
Vasculitis, systemic lupus erythematosus-related, 378
Vasoconstriction, pulse oximetry readings in, 23–24
Vasoconstrictor drugs, effect on denervated heart
  transplants, 465
Vasodilator drugs
  as aortic regurgitation treatment, 198–199
  as aortic stenosis treatment, 197
  classification of, 189
  as cor pulmonale treatment, 136
  effect on denervated heart transplants, 464
  as malignant hypertension treatment, 262
Vasopressors
  as hypotension treatment, 11
  as severe sepsis syndrome treatment, 209
Vasospasm, cerebral, 407–408
Vecuronium
  indications for, 470
  pharmacology of, 468
Venereal Disease Research Laboratory test, 228
Venous stasis, as venous thromboembolism risk factor,
  159
Venous wall injuries, as venous thromboembolism risk
  factor, 159
Ventilation. *See also* Mechanical ventilation
  in acute respiratory distress syndrome patients,
    145–146
  bag-valve-mask, 63
Ventilation-perfusion (V/Q) scan, 161